Minimally Invasive Uro-oncologic Surgery

Minimally Invasive Uro-oncologic Surgery

Edited by

Robert G Moore MD
Minimally Invasive Urology Institute of the Southwest
El Paso, Texas 79902 and
Department of Surgery, Division of Urology
Texas Tech Health Science Center, El Paso
El Paso, Texas
USA

Jay T Bishoff MD
Wilford Hall Medical Center
Department of Urology/MCSU
Lackland AFB
TX 78236
USA

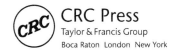

CRC Press
Taylor & Francis Group
Boca Raton London New York

CRC Press is an imprint of the
Taylor & Francis Group, an **informa** business

Contents

Contributors

Sidney C Abreu MD
Fellow, Section of Laparoscopic and Minimally Invasive
Surgery
Urological Institute
Cleveland Clinic Foundation
9500 Euclid Avenue
44195 Cleveland
Ohio
USA

Timothy D Averch MD FACS
Assistant Professor, Director of Endourology
Department of Urology
University of Pittsburgh Medical Center
3471 Fifth Ave
Kaufmann Bldg, Suite 700
Pittsburgh, PA 15213
USA

Sam B Bhayani MD
Instructor of Urology
4940 Eastern Avenue
A building, Room A347
Baltimore, MD 21237
USA

Jay T Bishoff MD
Wilford Hall Medical Center
Department of Urology/MCSU
Lackland AFB, TX 78236
USA

Moritz Braun MD
Assistant Professor
Department of Urology Medical Centre
University Cologne
Joseph-Stelzmann-Str. 9
50924 Cologne
Germany

Jeffrey A Cadeddu MD
Assistant Professor of Urology
Director, Clinical Center for Minimally
Invasive Urologic Cancer Treatment
University of Texas Southwestern Medical Center at
Dallas
Dallas, TX 75390–9110
USA

Christian G Chaussy MD FRCS
Professor of Urology Ludwig-Maximilian-University
Muenchen (Munich)
Chairman, Department of Urology
Staedtisches Krankenhaus Muenchen
Sanatoriumsplatz 2
81545 Muenchen
Germany

Steve Y Chung MD
Resident in Urology
Department of Urology
Cedars Sinai Medical Center
8635 W. 3rd street, Ste. 1070
Los Angeles, CA 90048
USA

John W Davis MD
Assistant Professor
Eastern Virginia Medical School
Norfolk, VA
USA

Serdar Deger MD
Assistant Professor, Department of Urology, CCM
Charité-University Medicine Berlin
10098 Berlin
Germany

Yoram Dekel
Department of Urology
SLK Kliniken Heilbronn
Am Gesundbrunnen 20
D 74078 Heilbronn
Germany

Thomas M Dykes MD COL USAF MC
Department of Radiology
Wilford Hall USAF Medical Center
Lackland AFB
TX 78236
USA

Mohamed El Ghoneimy
Fellow
Urology Department
KH der Elisabethinen
Fadingerstr. 1
Linz A 4020
Austria

Udo H Engelmann MD
Professor and Chairman
Department of Urology Medical Centre
University Cologne
Joseph-Stelzmann-Str. 9
50924 Cologne
Germany

Tibet Erdogru
Akdeniz University Faculty of Medicine
Department of Urology
Dumlupinar Bulvari, Kampüs
07059 Antalya
Turkey

Jeffrey Evans MD
Resident
Baylor College of Medicine
Scott Department of Urology
6560 Fannin, Suite 2100
Houston, TX 77030
USA

Thomas Frede MD
Assistant Professor
Department of Urology
SLK-Kliniken Heilbronn
University of Heidelberg
Am Gesundbrunnen 20
74078 Heilbronn
Germany

Inderbir S Gill MD MCh
Section of Laparoscopic and Minimally Invasive Surgery
Urological Institute, A 100
Cleveland Clinic Foundation
9500 Euclid Avenue, 44195
Cleveland, Ohio
USA

Mark L Gonzalgo MD PhD
Department of Urology
The James Buchanan Brady Urological Institute
The Johns Hopkins Medical Institutions
Baltimore, MD 21287–2120
USA

Kurt W Grathwohl MD FCCP
Assistant Professor of Medicine
Uniformed Services University of the Health Sciences
Edward Hebert School of Medicine
Bethesda, MD
USA

Bertrand Guillonneau MD
Professor of Urology
Weill Medical College of Cornell University
Head, Section of Minimally Invasive Surgery
Department of Urology
Memorial Sloan Kettering Cancer Center
Sidney Kimmel Center for Prostate & Urologic Cancers
353 East 68th Street
New York NY 10021
USA

Blake D Hamilton
Assistant Professor of Urology
Division of Urology
University of Utah
Salt Lake City, Utah
USA

Sean P Hedican MD
Assistant Professor of Surgery
University of Wisconsin Medical School
Department of Surgery, Division of Urology
G5/343 Clinical Science Center, 600 Highland Avenue
Madison, Wisconsin 53792–3236
USA

Stephen V Jackman MD
Associate Professor of Urology
University of Pittsburgh Medical Center
Pittsburgh, PA 15213
USA

Gunter Janetschek
Professor
Guenter Janetschek
Urology Department
KH der Elisabethinen
Fadingerstr. 1
Linz A 4020
Austria

Thomas W Jarrett MD
Chief
Division of Endourology
Johns Hopkins Medical Institutions
Brady Urological Institute
Baltimore, MD 21287
USA

Louis R Kavoussi
Patrick C Walsh
Distinguished Professor of Urologic Surgery
Vice Chairman of Urology
James Buchanan Brady Urological Institute
Johns Hopkins School of Medicine
Baltimore, MD
USA

Stefan Loening MD
Professor and Chief
Charité-Universitätsmedizin Berlin
Charité Campus Mitte
Klinik für Urologie
Schumannstrasse 20/21
10117 Berlin
Germany

Yair Lotan MD
Assistant Professor of Urology
Department of Urology
University of Texas Southwestern Medical Center
5323 Harry Hines Blvd
Dallas, TX 75390–9110
USA

Mani Menon MD
The Raj & Padma Vattikuti
Distinguished Professor and Director
Vattikuti Urology Institute
Henry Ford Health System
2799 W Grand Blvd. K-9
Detroit, MI 48202–2608
USA

Scott Miller MD
Staff Anesthesiologist
Assistant Director, Anesthesiology Residency Program
Wilford Hall Medical Center
Lackland AFB, TX
USA

Debora K Moore MD
President
Minimally Invasive Urology Institute of the Southwest
El Paso, Texas 79902
Assistant Professor of Surgery
Department of Surgery, Division of Urology
Texas Tech Health Science Center of the Southwest
El Paso, Texas
USA

Robert G Moore MD
Director
Minimally Invasive Urology Institute of the Southwest
El Paso, Texas 79902
Associate Professor of Surgery
Department of Surgery, Division of Urology
Texas Tech Health Science Center, El Paso
El Paso, Texas
USA

Stephen Y Nakada MD
Associate Professor of Surgery and Chairman of Urology
The David Theodore Uehling Professor of Urology
University of Wisconsin Medical School
Department of Surgery, Division of Urology
G5/339 Clinical Science Center
600 Highland Avenue
Madison, Wisconsin 53792–3236
USA

Alan W Partin MD PhD
Professor of Urology
The Johns Hopkins Brady Urological Institute
The Johns Hopkins Medical Institutions
Baltimore, MD 21287–2120
USA

Stephen E Pautler MD FRCSC
Fellow in Urology
Department of Urology
Urologic Oncology Branch
National Cancer Institute
Bethesda, Maryland
USA

Peter A Pinto MD
Clinical Instructor of Urology
Johns Hopkins Medical Institutions
Brady Urological Institute
Baltimore, MD 21287
USA

H J Porter II MD
Kansas University Medical Center
Division of Urology
Kansas City
KS 66160–7390
USA

Jens J Rassweiler
Professor, Doctor of Medicine
SLK-Kliniken Heilbronn
Am Gesundbrunnen 20
74078 Heilbronn
Germany

Jan Roigas MD
Associate Professor
Department of Urology, CCM
Charité-University Medicine Berlin
10098 Berlin
Germany

Steven J Shichman
Associate Clinical Professor of Urology
University of Connecticut Health Center
Senior Attending Urologist
Hartford Hospital
USA

Michael Schulze
Department of Urology
SLK Kliniken Heilbronn
Am Gesundbrunnen 20
D 74078 Heilbronn
Germany

Thomas M Seay MD LTCOL USAF MC FS
Department of Radiology
Wilford Hall Medical Center
Lackland AFB
TX 78236
USA

Robert J Stein MD
Resident in Urology
Department of Urology
University of Pittsburgh Medical Center
3471 Fifth Ave
Kaufmann Bldg, Suite 700
Pittsburgh, PA 15213
USA

Dan Stoianovici PhD
Assistant Professor of Urology and Mechanical
Engineering
Director, Robotics Program
James Buchanan Brady Urological Institute
Johns Hopkins University
Baltimore, MD 21224
USA

Li-Ming Su MD
Department of Urology
The James Buchanan Brady Urological Institute
The Johns Hopkins Medical Institutions
Baltimore, MD 21287–2101
USA

Tullio Sulser MD
Professor of Urology
Department of Urology
University Hospital Basel
Spitalstrasse 21
CH 4031 Basel
Switzerland

Chandru P Sundaram MD FRCS
Associate Professor and
Director of Minimally Invasive Surgery
Department of Urology
Indiana University School of Medicine
535 N Barnhill Drive, Suite 420
Indianapolis, IN 46202
USA

Dogu Teber MD
Assistant Professor
Department of Urology
SLK-Kliniken Heilbronn
University of Heidelberg
Am Gesundbrunnen 20
74078 Heilbronn
Germany

Ashutosh Tewari MD
Chief Resident in Urology
Josephine Ford Cancer Center Scholar
Vattikuti Urology Institute
Henry Ford Health System
2799 W. Grand Blvd. K-9
Detroit, MI 48202–2608
USA

J Brantley Thrasher MD
Kansas University Medical Center
Division of Urology
Kansas City
KS 66160–7390
USA

Stefan Thüroff MD
Vice Chairman Department of Urology
Staedtisches Krankenhaus Muenchen
Sanatoriumsplatz 2
81545 Muenchen
Germany

Ingolf Arthur Tuerk MD
Professor
Director of Minimally Invasive Urologic Surgery
Lahey Clinic
Boston, MA
USA

Joseph R Wagner MD
Assistant Clinical Professor of Urology
Urologic Oncology and Minimally Invasive Surgery
Connecticut Surgical Group
85 Seymour Street, Suite 416
Hartford CT 06106
USA

McClellan M Walther MD FACS
Staff Physician
Urologic Oncology Branch
National Cancer Institute
Bethesda, Maryland
USA

David S Wang
Fellow, Endourology and Laparoscopic Surgery
Department of Urology
University of Iowa Hospitals and Clinics
Iowa City, Iowa
USA

Robert Webster
Graduate Student
Whiting School of Engineering
Johns Hopkins University
223 Latrobe Hall
Baltimore MD 21218
USA

Howard N Winfield MD
Professor of Urology
Director of Endourology and Minimally Invasive Surgery
Department of Urology
University of Iowa Hospitals and Clinics
Iowa City, Iowa
USA

J Stuart Wolf Jr MD
University of Michigan, Department of Urology
1500 East Medical Center Drive
Ann Arbor
MI 48109
USA

Stefan Wolter MD
Department of Urology Medical Centre
University Cologne
Joseph-Stelzmann-Str. 9
50924 Cologne
Germany

Preface

Acceptance of creative ideas, theories and even surgical techniques has often been met with scepticism and, at times, even outrage. This was certainly the case in the seventeenth century when Galileo asserted that the earth was round. The invention of laparoscopic urological techniques in the early 1990s was not received with enthusiasm by the urological community. Urologists appropriately demanded that laparoscopic techniques prove themselves with surgical outcomes measured by the success of the procedure on the disease entity as well as associated morbidity, complication rates and affects on convalescences. All of the above variables were compared to the gold standard of 'open' surgical procedures. Laparoscopic techniques proved very quickly to have equal outcomes while significantly decreasing the postoperative morbidity and complication rate when compared to their open counterparts, and over time have gained acceptance through reproducible and durable outcomes.

In the area of urologic oncology, laparoscopic techniques were met with a 'wait and see attitude.' Only recently have outcome data exceeding five years become available, solidifying the place of laparoscopy in treating genitourinary malignancy. Laparoscopic radical nephrectomy was the first urologic laparoscopic procedure for cancer to significantly decrease the side effects of open surgery while giving equivalent or improved disease specific outcomes. Scepticism about cancer control and difficulty in learning the procedure delayed the dissemination of these techniques to the patient and limited laparoscopic teaching to a few academic laparoscopic centers of excellence.

The purpose of this new surgical text is to share the experience gained by experts of urologic laparoscopy in teaching techniques found to be effective and reproducible. It is our hope that this book will propagate the educational waves started by innovative, courageous surgeons who questioned long-standing, deeply rooted beliefs about surgical norms in order to decrease patient morbidity—before most urologists were ready to embrace those changes.

1

Evaluation, perioperative, and postoperative care of the endourologic/laparoscopic patient

Robert J Stein, Steve Y Chung, and Timothy D Averch

Before performing an endourologic or laparoscopic procedure, it is important to evaluate the patient in depth and plan for each stage of their care. This includes preoperative assessment with special attention to comorbidities, close perioperative monitoring in conjunction with anesthesia, and postoperative management according to specific patient needs. This chapter serves as a basic guideline for this planning and provides recommendations for management of patients undergoing minimally invasive surgery.

Preoperative evaluation

History and physical

The assessment of a patient begins with a thorough history and physical examination. The history should include a history of present illness, comorbidities, past surgeries, social history, medications, and pertinent review of systems. The physical examination should include auscul-

tation of the heart and lungs as well as an inspection for previous surgical scars. A full genitourinary and rectal examination should be performed, and note should be taken of umbilical or inguinal hernias.

Laboratory studies

Table 1.1 provides general guidelines when choosing preoperative laboratory and radiographic studies. In urologic surgery, baseline creatinine is checked in the majority of patients. Other laboratory values are checked preoperatively before specific operations, e.g. serum prostate-specific antigen (PSA) prior to transurethral resection of the prostate. If the PSA is elevated, a preoperative prostate biopsy should usually be performed. If a patient has diabetes, a fingerstick blood glucose determination should be performed preoperatively and perioperatively. An elevated blood glucose should prompt an investigation for possible infection. A preoperative

Table 1.1 *Suggested preoperative laboratory and radiographic studies*

Test	Indication
Complete blood count	Anticipation of significant blood loss, chronic illness
Electrolytes, creatinine	Renal disease, age >60, diabetes, liver disease
Urinalysis	Voiding complaints, genitourinary surgery, possible use of prosthetics
Coagulation studies	History of bleeding disorder, liver disease, anticoagulant use, family history of bleeding disorder
Pregnancy testing	Any woman of childbearing age
Chest X-ray	Risk of pulmonary complications, history of pulmonary disease
Electrocardiography	Men > age 40, women > age 50, cardiac history, diabetes
Type + cross/screen	Anticipation of significant blood loss

urinalysis can be helpful prior to endourologic procedures in order to recognize an occult urinary tract infection. A urine culture should be collected prior to an endourologic procedure in patients with chronic catheters in order to give directed antibiotic prophylaxis preoperatively and postoperatively.

Medications

Most medications can be continued perioperatively, exceptions include:

Diabetic medications

If the diabetes is diet-controlled, no medication changes are necessary. If oral hypoglycemics are being used, they should be held the night before or if long half-life medications are used, e.g. glyburide, they should be held two nights prior to surgery. If the patient is insulin-dependent, half the usual dose of insulin the morning of surgery is usually sufficient.

Anticoagulants

It is generally accepted that an international normalized ratio (INR) of 1.5 or less is adequate to avoid increased surgical hemorrhage. Preoperative anticoagulation with heparin while warfarin is being held is often necessary in patients with artificial cardiac valves or a diagnosis of deep vein thrombosis (DVT)/pulmonary embolism (PE) within the last month. Warfarin should be held for approximately 4 days prior to surgery and an INR determination can be performed on the day before or the day of surgery. If the INR does not appear to be decreasing in a reasonable amount of time, a small dose of vitamin K (1 mg subcutaneously) may be considered. If intravenous (IV) heparin is to be used postoperatively, it is often started 12 hours after surgery. Warfarin can routinely be given immediately as it takes several days for its anticoagulant effect to reach therapeutic levels.

With the current patient interest in alternative remedies, a comment should be made concerning the anticoagulant potential of the following medications. Saw palmetto (*Sabal serrulata*) inhibits cyclooxygenase, causing platelet dysfunction and increased bleeding time.[1] Garlic has also been associated with platelet dysfunction and may lead to increased INR in patients taking Coumadin.[2] Therefore, patients should be advised to stop these medications 7 days preoperatively.

Aspirin is an irreversible cyclooxygenase-1 inhibitor and a thromboxane A2 inhibitor. Discontinuation of aspirin at least 7 days prior to surgical procedures allows for new platelet production. Nonsteroidal anti-inflammatory drugs (NSAIDs) are reversible inhibitors of cyclooxygenase and therefore do not have to be stopped as early as does aspirin.

Other antiplatelet agents are not as well studied. Ticlodipine and clopidogrel inhibit ADP-induced platelet aggregation. Manufacturers recommend stopping ticlodipine 10 days and clopidogrel 7 days preoperatively.[3]

Statins

It is recommended that all HMG-CoA reductase inhibitors (e.g. atorvastatin, simvastatin) be held at least 1 day prior to surgery because of rare case reports of associated perioperative rhabdomyolysis. Some of the cases were severe and resulted in death.[4]

Bowel preparation and antibiotics

In surgery involving entrance into the bowel or when bowel perforation is considered a significant risk, a full bowel preparation with 4 liters of GoLYTELY solution can be used. In addition, preoperative oral antibiotics to cleanse the bowel contents are often used. One popular antibiotic regimen is 1 g of erythromycin and 1 g of neomycin at 1, 2, and 11 p.m. the day before surgery.[5]

Endourologic procedures are especially high risk for causing bacterial seeding of abnormal or artificial cardiac valves. Ampicillin 2 g IV and gentamicin 1.5 mg/kg IV should be given 30 min prior to surgery. Six hours postoperatively, amoxicillin 1.5 g orally or ampicillin 1 g IV completes the endocarditis prophylaxis. If the patient is allergic to penicillin, vancomycin 1 g IV before surgery and repeated in 8 hours can be used instead of ampicillin/ amoxicillin.[6]

Radiology A preoperative chest radiograph can help to discover any pleural or parenchymal abnormality and provides a useful baseline for future postoperative studies. Beyond this, other studies should be performed when indicated, e.g. 3-D computed tomography (CT) when trying to define vasculature before donor nephrectomy or to demonstrate a crossing vessel in ureteropelvic junction obstruction, or magnetic resonance imaging or inferior vena cavagram to image renal tumor thrombus.

Preoperative risk stratification
Cardiac risk stratification

Patients and procedures can be separately categorized as either low, intermediate, or high risk. Endourologic procedures are usually felt to be low-risk procedures, except for percutaneous nephrolithotomies, which are low-to-intermediate risk. Laparoscopic cases are considered low- to intermediate-risk procedures. Criteria for patients at increased cardiac risk include:

1. age > 70 years
2. angina
3. prior myocardial infarction (MI)
4. diabetes mellitus
5. history of ventricular ectopy requiring treatment
6. history of congestive heart failure (CHF).[7]

Further major predictors of cardiac risk include:

1. recent MI
2. unstable/severe angina
3. decompensated CHF
4. significant dysrhythmias (high-grade A-V block, symptomatic dysrhythmia, or supraventricular tachycardia with uncontrolled ventricular rate)
5. severe valvular disease.[8]

For low- to intermediate-risk procedures, if patients do not have one of the five major predictors of severe cardiac risk, further cardiac testing is not necessary, but if a patient has any of the six criteria for increased cardiac risk, a perioperative β-blocker should be used. β-blockers have been shown to decrease perioperative MI rates from 18% to 3% in abdominal aortic aneurysm repairs.[9] Postoperative mortality is also decreased in patients using β-blockers, from 14% to 3% in the first postoperative year and from 21% to 10% within 2 years.[10]

Pulmonary risk stratification

Laparoscopic procedures with CO_2 gas insufflation place patients with marginal pulmonary function at risk. Pneumoperitoneum places pressure on the diaphragm, causing increased intrathoracic pressure and work of breathing. With insufflation, CO_2 dissolves in the bloodstream and is buffered. When circulating buffers are exhausted, acidosis can be controlled with adequate respiration. If a patient has poor baseline respiratory function, severe acidosis and hypercarbia with possible arrhythmia or effects on various other organ systems can result.

If a patient has severe chronic obstructive pulmonary disease, heavy smoking history, poor activity tolerance, obesity, or neuromuscular/chest wall disease, pulmonary function tests and a pulmonary medicine consult should be considered. A preoperative arterial blood gas is also helpful to provide a baseline value.

Hepatic risk stratification

Indicators of high surgical risk are severe liver disease, bacterial contamination of ascites, bilirubinemia >3 mg/dl,

and albumin level <3 mg/dl. If the patient has a temporary hepatitis, the liver enzymes should be given time to return to normal. If a procedure is considered elective, encephalopathy and ascites should be optimally controlled and nutritional status should be improved as much as possible. When considering laparoscopic surgery, it is important to realize that ascites can cause the intestines to lie closer to the anterior peritoneum, making them more vulnerable to injury when using the Veress needle for access. A Hasson technique should be considered in this situation, and, when closing, the peritoneum should be sutured in a watertight fashion to prevent ascites leak.

Contraindications to laparoscopic surgery
Absolute contraindications

These include uncorrectable coagulopathy, peritonitis, or malignant ascites.

Relative contraindications

These include the following:

Extensive prior surgery or pelvic fibrosis. From pelvic inflammatory disease, for example, where a Hasson technique to gain access should be considered.

Organomegaly. The surgeon should avoid the enlarged viscera or consider a Hasson technique for access.

Obesity. In laparoscopy, obesity increases the technical difficulty of a procedure due to instruments being too short, difficulty in maneuvering the instruments with a large layer of subcutaneous fat, and difficulty in defining the internal anatomy as a result of too much peritoneal fat. A multi-institutional study of 125 obese patients undergoing laparoscopic urologic procedures showed that 30% of patients experienced a complication, including 15 patients (12%) who required open conversion.[11]

However, several studies have demonstrated a benefit of laparoscopic vs open surgery in obese patients.[12–16] Forty-two obese patients undergoing renal and adrenal surgery were randomized to laparoscopic or open approaches. The laparoscopic group had longer operating times but had less blood loss (100 vs 350 ml), quicker resumption of oral intake and ambulation (1 vs 5 days), less narcotic requirement (12 vs 279 mg), shorter hospital stay (1 vs 5 days), and quicker convalescence (3 vs 9 weeks). They also found a similar complication rate between the two groups.[12] Doublet and Belair reported on 55 patients undergoing retroperitoneal laparoscopic nephrectomy. The operative time was higher among obese patients (100 min vs 70 min) but otherwise there was a similar complication rate and length of stay between obese and non-obese patients. There were three open conversions in the non-obese patients and none in the obese patients.[13]

A comparison of obese and non-obese patients undergoing laparoscopic donor nephrectomy showed a higher conversion rate for the obese patients but otherwise a similar complication rate and postoperative graft function.[14] Another study included a comparison of 12 obese and 28 non-obese patients undergoing laparoscopic donor nephrectomy. There was no difference between these groups in conversion rate, complications, length of stay, or convalescence.[15] It appears that laparoscopic donor nephrectomy can be carried out safely in obese patients.

Contraindications to endourologic surgery

Absolute contraindications

These include uncorrectable coagulopathy, which is an absolute contraindication for percutaneous nephrolithotomy.

Relative contraindications

These include the following:

Stone management in pregnancy. This has been a controversial endourologic topic in recent years. A pregnant woman with flank pain should undergo ultrasound first to check for a stone or hydronephrosis. An intravenous urogram with a single 20 min post-injection film can be performed if additional information is needed.

In the past, stenting the ureter or performing percutaneous nephrostomy during pregnancy was recommended. If a stent or percutaneous nephrostomy is placed, it should usually be changed frequently since encrustation is thought to occur faster in pregnant women. This phenomenon of accelerated encrustation is thought to be due to a combination of hyperuricosuria, absorptive hypercalciuria, and increased incidence of infection during pregnancy.

There are several reports of rigid and flexible ureteroscopy with a combination of stone basketing, holmium laser, pulsed-dye laser, and ultrasonic lithotripsy.[16–25] No obstetric complications except for premature contractions in one patient have been described. In addition, there are reports of encrusted stents being removed using ureteroscopy and one pregnant patient undergoing percutaneous nephrolithotomy for stone disease in the setting of an existing nephrostomy tube.[25] The advantages of ureteroscopy in a pregnant woman include physiologic dilatation of the ureter during pregnancy as well as avoidance of multiple stent or nephrostomy changes.

The theoretical risks of endourologic stone management in pregnant women include premature labor (although no case has yet been reported), transmission of energy to the gravid uterus from laser or other lithotripter devices, and possible release of cyanide as a reaction product during holmium laser lithotripsy of a uric acid stone. Despite these possible risks, the success of multiple reports of ureteroscopy and even percutaneous nephrolithotomy suggest that these approaches are acceptable options in pregnant women.

Other preoperative considerations

Stent placement

Ureteral stent placement should be considered preoperatively for easier location of the ureter during laparoscopic surgery.

Transfusion

Blood transfusion should be considered in surgical patients preoperatively when the hemoglobin is less than 10 g/dl, especially when significant blood loss is likely. Special consideration should be given to patients with cardiac history, who are at higher risk of adverse events at low hemoglobin levels. Carson et al[26] studied 1958 patients postoperatively who were unable to obtain a blood transfusion for religious reasons. Mortality within 30 days correlated directly with preoperative hemoglobin values, as patients with hemoglobin greater than 12 g/dl had a 1.3% risk of death whereas those with a hemoglobin less than 6 g/dl had a 33.3% risk of death. Patients with a history of cardiovascular disease had an increased risk of death in all hemoglobin categories.[26]

Postoperative transfusion has also been investigated. A total of 838 patients in the intensive care unit were split into two groups. Patients in one group were maintained at a hemoglobin level of 7–9 g/dl and patients in the other group at a hemoglobin level of greater than 10 g/dl. The group maintained at a hemoglobin of 7–9 g/dl had a trend of decreased mortality compared with patients with the higher hemoglobin. This decreased mortality became significant when patients were not critically ill or were less than 55 years old.[27] This study seems to suggest that postoperative blood transfusions should be given only in the setting of ischemic heart disease when patients' hemoglobin values rest in the 7–9 g/dl range. The adverse effects of transfusion may possibly, but not necessarily, be due to increased blood viscosity.

In urologic patients it is recommended that transfusion be used to maintain hemoglobin at 7–8 g/dl except in the case of ischemic heart disease. A cardiac history should prompt an effort to maintain the hemoglobin between 9 and 10 g/dl.[28]

Antibiotic prophylaxis

For wound infection prophylaxis, administration of antibiotics 30 min to 2 hours prior to the procedure provides maximum prevention. Additional doses of antibiotics are of no benefit in uncomplicated patients.[29]

For prophylaxis against urinary tract infection (UTI) after endourologic procedures, the recommendations are less strict. There was no difference found in UTI incidence if antibiotics were given 2 hours before or 6 hours after a procedure. Therefore it is acceptable for a patient to take an antibiotic several hours after a cystoscopy is performed in the office.[30] If an endourologic procedure is performed on a patient with an indwelling catheter, special care should be taken to ensure that the patient is on proper antibiotics to target any colonizing organisms. A urine culture is an important part of the preoperative evaluation.

The need for prophylactic antibiotics in percutaneous nephrolithotomy has been investigated.[31,32] In one series, 107 patients were not given any prophylactic antibiotics around the time of their procedure: 35% were found to have postoperative bacteriuria, 10% with temperature >38.5°C.[31] Another group reported a 2% UTI rate for patients who received antibiotics perioperatively for percutaneous nephrolithotomy vs a 12% rate in patients who had not received antibiotics.[32] Indeed, the evidence seems to suggest that prophylactic antibiotics are indicated for percutaneous nephrolithotomy.

Several studies have addressed the need for prophylactic antibiotics with transurethral resection or cystoscopy.[33–42] Of 1249 patients undergoing urethral manipulation, 5/790 (0.6%) with 3-day prophylactic antibiotics and 16/459 (3.5%) without antibiotics developed a UTI. There was found to be an even greater risk for older patients not using antibiotics.[33] In another study, cefoxitin was administered from the time of surgery until catheter removal (mean 3.8 days) in patients undergoing transurethral resection of the prostate (TURP). At 3 days postoperatively the rate of UTI decreased from 26.4% in a placebo arm to 3.9% and at 7 days postoperatively the rate of UTI decreased from 42% in the placebo to 6.5%.[34] A separate group of patients received nitrofurantoin for 10 days after TURP. The catheters were usually removed 3 days postoperatively and urine cultures collected 24 hours later showed no bacteriuria in patients treated with antibiotics vs a 25% bacteriuria rate in the control group. Furthermore, 47% of controls developed bacteriuria 1 month later vs only 10% of treated patients.[35] Similarly,

other studies document an advantage from prophylactic antibiotics in patients undergoing TURP.[36–38] Although one group reported no difference in bacteriuria between patients treated with antibiotics (14%) vs those left untreated (11%), most practitioners believe that the Foley catheter is associated with bacterial colonization and therefore recommend continuing antibiotics until the catheter is removed or resuming antibiotics around the time of Foley catheter removal.[39]

The need for perioperative antibiotics around the time of cystourethroscopy or transurethral resection of bladder tumor (TURBT) is more controversial. Several studies document no advantage to using prophylactic antibiotics with these procedures if no bacteriuria is documented preoperatively.[40–42] Out of 138 patients undergoing outpatient diagnostic cystourethroscopy, 1.5% of those treated with antibiotics and 2.8% left untreated developed bacteriuria.[41] Another group of 30 patients undergoing TURBT were treated with carbenicillin or no antibiotics at all. One patient in the treated group vs no patients in the untreated group developed UTI.[42] It seems that use of prophylactic antibiotics for uncomplicated endoscopic procedures may sometimes be unnecessary; nevertheless, lack of bacteriuria should be documented before choosing to forego antibiotics perioperatively.

The use of antibiotics prior to extracorporeal shock wave lithotripsy (ESWL) has also been evaluated. A meta–analysis involving more than 800 patients demonstrated a reduction in postoperative UTI from 7% to 2% with one dose of prophylactic antibiotics.[43] Therefore, a dose of antibiotics is recommended when performing ESWL.

Recommended prophylactic antibiotics for some minimally invasive procedures are listed in Table 1.2.[44]

Informed consent

Risks of laparoscopic procedures must be discussed in full, including the possibilities of hemorrhage, infection, bowel injury, death, and any other more specific risks depending on which procedure is to be performed. Also complications unique to laparoscopy should be mentioned, including failure to progress and possible need to convert to open surgery. Medical or other surgical alternatives should also be discussed.

With endoscopic surgery, consent should also involve discussion of risks, including hemorrhage, hematuria, infection, and death, and more procedure-specific risks such as ureteral injury, bladder perforation, or pneumothorax. Open surgery in case of bladder perforation or chest tube placement in case of pneumothorax should be addressed. Possible inability to progress or ureteral injury requiring a stent or percutaneous nephrostomy should be explained as well.

Table 1.2 *Suggested antibiotics for laparoscopic and endourologic procedures*

Procedure	Antibiotic
Laparoscopic nephrectomy, adrenalectomy, prostatic brachytherapy	First-generation cephalosporin. Alternative, penicillinase-resistant penicillin, clindamycin, vancomycin (if MRSA is suspected)
Laparoscopic cystectomy, prostatectomy, ureteral reimplant, nephroureterectomy, pyeloplasty, percutaneous renal surgery	Cephalosporin or ampicillin $+/-$ aminoglycoside, ampicillin–sulbactam. Alternative, levofloxacin, vancomycin/aminoglycoside (if MRSA suspected)
Prostate needle biopsy	Fluoroquinolone

MRSA, methicillin-resistant *Staphylococcus aureus*.

Postoperative care of the laparoscopic, endourologic patient

Postoperative care should include resumption of activity within 1 day of surgery and supportive measures, e.g. pain control, IV fluids, when necessary. Specific recommendations concerning nasogastric tubes, nephrostomy tubes, Jackson–Pratt drains, etc., vary with the type and extent of surgery.

With the rapid expansion of laparoscopic capability, more complicated surgeries are being successfully performed. Vigilant postoperative management is essential, and it is important not to discharge patients too soon with the belief that all patients should return home on postoperative day 1 or 2. Vital signs and a physical examination should be performed regularly. Urine output should return to adequate levels postoperatively (>0.5 ml/kg/h) even though intraoperative urine output in laparoscopic surgery is usually decreased, perhaps secondary to decreased renal vein blood flow and direct compression of renal parenchyma.

On discharge, patients should be provided prescriptions for adequate pain medication, stool softener, and antibiotic if indicated. They should be cautioned not to operate a motor vehicle while in significant pain or while using narcotics. Follow-up in the office should include a wound-check and review of any pathology results. The section to follow includes some complications occasionally seen during the postoperative period.

Other postoperative considerations

Postoperative myocardial infarction

Chest pain in association with hypoxia, hypotension, and arrhythmia can suggest an MI or PE. In order to rule out an MI, a daily electrocardiogram (ECG) should be checked for 2 days, a serum troponin I level should be checked every 12 hours for a total of three determinations, and the patient should be moved to a monitored setting. Troponin I levels are more sensitive and specific for detecting MI compared with creatinine phosphokinase.[45] As soon as suspicion is raised for possible MI, the patient should be placed on 2 liters of oxygen and an aspirin should be given, as it has been shown to decrease mortality in acute MI.[46] Furthermore, chest discomfort should be controlled with a combination of narcotics and nitrates, and a cardiology consultation as well as intensive care monitoring should be considered.

Deep vein thrombosis

Surgical patients are at higher risk for DVT due to the three components of Virchow's triad: stasis, hypercoagulability, and venous injury. Perioperatively, episodes of stasis are common as patients are immobile on the operating room table and on bedrest for the first 1 to 2 days postoperatively. In addition, states of hypercoagulability and increased venous injury may exist due to the release of cellular mediators which affect clotting and the vascular endothelium. If the proper precautions are taken, perioperative DVT has a low incidence (0.8%).[11] In urologic patients, sequential compression devices (SCD) have been recommended for DVT prophylaxis, and it is strongly urged that laparoscopic patients wear SCD perioperatively.[47] Prophylactic doses of heparin or low-molecular-weight heparin injected subcutaneously can be considered in patients with additional risk factors, including age >40 years, obesity, malignancy, or previous history of DVT/PE.

Physical examination findings that suggest DVT include unilateral leg edema, erythema, tenderness with dorsiflexion (Homan's sign), or a palpable cord in the groin. A Doppler ultrasound should initially be performed. If the Doppler test is negative or nondiagnostic and suspicion remains high, contrast venography (the radiologic gold standard) may be performed. A diagnosed or highly suspected DVT should be treated with unfractionated IV heparin. Coumadin should be started upon confirmation of the DVT diagnosis, and a goal INR of 2–3 should be targeted. In isolated DVT, subcutaneous injections of low-molecular-weight heparin can be used while the patient's INR rises to a therapeutic level.[48]

Pulmonary embolism

Acute onset of chest pain and dyspnea should alert the physician to consider a diagnosis of PE. Diagnostic studies include ECG, which may show right ventricular hypertrophy with strain, right bundle branch block, and T-wave inversion in leads V_1 and V_4. Chest radiograph is not a very sensitive test for PE but may demonstrate a Westermark sign, which appears as decreased peripheral pulmonary vascular markings. An arterial blood gas classically shows a low PaO_2 and a large A-a gradient. In recent years, helical CT scan with IV contrast has emerged as a sensitive and noninvasive imaging modality for PE. Studies showed 91% sensitivity and 78% specificity for emboli in main pulmonary arteries, but decreased sensitivity (63%) when the emboli were in more peripheral subsegmental arteries.[49,50] If suspicion is high and a helical CT is non-diagnostic, a pulmonary angiogram, the gold standard, may be performed. When IV contrast infusion is contraindicated, a ventilation perfusion scan is an option but is neither as sensitive nor specific as helical CT. Once PE is discovered, the treatment is similar to that of DVT with IV heparin and long-term anticoagulation using Coumadin. Contrary to DVT management, low-molecular-weight heparin has not been approved for use in PE.

Conclusions

Successful minimally invasive urologic surgery can provide a patient with multiple benefits compared with an open approach. This success starts with a thorough evaluation of the patient and careful planning of every aspect of the clinical course. Minimally invasive surgeries cannot be treated as procedures without significant risk, and therefore the evaluation and preparation must be complete in order to avoid troublesome results. This chapter aims to provide guidelines for performing successful laparoscopic and endourologic procedures and to facilitate the decision making in the preoperative, perioperative, and postoperative courses.

Acknowledgments

We are indebted to Teuta Doko for her help and support on this project.

References

1. Chung KF, Dent G, McCusker M, et al. Effect of a ginkgolide mixture (BN 52063) in antagonising skin and platelet responses to platelet activating factor in man. Lancet 1987; 1:248–51.

2. Bordia A. Effect of garlic on human platelet aggregation in vitro. Atherosclerosis 1978; 30:355–60.

3. Stables G, Lawrence CM. Management of patients taking anticoagulant, aspirin, non-steroidal anti-inflammatory and other anti-platelet drugs undergoing dermatological surgery. Clin Exp Dermatol 2002; 27:432–5.

4. Forestier F, Breton Y, Bonnet E, Janvier G. Severe rhabdomyolysis after laparoscopic surgery for adenocarcinoma of the rectum in two patients treated with statins. Anesthesiology 2002; 97:1019–21.

5. Nichols RL, Condon RE, Gorback SL, Nyhus LM. Efficacy of preoperative antimicrobial preparation of the bowel. Ann Surg 1972; 176:227–32.

6. Dajani AS, Taubert KA, Wilson W, et al. Prevention of bacterial endocarditis, recommendations by the American Heart Association. JAMA 1997; 277:1794–801.

7. Eagle KA, Coley CM, Newell JB, et al. Combining clinical and thallium data optimizes preoperative assessment of cardiac risk before major vascular surgery. Ann Intern Med 1989; 110:859–66.

8. Romero L, de Virgilio C. Preoperative cardiac risk assessment: an updated approach. Arch Surg 2001; 136:1370–6.

9. Pasternack PF, Imparato AM, Baumann FG, et al. The hemodynamics of beta-blockade in patients undergoing abdominal aortic aneurysm repair. Circulation 1987; 76:1111–17.

10. Mangano DT, Layug EL, Wallace A, Tateo I. Effect of atenolol on mortality and cardiovascular morbidity after noncardiac surgery. N Engl J Med 1999; 341:1789–94.

11. Mendoza D, Newman RC, Albala D, et al. Laparoscopic complications in markedly obese urologic patients (a multi-institutional review). Urology 1996; 48:562–7.

12. Fazeli-Matin S, Gill IS, Hsu TH, et al. Laparoscopic renal and adrenal surgery in obese patients: comparison to open surgery. J Urol 1999; 162:665–9.

13. Doublet J-D, Belair G. Retroperitoneal laparoscopic nephrectomy is safe and effective in obese patients: a comparative study of 55 procedures. Urology 2000; 56:63–6.

14. Jacobs SC, Cho E, Dunkin BJ, et al. Laparoscopic nephrectomy in the markedly obese living renal donor. Urology 2000; 56:926–9.

15. Kuo PC, Plotkin JS, Stevens S. Outcomes of laparoscopic donor nephrectomy in obese patients. Transplantation 2000; 69:180–3.

16. Rittenberg MH, Bagley DH. Ureteroscopic diagnosis of urinary calculi during pregnancy. Urology 1988; 32:427–8.

17. Rodriguez PN, Klein AS. Management of urolithiasis during pregnancy. Surg Gynecol Obstet 1988;166:103–6.

18. Vest JM, Warden SS. Ureteroscopic stone manipulation during pregnancy. Urology 1990; 35:250–2.

19. Ulvik NM, Bakke A, Hoisaeter PA. Ureteroscopy in pregnancy. J Urol 1995; 154:1660–3.

20. Carlan SJ, Schorr SJ, Ebenger MF, et al. Laser lithotripsy in pregnancy. J Reprod Med 1995; 40:74–6.

21. Carringer M, Swartz R, Johansson JE. Management of ureteric calculi during pregnancy by ureteroscopy and laser lithotripsy. BJU Int 1996; 77:17–20.

22. Scarpa RM, De Lisa A, Usai E. Diagnosis and treatment of ureteral calculi during pregnancy with rigid ureteroscopes. J Urol 1996; 155:875–7.

23. Shokeir AA, Mutabagani H. Rigid ureteroscopy in pregnant women. BJU Int 1998; 81:678–81.

24. Watterson JD, Girvan AR, Beiko DT, et al. Ureteroscopy and holmium:YAG laser lithotripsy: an emerging definitive management strategy for symptomatic ureteral calculi in pregnancy. Urology 2002; 60:383–7.

25. Lifshitz DA, Lingeman JE. Ureteroscopy as a first-line intervention for ureteral calculi in pregnancy. J Endourol 2002; 16:19–22.

26. Carson JL, Duff A, Poses RM, et al. Effect of anaemia and cardiovascular disease on surgical mortality and morbidity. Lancet 1996; 348:1055–60.

27. Hebert PC, Wells G, Blajchman MA, et al. A multicenter, randomized, controlled clinical trial of transfusion requirements in critical care. N Engl J Med 1999; 340:409–17.

28. Gilbert WB, Smith JA. Blood use strategies in urologic surgery. Urology 2000; 55:461–7.

29. Burke JF. The effective period of preventive antibiotic action in experiments in dermal lesions. Surgery 1961; 50:161–8.

30. Nielsen KT, Madsen PO. Quinolones in urology. Urol Res 1989; 17:117–24.

31. Charton M, Vallancien G, Veillon B, Brisset JM. Urinary tract infection in percutaneous surgery for renal calculi. J Urol 1986; 135:15–17.

32. Inglis JA, Tolley DA. Antibiotic prophylaxis at the time of percutaneous stone surgery. J Endourol 1988; 2:59–62.

33. Fujita K, Matsushima H, Nakano M, et al. Prophylactic oral antibiotics in urethral instrumentation. Nippon Hinyokika Gakkai Zasshi 1994; 85:802–5.

34. Nielsen OS, Maigaard S, Frimodt-Moller N, Madsen PO. Prophylactic antibiotics in transurethral prostatectomy. J Urol 1981; 126:60–2.

35. Matthew AD, Gonzalez R, Jeffords D, Pinto MH. Prevention of bacteriuria after transurethral prostatectomy with nitrofurantoin macrocrystals. J Urol 1978; 120:442–3.

36. Hargreave TB, Hindmarsh JR, Elton R, et al. Short-term prophylaxis with cefotaxime for prostatic surgery. BMJ 1982; 284:1008–10.

37. Lacy SS, Drach GW, Cox CE. Incidence of infection after prostatectomy and efficacy of cephaloridine prophylaxis. J Urol 1971; 105:836–8.

38. Morris MJ, Golovsky D, Guiness MD, Maher PO. The value of prophylactic antibiotics in transurethral prostatic resection: a controlled trial, with observations on the origin of postoperative infection. Br J Urol 1976; 48:479–84.

39. Gibbons RP, Stark RA, Correa RJ, et al. The prophylactic use- or misuse- of antibiotics in transurethral prostatectomy. J Urol 1978; 119:381–3.

40. Ohishi Y, Machida T, Akasaka Y, et al. Treatment and prophylaxis for urogenital infections occurring after urethrocystoscopy. Hinyokika Kiyo 1988; 34:1601–5.

41. Manson AL. Is antibiotic administration indicated after outpatient cystoscopy? J Urol 1988; 140:316–17.

42. Upton JD, Das S. Prophylactic antibiotics in transurethral resection of bladder tumors: are they necessary? Urology 1986; 27:421–3.

43. Pearle MS, Roehrborn CG. Antimicrobial prophylaxis prior to shock wave lithotripsy in patients with sterile urine before treatment: a meta-analysis and cost-effectiveness analysis. Urology 1997; 49:679–86.

44. Terris MK. Recommendations for prophylactic antibiotic use in GU surgery. Contemp Urol 2001; 9:12–27.

45. Rice MS, MacDonald DC. Appropriate roles of cardiac troponins in evaluating patients with chest pain. J Am Board Fam Pract 1999; 12:214–18.

46. ISIS-2 Collaborative Group. Randomised trial of intravenous streptokinase, oral aspirin, both, or neither among 17,187 cases of suspected acute myocardial infarction: ISIS-2. Lancet 1988; 2:349–60.

47. Hyers TM, Hull RD, Weg JG. Antithrombotic therapy for venous thromboembolic disease. Chest 1989; 95(Suppl 2):37S–51S.

48. Lensing AW, Prins MH, Davidson BL, Hirsh J. Treatment of deep venous thrombosis with low-molecular-weight heparins: a meta-analysis. Arch Intern Med 1995; 155:601–7.

49. Remy-Jardin M, Remy J, Deschildre F, et al. Diagnosis of pulmonary embolism with spiral CT: comparison with pulmonary angiography and scintigraphy. Radiology 1996; 200:699–706.

50. Goodman LR, Curtin JJ, Mewissen MW, et al. Detection of pulmonary embolism in patients with unresolved clinical and scintigraphic diagnosis: helical CT versus angiography. AJR 1995; 164:1369–74.

2

Laparoscopic instrumentation and equipment

Stephen V Jackman and Jay T Bishoff

The advancement of laparoscopic surgical technique goes hand in hand with the development of laparoscopic instrumentation. Only the surgeon's imagination and the willingness of industry to produce innovative equipment limit the development and application of new devices. In this chapter we describe the current state of the art in laparoscopic instrumentation with the goal of increasing surgeons' knowledge of the devices available to assist them in their laparoscopic surgical procedures. Many instruments, although not essential, are advantageous in condensing the learning curve, shortening procedure times, and improving outcomes.

Access

A significant number of complications during laparoscopic surgery occur at the time of initial access to the peritoneal cavity.[1] The traditional method of Veress needle insufflation followed by blind insertion of a cutting trocar is being replaced by numerous more controlled and theo-

retically safer techniques. These include use of dilating-tip trocars, visual obturators, and variations on the open Hasson technique. Balloon inflation may be used to rapidly develop the retroperitoneal or retropubic spaces.

Blind-cutting trocars offer rapid access to the peritoneal cavity. Their sharp blades require less force than blunter options. However, their safety has been questioned for initial port placement, especially in the non-virgin abdomen. Even utilizing these trocars during secondary trocars placed under direct internal vision, the risk of laceration of body wall blood vessels and muscle exists. Transillumination of the abdominal wall is seldom useful for locating blood vessels, except in thin patients. Finally, cutting trocars ≥ 10 mm make incisions in the fascia that require closure. For these reasons, dilating-tip or non-bladed trocars were developed. Many manufacturers offer versions of this style of trocar (Figure 2.1). The tips are typically cone-shaped, often with laterally placed fins to assist in the dilation. The fins can vary from sharp to dull. Advantages include smaller fascial openings after port removal that do not require closure and a higher likelihood of pushing aside rather than lacerating blood vessels and

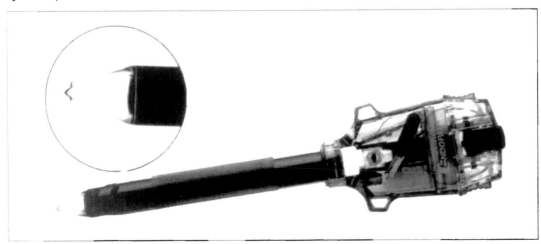

Figure 2.1
The 10/12 mm bladeless trocar with tip close-up (Ethicon Endo-Surgery, Cincinnati, Ohio). (Composite of photos courtesy of Ethicon Endo-Surgery.)

muscle.[2] This technology may be combined with direct visualization as described below. Disadvantages include a higher insertion force and increased difficulty penetrating compliant structures such as the peritoneum and bladder.[3]

Visual obturators or direct-view trocars are systems combining sheath, cutting, or dilating elements and laparoscope. These systems allow direct visualization of the layers and blood vessels of the body wall during entry. These devices are typically used after insufflation. However, with experience, they may be used for both initial access and insufflation. Two disposable instruments in this category are the Visiport RPF Optical Trocar (USSC, Norwalk, Connecticut), shown in Figure 2.2, and the Optiview Non-bladed Obturator (Ethicon Endo-Surgery, Cincinnati, Ohio), (shown in Figure 2.3). The Visiport uses a trigger-activated cutting blade to enter the abdomen, whereas the Optiview has two dilating fins. The Optiview requires more pressure and rotation to enter the abdomen but

retains the advantages of non-bladed instruments, including smaller fascial defects that may not require closure. The EndoTIP system (Karl Storz GmbH & Co. KG, Tuttlingen, Germany) is a reusable threaded screw-in trocar that allows visualization and also incorporates a dilating tip.

Arguably the safest method for entrance to the peritoneal cavity is by the open Hasson technique. Open access is particularly important in children, in whom standard-sized laparoscopic trocars may be more likely to damage vital structures. Disadvantages of the Hasson technique include the need for a larger incision, more cumbersome trocar systems that may leak gas if not well-secured, and increased difficulty in obese patients. The Step System (formerly InnerDyne, Inc.; now USSC, Norwalk, Connecticut) is a modification of this method that solves some of these problems (Figure 2.4). Through a small skin incision, the fascia and peritoneum are opened 2–3 mm

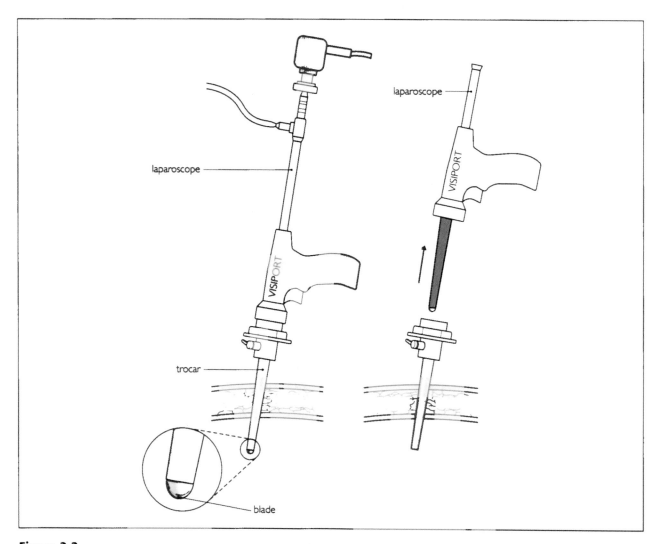

Figure 2.2

The Visiport (USSC, Norwalk, Connecticut) uses a recessed blade that extends out of the end of the obturator as the surgeon fires a trigger.

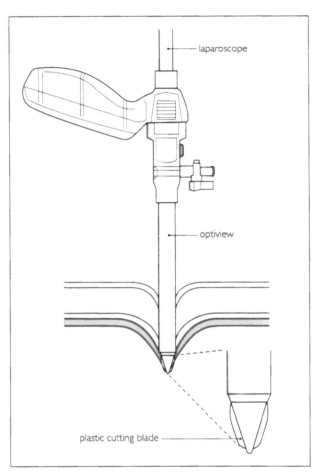

Figure 2.3
The Optiview (Ethicon Endo-Surgery, Cincinnati, Ohio) uses two sharpened plastic fins on the tip of the trocar.

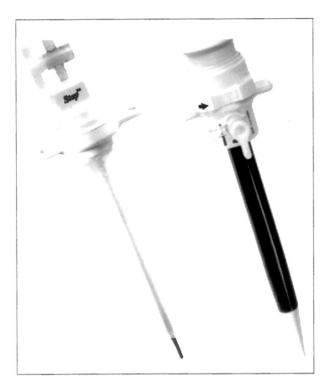

Figure 2.4
The Step System (USSC, Norwalk, Connecticut). The mesh sleeve can be placed in an open fashion or used with a Veress needle as shown. The cannula and dilator is then passed through the sleeve. (Photos courtesy of United States Surgical, a division of Tyco Healthcare.)

under direct visualization. The mesh sleeve is then inserted and dilated with a rigid cannula and dilator to the desired size (5–12 mm). This radial dilation both fixes the sheath in place and seals the peritoneal cavity, preventing gas leakage. The access may also be conveniently upsized if needed by inserting a larger rigid sheath and dilator. The entire system can also be used over a Veress needle. However, the advantages of open insertion are lost. The fascial defect left after removing a Step trocar has been shown to be 50% smaller than that associated with a conventional cutting trocar.[4] Overlying tissue and muscle planes return to their preoperative location after removal and provide further closure of the wound. A prospective randomized trial in 250 patients showed that the Step system results in significantly less intraoperative cannula site bleeding and fewer postoperative wound complications than conventional cutting trocars.[5] Furthermore, no port-site hernias were seen despite not closing any of the Step port sites.

Another modification of the Hasson technique for access to non-peritoneal locations is use of a balloon to rapidly develop the space. This was initially done using a red-rubber catheter with a glove finger secured to the end. More convenient commercial products that perform the same task are now available. A useful combination of balloon and visual obturator, the Preperitoneal Distention Balloon System (PDB; formerly Origin Medsystems; now USSC, Norwalk, Connecticut) or Spacemaker II Balloon Dissector (formerly GSI, Inc.; now USSC, Norwalk, Connecticut) is available to allow direct observation during space creation (Figure 2.5). A balloon-tipped or Hasson trocar is required to seal the initial incision. The Blunt-tipped Trocar (USSC, Norwalk, Connecticut) is a significant advance over the standard Hasson trocar. It has a balloon at the distal end to hold it in place and a sliding foam ring proximally to seal it to the abdomen. This allows full 360° motion without leakage in a small footprint device.

Retraction

Prolonged retraction of organs such as the liver and bowel is often necessary for access to the operative site. When adequate gravity retraction is not possible, numerous

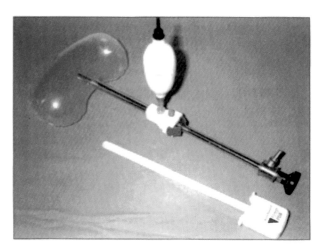

Figure 2.5
The PDB System (USSC, Norwalk, Connecticut). The retroperitoneal space can be balloon developed under direct vision.

instruments are available. The ideal retractor would fit through a small trocar, hold the target organ securely and atraumatically, remain exactly where it was placed, and be either reusable or inexpensive. Most current instruments accomplish the first two conditions with reasonable success. They are typically variations on the design of a straight 5 or 10 mm instrument that transforms into a wider configuration once inserted.

An innovative reusable device is the Diamond Flex 80 mm Angled Triangular Liver Retractor (Genzyme Surgical Products Corp., Tucker, Georgia) (Figure 2.6). This long multi-jointed instrument passes through a 5 mm port and then transforms into a rigid triangular shape after its knob is tightened. Other sizes and configurations exist.

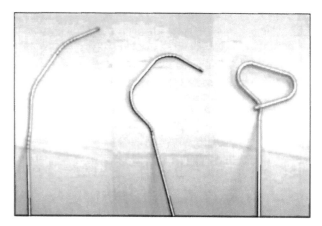

Figure 2.6
The Diamond Flex 80 mm Angled Triangular Liver Retractor (Genzyme Surgical Products Corp., Tucker, Georgia) fits through a 5 mm cannula and converts to a rigid angled triangular shape.

Disadvantages include the initial expense and the metal construction that does not hold organs as securely as some disposable fabric devices. The PEER retractor (Jarit Surgical Instruments, Hawthorne, New York) is another reusable device that opens to provide retraction in a variety of situations. It is available in 5 and 10 mm sizes.

Fan retractors are available from several manufacturers in either a reusable or disposable form. They typically fit through a 10 mm port and 'fan' open into a triangular shape. Other common variations include balloons and fabric that expand after insertion. One significant disadvantage of the previously described instruments is that they require an assistant to reliably hold them in position. This introduces the human factors of fatigue and inattention, which can cause lack of retraction, often at the worst possible moment. In addition, the assistant takes up space at the side of the table and can hinder the optimal movement and positioning of the surgeon. Several mechanical instrument holders have been developed to take the place of the assistant. The instrument is then positioned and locked in place by one of several methods. The basic Martin Arm (Mick Radio-Nuclear Instruments, Inc., Mount Vernon, New York) is a multi-jointed stainless steel arm that requires each joint to be positioned and hand-tightened. The Unitrac Retraction System (Aesculap, Center Valley, California) is an advanced version of the Martin Arm that uses compressed air to allow pneumatic locking and unlocking with a single button (Figure 2.7). The Endoholder (Codman Inc., Cincinnati, Ohio) is an innovative device with a flexible gooseneck that can be quickly bent into position.[6] The TISKA Endoarm is a system developed to assist with trocar and instrument positioning (TISKA Endoarm, Karl Storz, Endoskope, Tuttlingen, Germany). This device maintains the position of the trocar sheath at a fixed point at the trocar puncture site, while instruments or laparoscopes are changed or removed. Routine laparoscopic needs such as tissue retraction can easily be performed with this system. When combined with a robotic camera holder, these instrument holders permit many procedures to be done completely without assistance.

Hand-assist devices

The merits of hand-assisted laparoscopy (HAL) vs pure laparoscopy in urology are a matter of significant current debate. Proponents point to the proven ability to decrease operative times, allow performance of complex procedures, and aid in resident teaching.[7] This is achieved with a slight increase in postoperative pain but no significant increase in recovery times.[8] The issue of cost can be balanced by shorter operating room times and decreased need for other disposables such as trocars and entrapment

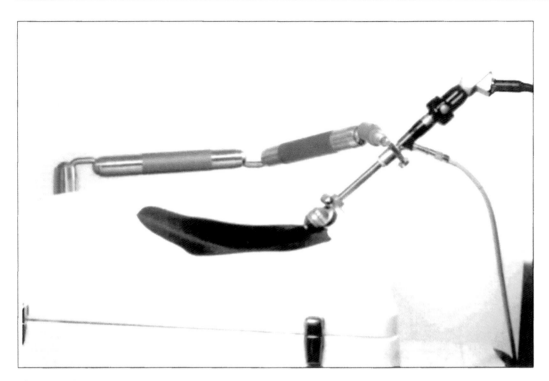

Figure 2.7
The Unitrac Retraction System (Aesculap, Inc., Center Valley, California) is locked in place with compressed air. It can hold various instruments for retraction. (Photo courtesy of Aesculap, Inc.)

bags. Furthermore, injuries related to Veress needle and initial trocar access should be eliminated, as all of the HAL devices except the Pneumo Sleeve can be used for primary insufflation. The GelPort and Lap Disc also allow airtight passage of the laparoscope to visually direct subsequent port placement.

Opponents object to hand-assisted techniques because they are not actually minimally invasive since HAL requires an incision large enough to allow placement of the surgeon's hand into the abdomen. The same complex cases are being done 'purely laparoscopically' by experts, often in shorter times than those reported in hand-assisted series. These experts argue that use of the hand is a 'crutch' rather than a 'bridge' to improved surgical ability.[9] Other disadvantages of HAL include device failure, air leakage, hand pain and fatigue with extended dissection or tight incisions, decreased view and working room due to the intra-abdominal placement of the surgeon's hand, and cosmetic concerns created by the larger incision.

Currently, there are six FDA-approved devices available for HAL surgery (Table 2.1). They all incorporate two basic features: an airtight seal between the device and the incision and a second seal between the device and the surgeon's arm (Figure 2.8). In general, devices using adhesive to seal the incision require a larger footprint and may offer more interference with choice of port-site locations. They also will not provide a reliable seal when placed so that the adhesive is near the umbilicus. An Ioban drape (3M Health Care, St. Paul, Minnesota) may be helpful in improving the durability of the adhesive seal. Regardless of the device chosen, some gas leakage can be expected, especially in longer operations. A high-flow or dual insufflation system is desirable.

Little data exist comparing the different HAL devices. A recent prospective evaluation of three HAL devices (HandPort, Intromit, and Pneumo Sleeve) showed highest overall satisfaction with the Intromit.[10] It was easier to exchange hands or lap pads with the Intromit or HandPort than with the Pneumo Sleeve. The HandPort was the easiest to set up but also had the highest failure rate. Surgeons are encouraged to try several devices before selecting one for routine use.

Hemostasis

Some of the most significant advances in laparoscopic instrumentation have been achieved in hemostasis. Excessive bleeding from even small venous vessels can

Table 2.1 *Hand-assisted laparoscopic devices*						
	Pneumo Sleeve	Omniport	HandPort	GelPort	Intromit	Lap Disc
Company	Weck Closure Systems, Research Triangle Park, North Carolina	Weck Closure Systems, Research Triangle Park, North Carolina	Smith & Nephew, Inc., Andover, Massachusetts	Applied Medical, Rancho Santa Margarita, California	Applied Medical, Rancho Santa Margarita, California	Ethicon Endo-Surgery, Cincinnati, Ohio
Seal to incision	Adhesive	Inflation/wound retractor	Inflation/wound retractor	Wound retractor	Adhesive	Wound retractor
Seal to arm	Sleeve	Inflation	Sleeve	Gel	Inflation	Iris
Cost	$495	$440	$375	$725	$495	$440

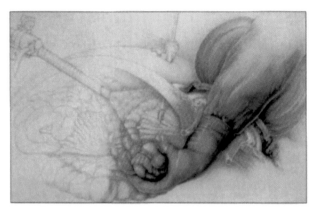

Figure 2.8
The Pneumo Sleeve (Weck Closure Systems, Research Triangle Park, North Carolina) in cross section showing the airtight seals between the device and abdominal wall and the device and the surgeon's arm. (Photo courtesy of Weck Closure Systems.)

quickly obscure the surgical field, making it difficult to find the correct planes of dissection. The availability of new delivery systems for electrocautery, ultrasound, clips, staples, clamps, and fibrin products has allowed laparoscopy to approach open surgery in even the most challenging cases.

Electrocautery

Monopolar electrocautery has been the mainstay for hemostasis of small vessels during dissection. In the monopolar circuit the active electrode is in the surgical site and the return electrode is the grounding pad. Consequently, the current passes through the body of the patient to complete the circuit. The waveform can be continuous or intermittent (cut or coagulation) and is low current with high voltage.

When monopolar electrocautery is used, the current is not localized to the visible portion of the instrument. Since only 15% of the entire length of the electrocautery instrument is seen with the laparoscope at any given time, injuries from stray energy can occur out of the surgeon's field of view.[11] More than half of laparoscopic bowel injuries reported in the literature result from monopolar electrocautery.[12] Application of monopolar electricity to duct-like strands of tissue attached to the bowel, even during a short burst of energy, can result in tissue death at the bowel segment.[13] Unrecognized bowel injuries can also occur from the use of monopolar electrocautery when stray energy is released from unrecognized breaks in the integrity of the insulated coating or from capacitive coupling along the shaft of the monopolar instruments or trocar.

The occurrence of cautery injury can be minimized through the use of active electrode monitoring (AEM) devices or insulation scanners for monopolar instruments and bipolar electrocautery. The Electroscope AEM system (Electroscope, Inc., Boulder, Colorado) includes a unique set of laparoscopic instruments that are simultaneously connected to a standard electrocautery machine and to a separate device that continuously searches for stray energy escaping along the shaft of the instrument. When stray energy is detected, the AEM system deactivates the electrosurgical generator before injury can occur. The integrity of the insulated coating on the shaft of laparoscopic instruments can also be determined on the back table, prior to placing the instrument into the patient, using the InsulScan (Medline Industries, Inc., Mundelein, Illinois). Both disposable and reusable instruments can be tested for visually undetectable holes in the insulation sheath.

In bipolar electrocautery, the active electrode and the return electrode functions are performed at the site of surgery between the tips of the instrument. The waveform is continuous, low current, and low voltage. Since the flow of current is restricted between the contact points of the instrument tip, only the tissue grasped is included in the electrical circuit, minimizing the risk of injury from stray surgical energy. Thermal injury can be prevented by vigilant surveillance of monopolar contact points during dissection.

The Ligasure is a specialized electrosurgical generator/instrument system that has been developed (Valleylab, Boulder, Colorado) to reliably seal tissue and blood vessels up to 7 mm in diameter during laparoscopic or open surgery. The electrical generator delivers a continuous waveform of low-voltage, high-current flow and pulsed electrosurgical energy to tissue between the jaws of the instrument. The tissue is under a predetermined amount of pressure set by the unique locking jaws of the instrument. The vessel lumen is obliterated as collagen and elastin in the vessel wall fuse to form a permanent seal. The seal zone is then divided with standard laparoscopic scissor. The newest version (Ligasure Atlas, Valleylab, Boulder, Colorado) is a 10 mm instrument that incorporates a blade in the jaws of the instrument to divide the obliterated tissue safely.

Argon gas coagulation

Argon gas enhanced coagulation is useful in partial nephrectomy and in the treatment of injury to the liver and spleen. This system uses the properties of electrosurgery and a stream of argon gas to improve the delivery of the electrosurgical current. Argon gas is noncombustible and inert, making it a safe gas to use in the presence of electrosurgical current. The argon gas is ionized by the electrical current, making it more conductive than air. The highly conductive stream of argon gas provides an efficient pathway for delivering the current to tissue, resulting in hemostasis. The flow of argon gas also disperses blood, improving visualization during coagulation. During argon beam coagulation, the pressure inside the abdomen can quickly rise above the preset level. Consequently, an insufflation port should be opened during coagulation and the intra-abdominal pressure carefully monitored.

Ultrasound

A relatively new tool for laparoscopic dissection uses ultrasonic energy to achieve precise cutting and coagulation. Three devices are currently available (The UltraCision System, Ethicon Endo-Surgery, Cincinnati, Ohio; The AutoSonix System, USSC, Norwalk, Connecticut; and SonoSurg, Olympus America, Inc., Melville, New York). Energy is delivered using a laparoscopic 5 mm or 10 mm handpiece with a shaft tuned to conduct the ultrasonic vibration at the rate of approximately 55,000 cycles/s. The vibration causes heat, which is more precisely located at the vibrating tip, and, at 50–100°C, is much lower than

conventional electrocautery. Different tip configurations are available, including hooks, shears, and blunt probes. As the tissue is compressed between the jaws of the shears, blood vessels are occluded and the vibration causes intracellular water vaporization. Proteins are denatured in the tissue and protein coagulum forms, sealing blood vessels while tissue is divided. Hemostasis and division of tissue occur at temperatures less than conventional cautery, without the wide dispersion of heat, creating a small band of tissue necrosis. Water vapor is emitted in the abdomen instead of smoke. While the cords are reusable for all three systems, only the Olympus SonoSurg offers an autoclaveable, reusable handpiece.

Temporary vessel occlusion

Laparoscopic partial nephrectomy is now possible due to instruments that allow temporary occlusion of the renal hilar vessels. Two manufacturers offer bulldog clamps that are endoscopically applied through a 10 mm trocar. The jaws range in size from 17 to 45 mm, and come in curved and straight configurations (Klein Surgical Systems, San Antonio, Texas; Aesculap, Inc., Center Valley, Pennsylvania) (Figure 2.9). A 5 mm laparoscopic Statinsky clamp is also available but requires the placement of an additional trocar (Klein Surgical Systems, San Antonio, Texas).

Surgical clips

Occlusive clips are useful for small veins and arteries, and have become standard equipment in most laparoscopic cases. As in open surgery, clips provide a rapid alternative for hemostasis. Most endoscopic clips today are made of titanium, and vary in size from 5 to 12 mm. Nonabsorbable polymer locking clips are also available and offer the advantage of being radiolucent (Weck Closure

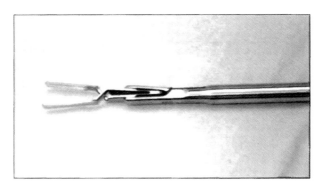

Figure 2.9
Laparoscopic bulldog clamp and applier (Klein Surgical Systems, San Antonio, Texas).

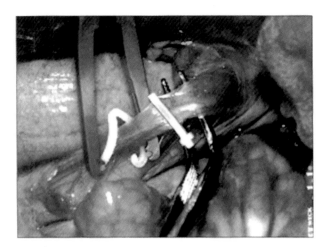

Figure 2.10
Hem-o-lok polymer clips (Weck Closure Systems, Research Triangle Park, North Carolina). (Photo courtesy of Weck Closure Systems.)

Systems, Research Triangle Park, North Carolina) (Figure 2.10). However, each clip is loaded separately on a reusable 10 mm applier. There are absorbable clips, and some research shows no difference in adhesion formation between metallic and absorbable clips.[14]

Most laparoscopic clip appliers are single use and multi-load, carrying between 15 to 30 clips per unit (Table 2.2). The ability to fire multiple clips without exiting the abdomen to reload can save significant time and decrease blood loss. In general, the diameter of the shaft depends on the size of clips. The Endoclip (USSC, Norwalk, Connecticut) 5 mm shaft single-use clip applier can deliver a slightly larger clip than other 5 mm clippers: its hinged jaws are normally retracted within the shaft, but upon squeezing the handles they advance and expand and a clip is automatically loaded. Most disposable clip appliers have 360° rotating shafts, allowing the handle of the instrument

to rest comfortably in the hand while placing the tips around the target tissue at an ideal angle. Right angle clip appliers (USSC, Norwalk, Connecticut) are also available and can offer a visual advantage in situations where the tips of straight appliers are not well seen.

Tacking staples

The laparoscopic biting stapler was originally developed for laparoscopic hernia repair with mesh, but these devices are also useful in refashioning the peritoneum in laparoscopic ureterolysis and fixing mesenteric defects in bowel resections. Much like the staplers used for skin wound closure, laparoscopic staplers fire titanium staples with sharp ends that enter the tissue and then undergo deformation into a rectangular shape. Most contemporary devices are single use and multi-load, with 15–30 staples/unit. A 360° rotating shaft allows accurate placement of the staple. Some devices also come with a 60–65° distal articulating head, which permits tacking hard-to-reach areas like the anterior abdominal wall and deep pelvis.

Linear staplers

Laparoscopic linear staplers are essential for rapid, safe intracorporeal tissue division and reapproximation of visceral structures. With a squeeze of a handle, these devices deploy multiple, closely spaced parallel rows of titanium staples. Staples come in three different 'loads' – thin/vascular, medium, and large/thick – and are color-coded for easy recognition. Thin staples penetrate tissue to a depth of 2–2.5 mm, deform to an exaggerated b-shape, and form a reliably hemostatic staple line. These staples are

Table 2.2 *Clip appliers (multi-load, single use)*					
	Ligaclip Allport	Ligaclip ERCA	Right Angle AccuClip	Endoclip 5 mm	Endoclip II
Company	Ethicon	Ethicon	USSC	USSC	USSC
Port size	5 mm	10 and 12 mm	8 mm	5 mm	10 mm
Clips	20	20	20	12	20
Clip sizes	Medium, medium/large	Medium, medium/large, large	Medium/large	Medium/large	Medium/large, large
Clip load	Automatic	Automatic	Automatic	Separate lever	Automatic
Cost	$288	$218	$210	$327	$236

Ethicon = Ethicon Endo-Surgery, Cincinnati, Ohio; USSC = USSC, Norwalk, Connecticut

ideal for rapid division of vascular pedicles. Medium-to-large staples are 3.0–4.8 mm thick in their closed form, and are useful in securing thicker tissues like bowel, bladder, and ureter. The larger staples do not fold to the same tight shape as small staples and should not be used for primarily hemostatic ligation. Staplers today allow the same instrument to fire between 8 and 25 separate loads before stapler disposal.

Linear staplers can be broadly classified into cutting and non-cutting. Cutting versions deploy loads with six intercalated parallel rows of staples. As the staples are fired, a knife follows closely behind and incises the tissue between the staples, leaving three rows of staples on each side. The staple line extends past the range of the cutting knife by one or two staples to avoid incising non-secured tissue. Once the staples are fired, a safety feature on all devices prevents accidental re-deployment of the cutting knife until a new load with staples is in place. Non-cutting staplers simply fire three to four parallel rows of staples, and are useful for closing enterotomies and repairing bladder injuries.

Laparoscopic linear cutting staplers are further distinguished by the length of their staple line (30/35, 45, and 60 mm), and whether their firing heads are articulated or not (Table 2.3). An articulating head gives a greater range of motion from a fixed trocar but also adds to the price. All devices offer a rotating shaft, which allows proper visualization of the tips during firing. On most models, a replacement load consists of a fresh six rows of staples but uses the same knife and anvil inherent to the actual stapling device. The Endo GIA Universal linear cutting stapler is a universal firing device that accommodates both articulating and non-articulating loads of varying lengths (30,

45, and 60 mm) (USSC, Norwalk, Connecticut). The stapler is unique in that the jaws, anvil, and knife are inherent to the load and not part of the actual base unit; i.e. each re-load comes with a new knife. Also, this system allows the surgeon to use loads (articulating or fixed) of varying lengths without having to open a new stapler. The minimum-size limitation posed by the width of the staple load requires use of a 10 mm or larger port for all currently available staplers.[15]

Loop ligation

Loop ligatures are valuable in securing an already transected pedicle. A length of suture with a pre-formed sliding, locking knot is passed intracorporeally. The structure to be ligated is then retracted through the loop with a grasper, and the loop cinched down with a knot pusher. Two loop ligature systems are available with both 0 and 2-0 plain gut, chromic gut, polyester, and synthetic absorbable varieties (Surgitie, USSC, Norwalk, Connecticut; Endoloop, Ethicon, Cincinnati, Ohio). The plastic knot pusher is only available in one length, and may be too short to reach the target site if the wrong port is chosen. Two hands are needed to cinch the knot, requiring an assistant to grasp the tissue and hold it still.

Fibrin products

Fibrin tissue adhesive (FTA) has gained widespread acceptance in a variety of surgical procedures as an adhesive,

Table 2.3 *Linear staplers*						
	Endopath ETS	Endopath ETS/flex articulating	Endopath EZ45: cutter	Multifire Endo GIA 30	Multifire Endo TA	Endo GIA Universal
Company	Ethicon	Ethicon	Ethicon	USSC	USSC	USSC
Port size	12 mm	12 mm	18 mm	12 mm	12 mm	12 and 15 mm
Staple size	2.5, 3.5, and 4.1 mm	2.5, 3.5, and 4.1 mm	3.8 and 4.5 mm	2.0, 2.5, and 3.5 mm	2.5 and 3.5 mm	2.0, 2.5, 3.5, and 4.8 mm
Staple length	35 and 45 mm	35 and 45 mm	45 mm	30 mm	30 mm	30, 45, and 60 mm
Rotating shaft	Yes	Yes	Yes	Yes	Yes	Yes
Articulating	No	Yes	No	No	No	Yes
Cost	$399	$498	$495	$433–500	$433–500	$433–500

Ethicon = Ethicon Endo-Surgery, Cincinnati, Ohio; USSC = USSC, Norwalk, Connecticut.

sealant, hemostatic agent, or carrier for growth factors or antibiotics. Fibrin products have been used in many different urologic procedures to assist with hemostasis and tissue adhesion.[16,17] FTA can also be valuable in treating complications of laparoscopic surgery, including spleen and liver injury, urinary fistula formation, and wound dehiscence.[18] Presently, FTA is made from autologous preparations using a patient's own blood or from homologous sources using a single donor or pooled samples.

Concentrates of coagulation factors are known for their adhesive and coagulation properties. In addition, fibrin in surgical wounds promotes healing by supplying a network for the growth of fibroblasts and activating macrophages.[19] Surgeons have prepared their own fibrin sealants for many years. However, these locally prepared products are not standardized and the sources of fibrinogen are not virally inactivated. Commercially available blood-derived products are now available for topical application to control bleeding and seal tissue. The basic principle is the same for these kits. Human thrombin and fibrinogen are applied separately to a bleeding site, resulting in formation of a layer of fibrin that controls the bleeding and seals tissue. Eventually, the fibrin film is reabsorbed.

Commercial preparations reproduce the final stage of coagulation, resulting in their adhesive, hemostatic, and healing effects through the polymerization of fibrin chains with collagen of adjacent or damaged tissue. These fibrin sealants are made from different combinations of fibrinogen and thrombin derived from human plasma and fibrinolysis inhibitor, a substance of bovine origin. As part of normal coagulation, fibrinogen undergoes proteolysis by the enzyme thrombin to form a fibrin monomer that polymerizes into fibrin strands, making up a major component of the actual clot. Thrombin also activates clotting factor XIII, promoting cross-linking of the fibrin monomer to stabilize the fibrin network. Thrombin is found in the plasma as an inactive precursor – prothrombin. After proteolysis, the active enzyme thrombin is formed. Proteolysis occurs as a result of tissue damage to cell membranes (extrinsic pathway) or trauma to the blood vessel walls, exposing collagen (intrinsic pathway), which results in the activation of thrombin followed by fibrin clot formation. The clotting time of fibrin sealant is dependent on the concentration of thrombin in the sealant.

Commercial fibrin sealants are typically packaged as freeze-dried concentrates of human fibrinogen and thrombin in separate containers. The powders are reconstituted and bovine fibrinolysis inhibitor (aprotinin) is added to the liquid fibrinogen. When the fibrinogen and thrombin solutions are mixed, they become active, forming a clot of adhesive (Haemacure Corp., Sarasota, Florida; Tisseel, Baxter Healthcare Corporation, Glendale, California). Another product currently available uses the patient's own plasma mixed with bovine thrombin and bovine collagen (CoStasis, US Surgical, Norwalk, Connecticut) but is FDA approved for hemostasis alone and not for tissue sealing or tissue adhesion.

The American Red Cross has developed a lyophilized fibrinogen and thrombin product that is combined on a prepackaged absorbable backing (similar to a 4×4 sponge) or a powder spray. The 4×4 bandage is designed to be applied directly to the wound in open cases, while the powder formulation is readily delivered laparoscopically.[20–23] When these products contact the surgical site or blood, they are activated and rapidly form a dense synthetic clot. The lyophilized formulation is currently under investigation and not FDA approved for human use.

Since fibrin sealants commonly consist of human and bovine products, there is a theoretical risk of viral transmission, anaphylaxis, and coagulopathy. Viral transmission is of great concern since pooled human plasma is used to make the sealant. Donor screening, heat treatment of tissue, and solvent/detergent treatment seem to be effective in maintaining the safety of these products by preventing the transmission of HIV, Epstein–Barr virus, cytomegalovirus, and hepatitis.[24] However, four patients are known to have been infected with parvovirus B19 following treatment with fibrin sealant.[25,26] Infection with parvovirus B19 is usually asymptomatic or may present with a minor febrile illness. Rarely, transient aplitic crisis with rapid red blood cell turnover can occur. There is an isolated report of a patient who developed rash, bronchospasm, and circulatory collapse following use of fibrin sealant to close an enterocutaneous fistula. A complete investigation showed her to have aprotinin-specific antibodies, which were the most likely cause of the severe anaphylactic reaction.[27] Fibrin sealants are designed for topical use and are not designed for systemic injection. Intravenous injection could result in systemic activation of the coagulation cascade and fatal thrombosis. No systemic effects have been reported using sealants on surgical bleeding sites.

Suture assist

Given the complexity of suturing in the laparoscopic environment, the majority of early laparoscopic urologic cases were extirpative and required little to no reconstruction. Unique demands to be overcome include a fixed center of motion, limited needle and suture handling ability, lack of three-dimensional perspective, and intracorporeal knot tying. Today, with the increasing interest in laparoscopic radical prostatectomy, more urologists are becoming proficient in free-hand suturing. This technique is applicable to most situations and offers the greatest flexibility with respect to suture and needle choices as well as the angle at which a needle may be held. For special circumstances and for those less experienced in free-hand techniques, several instruments have been developed to facilitate laparoscopic suturing.

The EndoStitch (USSC, Norwalk, Connecticut) is an innovative device that passes a small needle back and forth between jaws, allowing both running and interrupted suturing techniques without the need to worry about reloading the needle. It also facilitates rapid intracorporeal knot tying (Figure 2.11). Limitations of the EndoStitch include its 10 mm width and short dull needle that cannot be passed through thick tissue and is more traumatic than a similar-sized swedged-on suture. The needle can only be passed perpendicularly from jaw to jaw and may require excess tissue manipulation for proper suture placement. Finally, the device is disposable and reloads are costly, adding to the expense of a case. Despite these disadvantages, the EndoStitch has been used very successfully, even in cases requiring delicate reconstruction such as laparoscopic pyeloplasty.[28]

The Suture Assist (Ethicon Endo-Surgery, Cincinnati, Ohio) is a 5 mm instrument designed to place a pretied knot quickly after using either the device or a needle driver to place a single or figure-of-eight throw. Running sutures

are not possible without using an alternative knot-tying method for the second knot. Like the EndoStitch, the Suture Assist is disposable and relies on reloads.

A newer 5 mm instrument, the Sew-Right SR5 (LSI Solutions, Rochester, New York), uses two built-in needles to place a simple suture precisely through even relatively thick tissue. Advantages include its 5 mm size and needle passage parallel to the device, which may be better for some applications. With tenacious tissue, if the needle deviates or does not fully penetrate the tissue, it may miss or not engage the suture at the distal jaw. Again, this is a disposable instrument and only a single simple suture may be placed per load.

A final device, the Quik-Stitch (Pare Surgical, Englewood, Colorado) is available in 3, 5, 10, and 12 mm versions. This system consists of a proprietary needle driver passed through a spool containing a pretied knot. A single or figure-of-eight suture is placed or passed, followed by release, setting, and advancement of the knot. The device and needle driver are reusable, making it economical. Straight, curved, and blunt needles are available on absorbable and nonabsorbable sutures.

Intracorporeal knot tying, especially the second knot of a running suture, can be complicated. This is due to the short suture length often available for tying, the need to tie a single strand to a loop, and difficulty in maintaining constant tension on a knot. Two instruments are available to assist with this task. The Lapra-Ty (Ethicon Endo-Surgery, Cincinnati, Ohio) places a resorbable polyglycolic acid clip on the tail or tails of a suture to secure a running or simple suture. This allows precise tensioning of the suture with another instrument during 'tying'. The instrument is reusable and clips come six to a pack, making it economical. A concern is that a large number of clips may incite an inflammatory reaction or fistula. It is therefore most valuable for the final 'knot' of running sutures.

A second 'knot-tying' instrument is the Ti-Knot TK5 (LSI Solutions, Rochester, New York). This device is designed to replace extracorporeal knot tying. Once the two suture ends have been brought out through the trocar, they are snared and fed through a titanium cylinder at the end of the device. While holding the sutures under the proper tension, the instrument is advanced to the closure site and fired. This crimps the titanium knot onto the suture and trims the extra. Advantages promoted by the manufacturer include precise tensioning, one-step suture tying and cutting, and titanium's nonreactivity. Disadvantages are the need for extracorporeal loading of the suture into the device and the costs of a disposable instrument.

With experience, surgeons will find most suturing and knot tying is best done with a simple needle driver and curved graspers. However, the above instruments may be useful early in one's experience and in special circumstances.

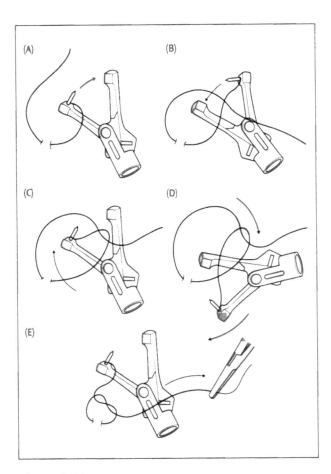

Figure 2.11
Knot tying with the EndoStitch (USSC, Norwalk, Connecticut).

Tissue retrieval

Anyone who has struggled to place an organ or tissue in a bag can immediately appreciate new advances in retrieval technology. The Endocatch (USSC, Norwalk, Connecticut) is a self-opening bag, which comes in several sizes, including 10 mm and 15 mm. Once the instrument is placed through a trocar or directly through the skin, the inner core handle slides forward, advancing the bag. A metal band automatically opens the bag and can be used to scoop up the tissue to be removed. A separate string is pulled, closing the bag and tearing it away from the metal ring. The ring is pulled back into the handle and the device removed, leaving the closed bag and string in the working space. The current bags are not strong enough to withstand automated tissue morcellation, but are useful when intact removal of specimens is required.

If the specimen is to be morcellated, a LapSac (Cook Urological, Inc., Spencer, Indiana) fabricated from a double layer of plastic and nondistendable nylon must be used. This device has been shown to withstand morcellation and remain impermeable to bacteria and tumor cells.[29] In the past, placing large specimens in the LapSac was often a consuming and frustrating experience. Using several simple tricks the bag can now be modified to allow rapid entrapment of specimens. A stiff hydrophilic wire can be double passed through the holes in the LapSac, creating a rigid opening. The bag and wire can be rolled up and inserted through an 11 mm trocar site with the trocar removed. Replacing the trocar alongside the protruding ends of the wire allows the pneumoperitoneum to be reestablished. The modified LapSac opens easily and the rigid wire maintains the mouth of the sac open. Once the specimen is entrapped, the wire can be pulled from the holes in the sac and the mouth of the sac brought out through a trocar site.

Morcellation

At the conclusion of any extirpative laparoscopic procedure, the organ must be removed from the patient. When malignancy is not involved and an incision is otherwise not required, morcellation and removal through the largest port site is ideal. This requires entrapment in a suitably sized pouch and mechanical reduction in size to allow passage through the port site. Morcellation of malignant lesions continues to be controversial.[30,31] There is clear cosmetic benefit and possibly a small decrease in postoperative morbidity with morcellation. Computed tomography (CT) has been proven to be an effective tool for planning surgery and predicting pathologic findings.[32] To date, there have been no reports of peritoneal seeding or local tumor recurrence in the renal fossa following laparoscopic nephrectomy with specimen morcellation. There have been two reports of trocar site seeding after radical nephrectomy. In one of the two patients it is likely that he had metastatic ascites at the time of nephrectomy.[33,34] No study to date has directly compared morbidity between use of morcellation vs use of an incision for specimen removal. One study compared pain and hospital stay in patients after morcellation vs those requiring conversion to an open procedure by subcostal incision.[35] Not surprisingly, there was less narcotic analgesic use and a shorter stay in the morcellation group. A more equal comparison would be that of HAL nephrectomy vs laparoscopic nephrectomy with morcellation. This has not shown a morbidity advantage for morcellation.[8] On the other hand, there has been only one reported port-site recurrence.[36] This was not clearly related to a morcellation accident but occurred at the appropriate port site. Finally, pathologic staging is rarely needed for treatment decisions after nephrectomy for renal cell carcinoma given excellent CT staging and the lack of effective adjuvant treatment options. This is not the case for transitional cell carcinoma, where morcellation is not recommended. In either case, prognostic information is lost with morcellation.

Once the decision has been made to morcellate an organ, it must first be placed in an impermeable bag (LapSac, Cook Urological, Inc., Spencer, Indiana). Once closed, the strings of the bag are removed through the chosen port site, removing the trocar at the same time. The area is then carefully draped with towels to prevent tumor contamination. The simplest, cheapest, and quickest option is to extend the fascial incision to 20 mm to allow manual fragmentation and extraction of the tissue using a combination of ring forceps, Kocher clamps, etc. The laparoscope should be used throughout this process to visually confirm bag integrity from inside the abdomen. The advantage of this technique is that it creates relatively large pieces of tissue and with the addition of India ink may allow preservation of much staging and margin information.[37]

Several instruments have been developed in an attempt to assist in the morcellation process, specifically to eliminate the need for port-site enlargement. Each is a combination of a rotating cylindrical blade with a mechanism for drawing the tissue into the device (Table 2.4). None is ideal and only one ex-vivo comparison trial exists, which attempts to quantitate morcellation time, bag integrity, and mean specimen weight.[38] Three morcellators were tested on human-sized kidneys without any perirenal tissue. This showed that the standard high-speed electrical laparoscopic (HSEL) morcellator (Cook Urological, Inc., Spencer, Indiana) performed the task acceptably in approximately 15 min. It was also the most economical. The Steiner morcellator (Karl Storz, Culver City, California) was twice as fast and provided specimen fragments 5 times larger (about 3 g), which may be more useful for pathologic evaluation. The Gynecare X-Tract (Ethicon

Table 2.4 *Comparison of laparoscopic tissue morcellators*

	HSEL	Steiner electromechanical	Gynecare X-Tract	RIWO CUT
Company	Cook Urological, Inc., Spencer, Indiana	Karl Storz, Culver City, California	Ethicon Inc., Somerville, New Jersey	Richard Wolf Medical Instrument Corp., Vernon Hills, Illinois
Mechanism	Suction	Forceps	Forceps	Forceps
Blade	Recessed	Protrudes ~2 mm	Recessed with manual blade guard	Reusable bare blade, no sheath

Inc., Somerville, New Jersey) and RIWO CUT (Richard Wolf Medical Instrument Corp., Vernon Hills, Illinois) devices are likely to perform similarly, given their modes of action. The modified electrical prostate morcellator (Coherent, Sturbridge, Massachusetts) was slow and expensive. A recommendation was additionally made that the use of a shortened trocar may provide increased safety by protecting the bag neck from heat and mechanical stress.

In conclusion, if the choice is made to morcellate a specimen, no current device offers a large advantage over the manual method. The Cook morcellator is currently unavailable. Use of one of the other morcellators may be time- and cost-efficient in high-volume programs and when already available in the operating room, usually as part of the gynecology instrumentation.

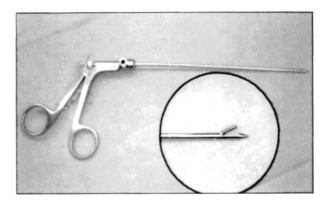

Figure 2.12
Berci fascial closure device (Karl Storz GmbH & Co. KG, Tuttlingen, Germany) with tip close-up.

Closure

Exiting the abdomen consists of visually controlled port removal and purging the carbon dioxide gas. Port sites 10 mm in size or larger have traditionally been closed to prevent port-site hernias. These have been reported to happen in up to 3% of cases.[39] Despite newer-style trocars that may not require fascial closure up to 12 mm, most surgeons continue to close ports ≥ 10 mm in adults and 5 mm sites in children.

Conventional open suture closure of port sites can be difficult, especially in obese patients. Multiple instruments have been developed to simplify and expedite this task. Most follow the same basic principle of suture passage through the fascia and into the peritoneal cavity under direct vision followed by suture retrieval with a second pass through the opposite side of the fascia. The Carter–Thomason needle-point suture passer (Inlet Medical Inc., Eden Prairie, Minnesota) and Berci fascial closure device (Karl Storz GmbH & Co. KG, Tuttlingen, Germany) are two commonly used nondisposable instruments based on this model (Figure 2.12). Both have a sharp beak which punctures the fascia and then opens to capture or release the suture. The EndoClose (USSC, Norwalk, Connecticut) is a similar disposable device. Its rigidity is less and suture capture opening smaller, making it somewhat more difficult to use.

Robotic-assisted surgery

Once a mere fantasy, robotic-assisted surgery is now reality. Currently available robots vary in complexity and degree of involvement in the procedure. Simple robots are used for laparoscope holding and direction, while others are more directly involved in tissue manipulation at the surgeon's direction. The automated endoscopic system for optimal positioning or AESOP robotic device (Computer Motion, Inc., Santa Barbara, California) was the first FDA-cleared surgical robot. The AESOP system attaches to the side of the operating room table and incorporates a 7-degree of freedom robotic arm to hold and position the endoscope during laparoscopic surgery. The robot is voice-activated, allowing control by the operating surgeon, eliminating unintentional movement, and ensuring a stable surgical image (Figure 2.13).

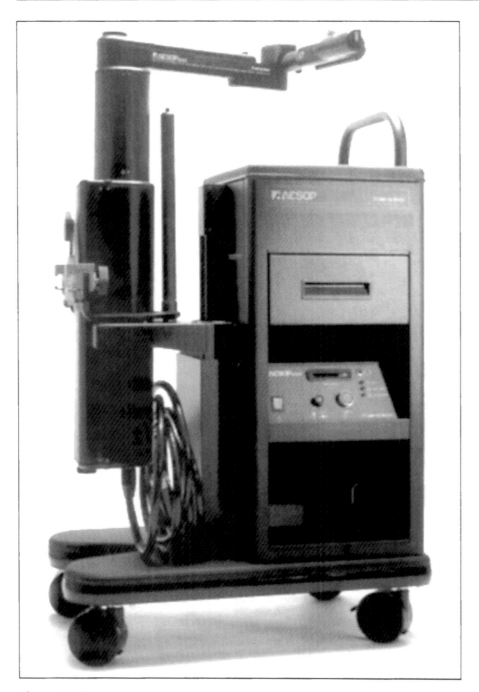

Figure 2.13
The AESOP robot (Computer Motion, Inc., Santa Barbara, California). (Photo courtesy of Computer Motion, Inc.)

Currently two robotic systems are FDA-cleared for tissue manipulation during laparoscopic surgery. Since the surgeon actually performs the procedure with the assistance of the mechanical device, these systems are not purely robotic. The ZEUS robotic surgical system (Computer Motion, Inc., Santa Barbara, California) consists of a surgeon's control console and three table-mounted robotic arms (Figure 2.14). Two arms are used for instrument manipulation and one for control of the endoscope. The da Vinci Surgical System (Intuitive Surgical, Inc., Mountain View, California) is a master–slave system that uses robotic technology with 3-dimensional visualization (Figure 2.15). The surgeon operates while seated at a console, viewing the surgical field. At the

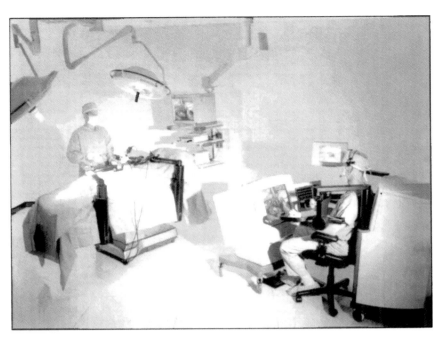

Figure 2.14
The ZEUS robotic surgical system (Computer Motion, Inc., Santa Barbara, California). (Photo courtesy of Computer Motion, Inc.)

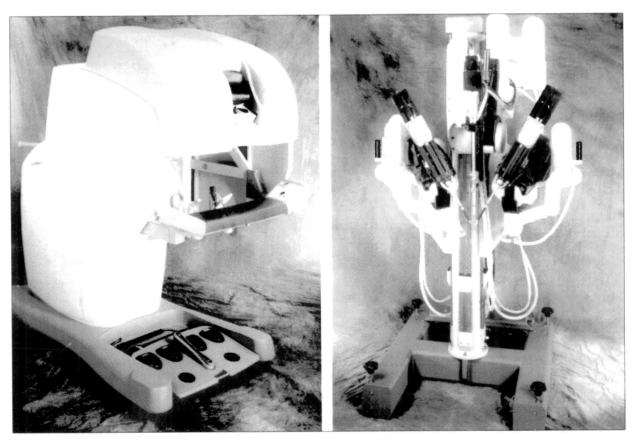

Figure 2.15
The da Vinci Surgical System (Intuitive Surgical, Inc., Mountain View, California) consists of the surgeon console and the patient side cart that provides the two robotic arms and one endoscope arm. (Photos courtesy of Intuitive Surgical, Inc.)

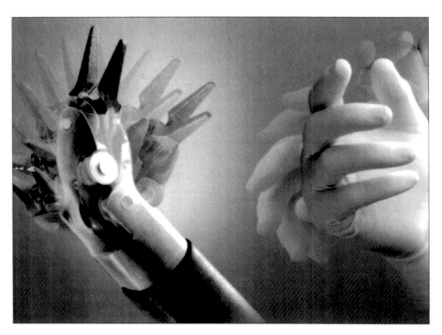

Figure 2.16
The 7 degrees of freedom Endowrist (Intuitive Surgical, Inc., Mountain View, California) end-effector of the da Vinci Surgical System. (Photo courtesy of Intuitive Surgical, Inc.)

patient's side, three robot arms position and maneuver the Endowrist endoscopic instruments and laparoscope with a wide range of movements and 360° maneuverability through laparoscopic trocars. The instruments are capable of delivering 7 degrees of freedom, like the human wrist (Figure 2.16). The surgeon's movements are translated into movements of the instruments, allowing precise dissection, manipulation, and suturing. The da Vinci Surgical System has received FDA market clearance for use in performing many different laparoscopic procedures. In the field of urology, it has received FDA clearance for use in radical prostatectomy, and several different studies have shown the feasibility of its use in this procedure.[40–42]

Robotic assistance has the potential to enhance the surgeon's capabilities. The machine translates the surgeon's movements into more steady and precise results at the end of laparoscopic instruments. With these new devices there is potential to decrease the learning curve associated with traditional laparoscopic surgery where instrument movements and degrees of freedom are limited. Motion scaling allows for more precise movements from the surgeon's hand. Intention and resting hand tremor are considerably diminished compared with open surgery, but are virtually eliminated with robotics.

References

1. Bhoyrul S, Vierra MA, Nezhat CR, et al. Trocar injuries in laparoscopic surgery. J Am Coll Surg 2001; 192:677–83.

2. Liu CD, McFadden DW. Laparoscopic port sites do not require fascial closure when nonbladed trocars are used. Am Surg 2000; 66:853–4.

3. Bohm B, Knigge M, Kraft M, et al. Influence of different trocar tips on abdominal wall penetration during laparoscopy. Surg Endosc 1998; 12:1434–8.

4. Bhoyrul S, Mori T, Way LW. Radially expanding dilatation. A superior method of laparoscopic trocar access. Surg Endosc 1996; 10:775–8.

5. Bhoyrul S, Payne J, Steffes B, et al. A randomized prospective study of radially expanding trocars in laparoscopic surgery. J Gastrointest Surg 2000; 4:392–7.

6. Dunn MD, McDougall EM, Clayman RV. Laparoscopic radical nephrectomy. J Endourol 2000; 14:849–55.

7. Wolf JS. Hand-assisted laparoscopy. Pro. Urology 2001; 58:310–12.

8. Wolf JS, Moon TD, Nakada SY. Hand assisted laparoscopic nephrectomy: comparison to standard laparoscopic nephrectomy. J Urol 1998; 160:22–7.

9. Gill IS. Hand-assisted laparoscopy: Con. Urology 2001; 58:313–17.

10. Stifelman M, Nieder AM. Prospective comparison of hand-assisted laparoscopic devices. Urology 2002; 59:668–72.

11. Grosskinsky CM, Hulka JE. Unipolar electrosurgery in operative laparoscopy. Capacitance as a potential source of injury. J Reprod Med 1995; 40:549–52.

12. Bishoff JT, Allaf ME, Kirkels W, et al. Laparoscopic bowel injury: incidence and clinical presentation. J Urol 1999; 161:887–90.

13. Saye WB, Miller W, Hertzman P. Electrosurgery thermal injury: myth or misconception. Surg Laparosc Endosc 1991; 4:223–8.

14. Ling FW, Stovall TG, Meyer NL, et al. Adhesion formation associated with the use of absorbable staples in comparison to other types of peritoneal injury. Int J Gynecol Obstet 1989; 30:361–6.

15. Tierney AC, Nakada SY. Laparoscopic stapling and reconstruction. In: Bishoff JT, Kavoussi LR, eds. Laparoscopic retroperitoneal surgery. Philadelphia: WB Saunders, 2000: 33–56.

16. Shekarriz B, Stoller ML. The use of fibrin sealant in urology. J Urol 2002; 167:1218–25.

17. McDonough RC, Morey AF. Urologic applications of fibrin sealant bandage. In: Lewandrowski KU, Tantolo DJ, Gresser JD, Yaszemski MJ, Altobelli DE, eds. Tissue engineering and biodegradable equivalents: scientific and clinical applications. New York: Marcel Dekker, 2002.

18. Canby E, Morey AF, Jatoi I, et al. Fibrin sealant treatment of splenic injury during open and laparoscopic left radical nephrectomy. J Urol 2000; 164:2004–5.

19. Leibovich SJ, Ross R. The role of macrophages in wound repair. Am J Pathol 1975; 78:71–100.

20. Cornum RL, Morey AF, Harris R, et al. Does the absorbable fibrin adhesive bandage facilitate partial nephrectomy? J Urol 2000; 164:864–7.

21. Morey AF, Anema JG, Harris R, et al. Treatment of grade 4 renal stab wounds with absorbable fibrin adhesive bandage in a porcine model. J Urol 2001; 165:955–8.

22. Cornum R, Bell J, Gresham V, et al. Intraoperative use of the absorbable fibrin adhesive bandage: long term effects. J Urol 1999; 162:1817–20.

23. Perahia B, Bishoff JT, Cornum RL, et al. The laparoscopic hemi-nephrectomy: made easy by the new fibrin sealant powder. J Urol 2002; 167:suppl 2 (abst).

24. Greenhalgh DG, Gamelli RL, Lee M, et al. Multicenter trial to evaluate the safety and potential efficacy of pooled human fibrin sealant for the treatment of burn wounds. J Trauma 1999; 46:433–40.

25. Morita Y, Nishii O, Kido M, Tsutsumi O. Parvovirus infection after laparoscopic hysterectomy using fibrin glue hemostasis. Obstet Gynecol 2000; 95:1026.

26. Hino M, Ishiko O, Honda K, et al. Transmission of symptomatic parvovirus B19 infection by fibrin sealant used during surgery. Br J Haematol 2000; 108:194–5.

27. Scheule AM, Beierlein W, Lorenz H, Ziemer G. Repeated anaphylactic reactions to aprotinin in fibrin sealant. Gastrointest Endosc 1998; 48:83–5.

28. Bauer JJ, Bishoff JT, Moore RG, et al. Laparoscopic versus open pyeloplasty: assessment of objective and subjective outcome. J Urol 1999; 162:692–5.

29. Urban DA, Kerbl K, McDougall EM, et al. Organ entrapment and renal morcellation: permeability studies. J Urol 1993; 150:1792–4.

30. Bishoff JT. Laparoscopic radical nephrectomy: morcellate or leave intact? Definitely morcellate! Rev Urol 2002; 4:34–7.

31. Kaouk JH, Gill IS. Laparoscopic radical nephrectomy: morcellate or leave intact? Leave intact. Rev Urol 2002; 4:38–42.

32. Shalhave AL, Leibovitch I, Lev R, et al. Is laparoscopic radical nephrectomy with specimen morcellation acceptable cancer surgery? J Endourol 1998; 12:255–7.

33. Fentie DD, Barrett PH, Taranger LA. Metastatic renal cell cancer after laparoscopic radical nephrectomy: long-term follow up. J Endourol 2000; 14:407–11.

34. Castilho LN, Fugita OE, Mitre AI, Arap S. Port site tumor recurrences of renal cell carcinoma after videolaparoscopic radical nephrectomy. J Urol 2001; 165:519.

35. Walther MM, Lyne JC, Libutti SK, Linehan WM. Laparoscopic cytoreductive nephrectomy as preparation for administration of systemic interleukin-2 in the treatment of metastatic renal cell carcinoma: a pilot study. Urology 1999; 53:496–501.

36. Fentie DD, Barrett PH, Taranger LA. Metastatic renal cell cancer after laparoscopic radical nephrectomy: long-term follow-up. J Endourol 2000; 14:407–11.

37. Meng MV, Koppie TM, Duh QY, Stoller ML. Novel method of assessing surgical margin status in laparoscopic specimens. Urology 2001; 58:677–81.

38. Landman J, Collyer WC, Olweny E, et al. Laparoscopic renal ablation: an in vitro comparison of currently available electrical tissue morcellators. Urology 2000; 56:677–81.

39. Bowrey DJ, Blom D, Crookes PF, et al. Risk factors and the prevalence of trocar site herniation after laparoscopic fundoplication. Surg Endosc 2001; 15:663–6.

40. Abbou CC, Hoznek A, Salomon L, et al. Laparoscopic radical prostatectomy with a remote controlled robot. J Urol 2001; 165:1964–6.

41. Binder J, Kramer W. Robotically-assisted laparoscopic radical prostatectomy. BJU Int 2001; 87:408–10.

42. Sung GT, Gill IS. Robotic laparoscopic surgery: a comparison of the da Vinci and Zeus systems. Urology 2001; 58:893–8.

3

Imaging in minimally invasive urologic surgery*

Thomas M Seay and Thomas M Dykes

Urology is only second to orthopedics as a specialty that has made extensive use of imaging in diagnosis and operative planning. Because of this reliance on imaging, rare is the situation where the urologic surgeon enters into an operation with exploration being the initial indication. Urologists, as part of their training, develop an intimate knowledge of those imaging techniques that have become essentials of their diagnostic armamentarium. Indeed, in the United States, part of the Board certification process in urology requires adeptness at specific image interpretation. That said, as surgical techniques have progressed in the last decade, so too has imaging technology. Beyond the intravenous pyelography/excretory urography (IVP/EXU), retrograde pyelogram, and cystogram, urologists of the 21st century require knowledge of ultrasound (US), new-generation computed tomography (CT), and magnetic resonance imaging (MRI) to such a degree as never before.

The purpose of this chapter is to briefly discuss those imaging techniques which are specifically of interest to the laparoscopic urologic surgeon. Briefly discussed will be current imaging evaluation of hematuria, specifically as regards renal cell carcinoma (RCCa), adrenal lesions, preoperative imaging evaluation of ureteropelvic junction obstruction (UPJO) in adults, and preoperative imaging evaluation of patients being considered as renal donors. The chapter is by no means all inclusive, but is meant as a practical review of what issues and studies are encountered on a day-to-day basis.

Hematuria

The major urologic problems for which the patient seeks evaluation are hematuria, either gross – causing distress in the patient – or microscopic – causing concern in the referring provider – and obstruction. The majority of clinicians mandate work-up for gross hematuria, with the indica-

tions for work-up of microhematuria a matter of debate, usually centering on a discussion as to what 'significant' microhematuria is to be defined as. The definition of 'significant', cognizant that up to 18% of individuals have some degree of hematuria, is usually based upon the number of red blood cells (RBCs) in centrifuged urinary sediment per high-power field (HPF). The upper limit of normal is quoted as 2–3 RBCs/HPF; this cutoff has also been raised to up to 5 RBCs/HPF and also lowered to considering the presence of any RBCs at all as an indication for evaluation.[1] Nonetheless, the three *major* entities of concern, which asymptomatic microscopic hematuria may be a harbinger of, are RCCa, transitional cell carcinoma, and urinary stone disease. While imaging may suggest transitional cell carcinoma in a particular patient, it is an endoscopically obtained diagnosis, whereas the clinician is on firmer ground with imaging studies demonstrating a urinary calcification or a solid renal mass.

Grossfeld et al have stratified patients based upon 'high-risk' vs 'low-risk' criteria (Table 3.1) and have consequently

Table 3.1 *Risk factors for significant disease in patients with microscopic hematuria: the 'high-risk' patient*

Smoking history
Occupational exposure to chemicals or dyes (benzenes or aromatic amines)
History of gross hematuria
Age > 40 years
Previous urologic history
History of irritative voiding symptoms
History of urinary tract infection
Analgesic abuse (e.g. phenacetin)
History of pelvic irradiation
Cyclophosphamide exposure

Reproduced with permission from Grossfeld et al.[2]

* The opinions expressed herein are those of the authors and are not to be construed as those of the United States Air Force or the Department of Defense of the United States of America.

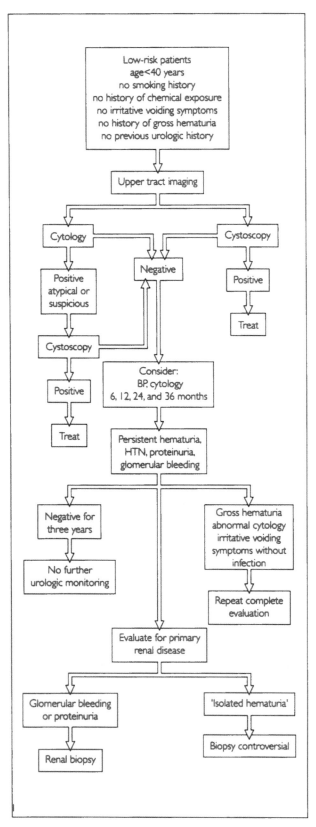

proposed algorithms for evaluation based upon this stratification (Figures 3.1 and 3.2).[1,2] Prudence, based upon the history of the patient, is in order. Patients with microscopic hematuria that can be surmised to be due to some activity or a urinary tract infection can be reassessed with urinalysis after cessation of that activity or resolution/treatment of the presenting clinical syndrome. A period of follow-up (at 6, 12, 24, and 36 months) is also recommended as

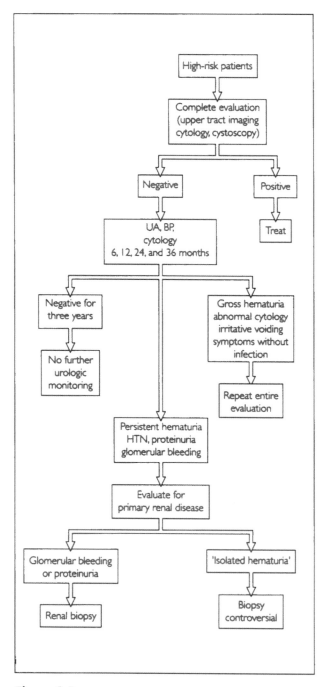

Figure 3.1
Suggested regimen for 'low-risk' patients with asymptomatic microhematuria. Reproduced with permission from Grossfeld et al.[2]

Figure 3.2
Suggested regimen for 'high-risk' patients with asymptomatic microhematuria. Reproduced with permission from Grossfeld et al.[2]

microscopic hematuria due to a significant cause may be intermittent.

Taking the algorithms above at face value, there does not seem to be discrimination between the initial work-up between the two groups. Upper tract imaging does play a paramount role in both populations. Upper tract imaging may be performed using IVP/EXU, CT, or CT urography.

IVP is widely available, and has served for decades as the standard initial imaging modality in the work-up of hematuria. However, if one is to treat in a minimally invasive manner, one hopes to discover the disease at a stage when such treatment is still feasible and effective. As regards renal cell carcinoma, IVP, while identifying patients with larger tumors (>3 cm), is found wanting in the detection of those lesions that are best served by laparoscopy or open partial nephrectomy (Figures 3.3, 3.4, and 3.5). CT is becoming more available, and in combination with a

limited IVP – which can be performed in any facility where the two modalities are physically in close proximity – complete assessment of both parenchymal and urothelial disease, as well as local staging, can be immediately obtained. The patient that is so evaluated has no need to return for a CT or US when an isolated IVP detects a contour abnormality.

Optimal evaluation of the renal mass: intravenous pyelography, computed tomography – intravenous pyelography

Survival from RCCa is intimately related to presenting stage.[3,4] This is indirectly a function of the size of the primary tumor. Limiting discussion to a T1 lesion (which under the 1997 TNM (tumor–node–metastasis) classification includes organ-confined tumors up to 7 cm in size),[5] further stratification has suggested a significant breakpoint in prognosis between those patients with tumors less than 4.5 cm in size and those between 4.5 and 7 cm.[6] Additionally, DNA content, ploidy versus nonploidy, correlates with tumor size, with one series demonstrating that 100% of tumors < 3 cm, 88% of tumors > 3 and < 5 cm, and 28% of tumors > 5 cm being diploid.[7] A patient with a diploid tumor less than 3 cm had a 4% risk of progression vs 43% for a diploid 10 cm tumor. Tumor size and DNA ploidy were independent factors of progression in this series, with size contributing the greater relative risk (9.32 vs 1.45, respectively) to progression. Based upon the above, it would seem that the ideal situation would be detection of the lesion when it is 3 cm or less in size.

Using CT as a reference standard, intravenous pyelography with plane tomography has been shown to be able to detect 85% of parenchymal lesions ≥ 3 cm, with a decline to 52% for those lesions ≥ 2 but < 3 cm, to 21% for those lesions ≥ 1 but < 2 cm and 10% for those lesions less than 1 cm.[8] Comparative numbers using ultrasound were 85%, 82%, 60% and 26%, respectively (Figure 3.6). An earlier retrospective study of patients with a solitary lesion less than 3 cm found that initial screening urography failed to identify the lesion in 66% of cases.[9] While these data were generated in the late 1980s, one has to remember that the basic means of performing and interpreting an IVP have not changed. Additionally, IVP, though standardized at most facilities, is subject to great variability in quality due to patient variation in preparation and habitus. Finally, while a substantial cortical lesion along the lateral surface of the kidney may be amenable to detection, lesions that are arising from the anterior or posterior surface of the kidney, or near the hilum without any discernible effacement of the collecting system, may easily escape notice.

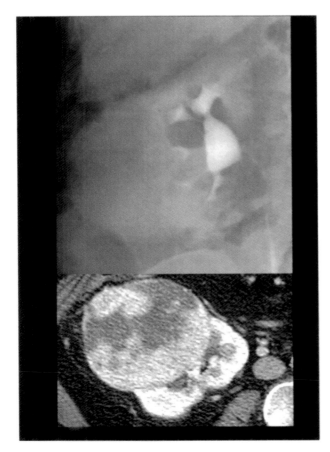

Figure 3.3
Selected image from IVP-correlated CT image with contrast from same patient demonstrates large right renal mass that is readily observable on IVP.

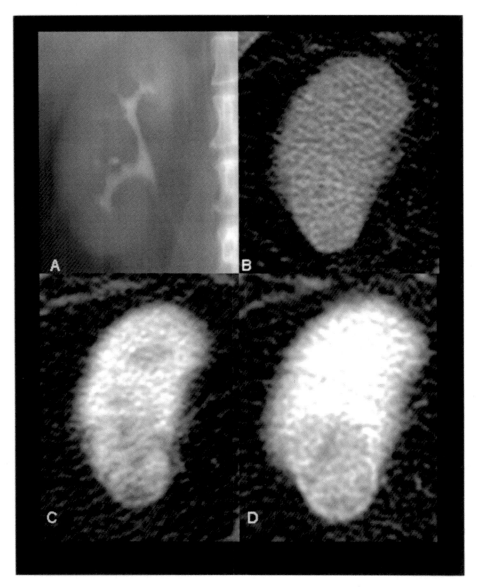

Figure 3.4
(A) Selected image of right kidney from an IVP obtained for microhematuria in a 45-year-old male. (B–D) Subsequent CT images show lower pole 2 cm renal cell mass. Lesion was not appreciated on IVP.

CT has been established as the most sensitive and specific modality in the detection and staging of RCCa.[10–13] Indeed, the ubiquitous use of CT scanners in the United States for diagnosis of various complaints has led to an artificial increase in the incidence of RCCa.[14,15] From 1935 to 1965 only 7% of RCCa were found incidentally, 13% from 1961 through 1973, 48% from 1980 through 1984, with now 60–81% being discovered incidentally.[14,16–18] Due to the advances in imaging, up to 38% of lesions are now detected when they are 3 cm or less in size.[11] Such early detection has seemingly led to an improvement in survival, although lead time bias may play a role. Thompson et al found that 90% of patients with incidentally discovered

tumors were alive at 10 years, vs only 30% of patients with symptomatic tumors.[19] Such early detection has also expanded the options for patients as regards radical nephrectomy vs open nephron-sparing surgery vs laparoscopic radical or partial nephrectomy. Patients with low-grade, small (i.e. < 4 cm) tumors having nephron-sparing surgery seem to have an outcome equivalent to that obtained via radical nephrectomy.[20]

At our institution we evaluate all adult patients referred with hematuria using a combination of helical triphasic CT and IVP (Table 3.2). To summarize, patients have a routine KUB (kidney, ureter, and bladder) performed, followed by noncontrast CT through the abdomen and

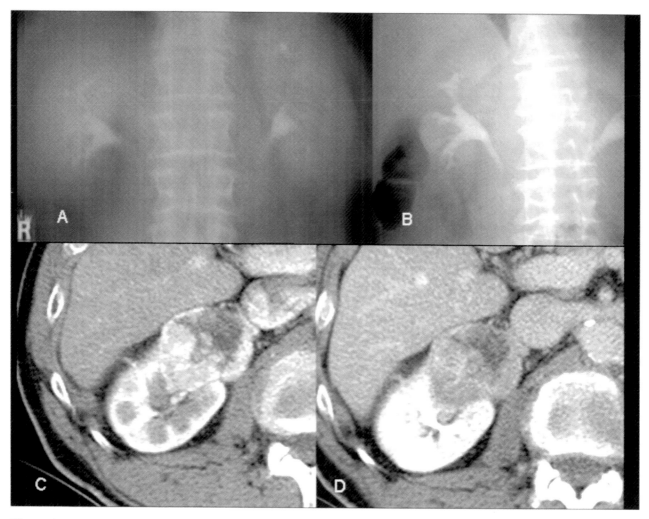

Figure 3.5
(A and B) Selected images obtained from IVP performed in a patient with microhematuria. (C and D) Subsequent CT images demonstrate large mass arising from medial upper pole of right kidney. Note that this large lesion is not readily apparent on the IVP.

pelvis, followed by image acquisition during a cortico-medullary phase at 90 s after contrast injection to assess the parenchyma, followed by an excretory delayed phase at 5 min to assess the collecting system. The last phase is also obtained from the top of the kidneys through the entire abdomen and pelvis. After the last phase there is excellent opacification of the collecting system and a compression device is applied to the lower abdomen. The collecting system is thus distended and the patient removed to the routine radiography suite for anteroposterior (AP), prone, and oblique views to assess the ureters and finally a post-void image of the pelvis. Each request is reviewed by a radiologist days in advance, with the protocol being easily adaptable for the question to be answered. The nephrographic phase demonstrates the highest sensitivity for parenchymal lesion detection, whereas the cortico-medullary phase is best for assessing the renal vasculature and surrounding organs for metastatic disease or coexisting pathology.[21]

The use of helical CT allows high resolution due to rapid acquisition of the images.[12] First, each phase of the CT portion of the protocol can be obtained in a standard single breath hold, which is comfortable for the majority of patients. This minimizes mis-registration between individual slices due to respiratory variation. Also, each phase can thus be obtained with a similar breath-hold maneuver, which allows a slice-by-slice comparison as regards enhancement of any lesion being assessed (Figure 3.7). Such comparison is facilitated by use of a multipanel computer workstation (PACS – picture acquisition and communication system) (Figure 3.8), which allows side-by-side evaluation of each phase. The radiologist can also

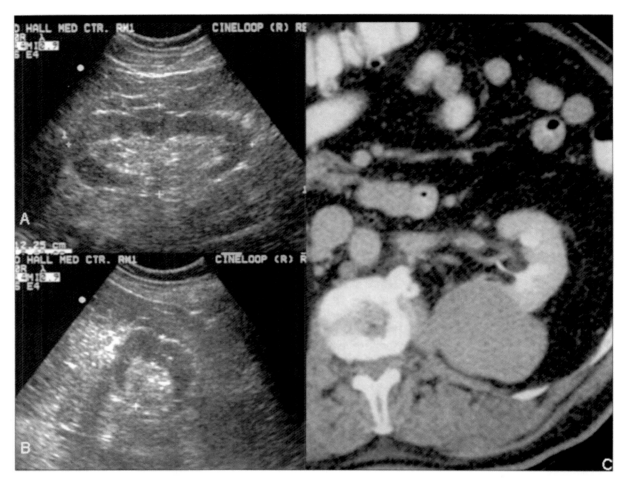

Figure 3.6
(A and B) Longitudinal and transverse ultrasound images of left kidney obtained in a patient with microhematuria. (C) Correlating CT image demonstrates large left renal mass. Mass was not initially appreciated on US.

apply region of interest (ROI) boxes of any desired size to assess relative attenuation – application of Hounsfield units (HU) – of the tissues, pre- and post-contrast.

Renal masses: cystic and otherwise

Fortunately, the majority of renal 'masses' are not malignant.[11] The differential diagnosis includes benign cysts, angiomyolipoma, lymphoma, metastases, oncocytomas, abscesses, and hematomas. History and ancillary studies may help narrow the diagnosis in the particular patient. Simple renal cysts are extremely common, being seen in over half of the population over the age of 50 years.[22] CT criteria for a simple benign cyst include:

1. sharp margination with the surrounding renal parenchyma

2. no perceptible wall
3. homogenous attenuation near water density (-10 to 15 Hounsfield units)
4. no enhancement after administration of contrast.[23]

Indeterminant cystic masses may represent cystic RCCa, or a simple cyst that has been complicated by infection or hemorrhage (Figure 3.9). A cyst cannot be assessed as simple if:

1. there is a perceptible wall with either regular or irregular thickening of the wall
2. solid components within a cystic mass
3. enhancement of the wall or septations
4. irregular margins
5. inhomogeneous cyst fluid.

However, cysts which are < 3 cm which have high attenuation values, commonly termed 'hyperdense' cysts, may be considered benign provided that other criteria of

Table 3.2 *CT/IVP protocol*

Position: supine
Scout: AP
Pitch: 1.5
KVP: 120
MA: 250
Rotation time (s): 1
Injection rate: 2 ml/s
IV contrast: 125 ml non-ionic

	Phase 1 (NONCON)	Phase 2	Phase 3
Slice thickness	5 mm	5 mm	5 mm
Slice increment	5 mm	5 mm	5 mm
Scan delay	N/A	90 s	5 min
Scan area	ABD/PLV	KIDS	ABD/PLV

Scanogram (topogram of ABD/PLV after the 90 s and 5 min scans).

Compression applied to lower abdomen immediately after 5 min scan and patient taken to standard radiography suite for completion of IVP portion of examination.

Assumes single-detector helical system with pitch = distance couch moves during one revolution of the X-ray tube.

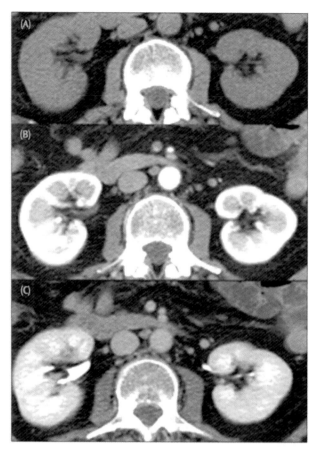

Figure 3.7
Three-phase CT as part of CT-IVP, demonstrating co-registration of images in noncontrast (A), nephrogram (B), and excretory phases (C).

simplicity are met, most notably lack of enhancement.[23] Approximately one-third of RCCas are hyperdense relative to the surrounding parenchyma on noncontrast CT.[24] A lesion with CT characteristics suggesting a hyperdense cyst may be further evaluated with ultrasound, in which 50% will meet criteria of a simple cyst.[25]

In 1986 Bosniak proposed a classification system of renal cystic lesions to allow stratification into management groups. Category 1 includes the purely simple cyst in which no further management is necessary unless symptomatic due to pure mass effect. Category 2 comprises minimally complicated cysts in which there are fine septations and minimal wall (i.e. rim) calcifications. This category includes hyperdense cysts. Category 3 comprises moderately complicated cysts that cannot be dismissed as benign by radiologic studies. Such lesions may be grossly hemorrhagic, have thick septations, dense calcifications, etc. As these lesions cannot be safely characterized as benign, excision is mandatory (Figure 3.10). Category 4 implies cystic RCCa until proven otherwise.[26] Finally, a last category, 2F, was devised, comprising minimally complicated cysts that require follow-up. This 'gray zone' between categories 2 and 3 is left to the judgment of the radiologist in concert with the urologic surgeon. Stability implies benignity, and such patients should be monitored with repeat studies at 3 months, 6 months, and 1 year.[25] Subsequent yearly monitoring out to 5 years would seem an acceptable and conser-

vative extension to this regimen. Prolonged monitoring of a suspicious lesion must take into account the concerns of the patient, and the reliability of the patient as regards return for follow-up.

The use of, and reliance upon, the Bosniak classification must be tempered with an understanding of the limits of interobserver variability. Siegel et al demonstrated in one series that 16% of lesions thought to be Bosniak category 1 or 2 by one radiologist were upgraded by a another radiologist to category 3 or 4.[27] Based upon pathologic verification, the incidences of malignancy in this series correlated to the respective categories and were 0%, 13%, 45%, and 90%.

Non-RCCa masses include angiomyolipomas (renal hamartoma), metastatic disease, and lymphomas, either primary or secondary. The sine qua non of radiologic diagnosis of angiomyolipoma (AML) is the presence of macroscopic fat within the lesion (Figure 3.11). Ninety percent of AMLs have sufficient fat to make the diagnosis on CT, with the remainder termed angiomyomas as they lack the lipomatous component.[28] Twenty percent of patients with

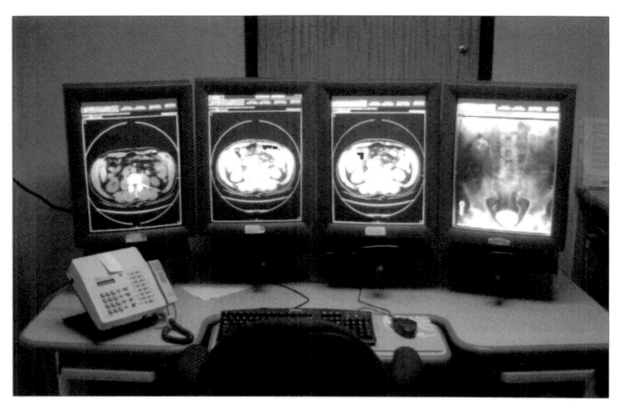

Figure 3.8
PACS (Picture archiving and communication system) workstation. A computerized workstation facilitates direct comparison between phases of triphasic CT during CT-IVP. The system allows rapid scrolling through images. Note that the far right panel may be used to correlate IVP images with CT images on other panels.

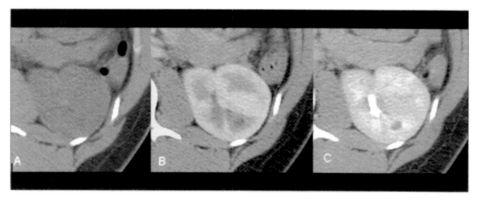

Figure 3.9
CT-IVP small renal cell carcinoma. A 35-year-old male with persistent microhematuria had negative evaluation with IVP and cystoscopy several months before. Repeat evaluation with triphasic CT demonstrates small lesion that is inconspicuous on noncontrast image (A), but is identified on the nephrogram/cortical phase (B), and excretory phase (C). The lesion, removed with partial nephrectomy, was a small renal cell carcinoma.

AML, predominantly males, suffer from tuberous sclerosis, a phakomatosis characterized by the constellation of adenoma sebaceum of the face, cerebral cortical tubers predisposing the patient to seizures, mental retardation, and giant cell astrocytomas.[29] However, 80% of cases, predominantly middle-aged women, have sporadic AMLs that are not related to any syndrome. The predominant clinical manifestation of AML is hemorrhage, with the risk increasing markedly after a size of 4 cm is reached.[30] While histologically benign, AMLs do grow over time, with up to 50% of AMLs < 4 cm and 75% > 4 cm demonstrating growth over a 4-year period.[31,32] Seventy percent of patients eventually become symptomatic once tumor size exceeds 4 cm; 20% of patients present in shock due to

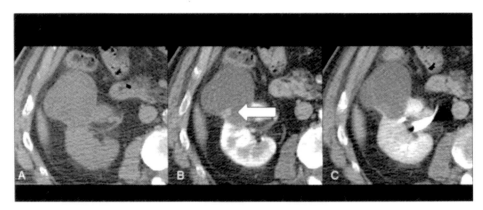

Figure 3.10
Cystic renal cell carcinoma. A 48-year-old patient with microhematuria. A noncontrast image (A) suggests the presence of a simple cyst, arising from anterior surface of the right kidney. Nephrographic (B) and excretory (C) phases demonstrate a nodule (arrow) within the cyst as well as enhancement of a septum. It was classified as a Bosniak category 3 lesion, and exploration revealed a cystic renal cell carcinoma.

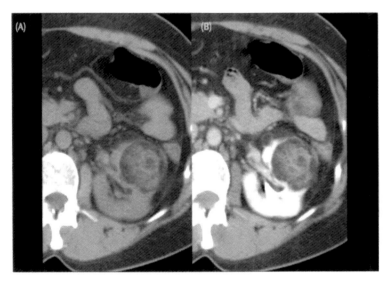

Figure 3.11
Angiomyelolipoma. A 34-year-old female presented to the emergency department, complaining of left flank pain. Noncontrast CT (A) was requested to rule out ureteral calculus. Incidental finding of angiomyelolipoma. Note the macroscopic fat within the lesion in comparison to retroperitoneal fat. (B) Contrast enhanced CT at the same level.

hemorrhage.[33] Once diagnosis is made for those tumors less than 4 cm, a period of yearly observation, via ultrasound, is recommended. For those patients with tumors greater than 4 cm, excision should be considered, or, if comorbidity prohibits surgery, transcatheter angiographic embolization is an option.[34]

Metastatic disease to the kidney, while often not symptomatic, is sometimes discovered due to the frequent CTs cancer patients receive. The most common lesion is secondary to a lung primary. Metastases to the kidney can be expansile and 'ball' shaped or infiltrative, a pattern seen in squamous cell carcinomas and lymphomas.[35]

Additionally, infiltration of renal pelvic transitional cell carcinoma into the parenchyma needs to be considered (Figure 3.12). Usually there is a history of a primary malignancy, and, if the renal lesion seems to be the only lesion present, consideration should be made regarding biopsy so the proper therapy is rendered. However, in the majority of patients with a history of malignancy who have an isolated renal lesion the pathology will reveal primary RCCa.[25] Lymphoma, while predominantly infiltrative, can also present as a solitary renal mass or diffuse involvement of both kidneys. The most common lymphoma to involve the kidneys is of the non-Hodgkin's variety. Lymphoma may

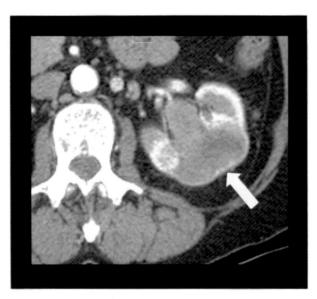

Figure 3.12

Transitional cell carcinoma infiltrating the kidney. A 68-year-old male with a history of prior muscle invasive bladder transitional cell carcinoma with gross hematuria from ileal conduit diversion. This CT image with contrast reveals diffuse infiltration of renal parenchyma (arrow) with disease that has already filled the collecting system. Note that primary or secondary renal lymphoma can have a similar appearance.

also involve the perirenal space, with direct spread from primary retroperitoneal disease.[35] Bulky retroperitoneal adenopathy with an infiltrative renal lesion suggests the diagnosis.

Use of magnetic resonance imaging

MRI in the evaluation of the renal mass for the most part is not necessary given the advances in CT technique. However, MRI is a consideration for those patients with an allergy to iodinated contrast or with pre-existing renal insufficiency which may be worsened with a contrast load. This is of special import in those patients that have had prior nephrectomy and are now faced with a metachronous lesion of the remaining kidney. The immediate advantage of MRI is in multiplanar imaging and in assessment of venous involvement (Figure 3.13).[36] Additionally, gadolinium contrast may be used with safety in patients with renal insufficiency and has an extremely low risk of inducing an allergic response.[37]

As with CT, simple cysts should be well circumscribed, with homogenous decreased signal intensity on T1-weighted imaging and increased intensity on T2 (usually isointense to the cerebrospinal fluid (CSF) in the spinal canal, a useful internal reference for comparison).

Hemorrhagic cysts will demonstrate variable T1-signal intensity, depending upon the protein content of the fluid and/or the age of the hemorrhagic components in the cyst. Similar variability is also seen on T2-weighted images. With continued evolution, hemorrhagic cysts become of low signal intensity in both T1 and T2 as the hemoglobin within the cyst breaks down and eventually becomes replaced with hemosiderin. Wall calcification in a cyst is poorly appreciated by MRI. The principal criterion of differentiation between a benign complex cyst and a cystic neoplasm is lack of enhancement of the former entity. However, some benign lesions will demonstrate variable enhancement with gadolinium, to include traumatic hematomas, infectious processes such as infected cysts and abscesses, and xanthogranulomatous pyelonephritis.[38] Again, clinical history is indispensable in this regard.

While considerable variability exists, RCCa appears heterogeneous on T1-weighted sequences and becomes hyperintense on T2-weighted sequences.[39] However, some investigators have abandoned T2-weighted images in their 'renal mass' protocols as it is felt that lesion characterization with this pulse sequence is not necessary for a solid mass.[40] Instead, reliance is on rapid T1-weighted gradient echo (GRE) sequences with fat suppression. T2-weighted images require several seconds for acquisition, whereas T1-GRE images can be obtained in milliseconds. Such rapidity allows minimization of motion-related artifacts due to breathing or vasculature pulsation. Fat-suppressed images also assist in evaluating the perirenal space for involvement. Evaluation of indeterminant lesions may be evaluated with T1, T2 (still useful, in our opinion, for cystic lesions), and T1-GRE fat-saturated post-gadolinium contrasted images, again with the determination of possible malignancy based upon enhancement. However, due to the expense of MRI, in the absence of the contraindications above, it is recommended that most patients be evaluated with dynamic enhanced CT due to its wide availability and accuracy.[36]

Multidetector computed tomography

While, as discussed above, the IVP has limitations assessing parenchymal lesions, it remains the mainstay of assessing the collecting system and ureters. Recently, however, the use of multidetector CT (MDCT) has begun to challenge the seeming monopoly on the collecting system that IVP has held for decades. The majority of helical CT scanners in use in the United States are currently those employing single-detector technology. A single spiral or helical plane of data is generated with each rotation of the X-ray tube and detector as the patient is moved through the gantry.[41] The images eventually created at each axial plane are

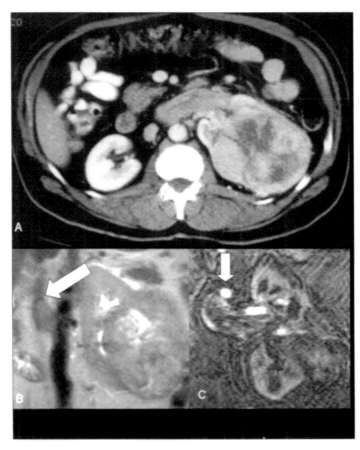

Figure 3.13

Tumor thrombus. A 56-year-old male presenting with asymptomatic gross hematuria. Contrast CT (A) reveals a large left renal mass with markedly engorged left renal vein. This T2-weighted coronal MR image (B) suggests the presence of a tumor thrombus just within inferior vena cava (arrow). A gradient recall image (C) confirms the thrombus within the left renal vein, extending into the inferior vena cava (IVC) (arrow on superior mesenteric artery origin).

actually *an estimate*, or interpolation, of the information (specifically of the portions of the patient between the helical imaging 'slices') that would have been obtained had the gantry made an entire revolution at each particular axial position (the 'old' stop and image in each plane method). Slice thickness is determined by the collimation of the X-ray beam before imaging acquisition. With MDCT, multiple helical scan planes are obtained simultaneously and slice thickness is determined by the configuration of the detector row and the pre-selected X-ray beam collimation. To use a simplified example, with a 4 detector bank, 4 times the information is obtained (4 times the number of slices) with a single pass through the scanner compared to a single detector system in the same amount of time. Consequently, more refined post-acquisition image reconstruction can be done, in any plane, with very little loss of resolution, as the originally imaged planes obtained overlap. Additionally, post-acquisition slice thickness reconstruction can be done down to the size of the smallest detector without having to re-scan the patient and reset the beam collimation. The amount of information

acquired not only allows multiplanar reconstruction but also allows smooth 3D volume-rendered images to be reconstructed. This is of benefit in situations where detailed imaging of vascular anatomy is requested prior to minimally invasive surgery such as with living related renal donors and correction of ureteropelvic junction obstruction.[21,42,43] Evaluation of such patients is discussed later in this chapter.

Computed tomographic urography

Three types of 'CT urography' have been described:

1. standard axial CT, with scout images of the abdomen (the 'scanogram') pre- and post-contrast using the CT scan dataset obtained during axial acquisition
2. hybrid examinations that combine CT and IVP (used at our institution)

3. MDCT with subsequent 3D reconstructed images in the coronal plane from the data set.[44]

For those institutions with MDCT technology, complete imaging evaluation of the urinary tract may be performed in the CT suite. Reportedly, there is no significant difference in the opacification of the collecting system as regards conventional urography and reconstructed MDCT urography.[45] However, there has yet been no comparison of MDCT urography with conventional urography as regards small-volume upper-tract urothelial (i.e. transitional cell carcinoma) disease. MDCT urography does have utility, however, in localizing urolithiasis, defining collecting system anatomy and anomalies, and assessing intravesicle pathology.[46] The use of MDCT urography to produce detailed images of the bladder has led to 3D reconstructed images yielding the so-called 'virtual cystoscopy'. While polypoid lesions are ideal for detection with the 3D reconstructed images, detection of bladder wall thickening requires detailed assessment of the axial views. Recently reported, however, is a series in which 88% of bladder urothelial lesions less than 0.5 cm in size were detectable with an overall sensitivity and specificity of 95 and 87%, respectively.[47] While MDCT may demonstrate ureteral obstruction and narrowing, concentric wall narrowing due to urothelial disease is not well appreciated on the reconstructed images, whereas with standard urography small mucosal abnormalities that may indicate a need for ureteroscopic evaluation may be easily detected.[44] Using a phantom, screen-film systems and computerized radiography have been demonstrated to maintain higher resolution in regards to line pairs per millimeter, whereas CT offers better contrast discrimination.[48] Although this is a technology that is in evolution and will, no doubt, improve, several investigators feel that due to limitations in spatial resolution MDCT urography has not yet reached a point where the standard intravenous urogram can be abandoned.[49–51] The main advantage of MDCT urography at this point is the ability to obtain a complete imaging package with 'one' study, i.e the patient has just the CT and does not require movement to another room for subsequent radiographic imaging.

Noncontrast computed tomography in evaluation of renal colic

Intravenous pyelogram/urography has ceded superiority to unenhanced helical CT (UHCT) in the diagnosis of acute renal colic due to ureterolithiasis. This paradigm shift began with the publication of Smith et al regarding direct comparison of UHCT with what was then the gold standard, IVP.[52] The efficacy of CT in this regard was further demonstrated by the study being terminated after only 22 patients when CT was found to be the profoundly more accurate modality. Advantages of UHCT included rapid acquisition of images, no need for contrast, lower dose of radiation (compared to IVP), and the ability to diagnose other causes of flank pain.[53] Disadvantages were misdiagnosis of urolithiasis due to surgical clips or pelvic phleboliths. A recent review of the world literature regarding UHCT for renal colic reveals the sensitivity and accuracy for calculus identification and diagnosis ranges from 94 to 100% and from 93 to 98%, respectively.[54] About 10% of patients thought to have a ureteral calculus were found in one series to have an alternative diagnosis which was felt to be the etiology of the patient's flank pain.[55] Thus, UHCT was felt to be a useful screening tool that allowed triaging the patient to either optimal therapy, or selection of additional imaging to further elucidate the problem (Figure 3.14).

Occasionally, identification of the actual calculus may be difficult, either due to small size, or the patient may be imaged immediately after stone passage. Additionally, calcification in the pelvis may be due to venous phleboliths or atherosclerotic disease. Thus, secondary signs of obstruction/inflammation are also of import in UHCT. Definitive identification of a ureteral stone is thought to require the calcification to have a surrounding rim of tissue – the edematous ureteral wall (Figure 3.15)[56] However, the so-called 'rim sign' is only observed in 50–80% of patients, and 8% of phleboliths may also have a soft tissue rim.[57,58] Attenuation of the calcification is also helpful, as in one series it was found that if the calcification had an attenuation of more than 311 Hounsfield units the probability of it being a phlebolith was only 0.03%.[59]

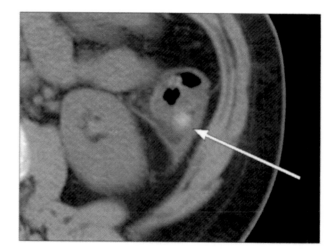

Figure 3.14
Diverticulitis. A 19-year-old female presenting to the emergency room with complaint of left flank pain was found instead to have diverticulitis of the descending colon. Note the surrounding inflammation and presence of a fecalith in the infected diverticulum (arrow).

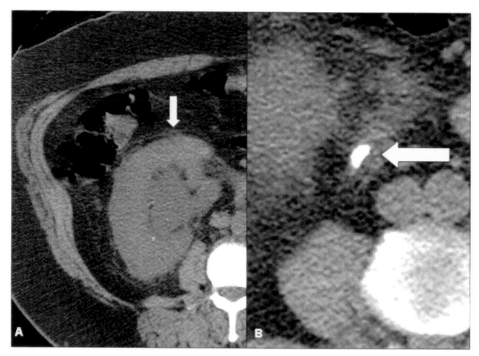

Figure 3.15
NECT (nonenhanced CT) for renal colic. A 55-year-old female presenting to emergency department with complaint of right flank pain. (A) NECT demonstrates an enlarged hydronephrotic right kidney with perinephric stranding (arrow). (B) Magnified image of proximal ureter demonstrates a calculus obstructing the ureter with surrounding soft tissue density, the 'rim' sign.

Hydronephrosis proximal to the stone is seen in almost 70% of patients, with perinephric stranding in 65% of patients (Figure 3.15).[60] Combination of unilateral hydronephrosis or ureteral dilatation with ipsilateral perinephric or periureteral stranding in one series had a positive predictive value of 98%:[61] absence, thereof, had a negative predictive value of 91%. Additionally, stones that are not readily seen by plain radiography are easily seen via unenhanced computed tomography (UECT) (Figure 3.16).

Rarely, the use of contrast may be required to make the definitive diagnosis. Older and Jenkins have proposed a management schema outlining UHCT findings and further diagnostic evaluation:[56]

1. Secondary signs positive: hydronephrosis and/or perinephric fluid, and definite stone (rim sign) or very likely stone in ureter. Diagnosis: ureteral stone – no contrast needed.
2. Secondary signs positive: hydronephrosis and/or perinephric fluid, and no ureteral stone definitively seen. Diagnosis: the stone has probably passed – no contrast needed.
3. Secondary signs negative: no hydronephrosis or

perinephric fluid, but definitive stone in ureter on side of flank pain (rim sign present). Diagnosis: ureteral stone – no contrast needed.
4. Secondary signs positive: hydronephrosis and/or perinephric fluid and probable stone in ureter. Diagnosis: ureteral stone – no contrast needed.
5. Secondary signs negative: no hydronephrosis or perinephric fluid, and no suspicious calcification. Diagnosis: no ureteral stone – no contrast needed.
6. Secondary signs negative: no hydronephrosis, no perinephric fluid; possible ureteral stone, but not definite. Diagnosis: indeterminant – contrast needed.

In the sixth scenario, definitive evaluation may be made by intravenous pyelography or retrograde pyelography. The advantage of the latter is that the urologist may immediately manage or temporize the problem with ureteroscopic removal or placement of a ureteral stent if felt to be clinically necessary. The CT protocol for renal colic used at our institution is provided in Table 3.3. Note that the patient may be scanned in the prone position to discriminate calculi that have passed into the bladder from those that remain lodged in the ureterovesical junction (Figure 3.17).

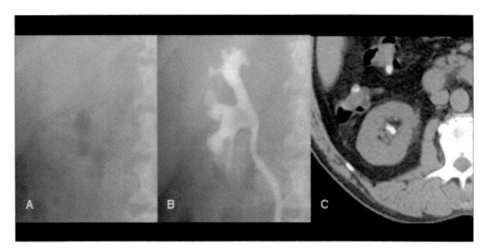

Figure 3.16
Radiolucent stone. (A) Coned down scout image of right renal fossa in a KUB obtained prior to retrograde pyelogram for gross hematuria in a 45-year-old male. (B) Coned down image obtained from retrograde pyelogram demonstrating radiolucent filling defect in renal pelvis. (C) Noncontrast CT reveals unsuspected calculus composed of uric acid. Retained enteric contrast in several colonic diverticula are also seen.

Table 3.3 *CT abdomen/pelvis (noncontrast) for urinary calculi*

Position: prone (allows any stones in posterior bladder
   to fall forward)
Scout: PA
Scan area: from just above diaphragm through
   symphysis pubis
Slice increment: 5.0 mm
Slice thickness: 6.5 mm
Field of view: varies with patient size
Pitch: 0.875
Rotation time (s): 0.75
KVP: 120
mA: 200–300
Algorithm: standard
Breath hold: 25–30 s inspiration

Assumes single-detector helical system with pitch = distance
couch moves during one revolution of the X-ray tube.

Preoperative evaluation of ureteropelvic junction obstruction in adults

The three goals of imaging of possible UPJO are:

1. determination of the presence and degree of renal obstruction
2. determination of residual renal function
3. determination of the cause of the obstruction.[62]

The most common complaint is pain, either constant or with diuretic states, with stones; microhematuria and pyelonephritis are also significant presenting signs.[63] Further evaluation may then be made with IVP, diuretic nuclear renography, retrograde pyelography, and a provocative assessment of intrapelvic pressures, the Whitaker test.[64]

After presenting symptoms and initial imaging suggest the possibility of UPJO, most authors state reliance upon diuretic nuclear renography for assessment of residual renal function and degree of obstruction due to the relative noninvasiveness of the test.[62] The agents used currently are technetium 99m diethylenetriamine pentaacetic acid (Tc99m–DTPA) and technetium 99m mercaptoacetyl-triglycine (Tc99m–MAG-3), with the former being predominantly excreted by glomerular filtration, the latter predominantly by tubular secretion. Tc99m–MAG-3 is currently felt to be the agent of choice as it is much less affected by impaired glomerular filtration, which may be significant in chronically obstructed kidneys.[65] Initial imaging, specifically the first 1–2 min after radiopharmaceutical injection, demonstrates renal blood flow and processing of the radiopharmaceutical through the parenchyma, thus assessing function. The peak cortical uptake of radiopharmaceutical in the obstructed side may be delayed, with the maximum parenchymal uptake rarely reaching that of the normal side. Filling of the collecting system is likewise delayed. However, due to the capacity of the dilated renal pelvis, the maximum activity in the affected collecting system frequently exceeds the normal side long after the normal side has cleared the radiopharmaceutical.[66] Usually, furosemide (40 mg) is administered either after a preset time during the protocol (15–30 min

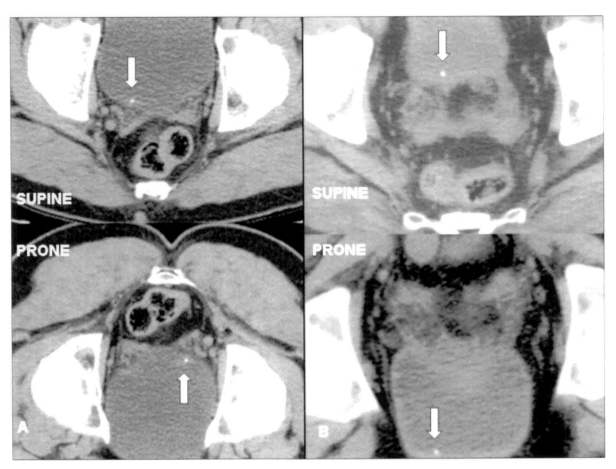

Figure 3.17
Effect of positioning in patients undergoing NECT (nonenhanced CT) for renal colic. Patients are placed in the prone position routinely. (A) A patient with a calculus at the ureterovesical junction, confirmed with stone remaining in position while prone. (B) Another patient with a posterior calculus, which, when in the supine position, may be trapped at the ureterovesical junction. In the prone position the stone is seen to fall forward, confirming that the stone is intravesical.

after radiopharmaceutical injection) or, more appropriately, after the collecting system on the obstructed side has reached maximum activity. In an obstructed system, washout of radiopharmaceutical from the collecting system is either unchanged with diuretic administration or significantly blunted. Quantification is done by calculating a $T_{1/2}$ value – the time that half the activity is lost from the drawn region of interest. While $T_{1/2}$ standards were first formulated in the pediatric population, most clinicians agree that a $T_{1/2}$ of less than 10 min indicates no significant obstruction, 10–20 min is equivocal, and more than 20 min is strongly suggestive of obstruction (Figure 3.18).[67]

False-positive results may occur in patients that are inadequately hydrated and may arise with kidneys that are extremely compromised and thus not able to respond adequately to furosemide (or due to an inadequate dose being given). Failure of the collecting system to fill with radiopharmaceutical within 1 hour or ipsilateral function

less than 20% of total renal function virtually guarantees prolonged excretion, even without significant obstruction. Also, induced diuresis may fail to clear a system of very large capacity. Finally, a *normal* kidney without any collecting system retention will produce a $T_{1/2}$ of greater than 20 min; thus, furosemide should not be administered unless radiopharmaceutical is demonstrated to be retained in the renal pelvis or ureter.[68] A false positive may be seen in over 10% of patients, even when no significant obstruction exists.[62] Despite limitations, with attention to technique and appropriate pre-study hydration, the incidence of a false-negative study is very low (<1%).[69] Studies that are discordant with other imaging studies, or the patient's symptoms, should be either repeated, or consideration given to performing a perfusion pressure, or Whitaker test. The Whitaker test does require percutaneous access of the collecting system, limiting enthusiasm for its use. Also, accumulated experience with diuretic nuclear renography

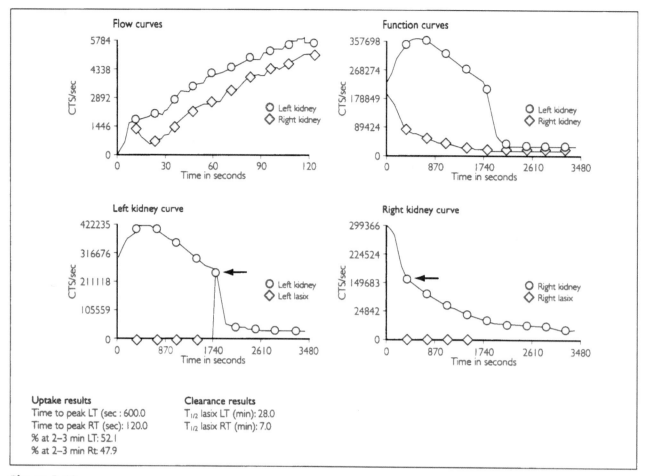

Figure 3.18

Diuretic renography. Tc99m–MAG-3 diuretic renogram in a 30-year-old female with symptomatic left ureteropelvic junction obstruction. Furosemide is administered intravenously when the collecting systems have reached maximum counts and $T_{1/2}$ calculated when counts in the collecting system reach half-maximum (black arrows). In this case the $T_{1/2}$ for the symptomatic left kidney is 28 min, which is indicative of significant obstruction.

has also made the Whitaker test a modality that is now infrequently used.

Once physiologic evidence of obstruction is established, anatomic imaging serves in selecting the operative modality that would best serve the patient. Specifically, the questions to be answered are:

1. How much residual function remains in the obstructed kidney or, more to the point, would the patient be better served with a nephrectomy?
2. Are there any stones in the collecting system? Is there a need for concomitant percutaneous or ureteroscopic stone removal?
3. What is the vascular anatomy of the kidney? How does it relate to the obstruction? How will the anatomy affect the modality selected?

During the diuretic renogram care is taken to draw the ROI area only over the renal parenchyma and not to include the area of the collecting system.[70] Also, as above,

functional imaging is obtained in the first 1–2 min for MAG-3 to avoid a spurious overassessment of functionality due to excretion into the collecting system. Each kidney, in the normal state, contributes between 45 and 55% of the total nephron mass/function. Poor renal function does play a role in the success of relief of UPJO by endoscopic/endourologic means. Success rates from antegrade pyelotomy in one large adult series were found to decrease from 92% to 54% when preoperative function in the affected kidney was less than 25%.[71] This has also been confirmed in the pediatric population, although such a decrease in success is not reported for open dismembered pyeloplasty.[72] Nakada and coworkers have recommended 20% function as a decision point in adults and also recommend a period of percutaneous drainage to allow any residual function to return prior to making a decision for nephrectomy.[64,73] Should diuretic renography be equivocal and a period of percutaneous drainage considered, a Whitaker test may be easily accomplished.

Calculi are present in the setting of UPJO in approximately 20% of patients.[63] Inflammation within the renal pelvis due to calculus disease may play a role in the etiology of the UPJO, although this is felt to be more a theoretical concern as no studies exist to suggest direct causation of submucosal fibrosis.[74] However, if a calculus is impacted at the site of the UPJO or has been so, there is some evidence to suggest that success of pyelotomy may be compromised due to underlying scarring.[75] Indeed, if a calculus was impacted at the UPJ, consideration may be given to stone removal and then reassessment of residual obstruction after a period of ureteral stenting and removal. However, non-impacted stones should be treated simultaneously with management of the UPJO to allow the patient to be managed with one procedure if at all possible.[64,74] Given the previous discussion as regards superiority of UHCT in the diagnosis of urolithiasis, any suspicion of a coexisting calculus may be assessed by that modality.

While in the pediatric population UPJO seems to be more related to intrinsic smooth muscle deficiency, the etiology of adult UPJO seems less well established.[76] Confounding the intrinsic muscular deficiency etiology in adults is the relatively late presentation in some patients,

cognizant that such muscle deficiency should have become manifest in childhood.[77] There is, however, compelling evidence of the role of vessels crossing the ureter either at or in close proximity to the UPJ. In a study of several hundred cadaver kidneys, Sampaio found large arteries or veins ventrally to the UPJ in 65% of kidneys, with 45% of UPJs being found in close proximity to the inferior segmental artery.[78] Inferior polar arteries (arteries directly entering the parenchyma, not the hilum) were found in 6.8%, and in 6.2% there was a dorsal artery in close relation to the UPJ. The majority of these polar arteries arise directly from the aorta. The incidence of a crossing vessel in adults with UPJO is from 50 to 80%.[77,79] In many cases it may be a direct cause of the obstruction; in others the aberrant vessel may be merely an innocent bystander. The vessel may exacerbate the problem as the dilated renal pelvis may, over time, drape over the vessel and compound the pre-existing obstruction.[80]

The initial implication of the crossing vessel seems to be decreased success with endopyelotomy; however, postoperative hemorrhage and segmental parenchymal infarction are also important considerations (Figure 3.19). Accordingly, some authors have proposed that patients

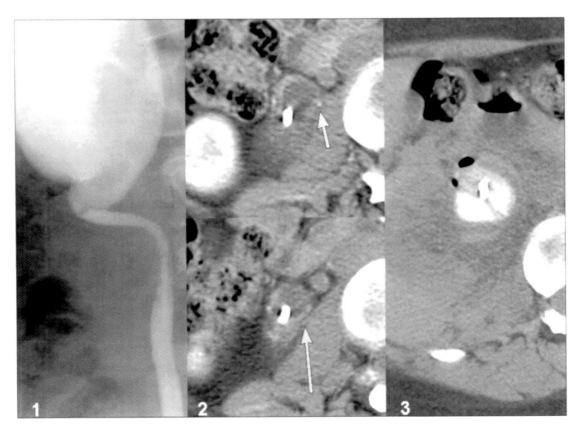

Figure 3.19
Crossing vessel on CT and postoperative hemorrhage. (1) A 24-year-old female with symptomatic left-sided ureteropelvic junction obstruction. (2) Contrast-enhanced CT demonstrates a small vessel abutting the area of the obstruction and passing anterior to it. This vessel was not recognized preoperatively. A ureteral stent is in place across the obstruction. (3) After endoscopic endopyelotomy, there is a large perinephric hematoma secondary to transection of this vessel.

with crossing vessels be offered open or laparoscopic pyeloplasty instead of endoluminal techniques such as endoscopic pyelotomy. Van Cangh et al found that the success rate of endopyelotomy was only 33% with a crossing vessel, vs 82% in those patients without.[81] Assessment of the perirenal vascular anatomy would seem essential regarding successful treatment of UPJO. A large inferior segmental artery or small parenchymal branch may play a role in the etiology of the UPJO, and may be problematic for endourologic treatment. Such a patient may require selection for laparoscopic or open pyeloplasty and thus may be appropriately counseled.[80,82] Vessels that cross the ureter within 1.5 cm of the UPJ are usually anterior; thus, most urologists, when performing endoscopic pyelotomy, make the ureteral incision posterolaterally.[79]

However, there is controversy regarding the import of crossing vessels in regards to success rates of endopyelotomy. A report in 1998 found that 80% of patients had a successful outcome regardless of the presence of a crossing vessel.[83] Questions regarding the additional expense of preoperative imaging (e.g. angiography, spiral CT, or endoluminal US) were raised. However, a later report from the same group 3 years later stated an institutional bias to perform preoperative imaging with spiral CT due to multiple reports of the deleterious effects upon the success rate of endopyelotomy due to crossing vessels.[80]

As regards appropriate imaging for crossing vessels, helical contrast-enhanced CT (HCECT) has replaced conventional intra-arterial digital subtraction angiography (DSA). Rouviere et al, using DSA as a reference standard, found HCECT to be 100% sensitive, and 97% specific for the detection of crossing vessels.[84] Additional information may be obtained from 3D reconstruction of the data obtained during the HCECT, with one study demonstrating 100% concordance between imaging evidence of a crossing vessel and intraoperative findings.[43] Compared to DSA, HCECT provides a relatively noninvasive means of evaluating renal vasculature and its relation to the collecting system. Patients undergoing evaluation with HCECT should first undergo, at the same setting, UECT, to assess for any simultaneous nephrolithiasis. A test injection of contrast (20 ml) may be done with an automated timing system in CT units that are so equipped to allow imaging of the arterial phase at the level of the kidneys during optimal opacification. Alternatively, a rough estimate may be obtained by imaging the aorta at the level of the kidneys every 2–4 s after the test injection to determine the delay from injection to maximal vessel opacification. This is followed by the full contrast injection (120 ml) for the vascular/arterial phase at a slice thickness of 3 mm and a table speed of 3–6 mm/s (with scanning commencing at the appropriate time after injection). A delayed parenchymal phase may then be obtained at 90–120 s after injection.[13] As with the previously described evaluation of the kidneys with CT, review of the study on a PACS workstation greatly facilitates image interpretation. For those patients with contrast allergy or impaired renal function, MR angiography using intravenously administered gadolinium may be a consideration, with the understanding that resolution of small accessory vessels may be limited (Figures 3.20 and 3.21).[85]

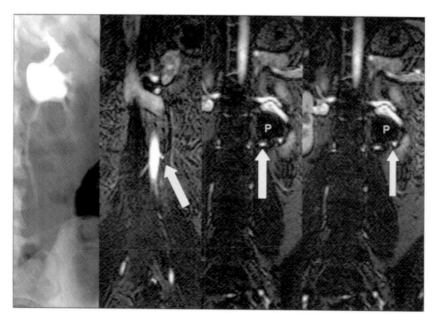

Figure 3.20
Crossing vessel on MR. Coronal gradient recall gadolinium-enhanced MR images demonstrate an accessory artery supplying the lower pole of the left kidney in a 30-year-old female with symptomatic ureteropelvic junction obstruction. The vessel abuts the lower aspect of the dilated renal pelvis (P).

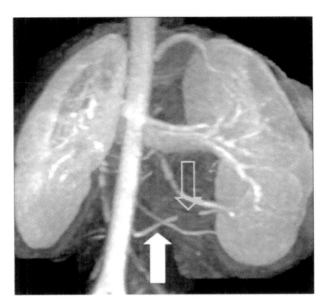

Figure 3.21
Crossing vessel on MR 2. 3D reconstructed image from gradient recall gadolinium-enhanced MR images (see Figure 6.20) demonstrate the accessory polar vessel is abutting the ureteropelvic junction (white arrow). Note the drop out in signal due to the overlying dilated renal pelvis, which is not imaged on the GRE pulse sequence (clear arrow).

Another modality for consideration in the assessment of crossing vessels is endoluminal ultrasound (EUS), either preoperatively, or at the time of planned endopyelotomy. A 6.2F over-the-wire US probe may be advanced to the level of the UPJO under fluoroscopic guidance after retrograde opacification of the collecting system.[86] Findings of a crossing vessel are suggested by a linear area of hypo-echogenicity in close proximity to the center of the tranducer sweep. Location of the vessel can be accurately assessed and orientation of the endoluminal incision can be optimally planned. Also, in those situations in which there is a high insertion of the ureter on the pelvis, a septum, representing the ureteral wall against the redundant renal pelvis, may be readily identified and alternative plans made for pyeloplasty. Direct comparison of EUS with helical CT in 20 patients with symptomatic UPJO found that the former modality was more sensitive in the detection of crossing vessels.[87] Crossing vessels were identified in 35% of patients via CT and in 70% by endoluminal US. Thirty-five percent of patients were found by EUS to have a septum, a finding not assessed by CT. Endoluminal US assisted in planning the orientation of endopyelotomy incision in 4 patients and changed the planned operation from endopyelotomy to pyeloplasty in another 4. Thus, almost half of the patients had treatment impacted by EUS findings.

Imaging in the work-up of the living renal transplant donor

The ultimate goal of laparoscopic renal donation is to expand the pool of potential donors available. Unfortunately, too many patients still die from complications of renal failure while on a waiting list to receive a kidney. With the decreased morbidity of laparoscopic donation, it is hoped that this trend will be ameliorated. Laparoscopic donor nephrectomy has marked advantages over conventional open nephrectomy such as at least a halving of the time of hospital stay and a more rapid return to full activity and employment.[88] Laparoscopic nephrectomy is, however, a challenge to the surgeon due to limitations in exposure, with clear understanding that the safety of the donor is of paramount concern. Essential to the evaluation of the potential laparoscopic renal donor is accurate delineation of the vascular anatomy of the renal allograft. Assessment of renal artery origin, length, branches, and accessory vessels was once obtained with the use of conventional arteriography.[89] Up to one-third of donors have variant renal arterial anatomy. Also to be considered are situations in which the donor has occult vascular disease, such as atherosclerosis or fibromedial disease. Standard IVP was also obtained to evaluate the collecting system for anomalies such as duplications (Figure 3.22). Aberrant anatomy in either case may disqualify a donor, or at the very least may alter the approach at harvest from the donor, or instillation in the recipient.

Conventional arteriography and IVP can now be replaced with helical or multidetector CT, which except for intravenous access for contrast administration, has

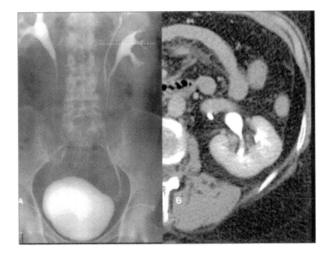

Figure 3.22
Duplication seen on CT-IVP. A 25-year-old female undergoing evaluation as a potential renal donor. (A) IVP demonstrates unsuspected complete duplication of left renal collecting system. (B) CT also demonstrates this duplication. Dashed line in A represents correlation with level of CT image.

become what one investigator has called 'The marriage of minimally invasive imaging with minimally invasive surgery'.[42] A three-phase protocol is recommended to include a noncontrast evaluation of the kidneys and abdomen at 2.5 mm slice thickness to assess for nephrolithiasis, followed by contrast-enhanced evaluation of the kidneys at 1 mm slice thickness at 25 s and 60 s after contrast administration to assess the arterial anatomy and the parenchyma, respectively (Table 3.4).[42,90] Imaging in the arterial phase should include levels down to the iliac bifurcation to assess for any accessory vessels (Figures 3.23 and 3.24). Venous drainage as regards circumaortic or retroaortic morphology on the left, and adrenal venous anatomy, can also be assessed (Figure 3.25). Three-dimensional images may then be reconstructed on a separate workstation to provide a more familiar product for reference by the surgeon. Finally, a conventional excretory urogram may be obtained several minutes after contrast administration to assess the collecting system, or a topogram may be obtained while the patient remains on the CT table.[90]

Aside from the obviation of the need for invasive arterial access, helical or MDCT evaluation may result in a 50% savings in imaging costs for the prospective renal donor.[91] The accuracy of CT-acquired images in assessing renal arterial anatomy is essentially equal to conventional angiography and superior in assessment of parenchymal and venous anatomy.[92] Because of these advantages, helical CT angiography has been proposed as the initial imaging modality of choice in the evaluation of the potential renal donor.[93]

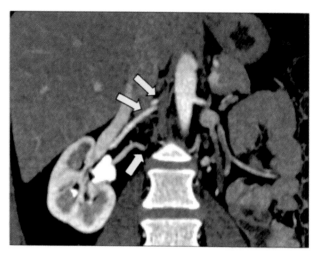

Figure 3.23
Multiple right renal arteries detected using multidetector CT angiography. A 25-year-old female undergoing evaluation as a potential renal donor. Note extreme detail provided by multidetector technology. Each artery had a separate origin from the aorta.

Imaging of adrenal lesions

Up to 5% percent of patients undergoing abdominal CT for any indication are found to harbor an adrenal lesion, with the autopsy incidence being up to 8%.[94,95] Despite their small size, the adrenals however are the fourth most common site for metastases from tumors of epithelial origin, with an autopsy incidence of 27%.[96,97] The majority of masses are benign adenomas, even in the setting of known extra-adrenal malignancy. Adenomas tend to be smaller than 3 cm, whereas metastases tend to be multiple and larger. The differential diagnosis of an adrenal lesion includes adenomas, metastases, pheochromocytomas, hemorrhage, myelolipoma, and adrenocortical carcinoma. The role of imaging for the laparoscopic surgeon is to characterize the lesion as benign or potentially malignant, thus providing or refuting a rationale for intervention.

The initial evaluation begins with review of the medical history.[98] Does the patient have hypertension? If so, is the hypertension sustained or episodic? Are aldosterone levels elevated; are serum renin levels low? Is there evidence of hypokalemia? Are there elevations of urinary catecholamines? Such inquiries may help make the diagnosis of Conn's syndrome (due to a functioning adenoma producing aldosterone) or a pheochromocytoma, respectively. Does the patient have a physical examination suggesting hypercortisolism, such as truncal obesity, or hirsutism, seen in Cushing's syndrome from a hyperfunctioning cortisol adenoma? Is there a history of malignancy suggesting metastasis?

In the majority of cases, subsequent CT evaluation can establish a diagnosis. Most adenomas are of low density

Table 3.4 *CT for assessment of renal vasculature*

Position: supine
Scout: AP
Scan area: 2 cm above celiac artery to the bifurcation
Slice increment: 2 mm
Slice thickness: 2 mm
Field of view: varies with patient size
Pitch: 1.5
Rotation time (s): 1
KVP: 120
MA: 225
IV contrast: 125 ml nonionic
Injection rate: 3 ml/s via 20GA angiocath antecubital vein
Scan delay: 25 s after injection or greater, depending on test dose; delayed scans through kidneys to assess parenchyma and veins

Assumes single-detector helical system with pitch = distance couch moves during one revolution of the X-ray tube.

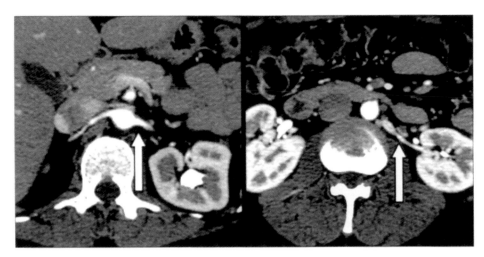

Figure 3.24
Multiple left renal arteries detected using multidetector CT angiography. A 25-year-old female undergoing evaluation as a potential renal donor. Note extreme detail provided by multidetector technology. Each artery had a separate origin from the aorta.

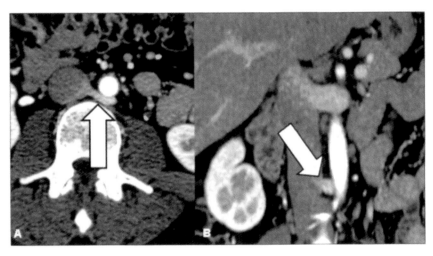

Figure 3.25
Circumaortic left renal vein detected using multidetector CT angiography. (A) Axial source images. (B) Coronal reconstructed images. A 25-year-old female undergoing evaluation as a potential renal donor. Normal main left renal vein is seen more cephalad overlying the aorta. Note extreme detail provided by multidetector technology.

due to intracytoplasmic lipid. A small well-circumscribed lesion with Hounsfield units on unenhanced CT equal to or less than 10 is of such specificity for the diagnosis of adenoma that no further imaging is felt to be warranted (Figure 3.26).[99] In a meta-analysis of multiple series, Boland et al found that using ≤10 HU as a demarcation point yielded a sensitivity of 78% and a specificity of 98% for diagnosis of benign adenoma.[100] Such lesions are termed 'lipid-rich' adenomas.

Difficulty arises for those lesions with attenuation values greater than 10 HU. Is the lesion a 'lipid-poor' adenoma or some other entity? Efforts have been made to establish criteria using the contrast washout characteristics of adrenal lesions. A suggested protocol involves directed CT of the adrenal glands at 3–5 mm collimation first unen-hanced, repeated 60 s after contrast administration, and finally 15 min later.[101] Identical ROI areas are drawn over the adrenal lesion in question and attenuation values obtained in each phase. Percentage of contrast washout is calculated by the equation:

$$\frac{HU_{enhanced} - HU_{delayed}}{HU_{enhanced} - HU_{unenhanced}} \times 100\%$$

Well-circumscribed homogenous lesions with contrast washout greater than 60% at 15 min are felt to meet criteria for an adenoma (Figure 3.27, Table 3.5). Using such a standard and based upon either percutaneous biopsy results or stability over a period of surveillance, Caoili et al were able to correctly characterize 96% of 166 adrenal

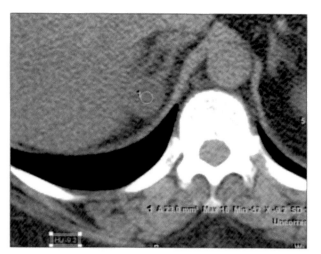

Figure 3.26
Adrenal adenoma on NECT (nonenhanced CT). This 2 cm right adrenal mass was incidently discovered in a 55-year-old female. The region of interest (ROI) circle was drawn within the lesion, with subsequent densitometry yielding a Hounsfield unit of −9.2, indicating a benign adenoma.

Table 3.5 *Adrenal CT protocol*

Position: supine
Scout: AP
Pitch: 0.875
KVP: 120
MA: 300
Rotation time (s): 0.750
Field of view: 300 mm
Scan area: 2 cm above kidneys through bottom of kidneys
Contrast: nonroutinely used (see below)
Noncontrast scan done first and reviewed by radiologist. If adrenal mass has attenuation < 10 HU, no further imaging required (adenoma). If > 10 HU, administer IV contrast and time for arterial phase. Delayed images at 15–20 min to evaluate for contrast washout (see text).

Assumes single-detector helical system with pitch = distance couch moves during one revolution of the X-ray tube.

masses, yielding a sensitivity and specificity of 98 and 92%, respectively.[101] If there has not been a corresponding unenhanced CT obtained, a relative percent washout equation may be used:

$$\frac{HU_{enhanced} - HU_{delayed}}{HU_{enhanced}} \times 100\%$$

with values greater than 40% suggesting adenoma.[102]

For those patients in whom renal insufficiency or iodinated contrast allergy is a problem, MR may be of benefit. Using T1-weighted GRE techniques there are different reso-nant frequency peaks, and thus different signal intensities generated by protons in water molecules of the tissues in nonadenomas vs those in the cytoplasmic triglycerides found in adenomas (Figure 3.28).[103] In initial reports 95% of adenomas were accurately characterized by loss of signal in the adenoma on out-of-phase images (see Figure 3.28). Later reports have reported sensitivities of 81–87% and specificities of 92–100% for accurate characterization of adenomas.[104,105] Gadolinium enhancement or washout has not been found to be of benefit in lesion characterization.[99]

Other lesions of note include pheochromocytomas, myelolipomas, cysts, and carcinomas. Pheochromo-

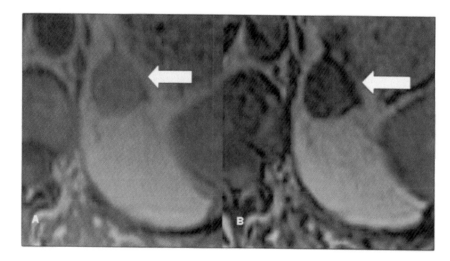

Figure 3.27
Opposed-phase MR imaging in assessment of possible adrenal adenoma. A 58-year-old female with lung carcinoma found to have left adrenal mass on staging chest CT. Noncontrast CT HU was 25. (A) T1-weighted in-phase axial image demonstrates left adrenal mass (arrow). (B) T1-weighted out-of-phase image demonstrates signal drop out in the left adrenal due to high concentration of intracellular lipid in adrenal cortical tissue. Consistent with benign adenoma.

cytomas are usually suggested clinically by episodic hypertension, tachycardia, sweating, and headache. The majority in adults are of adrenal medullary origin, whereas 10% are found to be extra-adrenal and are found near the origin of the inferior mesenteric artery/aortic bifurcation (the organ of Zuckerkandl) or, less commonly, along the sympathetic chain from the thoracic inlet to the pelvis.[106] Evaluation is usually limited to assessment of urinary catecholamines and CT of the abdomen and pelvis. Should CT be non-diagnostic for an adrenal lesion, further evaluation for an extra-adrenal site using I-123 metaiodobenzylguanidine or In-111 octreotide may be of benefit for localization.[95] These adrenal lesions tend to be greater than 3 cm when discovered and tend to be of low signal intensity on T1-

weighted MR but are characteristically of high signal intensity on T2-weighted images (Figure 3.29).[97] There may be heterogeneity due to intralesional hemorrhage or necrosis, and there is avid gadolinium enhancement.

Myelolipomas are rare, benign, adrenal lesions containing mature adipose tissues and hematopoeitic elements, which, on histologic section, resemble bone marrow (Figure 3.30).[107] The specific finding is that of macroscopic fat, of similar density to the surrounding retroperitoneal fat, easily assessed on noncontrast CT (see Figure 3.30). Density may be variable due to mixed soft tissue density in 20% of cases.[102] Additional hemorrhage or necrosis may complicate imaging diagnosis. While usually an incidental finding, myelolipomas may present with

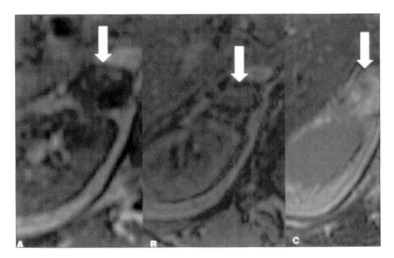

Figure 3.28
Pheochromocytoma. A 34-year-old female with episodic hypertension and elevated 24-hour urinary catecholamines. (A) Axial T1-weighted in-phase MR image demonstates left adrenal mass (arrow). (B) Axial T1-weighted out-of-phase MR image demonstrates no significant signal drop out, suggesting lesion is not a benign adenoma. (C) Axial T2-weighted image demonstrates characteristic hyperintensity of pheochromocytoma on T2 imaging.

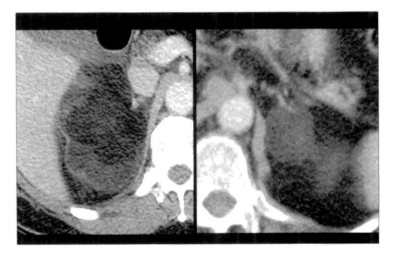

Figure 3.29
Adrenal myelolipoma. Representative lesions from two different patients; in each case the lesion was discovered incidentally. Lesions can attain large size, as seen in image on the left. Note the presence of macroscopic fat in the lesion as compared with the surrounding retroperitoneal fat.

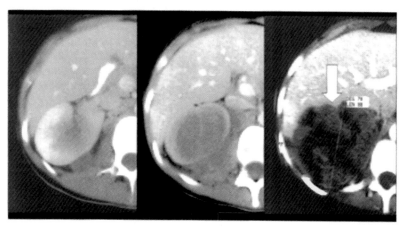

Figure 3.30
Adrenal cortical carcinoma. CT images of large mass arising near upper pole of right kidney in an 18-year-old female presenting with abdominal pain and stigmata of virilization. The mass involved both the upper pole of the right kidney and the right posterior segment of the liver.

flank pain due to large size, ranging from 2 to 20 cm.[108] On MR, myelolipomas are usually isointense with retroperitoneal fat on T1-weighted images and of intermediate signal intensity on T2-weighted images.[97] Subsequent fat-saturation T1-weighted imaging will demonstrate signal drop out. The differential of such a fatty lesion of the adrenal does include lipoma and liposarcoma, which are comparatively rarer still, although a large lesion may resemble the latter and thus require resection or biopsy even if asymptomatic.

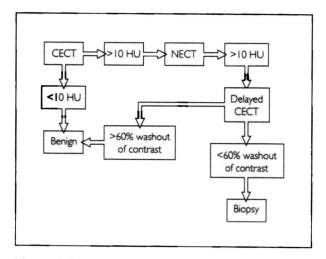

Figure 3.31
Proposed evaluation of an incidentally discovered solid adrenal lesion. Contrast washout calculated via

$$\frac{HU_{enhanced} - HU_{delayed}}{HU_{enhanced} - HU_{unenhanced}} \times 100\%$$

CECT = contrast enhanced CT; NECT = nonenhanced CT.

Adrenal cysts may be large, up to 20 cm, when discovered, and exhibit a 3:1 female-to-male predilection.[95] Four types are described: endothelial cysts with possible lymphangiomatous or angiomatous origin; pseudocysts from probable prior hemorrhage; parasitic cysts from echinococcal infection; and, finally, epithelial cysts.[97] Like their renal counterparts, cysts may be further characterized as: uncomplicated, requiring no further evaluation; complicated, requiring resection; and indeterminent, requiring further diagnostic maneuvers, including aspiration, biopsy, or ultimately resection.[108] Enhancement of the wall may merely represent normal adrenal tissue draped over the cyst. While septations may exist, cysts with thicknesses up to 3 mm are allowed to be considered to have benign characteristics.[95] A complicated cyst is defined by a nodular or thick (> 5 mm) wall, internal attenuation values greater than 30 HU, and stippled or rim calcifications. Such a cyst should be resected to rule out a cystic adrenal neoplasm.[109]

Adrenal carcinoma is rare (about 2000 cases reported) with approximately 50% of patients manifesting an associated endocrinopathy, usually Cushing's syndrome or a virilizing syndrome in females, feminization in males, or Conn's syndrome.[97,102] Almost 70% of patients present with symptomatic unresectable disease, and usually these patients have large hormonally silent tumors.[110] A solid unilateral adrenal mass larger than 5 cm is considered suggestive of carcinoma and resection of a mass larger than 6 cm is recommended for definitive diagnosis, as surgery provides the only durable treatment (Figure 3.31).[102] Carcinomas tend to be large, with areas of heterogeneity on CT suggesting necrosis; calcification may be seen in 30%.[97] Findings suggesting malignancy include direct involvement of adjacent organs, vena caval invasion and distant metastases. The multiplanar capabilities of MR, and now with MDCT, allow assessment of local invasion, and venous involvement.

References

1. Grossfeld GD, Litwin MS, Wolf JS Jr, et al. Evaluation of asymptomatic microscopic hematuria in adults: the American Urological Association Best Practice Policy – Part I: definition, detection, prevalence, and etiology. Urology 2001; 57:599–603.

2. Grossfeld GD, Litwin MS, Wolf JS Jr, et al. Evaluation of asymptomatic microscopic hematuria in adults: the American Urological Association best practice policy – Part II: patient evaluation, cytology, voided markers, imaging, cystoscopy, nephrology evaluation, and follow-up. Urology 2001; 57:604–10.

3. Levy DA, Slayton JW, Swanson DA, Dinney CPN. Stage specific guidelines for surveillance after radical nephrectomy. J Urol 1998; 159:1163–7.

4. Gilberti C, Oneto F, Martorana G, et al. Radical nephrectomy for renal cell carcinoma: long-term results and prognostic factors on a series of 328 cases. Eur Urol 1997; 31:40–8.

5. Sobin LH, Wittekind Ch. Kidney. In: TNM classification of malignant tumors, 5th edn. New York: International Union Against Cancer, 1997:180.

6. Zisman A, Pantuck AJ, Chao D, et al. Reevaluation of the 1997 TNM classification for renal cell carcinoma: T1 and T2 cutoff point at 4.5 rather than 7 cm better correlates with clinical outcome. J Urol 2001; 166:54–8.

7. Di Silverio FD, Casale P, Colella D, et al. Independent value of tumor size and DNA ploidy for prediction of disease progression in patients with organ confined renal cell carcinoma. Cancer 2000; 88:835–43.

8. Warshauer DM, McCarthy SM, Street L, et al. Detection of renal masses: sensitivities and specificities of excretory urography/linear tomography, US and CT. Radiology 1988; 169:363–5.

9. Curry NS, Schabel SI, Betsill WL. Small renal neoplasms: diagnostic imaging, pathologic features, and clinical course. Radiology 1986; 158:113–17.

10. Russo P. Renal cell carcinoma: presentation, staging, and surgical treatment. Semin Oncol 2000; 27:160–76.

11. Curry NS. Small renal masses (lesions smaller than 3 cm): imaging evaluation and management. AJR Am J Roentgenol 1995; 164:355–62.

12. Szolar H, Kammerhuber F, Altziebler S, et al. Multiphasic helical CT of the kidney: increased conspicuity for detection and characterization of small (<3-cm) renal masses. Radiology 1997; 202:211–17.

13. Herts BR. Helical CT and CT angiography for the identification of crossing vessels at the ureteropelvic junction. Urol Clin N Am 1998; 25:259–67.

14. Jayson M, Sanders H. Increased incidence of serendipitously discovered renal cell carcinoma. Urology 1998; 51:203–5.

15. Chow WH, Devesa SS, Warren JL, Fraumeni JF Jr. Rising incidence of renal cell cancer in the United States. JAMA 1999; 281:1628–31.

16. Skinner DG, Colvin RB, Vermillion CD, et al. Diagnosis and management of renal cell carcinoma: a clinical and pathologic study of 309 cases. Cancer 1971; 28:1165–77.

17. Konnak JW, Grossman HB. Renal cell carcinoma as an incidental finding. J Urol 1985; 134:1094–6.

18. Ozen H, Colowick A, Freiha FS. Incidentally discovered renal masses: what are they? Br J Urol 1993; 72:274–6.

19. Thompson IM, Peek M. Improvement in survival of patients with renal cell carcinoma – the role of the serendipitously detected tumor. J Urol 1988; 140:487–90.

20. Lerner SE, Hawkins CA, Blute ML, et al. Disease outcome in patients with low stage renal cell carcinoma treated with nephron sparing or radical surgery. J Urol 1996, 155:1868–73.

21. Sheth S, Scatarige JC, Horton KM, et al. Current concepts in the diagnosis and management of renal cell carcinoma: role of multidetector CT and three dimensional CT. Radiographics 2001; 21:S237–54.

22. Kissane JM. The morphology of renal cystic disease. In: Gardner KD Jr, ed. Cystic diseases of the kidney. New York: John Wiley & Sons, 1976:31.

23. Brant WE. Kidneys. In: Webb WR, Brant WE, Helms CA, eds. Fundamentals of body CT. St. Louis: WB Saunders, 1998:249.

24. Aslasken A, Gothlin JH. Imaging of solid renal masses. Curr Opin Radiol 1991; 3:654–62.

25. Bosniak MA. Problems in the radiologic diagnosis of renal parenchymal tumors. Urol Clin N Am 1993; 20:217–30.

26. Bosniak MA. Difficulties in classifying cystic lesions of the kidney. Urol Radiol 1991; 13:92–3.

27. Siegel CL, McFarland EG, Brink JA, et al. CT of cystic renal masses: analysis of diagnostic performance and interobserver variation. AJR Am J Roentgenol 1997; 169:813–18.

28. Bosniak MA, Megibow AJ, Hulnick DH, et al. CT diagnosis of renal angiomyolipoma: the importance of detecting small amounts of fat. AJR Am J Roentgenol 1988; 151:497–501.

29. Seidenwurm DJ, Barkovich AJ. Understanding tuberous sclerosis. Radiology 1992; 183:23–4.

30. Yamakado K, Tanaka N, Nakagawa T, et al. Renal angiomyolipoma: relationship between tumor size, aneurysm formation, and rupture. Radiology 2002; 225:78–82.

31. Steiner MS, Goldman SM, Fishman EK, Marshall FF. The natural history of renal angiomyolipoma. J Urol 1993; 150:1782–6.

32. Lemaitre L, Robert Y, Dubrulle F, et al. Renal angiomyolipoma: growth followed up with CT and/or US. Radiology 1995; 197:598–602.

33. Pode D, Meretik S, Shapiro A, Caine M. Diagnosis and management of renal angiomyolipoma. Urology 1985; 25:461–7.

34. Mourikis D, Chatziionnou A, Antoniou A, et al. Selective arterial embolization in the management of symptomatic renal angiomyolipomas. Eur J Radiol 1999; 32:153–9.

35. Hartman DS, Davidson AJ, Davis CJ Jr, Goldman SM. Infiltrative renal lesions: CT-sonographic-pathologic correlation. AJR Am J Roentgenol 1988; 150:1061–4.

36. Zagoria RJ, Bechtold RE, Dyer RB. Staging of renal adenocarcinoma: role of various imaging procedures. AJR Am J Roentgenol 1995; 164:363–70.

37. Rofsky NM, Weinreb JC, Bosniak MA, et al. Renal lesion characterization with gadolinium enhanced MR imaging: efficacy and safety in patients with renal insufficiency. Radiology 1991; 180:85–9.

38. Miller MA, Brown JJ. Renal cysts and cystic neoplasms. MRI Clin N Am 1997; 5:49–66.

39. Leder RA, Walther PJ. Radiologic imaging of renal cell carcinoma: its role in diagnosis, staging, and management. In: Vogelzang NJ, Scardino PJ, Shipley WU, Coffey DS, eds. Comprehensive textbook of genitourinary oncology. Philadelphia: Lippincott, Williams and Wilkins, 2000:150.

40. Rofsky NM, Bosniak MA. MR imaging in the evaluation of small renal masses. MRI Clin N Am 1997; 5:67–81.

41. Brink JA. Multidetector CT: general principles. In: Birnbaum BA, Brink JA, Johnson CD, Kazerooni EA, eds. Body CT: categorical course syllabus. Am Roentgen Ray Soc 2002:1.

42. Rydberg J, Kopecky KK, Tann M, et al. Evaluation of prospective living renal donors for laparascopic nephrectomy with multisection CT: the marriage of minimally invasive imaging with minimally invasive surgery. Radiographics 2001; 21:S223–6.

43. Farres MT, Pedron P, Gattegno B, et al. Helical CT and 3D reconstruction of ureteropelvic junction obstruction: accuracy in detection of crossing vessels. J Comp Assist Tomogr 1998; 22:300–3.

44. Caoili EM. Multidetector CT of the urinary tract. In: Birnbaum BA, Brink JA, Johnson CD, Kazerooni EA, eds. Body CT: categorical course syllabus. Am Roentgen Ray Soc 2002:67.

45. McNicholas MM, Raptopoulos VD, Schwartz RK, et al. Excretory phase CT urography for opacification of the urinary collecting system. AJR Am J Roentgenol 1998; 170:1261–7.

46. Caoili EM, Cohan RH, Korobkin M, et al. Urinary tract abnormalities: initial experience with multi-detector row CT urography. Radiology 2002; 222:353–60.

47. Kim JK, Ahn JH, Park T, et al. Virtual cystoscopy of the contrast material-filled bladder in patients with gross hematuria. AJR Am J Roentgenol 2002; 179:763–8.

48. McCollough CH, Bruesewitz MR, Vrtiska TJ, et al. Image quality and dose comparison among screen-film, computed, and CT scanned projection radiography: applications to CT urography. Radiology 2001; 221:395–403.

49. Dyer RB, Chen MYM, Zagoria RJ. Intravenous urography: technique and interpretation. Radiographics 2001; 21:799–821.

50. Hattery RR, King BF. Invited commentary to Dyer RB, Chen MYM, Zagoria RJ. Intravenous urography: technique and interpretation. Radiographics 2001; 21:799–821. Radiographics 2001; 21:822–3.

51. Becker JA, Pollack HM, McClennan BL. Urography survives (letter). Radiology 2001; 218:299–300.

52. Smith RC, Rosenfield AT, Choe KA, et al. Acute flank pain: comparison of non-contrast-enhanced CT and intravenous urography. Radiology 1995; 194:789–94.

53. Spencer BA, Wood BJ, Dretler SP. Helical CT and ureteral colic. Urol Clin N Am 2000; 27: 231–41.

54. Dalla Palma L, Pozzi Mucelli R, Stacul F. Present-day imaging of patients with renal colic. Eur Radiol 2001; 11:4–17.

55. Eshed I, Kornecki A, Rabin A, et al. Unenhanced spiral CT for the assessment of renal colic. How does limiting the referral base affect the discovery of additional findings not related to urinary tract calculi? Eur Radiol 2002; 41(1):60–4.

56. Older RA, Jenkins AD. Stone disease. Urol Clin N Am 2000; 27:215–29.

57. Heneghan JP, Dalrymple NC, Verga M, et al. Soft tissue 'rim' sign in the diagnosis of ureteral calculi with the use of unenhanced helical CT. Radiology 1997; 202:709–11.

58. Kawashima A, Sandler CM, Boridy IC, et al. Unenhanced helical CT of ureterolithiasis: value of the tissue rim sign. AJR Am J Roentgenol 1997; 168:997–1000.

59. Bell TV, Fenlon HM, Davidson BD, et al. Unenhanced helical CT criteria to differentiate distal ureteral calculi from pelvis phleboliths. Radiology 1998; 207:363–7.

60. Katz DS, Lane MJ, Sommer FG. Unenhanced helical CT of ureteral stones: incidence of associated urinary tract findings. AJR Am J Roentgenol 1996; 166:1319–22.

61. Smith RC, Verga M, Dalrymple N, et al. Acute ureteral obstruction: value of secondary signs of helical unenhanced CT. AJR Am J Roentgenol 1996; 167:1109–13.

62. Wolf JS Jr, Siegel CL, Brink JA, Clayman RA. Imaging for ureteropelvic junction obstruction in adults. J Endourol 1996; 10:93–103.

63. Clark WR, Malek RS. Ureteropelvic junction obstruction: I. Observations on the classic type in adults. J Urol 1987; 138:276–9.

64. Nakada SY, Johnson M. Ureteropelvic junction obstruction: retrograde endopyelotomy. Urol Clin N Am 2000; 27:677–84.

65. O'Reilly PH, Aurell M, Britton K, et al. Consensus on diuresis renography for investigating the dilated upper urinary tract. Radionuclides in nephrourology group. Consensus Committee on Diuresis Renography. J Nucl Med 1996; 37:1872–6.

66. Dunnick NR, Sandler CM, Amis ESJr, Newhouse JH. Ureter. In: Textbook of uroradiology. Baltimore: Williams and Wilkins, 1997:367–8.

67. Krueger RP, Ash JM, Silver MM, et al. Primary hydronephrosis: assessment of diuretic renography, pelvis perfusion pressure, operative findings, and renal and ureteral histology. Urol Clin N Am 1980; 7:231–42.

68. Taylor A, Ziffer J. Urinary tract. In: Early PJ, Sodee DB, eds. Principles and practice of nuclear medicine. St Louis: Mosby, 1995:593–6.

69. O'Reilly PH. Diuresis renography 8 years later: an update. J Urol 1986; 136:993–9.

70. Roarke MC, Sandler CM. Provocative imaging: diuretic renography. Urol Clin N Am 1998; 25:227–49.

71. Gupta M, Tuncay O, Smith A. Outcomes analysis of percutaneous antegrade endopylotomy. J Urol 1997; 157S:285.

72. Figenshau RS, Clayman RV. Endourologic options for the management of ureteropelvic junction obstruction in the pediatric patient. Urol Clin N Am 1998; 25:199–209.

73. Preminger GM, Clayman RV, Nakada SY, et al. A multicenter clinical trial investigating the use of a fluoroscopically

controlled cutting balloon catheter for the management of ureteral and ureteropelvic junction obstruction. J Urol 1997; 157:1625–9.

74. Rutchik SD, Resnick MI. Ureteropelvic junction obstruction and renal calculi. Urol Clin N Am 1998; 25:317–21.

75. Green DF, Lytton B, Glickman M. Ureteropelvic junction obstruction after percutaneous nephrolithotripsy. J Urol 1987; 138:599–602.

76. Cussen LJ. The morphology of congenital dilation of the ureter: intrinsic ureteral lesions. Austral NZ J Surg 1971; 41:185–94.

77. Janetscheck G, Peschel R, Franscher F. Laparoscopic pyeloplasty. Urol Clin N Am 2000; 27:695–704.

78. Sampaio FJ. The dilemma of the crossing vessel at the ureteropelvic junction: precise anatomic study. J Endourol 1996; 10:411–15.

79. Sampaio FJB, Favorito LA. Ureteropelvic junction stenosis: vascular anatomic background for endopyelotomy. J Urol 1993; 150:1787–91.

80. Rehman J, Landman J, Sundaram C, Clayman RV. Missed anterior crossing vessels during open retroperitoneal pyeloplasty: laparoscopic transperitoneal discovery and repair. J Urol 2001; 166:593–6.

81. Van Cangh PJ, Nesa S, Galeon M, et al. Vessels around the ureteropelvic junction: significance and imaging by conventional radiology. J Endourol 1996; 10:111–19.

82. Kumon H, Tsugawa M, Hashimoto H, et al. Impact of 3-dimensional helical computerized tomography on selection of operative methods for ureteropelvic junction obstruction. J Urol 1997; 158:1696–700.

83. Nakada SY, Wolf JS, Brink JA, et al. Retrospective analysis of the effect of crossing vessels on successful retrograde endopyelotomy outcomes using spiral computerized tomography angiography. J Urol 1998; 159:62–5.

84. Rouviere O, Lyonnet D, Berger P, et al. Ureteropelvic junction obstruction: use of helical CT for preoperative assessment – comparison with intraarterial angiography. Radiology 1999; 213:668–73.

85. Borello JA. Renal MR angiography. MRI Clin N Am 1997; 5:83–93.

86. Bagley DH, Liu J. Endoureteral sonography to define the anatomy of the obstructed ureteropelvic junction. Urol Clin N Am 1998; 25: 271–9.

87. Keeley FX Jr, Moussa SA, Miller J, Tolley DA. A prospective study of endoluminal ultrasound versus computerized tomography angiography for detecting crossing vessels at the ureteropelvic junction. J Urol 1999; 162:1938–41.

88. Ratner LE, Kavoussi L, Sroka M. Laparoscopic assisted live donor nephrectomy: comparison with the open approach. Transplantation 1997; 63:229–33.

89. Manu MA, Tanabe K, Ishikawa N, et al. Comparative study of helical CT scan angiography and conventional arteriography for evaluation of living renal transplant donors. Transplant Proc 1999; 31:2883–4.

90. Fishman EK. Multidetector CT of the kidneys: CT angiographic applications. In: Birnbaum BA, Brink JA, Johnson CD, Kazerooni EA, eds. Body CT: catagorical course syllabus. American Roentgen Ray Soc 2002:55–65.

91. Cochran ST, Krasny RM, Danovitch GM. Helical CT angiography for examination of living renal donors. AJR Am J Roentgenol 1997; 168:1569–73.

92. Lerner LB, Henriques HF, Harris RD. Interactive 3-dimensional computerized tomography reconstruction in evaluation of the living renal donor. J Urol 1999; 161:403–7.

93. Manu MA, Harza M, Manu R, et al. Comparative study of helical CT scan angiography, conventional arteriography and intraoperative findings for the evaluation of living renal transplant donors. Transplant Proc 2001; 33:2028–39.

94. Korobkin M, Francis IR, Kloos RT, Dunnick NR. The incidental adrenal mass. Radiol Clin N Am 1996; 34:1037–54.

95. Tung GA, Zagoria RJ, Mayo-Smith WW. Case review: genitourinary imaging. St. Louis: Mosby, 2000:8.

96. Choyke PL, Doppman JL. Adrenal glands. In: Stark DD, Bradley WG Jr, eds. Magnetic resonance imaging, Vol 2. St. Louis: Mosby Year-Book, 1992:1880–902.

97. Krebs TL, Wagner BJ. The adrenal gland: radiologic–pathologic correlation. MRI Clin N Am 1997; 5:127–46.

98. Dunnick NR. Question and Answer re appropriate strategy for dealing with incidentally found adrenal masses (< 5cm). AJR Am J Roentgenol 2002; 179:1344.

99. Korobkin M, Brodeur FJ, Yutzy GG, et al. Differentiation of adrenal adenomas from nonadenomas using CT attenuation values. AJR Am J Roentgenol 1996; 166:531–6.

100. Boland GW, Lee MJ, Gazelle GS, et al. Characterization of adrenal masses using unenhanced CT: an analysis of the CT literature. AJR Am J Roentgenol 1998; 171:201–4.

101. Caoili EM, Korobkin M, Cohan RH, et al. Adrenal masses: characterization with combined unenhanced and delayed enhanced CT. Radiology 2002; 222:629–33.

102. Dunnick NR, Korobkin M. Imaging of adrenal incidentalomas: current status. AJR Am J Roentgenol 2001; 179:559–68.

103. Mitchell DG, Crovello M, Matteucci T, et al. Benign adrenocortical masses: diagnosis with chemical shift MR imaging. Radiology 1992; 185:345–51.

104. Korobkin M, Lombardi TJ, Aisen AM, et al. Characterization of adrenal masses with chemical shift and gadolinium-enhanced MR imaging. Radiology 1995; 197:411–18.

105. Outwater EK, Siegelman ES, Radecki PD, et al. Distinction between benign and malignant adrenal masses: value of T1 weighted chemical shift MR imaging. AJR Am J Roentgenol 1995; 165; 579–83.

106. Atiyeh BA, Baraket AJ, Abumrad NN. Extra-adrenal pheochromocytoma. J Nephrol 1997; 10:25–9.

107. Francis IR, Korobkin M. Incidentally discovered adrenal masses. MRI Clin N Am 1997; 5:147–64.

108. Musante F, Derchi LE, Zappasodi F, et al. Myelolipoma of the adrenal gland: sonographic and CT features. AJR Am J Roentgenol 1988; 151:961–4.

109. Rosenblit A, Morehouse HT, Amis ES Jr. Cystic adrenal lesions: CT features. Radiology 1996; 201:541–8.

110. Wooten MD, King DK. Adrenal cortical carcinoma: epidemiology and treatment with mitotane and a review of the literature. Cancer 1993; 72(11):3145–55.

4

Anesthetic implications of minimally invasive urologic surgery

Kurt W Grathwohl and Scott Miller

Introduction

Minimally invasive surgery, specifically laparoscopy, has become increasingly more common because of reduced postoperative pain, shortened convalescence, decreased hospitalization, and significant cost savings.[1–4] The types of laparoscopic procedures and patient indications are also growing as technologies enhance the surgeon's abilities to perform these operations. In fact, the United Kingdom Department of Health predicted that 70–80% of surgical procedures would be performed endoscopically.[5] Consequently, laparoscopy is performed on elderly, pediatric, pregnant, and obese patients as well as those with significant comorbid diseases.

Currently, there are no studies evaluating anesthesia-related complications of newer minimally invasive laparoscopic surgery, although the incidence is extremely low.[1] Rose and associates in 1992, however, reported anesthetic-related complications of laparoscopic cholecystectomy, noting considerable perioperative morbidity that consisted of hypotension (12.9%), Post-Anesthetic Care Unit hypothermia (31.4%), nausea and vomiting (12.9%), and desaturation (10.9%).[4] More recently, in a 1995 multi-institutional study of 185 laparoscopic nephrectomy patients, Gill et al reported 1 case of intraoperative pneumothorax which was attributed to transpleural trocar placement.[6] Postoperative anesthetic-related complications included congestive heart failure (3), atrial fibrillation (2), myocardial infarction (1), pneumonitis (2), pulmonary embolism (1), brachial nerve palsy (1), lateral compartment syndrome (1), non-oliguric acute tubular necrosis (1), and confusion (1).[6] Kavoussi and associates evaluated 372 laparoscopic pelvic lymph node dissection patients at eight medical centers in 1993 and found anesthesia-related complications in 9 cases (2.4%): hypercarbia (1), prolonged sedation (1), obturator nerve palsy (2), and lower extremity deep venous thrombosis (5).[7] There were no deaths in either study.[6,7] The incidence of complications also varies widely, depending on the type of procedure and the experience of the surgeon.[1]

Despite improved outcomes and the minimally invasive title, laparoscopy can be associated with major cardiopulmonary perturbations and anesthesia-related complications (Table 4.1) that pose significant challenges to the anesthetist and surgical team. Subsequently, laparoscopy

Table 4.1 *Anesthetic-related complications of laparoscopic surgery*

Intraoperative
Gastroesophageal reflux/aspiration pneumonitis
Positioning-related nerve injury
Positioning-related physiologic effects
Hemorrhage from vascular injury
Fluid therapy overload
Hypothermia

Associated with insufflation/pneumoperitoneum
Vagal response
Cardiac arrhythmias
Hypercarbia
CO_2/gas embolism
Emphysema (subcutaneous, preperitoneal)
Pneumothorax/pneumomediastinum/
    pneumopericardium
Hypotension
Hypertension
Elevated peak airway pressures
Hypoxemia
Oliguria

Postoperative
Nausea/emesis
Abdominal/shoulder pain
Pulmonary impairment

mandates a vigilant knowledgeable anesthetist and communication with the entire surgical team.

The primary anesthetic goals for minimally invasive surgery include:

1. patient safety
2. avoidance or early treatment of pathophysiologic changes associated with laparoscopy
3. amnesia/analgesia
4. ideal surgical field, i.e. muscle relaxation, position, etc.
5. rapid recovery
6. therapy for adverse effects of anesthesia, i.e. nausea/ vomiting.

The aim of this chapter is to review, enhance, and facilitate the anesthetist and surgeon's appreciation of the unique anesthetic-related implications of minimally invasive urologic surgery to improve communication and patient safety.

Physiologic considerations unique to laparoscopy

Pneumoperitoneum after peritoneal insufflation and alterations in patient position causes several physiologic effects unique to laparoscopy. Hemodynamic changes during brief procedures in healthy patients are minimal; however, patients with preoperative cardiopulmonary disease demonstrate significant pathophysiologic changes.[8–10]

Relatively high solubility and lack of combustion make CO_2 the most common gas utilized for peritoneal insufflation, although N_2O or He can be used.[11,12] Carbon dioxide is also highly permeable, approximately 20 times that of O_2. Peritoneal insufflation pressures of 10–25 mmHg plus 100% CO_2 at atmospheric pressure (760 mmHg) creates a large gradient for CO_2 diffusion into the bloodstream (CO_2 partial pressure 40 mmHg). Most of the transperitoneally absorbed CO_2 is converted to bicarbonate for transportation in the blood until the oxidation of hemoglobin causes CO_2 to be released in the alveolar capillaries and expired. Absorption of CO_2 causes an increased arterial pressure of CO_2 ($PaCO_2$). This is easy to understand, since $PaCO_2$ is directly related to CO_2 production (VCO_2) – sum of metabolic CO_2 and adsorbed CO_2 – and inversely related to alveolar ventilation (VA) by the equation:

$$PaCO_2 = 0.863(VCO_2)/VA.$$

Furthermore, alveolar ventilation is determined by total minute ventilation (VE) minus dead space ventilation (VD):

$$VA = VE - VD.$$

The net effect, therefore, without a change in alveolar ventilation is an increase in $PaCO_2$. The elevation of $PaCO_2$ is unpredictable in patients with cardiopulmonary disease, but an average increase in $PaCO_2$ among 3 studies comparing laparoscopy of less than 30 min was 10.7 mmHg.[2,8,9] Consequently, patients also typically demonstrate mild respiratory acidosis.[2,8,9]

Carbon dioxide acts directly to inhibit the cardiovascular system, decreasing heart rate, cardiac contractility, and systemic vascular resistance (SVR) while increasing pulmonary artery pressures.[1,5,13,14] Stimulation of sympathetic nervous system efferents and increased circulating catecholamines from the adrenal medulla caused by CO_2, however, result in increased heart rate, contractility, and SVR, with net increases in cardiac output (CO) and blood pressure.[2,5,10] Cardiac arrhythmias are also frequently seen with hypercarbia.[2,13]

There are several mechanical effects of increased intra-abdominal pressure (IAP) from pneumoperitoneum. Compression of the abdominal aorta contributes to an increased SVR and afterload, which can result in decreased CO.[5,10] Venous compression, likewise, results in decreased CO secondary to an initial increased venous return to the heart followed by a significant decline in inferior vena cava flow and reduced cardiac preload.[15] Cephalad shift of the diaphragm increases intrathoracic pressures, resulting in elevated central venous pressures. Heart rate is also increased by IAP independent of CO_2.[2] Cephalad elevation of the diaphragm by IAP also results in several pulmonary effects including decreased functional residual capacity (FRC) and respiratory compliance, as well as increased pulmonary dead space, shunt, and peak airway pressure.[8,10,16] These effects are magnified or may be altered with the administration of anesthetic, in obese patients, lateral decubitus, and Trendelenburg positions, although the contribution of position is now debated.[2,16–18] The effects of position may be attenuated by peritoneal insufflation in the supine position prior to movement into Trendelenburg or reverse Trendelenburg positions.[16–18] As a consequence of these combined cardiopulmonary changes, oxygenation may worsen, although it is typically easily increased by raising the inspired O_2 concentration.[2,17,19] Table 4.2 summarizes the cardiopulmonary effects of IAP, although alterations are dependent on several patient and surgical interactions such as the chosen anesthetic, preoperative fluid balance, position, degree of IAP, type and duration of the procedure, etc. Furthermore, patients with underlying cardiopulmonary diseases may display accentuated responses to the laparoscopic-induced physiologic changes.[2,8]

Increased IAP and resultant cardiovascular changes also cause several regional circulatory and endocrine aberrations. Elevated CO_2 and IAP increase cerebral blood flow and intracranial pressure (ICP), although the clinical significance is not clear.[5,20] Splanchnic perfusion and hepatic blood flow are decreased, resulting in gastric mucosal hypoperfusion.[5] Both neurohumoral factors, such

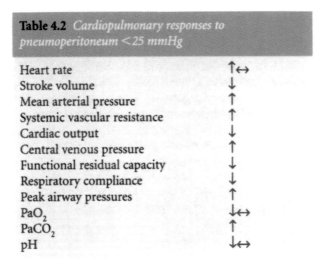

Table 4.2 *Cardiopulmonary responses to pneumoperitoneum <25 mmHg*

Heart rate	↑↔
Stroke volume	↓
Mean arterial pressure	↑
Systemic vascular resistance	↑
Cardiac output	↓
Central venous pressure	↑
Functional residual capacity	↓
Respiratory compliance	↓
Peak airway pressures	↑
PaO_2	↓↔
$PaCO_2$	↑
pH	↓↔

↑, increases; ↓ decreases; ↔ no change.

as increased antidiuretic hormone (ADH or vasopressin), and mechanical compression of the renal arteries and veins decrease renal blood flow, glomerular filtration rate (GFR), sodium excretion, and creatinine clearance.[5,15] Finally, decreased lower limb venous flow has been speculated to increase risk of deep venous thrombosis (DVT), although data are confounding.[5,7]

Helium peritoneal insufflation has been used to prevent the adverse physiologic sequelae of hypercarbia in patients with severe pulmonary disease and pheochromocytoma.[11,12] The lower solubility of helium, however, may theoretically worsen the outcome of venous gas embolism, which limits its use.[12]

Preoperative preparation

The potentially severe cardiopulmonary changes associated with minimally invasive surgery make it imperative that a thorough pre-anesthetic assessment is performed on every patient. Even though laparoscopy is not contraindicated in obesity, extremes of age, pregnancy, and those with severe cardiopulmonary disease, it is important to insure that the patient is medically maximized in order to safely tolerate the physiologic changes. Moreover, the potential for conversion to an open procedure necessitates that the patient be counseled appropriately and is medically ready to tolerate the surgical stress associated with these procedures. Standards for preoperative assessment have been outlined and should be adhered to.[21,22] The preoperative evaluation also allows the anesthetist to properly plan perioperative management and it serves to decrease patient anxiety. In one study, information obtained during the pre-anesthetic evaluation resulted in changes of care plans in 20% of all patients.[23] For instance, a patient may be found to have severe pulmonary disease

or pulmonary hypertension that may require the avoidance of CO_2 insufflation.[12]

Practice guidelines for preoperative fasting and the use of pharmacologic agents to reduce the risk of pulmonary aspiration have been published and, as with all surgical procedures, should be adhered to.[24]

The perioperative evaluation and management of patients with pheochromocytoma is well known and should not be different for laparoscopic adrenalectomy of pheochromocytoma. Increased release of catecholamines during anesthesia and tumor manipulation may exacerbate the pathophysiologic effects of CO_2-induced pneumoperitoneum, although reports have been conflicting.[11,12,25–27]

Monitoring considerations

Routine intraoperative monitoring should include electrocardiogram, noninvasive blood pressure, temperature sensor, concentration of oxygen in the patient's breathing system, pulse oximetry, and capnography. Mechanically ventilated patients should also have tidal volume and airway pressure monitoring. Urinary output is measured after bladder catheterization, which also serves to decompress the bladder prior to trocar placement.

Continuous capnography is useful in monitoring the effects of CO_2 absorption and the adverse cardiopulmonary effects of laparoscopy and anesthesia. Capnography measures exhaled CO_2 breath by breath, allowing for determination of end-tidal CO_2 ($ETCO_2$). Figure 4.1 shows a normal capnogram. Under normal physiologic conditions in healthy patients $ETCO_2$ approximates $PaCO_2$. A small gradient ($PaCO_2 - ETCO_2$) of approximately 5 mmHg exists because of dilution by dead space gases. End-tidal CO_2 is normally maintained between 35 and 40 mmHg to ensure $PaCO_2$ less than 45 mmHg. However, increased dead space ventilation in chronic obstructive pulmonary disease, acute respiratory distress syndrome, and acute decreases in cardiac output, etc., increases $PaCO_2 - ETCO_2$ and makes $ETCO_2$ unreliable as an estimate of $PaCO_2$ in these circumstances.[8,28] Arterial blood gas sampling therefore remains the gold standard for evaluation of unanticipated trends or changes.[8]

Arterial line placement for blood gas analysis allows close monitoring in prolonged procedures and in patients with severe cardiopulmonary diseases. Central venous pressure (CVP), pulmonary artery catheter (PAC) monitoring and transesophageal echocardiography (TEE) are also indicated in patients with severe cardiopulmonary diseases and pheochromocytoma.[26,29] Portera et al prospectively evaluated 10 cardiac patients and found that the PAC identified 2 patients who developed postoperative

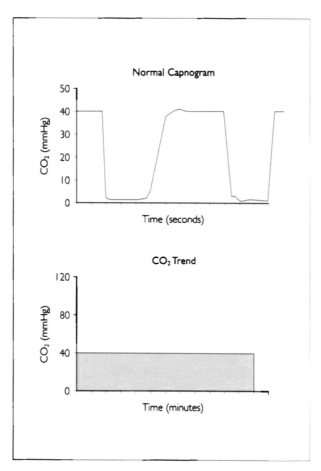

Figure 4.1

Normal capnogram. CO_2 reaches near 0 at the end of inspiration and beginning of expiration when dead space gas is exhaled. As expiration continues, CO_2 rises rapidly toward the alveolar plateau, which lasts for the greater part of the trace. $ETCO_2$ is measured immediately before inspiration begins the rapid downslope.

congestive heart failure.[29] Interpretation of CVP and PAC may be problematic, however, because IAP increases intrathoracic pressures, artificially elevating CVP, and pulmonary artery occlusion pressures.[28] Transesophageal echocardiography is useful for the evaluation of left ventricle regional wall motion abnormalities while continuous monitoring for the identification of gas embolism is not clinically practical. One recent study utilizing TEE identified unexpected increased regurgitant valvular lesions in 15 of 16 healthy laparoscopic donor nephrectomy patients, although the significance is not clear.[30]

Anesthetic techniques

General anesthesia is most commonly chosen for transretroperitoneal or retroperitoneal laparoscopic procedures because of positioning requirements, need for optimal muscle relaxation, time to accomplish the proce-

dure, patient discomfort associated with pneumoperitoneum, and the need to control ventilation in patients with cardiopulmonary diseases. Regional and even local anesthesia, however, is increasingly performed in non-urologic laparoscopy.[31] Advantages of regional techniques (subarachnoid, epidural block) includes less postoperative pain and decreased emesis.[31,32] Additionally, Chiu et al studied the cardiopulmonary effects of laparoscopic ligation of bilateral spermatic varices under epidural anesthesia and found decreased physiologic perturbations.[33] Further evaluation is necessary before this can be recommended for patients with severe comorbid conditions. Disadvantages of regional techniques include the requirement for a T4 block to allow adequate analgesia, which is associated with dyspnea and sympathetic blockade-mediated hypotension.[2,32] Subdiaphragmatic irritation from the insufflated gas also results in shoulder pain despite the high level of blockade.[32] Hyperbaric subarachnoid block may cause severe sympathectomy and hypotension when utilized in the Trendelenburg position and should be avoided while the risk with hypobaric solutions is reduced.[2,31,32]

General anesthesia and muscle relaxation afford the anesthetist and surgeon optimum conditions. Aspiration from positioning and peritoneal insufflation is reduced with cuffed endotracheal tube placement, although the laryngeal mask airway (LMA), which does not protect gastric content aspiration, has been utilized in shorter procedures.[3,32] Oro/nasogastric decompression after anesthetic induction further decreases aspiration risk and facilitates safe trocar placement.[33] Chiu and Ng reported two cases of gastric perforation secondary to trocar placement associated with gastric insufflation during anesthesia induction.[34] Mechanical ventilation allows adjustment of $ETCO_2 < 45$ mmHg. There are no clear differences in anesthetic agents, although DeGrood et al discovered that patients who received total intravenous anesthesia with propofol compared to isoflurane experienced less nausea and faster postoperative recovery.[35]

Nitrous oxide (N_2O) has several properties that make it a useful anesthetic. While not potent enough to be utilized alone, it decreases the minimum alveolar concentration (MAC) of the volatile anesthetic agents and its low solubility creates rapid induction and emergence. Nitrous oxide stimulates the sympathetic nervous system, which may exacerbate and confound the effects of peritoneal insufflation. Furthermore, N_2O is 35 times more soluble than nitrogen, which can produce bowel distention as well as worsen the effects of air embolism and pneumothorax.[36] During short procedures, there is little consequence; however, procedures lasting > 2–4 hours can cause significant bowel distention of over 100–200%.[36] Desflurane, a newer volatile anesthetic agent, obviates the need for N_2O since it has a blood–gas partition coefficient less than N_2O, resulting in very rapid induction and emergence when used as the sole anesthetic. Interestingly, despite these concerns, almost all of the reports we reviewed regarding laparoscopic surgery included N_2O as part of the anesthetic regimen.

Anesthetic-related complications

Intraoperative

Gastroesophageal reflux/aspiration pneumonitis

Several diseases such as diabetic gastropathy, hiatal hernia, and renal failure, as well as Trendelenburg position and IAP from peritoneal insufflation, theoretically predispose patients to an increased risk of aspiration during anesthesia. However, controversy currently exists regarding the effects of IAP.[3,37] One study found that increased IAP raised lower esophageal sphincter pressure to a greater degree than intragastric pressure, thereby actually decreasing the risk of regurgitation.[37] Additionally, studies evaluating the risk of aspiration utilizing the LMA during gynecologic laparoscopy failed to document clinically significant aspiration or reflux.[38] Realistically, the risk for laparoscopic procedures is probably not different from other intra-abdominal surgical procedure. Needless to say, the aspiration risk is significantly decreased after intubation with a cuffed endotracheal tube and when preoperative fasting guidelines are followed.[24] Oro/nasogastric decompression after intubation may further decrease the risk of large-volume gastric content aspiration.

Clinically, intraoperative findings of significant aspiration include hypoxemia, elevated peak airway pressures from bronchospasm, and, potentially, hypotension (see Tables 4.5, 4.7, and 4.8).

Positioning-related nerve injury

Care must be taken to avoid direct mechanical compression or excessive stretch on nerves. While the ulnar nerve is the most frequently injured nerve associated with anesthesia, the pathophysiologic mechanism remains elusive.[39] The lithotomy position has been associated with compression and resultant common peroneal nerve injury.[40]

Positioning-related physiologic effects

Position-related pulmonary and cardiovascular changes are common in lateral decubitus, and head up or down positions. Head-down position increases central venous pressure and CO. Usually, these changes are of minimal clinical significance, although patients with significant coronary artery disease may not tolerate increases in myocardial oxygen demand. As mentioned previously, pneumoperitoneum decreases FRC and pulmonary compliance, resulting in ventilation/perfusion (V/Q) mismatch and predisposing the patient to hypoxemia. Obese patients or those with coexisting respiratory disease exhibit marked responses that are magnified with increased head-down position. Pneumoperitoneum and the head-down position exacerbates raised ICP seen in patients with head trauma.[5] The head-up position and pneumoperitoneum usually results in a decrease in CO from a fall in preload,[5,41] while respiratory perturbations observed from pneumoperitoneum improve. Pneumatic compression stockings may attenuate impaired venous return by improving lower extremity venous blood flow.[42]

Hemorrhage from vascular injury

Fortunately, significant morbidity and mortality from vascular injury is rare, as is re-exploration from postoperative hemorrhage. Most injuries result from trochar or Veress needle insertion. However, as increasingly complex laparoscopic surgeries are being performed, requiring multiple ports, the risk of abdominal wall vessel injuries are becoming more common.[1] In some instances, particularly if an abdominal wall vessel or retroperitoneal vessel are injured, the bleeding can be concealed. One must have a high degree of suspicion for hemorrhage if the patient develops hypotension or has a falling hematocrit. In patients who have involved laparoscopic procedures or known bleeding diathesis, type and screen should be performed.

Fluid therapy overload

The hemodynamic effects of laparoscopy may be magnified by hypovolemia, necessitating adequate intravascular volume replacement; however, several cases of presumed volume overload have been reported during laparoscopic procedures.[6] One author suggests limiting intravenous fluid therapy rates to 3–5 ml/kg/h.[2] Insensible fluid losses and interstitial space requirements are significantly less during laparoscopic procedures compared to open laparotomy or retroperitoneal procedures, where fluid losses can exceed 8–12 ml/kg/h.[6] The oliguric state secondary to vena cava and renal vein compression also creates the impression of decreased intravascular volume, which may lead to overhydration.[43,44] Clinical findings associated with fluid therapy volume overload include hypertension and hypoxemia from pulmonary edema. Cardiac patients may also develop myocardial ischemia and congestive heart failure manifested by arrhythmias, oliguria, and hypotension.

Associated with insufflation/pneumoperitoneum

Vagal response

Insertion of the Veress needle or trocar, but more commonly peritoneal stretching from gas insufflation, can cause a profound vagal response manifested by hypotension, bradycardia, atrioventricular dissociation, and even asystole.[1,9,32] Correction is usually easily achieved by cessation of the surgical stimulation, release of the pneumoperitoneum, and the administration of atropine.[1,9,19,32]

Cardiac dysrhythmias

As mentioned earlier, the heart rate either does not change or slightly increases during insufflation and pneumoperitoneum. Bradydysrhythmias are common during insufflation.[1] Tachydysrhythmias occur less often but are common in the setting of hypercarbia, hypoxemia, acidosis, inadequate levels of anesthesia, and embolic events.

Hypercarbia

Hypercarbia is typically diagnosed intraoperatively when the $ETCO_2$ rises > 45 mmHg. While it is well known that the insufflation of CO_2 results in the elevation of $PaCO_2$ and its adverse physiologic consequences (see Physiologic considerations unique to laparoscopy section above), there are several other diagnostic considerations.[13] Hypercarbia typically occurs over the first 10 min of insufflation. Given the equation

$$PaCO_2 = 0.863(VCO_2)/VA$$

where

$$VCO_2 = \text{metabolic } CO_2 + \text{absorbed } CO_2$$

and

$$VA = VE - VD$$

elevations of $PaCO_2$ can arise from only four sources:

1. increased metabolic production of CO_2
2. increased absorbed CO_2

Table 4.3 *Differential diagnosis of elevated $PaCO_2$ during general anesthesia with mechanical ventilation*

	Effect on $ETCO_2$
Increased metabolic production	
Pyrexia	↑
Sepsis	↑
Malignant hyperthermia	↑
Shivering	↑
Thyroid storm	↑
Catecholamine release/pheochromocytoma	↑
Increased CO_2 absorption	
CO_2-induced pneumoperitoneum	↑
CO_2-induced subcutaneous emphysema/pneumomediastinum	↑
Capnothorax	↑
CO_2 rebreathing from failure of CO_2 absorber/breathing circuit valves	↑
Decreased alveolar ventilation	
Mechanical failure of endotracheal tube, breathing circuit, or ventilator	↑
Increased dead space ventilation	
Pulmonary thromboembolism	↓
Pulmonary gas embolism	↓
Increased positive end-expiratory pressure (PEEP)	↓
High peak/plateau airway pressure	↓
Pulmonary disease	↓↑
Hypotension	↓

↑, increased; ↓, decreased.
Increased dead space ventilation causes V/Q mismatch, which will increase the $PaCO_2$ − $ETCO_2$ gradient. Increased PEEP and high airway pressures distend normal alveoli and compress alveolar capillaries, increasing dead space ventilation. Pulmonary diseases such as bronchospasm, asthma, and chronic obstructive pulmonary disease may demonstrate elevations in $ETCO_2$ when $PaCO_2$ is dramatically elevated.

3. decreased alveolar ventilation or
4. increased dead space ventilation.

See Table 4.3 for the differential diagnosis of elevated $PaCO_2$ during general anesthesia with mechanical ventilation. Figure 4.2 demonstrates the gradual increase in $ETCO_2$ seen in these cases with the exception of increased dead space ventilation.

The $ETCO_2$ is a reliable intraoperative indicator of hypercarbia in healthy patients, although it may be unreliable in patients with cardiopulmonary disease secondary to V/Q mismatching from increased dead space ventilation.[1,8,28] Likewise, any cause of increased $PaCO_2$ from dead space ventilation will also cause an increased $PaCO_2$ – $ETCO_2$ gradient as a result of a concomitant decrease in $ETCO_2$. As a matter of fact, the $ETCO_2$ may dramatically decrease during pulmonary gas embolism, hypotension, etc. (Figure 4.3), despite significantly elevated $PaCO_2$, making capnometry a valuable diagnostic tool and monitor in laparoscopy. Arterial blood gas analysis, however, still remains the gold standard for evaluation of $PaCO_2$.[8]

In mechanically ventilated healthy patients the elevation of $ETCO_2$ and $PaCO_2$ is easily remedied by increasing alveolar ventilation through increased respiratory rate or secondly tidal volumes.[2] In rare circumstances or in patients with severe cardiopulmonary disease, increased ventilation may be prohibited or ineffective, necessitating conversion to an open procedure.[2] Wittgen and associates reported 10 patients for laparoscopic cholecystectomy with cardiac or pulmonary disease and recorded one case of conversion to an open procedure for severely elevated

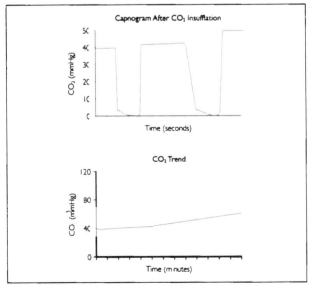

Figure 4.2
Capnogram after CO_2 insufflation. Capnometry demonstrating the slow increase in CO_2 seen with CO_2 absorption and other causes of increased CO_2 production or decreased alveolar ventilation.

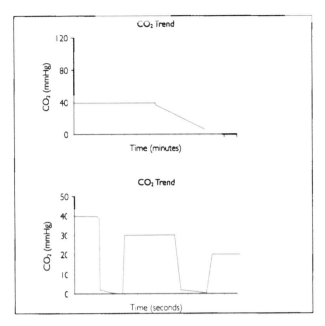

Figure 4.3
Capnogram with increased dead space ventilation. Capnometry demonstrating a decrease in $ETCO_2$ seen in cases of increasing dead space ventilation such as pulmonary embolism or decreased cardiac output. Bronchospasm, asthma, and chronic obstructive diseases demonstrate a characteristic upslope of the expired CO_2 without a plateau or identifiable end tidal point.

$PaCO_2$ and acidosis.[8] Table 4.4 lists the diagnostic and therapeutic maneuvers that should be performed when faced with severely increased $ETCO_2$. Life-threatening complications should be ruled out or treated before a diagnosis of CO_2 absorption is made. A decreasing $ETCO_2$ particularly in the face of unchanged ventilation, hypotension or oxygen desaturation should also prompt thorough diagnostic and therapeutic maneuvers to rule out pulmonary gas embolism or thromboembolism.

Carbon dioxide may be stored in tissues remaining persistently elevated even after desufflation.[2] Patients should therefore be monitored prior to and after extubation to ensure adequate minute ventilation.[2]

CO_2/gas embolism

Carbon dioxide embolism to the heart or pulmonary vessels has been observed in 69% of patients during laparoscopic cholecystectomy.[45] Fahy postulated, as have others, that gas embolism would be higher in laparoscopic nephrectomy because of associated renal vein manipulation.[1,30] Fahy's study, utilizing continuous TEE, documented only one episode of gas embolism, out of 16 cases (6%) which did not result in any hemodynamic instability.[30] The

Table 4.4 *Evaluation and management of elevated $ETCO_2$ during mechanical ventilation*

Evaluation	Therapy
1. Ensure adequate oxygenation	1. Place on 100% FiO_2

2. Auscultate for bilateral breath sounds:
    R/O mechanical malfunction
    capnothorax/endobronchial intubation
    wheezing
	2. Use alternative breathing circuit, decompress chest, reposition ETT, treat bronchospasm

3. Check inspired CO_2 level, > 2 mmHg indicates rebreathing	3. Change CO_2 absorber, inspiratory and expiratory valves, increase fresh gas flow

4. Associated with CO_2 insufflation	4. Increase alveolar ventilation:
	    tidal volumes 10–12 ml/kg or PAWP < 35
	    respiratory rate maximum 18–24
	    avoid PEEP if O_2 adequate
	    insure adequate intravascular volume

5. Check arterial blood gas:
    R/O causes of increased CO_2 production:
    pyrexia, malignant hyperthermia, etc.	

6. Palpate skin to R/O subcutaneous CO_2 emphysema	5. As indicated; cooling, dantrolene
	6. Create 'blow holes' to allow CO_2 escape
7. Other etiologies excluded $PaCO_2$ > 55 mmHg with acidosis	7. Limit intra-abdominal pressure, change patient position
8. Associated with hypotension, hypoxemia or severe elevations in PAWP	8. Convert to an open procedure

FiO_2, fractional inspired concentration of oxygen; R/O, rule out; ETT, endotracheal tube; PAWP, peak airway pressure; PEEP, positive end-expiratory pressure.

This is a suggested algorithm that can be followed to evaluate and treat severe increases in $ETCO_2$. The therapies are not intended to be mutually exclusive. Endobronchial intubation would be an uncommon cause of elevated CO_2 but can be seen in patients with cardiopulmonary diseases.

exact incidence of gas embolism is not known but it remains rare.[45,46] Unfortunately, gas embolism can be catastrophic resulting in severe cardiovascular collapse or death.[1,19,45,46]

During laparoscopy, initial insufflation of pressurized gas is the most common period to observe gas embolism.[2,45] Vascular injury or direct placement of the Veress needle/trocar into a vein or a highly vascularized parenchymal organ such as the liver can cause significant embolism if not detected early.[1,2,46,47] The high solubility of CO_2 means that significantly larger volumes of gas (> 25 ml/kg, 1200 ml, > 1 liter/min) are necessary compared to air (> 3–5 ml/kg, 240 ml), He, etc., to cause clinically significant embolism.[1,2,48] If an embolism does occur, its solubility results in rapid resolution.[1,46] The risk of embolism is decreased by mechanical ventilation with positive pressure, adequate hydration, limiting CO_2 insufflation pressure and volume to less than 30 mmHg and 3 liters.[45,46] Monitoring with precordial Doppler and TEE has been advocated for procedures with significant risk such as posterior fossa craniotomy in the sitting position but is not practical on a routine basis for laparoscopy.

Clinical signs include sudden hypotension, hypoxemia, tachycardia, and arrhythmias.[45,46] End-tidal CO_2 may initially increase, but if the embolism does not resolve quickly, it will fall dramatically (see Figure 4.3) from cardiovascular collapse and decreased pulmonary perfusion. The classical finding of a 'mill wheel murmur' is a late finding that is rarely appreciated in air embolism but has been appreciated in CO_2 embolism.[46] Therapy includes immediate cessation of pressurized gas, discontinuation of N_2O, administration of 100% O_2, Valsalva maneuver to prevent further gas entry into the heart and lungs, elevation of CVP by administration of intravenous (IV) fluids, and hemodynamic/cardiac support as needed. Nitrous oxide has been traditionally thought to not increase the size of CO_2 bubbles because of similar solubilities, but Junghans demonstrated in a recent study that the addition of N_2O did in fact worsen hemodynamics and cardiac function.[49] The optimum patient position to limit and treat gas embolism is currently controversial. Most authors recommend the position described by Durant over 50 years ago – Trendelenburg (head down), left lateral decubitus to trap air in the right ventricle – although recent animal studies do not support this.[50–52] Blood flow rather than buoyancy of the bubble determined the course of air emboli in one animal study.[50] Geissler et al studied venous air embolism with TEE, and found that body position did not benefit hemodynamic performance and that cardiac decompensation was not from air lock of the right ventricular outflow tract but rather the effects of right ventricular ischemia.[52] Trendelenburg position may also exacerbate the resultant cerebral edema, pulmonary mechanics, and hemodynamics seen with cephalad movement of the diaphragm.[46,52] Practically speaking, the supine position facilitates therapeutic intervention, i.e.

central venous access, cardiopulmonary resuscitation (CPR), etc., although further studies are needed to establish the optimum position for resuscitation. Clinically, placement of a central line if not already in situ, with aspiration of air, may take several minutes, and hyperbaric therapy, while controversial, may also not be readily available.[2] If cardiac arrest occurs and embolism does not correct quickly, thoracotomy with direct aspiration, internal cardiac massage, and cardiac bypass may be life saving. Up to 20% of adults have a probe patent foramen ovale which may result in right-to-left embolism and cerebral infarction.[2] Also, it is debatable if, like air, CO_2 initiates the release of inflammatory mediators, resulting in vascular endothelial damage and causing pulmonary edema and acute respiratory distress syndrome.

Emphysema (subcutaneous/preperitoneal)

Subcutaneous CO_2 emphysema may be appreciated by the surgical team or anesthetist as crepitance of the skin on the abdomen, thorax, neck, or face. Alternatively, elevations of the $ETCO_2$ may precipitate evaluation of the hypercarbia (see Table 4.4). While it can occur during removal of the insufflating trocar, it most commonly manifests during Veress needle/trocar insertion.[1,2,51] The Veress needle/trocar may be improperly placed or CO_2 may inadvertently leak around the trocar.[1,51] The surgical team should be well versed in recognition and malfunctions during insufflation.[51] Preperitoneal needle placement can result in penile and scrotum subcutaneous emphysema. Subcutaneous emphysema during laparoscopy may also result from pulmonary barotrauma associated with high tidal volumes or increased airway pressures. Clinically, hypercarbia from the subcutaneous absorption of CO_2 may become problematic, necessitating increased minute ventilation, although more frequently it looks worse than it is. No significant hemodynamic sequelae should result, although if accompanied by hypotension, increased airway pressure, or hypoxemia, pneumothorax should be ruled out. The emphysema rapidly resolves and no therapy is typically needed, although subcutaneous IV catheters can be placed or simple skin incisions, 'blow holes', may be created to allow the CO_2 to escape into the atmosphere. Figure 4.4 shows a chest radiograph of a patient with massive subcutaneous gas.

Pneumothorax/pneumomediastinum/ pneumopericardium

Subcutaneous CO_2 emphysema may occur as an isolated phenomenon or more ominously may be the harbinger of pneumothorax (PTX), pneumomediastium (PMD), or pneumopericardium (PPM). For example, the patient in

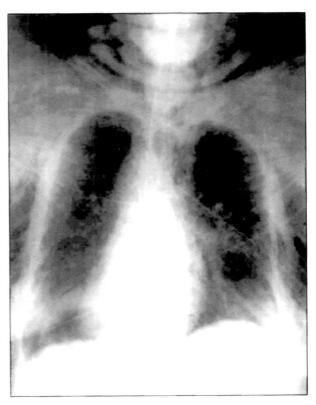

Figure 4.4
Massive subcutaneous emphysema. This patient developed massive subcutaneous emphysema, which was followed by hypotension and hypoxemia. Bilateral chest tubes were placed with gas release and immediate improvement in hemodynamics and oxygenation.

Figure 4.4 presented initially with massive subcutaneous emphysema but developed hypotension and hypoxemia suggestive of PTX, resulting in bilateral chest tube thoracostomy and subsequent hemodynamic improvement. Similarly, PTX, PMD, or PPM may occur without evidence of each other or subcutaneous emphysema. Isolated PMD and PPM do not typically have significant clinical effects and are found incidentally on postoperative chest X-ray or when patients complain of substernal chest pains.[53] Clinical signs include elevated $ETCO_2$, hypotension, hypoxemia, or elevated peak airway pressures (PAWPs), which should prompt the evaluation for potentially catastrophic complications such as a tension PTX. Decreased unilateral or bilateral breath sounds, neck vein distention, and tracheal deviation may not be very sensitive intraoperatively, so high clinical suspicion is needed.

Similar to subcutaneous emphysema, PTX, PMD, and PPM may be the result of pulmonary volume trauma or barotrauma from elevated pulmonary airway pressures. Patients typically have underlying pulmonary disease such as bullous emphysema, bleb disease, pulmonary cyst, or other underlying predisposing condition.

Insufflation of CO_2 can also cause PTX, PMD, and PPM via several mechanisms. Pneumothorax (capnothorax) results from either congenital defects in the diaphragm, diaphragm injury, dissection through fascial retroperitoneal planes, or inadvertent trocar placement into the pleural space.[6,54] Figure 4.5 demonstrates the continuity of the retroperitoneal spaces with the mediastinum, thorax, neck, and chest wall, which is one of the anatomic reasons that explains how CO_2 can dissect through tissue planes to cause PTX, PMD, and PPM. If discovered during posi-

tive pressure ventilation or with associated hemodynamic and respiratory compromise, 100% oxygen, discontinuing N_2O, IV fluid therapy, vasopressor support, hand ventilation, and immediate desufflation should relieve the capnothorax. Many authors note that a capnothorax will resolve within 30 min and no treatment is necessary; however, we believe that if immediate improvement is not seen, needle decompression or chest tube thoracostomy is indicated because pulmonary volume or barotrauma cannot be easily differentiated. Cessation of insufflation

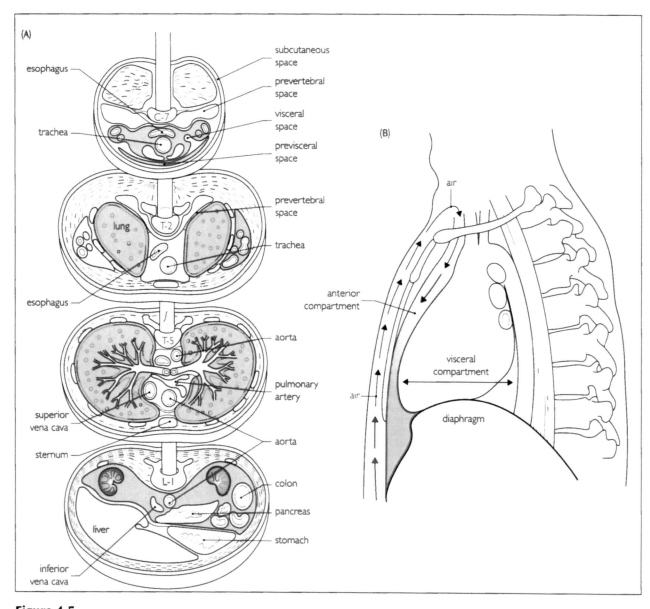

Figure 4.5

Anatomic fascial planes of the peritoneum, retroperitoneum, mediastinum, and thorax. Fascial planes separating these compartments allow gas to spread through them, depending on the quantity and rate of gas they are subject to as well as the individual integrity of the various layers. The visceral space extends from the retroperitoneum through the diaphragm, mediastinum, and neck. Air originating in any of these structures can dissect into any of the others. (Reproduced with permission from Maunder RJ, Pierson DJ, Hudson LD. Subcutaneous and mediastinal emphysema: pathophysiology, diagnosis and management. Arch Intern Med 1984; 144:1447–53.)

and evaluation prior to continuance is mandatory and conversion to an open procedure may be required. Postoperative discovery is not unusual and because the solubility of CO_2 typically results in rapid resolution mild–moderately symptomatic patients with PTX less than 20% can be managed with observation.[54]

Hypotension

Hypotension is defined as a fall in arterial blood pressure of more than 20% below baseline or an absolute value of systolic pressure below 90 mmHg or a mean arterial pressure (MAP) below 60 mmHg.[55] Hemodynamic perturbations are common during laparoscopy; however, the incidence of serious cardiovascular complications is low.[1] Hypotension is most frequently caused by a decrease in venous return during development of pneumoperitoneum.[56] However, a thorough differential diagnosis of hypotension in the anesthetized patient undergoing laparoscopic surgery should be considered (Table 4.5) with

Table 4.5 *Differential diagnosis of hypotension in the patient undergoing laparoscopic surgery*

Rate/rhythm
Bradydysrhythmias – CO_2 insufflation, traction on
    pelvic structures
Tachydysrhythmias – sinus tachycardia and ventricular
    dysrhythmias

↓ *Preload*
Hypovolemia
Caval compression
Vasodilatation
Excessive pneumoperitoneum
Abrupt change in patient position
Tension pneumothorax
Pericardial tamponade

↓ *Contractility*
Hypoxemia
Myocardial ischemia
Drug-induced myocardial depression
RV failure from embolic event
Acute valve dysfunction
Severe acidosis
Abrupt increase in SVR

↓ *Afterload (SVR)*
Drugs
Distributive mechanisms – sepsis, anaphylaxis,
    neurogenic, addisonian crisis, transfusion reaction
Histamine release

↓, decreased; RV, right ventricle; SVR, systemic vascular resistance.

treatment directed by the cause. Most frequently it involves release of the pneumoperitoneum. Vasopressor agents are commonly used to maintain perfusion to the heart and brain, although detrimental in the setting of hypovolemic or hemorrhagic shock. Therefore, vasopressors should be used only to temporize while volume resuscitation is in progress. Atropine is indicated for bradydysrhythmia, which is thought to be the cause of the hypotension.

Hypertension

Hypertension is typically defined as a systolic blood pressure >160 mmHg or diastolic blood pressure >90 mmHg, or both, regardless of age.[57] Severe intraoperative hypertension is rare during laparoscopy.[14] Pneumoperitoneum is the most likely cause and not hypercarbia.[58] Positioning in the head-down position is associated with increased systolic, diastolic, and mean arterial pressure.[59] Several other causes of hypertension such as hypoxemia, and inadequate depth of anesthesia, must always be in the differential diagnosis (Table 4.6). Pre-existing hypertension predisposes to an increased incidence of intraoperative hypertension. Treatment of intraoperative hypertension usually involves deepening the anesthetic but may require the use of sympatholytics. Severe unremitting hypertension may necessitate release of the pneumoperitoneum. Any evidence of ischemia during periods of hemodynamic perturbations should prompt a work-up for significant cardiovascular disease.

Table 4.6 *Differential diagnosis of intraoperative hypertension in the patient undergoing laparoscopic surgery*

Hypoxemia
Hypercarbia
Pneumoperitoneum
Light anesthesia
Pre-existing hypertension
    Primary
    Renovascular
Volume overload
Drugs
Elevated intracranial pressure
Autonomic hyperreflexia
Malignant hyperthermia
Endocrine
    Pheochromocytoma, carcinoid, glomus tumors,
    thyrotoxicosis

Reproduced with permission from Steven G Venticinque.

Elevated peak airway pressures

Functional residual capacity and lung compliance decrease with pneumoperitoneum.[5] Several studies have documented increased PAWPs during pneumoperitoneum.[2,14,16] The PAWPs increase approximately 50% above baseline values.[5] Interestingly, patients with documented cardio-respiratory disease did not appear to have significant elevation in PAWPs beyond patients with normal cardiopulmonary status.[8] Position changes such as head-up or head-down do not appreciably alter PAWPs.[16] Other airway misadventures must be in the differential diagnosis of increased PAWPs (Table 4.7). Patients with significant pulmonary disease may manifest marked elevations of $PaCO_2$ as a result of the ventilator limiting airway pressures, and in some circumstances may make maintaining a pneumoperitoneum difficult. Despite this, patients with significant pulmonary disease should not be summarily dismissed as potential candidates for laparoscopic surgery and they may benefit postoperatively. Fortunately, once the pneumoperitoneum is released, the inspiratory airway pressures return to baseline.

Hypoxemia

With the institution of the pneumoperitoneum, there is a drop in PaO_2. This decrease in the PaO_2 rarely results in hypoxemia in ASA I/II (American Society of Anesthesiology physical classification) patients.[5] There are a few reports that actually demonstrated an increased PaO_2 when local anesthesia was used.[60,61] When hypoxemia does occur, many potential etiologies should be considered (Table 4.8). Baseline decreases in PaO_2 may result in more significant decreases on insufflation. Patients who require home O_2 are at high risk for hypoxemia and may require periodic release of the pneumoperitoneum. Smokers may also be more prone to hypoxemia.[62] PEEP may be useful in increasing MAP, which may improve oxygenation. The immediate treatment of hypoxemia involves increasing the delivered O_2 to the patient. Some authors advocate a fractional inspired concentration of oxygen (FiO_2) of >50% to provide an added margin of safety during insufflation.

Oliguria

Oliguria is defined as urine production at a rate below 0.5 ml/kg/h. Decreased urine output is a common complication of pneumoperitoneum and pneumoretroperitoneum.[63] The mechanism for the decreased urine output cannot simply be explained by decreased venous return

Table 4.7 *Differential diagnosis of intraoperative increased peak airway pressure in the patient undergoing laparoscopic surgery*

Anesthesia circuit factors
Kink
Secretions
One-way valve malfunction

Endotracheal tube factors
Endobronchial intubation
Secretions
Kink or patient biting on endotracheal tube

Patient factors
Pneumoperitoneum
Bronchospasm
Mucous plug
Pneumothorax/hemothorax
Pulmonary edema
ARDS/pneumonia/aspiration
Poor baseline pulmonary compliance
    Restrictive lung disease
    Obesity
    Kyphoscoliosis

ARDS, acute respiratory distress syndrome.

Table 4.8 *Differential diagnosis of hypoxemia in the patient undergoing laparoscopic surgery*

Hypoventilation
Esophageal intubation
Mainstem intubation
Failure to ventilate
Airway obstruction
Pneumoperitoneum

V/Q mismatch
Mainstem intubation
Atelectasis
Pulmonary edema
Bronchospasm
Aspiration
ARDS
Pneumothorax
Embolic phenomena

Shunt
Intrapulmonary
Intracardiac

Diminished SVO₂
Shock
Decreased FRC when compared to CC

ARDS, acute respiratory distress syndrome; CC, closing capacity; FRC, functional residual capacity, SVO₂, mixed venous oxygen saturation; V/Q, ventilation/perfusion.

with subsequent decreased cardiac output. If this were the only factor, expansion of the blood volume should improve urine output. Animal studies have demonstrated that extrarenal pressures as low as 10 mmHg impair renal blood flow and urine production.[39]

Neurohormonal factors probably play a role in the decreased urine output observed clinically. With pneumoperitoneum, plasma renin activity is increased and ADH levels rise.[5] One study found warm CO_2 to be associated with greater urine output.[64]

Anesthetic drugs also decrease renal blood flow, glomerular filtration rate (GFR), and urine output.[65] The decrease in urine output due to anesthetic-related effects can be attenuated by perioperative hydration.[66]

Once the pneumoperitoneum or pneumoretroperitoneum is deflated, an increase in urine output should follow. If prompt improvement of urine output does not occur, a thorough search for other etiologies should be conducted (Table 4.9).

Postoperative

Nausea/emesis

Postoperative nausea and vomiting (PONV) is one of the most frequent complaints following laparoscopic procedures. Risks for PONV include laparoscopic surgery, female gender, history of PONV or motion sickness, postoperative opioid use, and nonsmoker.[67] An increased number of risk factors correlate with increased incidence of PONV.[68] While PONV is considered a minor complaint, it can be quite distressing to the patient and leads to an

increased length of stay in ambulatory surgical center and to decreased patient satisfaction.[66] Gan has provided useful guidelines for prophylactic antiemetic therapy based on multimodal therapy[67] (Figure 4.6). Other factors that may decrease PONV are stomach drainage[69] and possibly the avoidance of nitrous oxide.[3] Nonopioid analgesics may be beneficial in not only reducing the pain after laparoscopic surgery but may also decrease PONV by minimizing postoperative opioids.

Postoperative pain

Postoperative pain from laparoscopy is significantly less than laparotomy, although patients can have significant discomfort following laparoscopic procedures. Shoulder and neck pain is reported by a high percentage of patients following laparoscopic procedures.[69] Pain out of proportion to the procedure should prompt an investigation for possible surgical causes (e.g. hemorrhage, bladder perforation, bowel injury, nerve injury).

A variety of techniques are used to minimize discomfort after laparoscopic procedures, including opioids, nonsteroidal anti-inflammatory drugs (NSAIDs), local anesthetics, regional anesthesia, and combination therapy. Opioids are effective in alleviating postsurgical discomfort. However, these drugs, in larger doses, have side-effects (PONV, sedation, respiratory depression) that make their use less desirable. The most promising technique for reduction of postoperative pain appears to be multimodal therapy, whereby opioids, NSAIDs, and local anesthetics are used.[3] Other analgesics that can be considered include tramadol and acetaminophen.

Pulmonary impairment

Postoperative pulmonary complications (PPCs) are an important area of morbidity and mortality in clinical medicine. PPCs comprise a group of events such as pneumonia, respiratory failure, bronchospasm, atelectasis, and hypoxemia.[70] Risk factors for PPCs include surgery lasting over 3 hours, general anesthesia, upper abdominal surgery or thoracic surgery, and intraoperative use of pancuronium.[71] Potential patient-related risk factors include smoking, ASA class greater than II, age greater than 70 years, obesity, obstructive sleep apnea, and chronic obstructive pulmonary disease (COPD).[71] The risk of PPCs is lower in patients who underwent laparoscopic cholecystectomy than those undergoing open cholecystectomy.[71] There are a multitude of studies showing improved postoperative pulmonary function when comparing laparoscopy to laparotomy.[72] Strategies to improve postoperative pulmonary function have been outlined elsewhere.[70,71]

Table 4.9 *Differential diagnosis of oliguria in the patient undergoing laparoscopic surgery*

Prerenal
Hypovolemia
Decreased cardiac output
Hypotension

Intrinsic
ATN
Increased ADH
Glomerulonephritis

Postrenal
Obstruction
  Bladder catheter
  Ureteral

ADH, antidiuretic hormone.

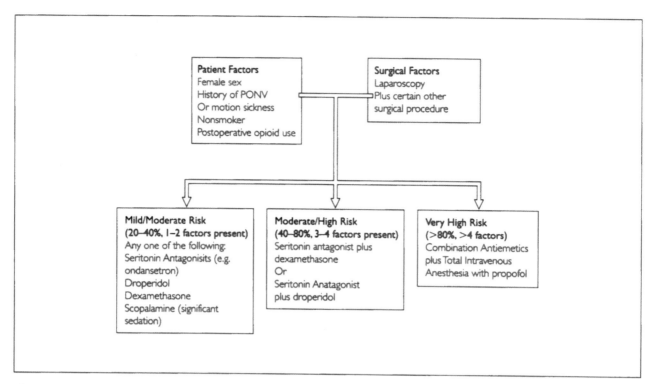

Figure 4.6
Risk factors for PONV and guidelines for prophylactic antiemetic therapy.
Adapted from Gan TJ, Postoperative nausea and vomiting – can It be eliminated? JAMA 2002; 287(10): 1233–6.

Conclusion

Minimally invasive urologic surgery is increasingly common. The postoperative benefits are less pain, shorter hospital stays, and better postoperative pulmonary function. As more procedures are performed laparoscopically, the anesthesiologist and urologist need to have an understanding of the unique physiologic events that occur as a result of laparoscopy. For the healthy patient undergoing laparoscopy, the cardiorespiratory events are usually little more than minor intraoperative issues. However, for the patient with cardiac or pulmonary compromise the physiologic perturbation can be more severe and requires more preoperative planning.

References

1. Joshi GP. Complication of laparoscopy. Anesth Clin N Am 2001; 19:89.

2. Stoller ML, Wolf JS, Jr. Physiologic considerations in laparoscopy. In: Clayman RV, McDougall EM, eds. Laparoscopic urology. St. Louis: Quality Medical Publishing, 1993:17–34.

3. Smith I. Anesthesia for laparoscopy with emphasis on outpatient laparoscopy. Anesth Clin N Am 2001; 19:89.

4. Rose KD, Cohen MM, Soutter DI. Laparoscopic cholecystectomy: the anaesthetist's point of view. Can J Anaesth 1992; 39:809.

5. O'Malley C, Cunningham AJ. Physiologic changes during laparoscopy. Anesth Clin N Am 2001; 19:1.

6. Gill IS, Kavoussi LR, Clayman RV, et al. Complications of laparoscopic nephrectomy in 185 patients: a multi-institutional review. J Urol 1995; 154:479.

7. Kavoussi LR, Sosa E, Chandhoke P, et al. Complications of laparoscopic pelvic lymph node dissection. J Urol 1993; 149:322.

8. Wittgen CM, Andrus CH, Fitzgerald SD, et al. Analysis of the hemodynamic and ventilatory effects of laparoscopic cholecystectomy. Arch Surg 1991; 126:997.

9. Motew M, Ivankovich AD, Bieniarz J, et al. Cardiovascular effects and acid-base and blood gas changes during laparoscopy. Am J Obstet Gynecol 1973; 115:1002.

10. Girardis M, Ugo DB, Guglielmo A, Pasetto A. The effect of laparoscopic cholecystectomy on cardiovascular function and pulmonary gas exchange. Anesth Analg 1996; 83:134.

11. Fernandez-Cruz L, Taura P, Saenz A, et al. Laparoscopic approach to pheochromocytoma: hemodynamic changes and catecholamine secretion. World J Surg 1996; 20:760.

12. Wolf JS Jr, Clayman RV, McDougall EM, et al. Carbon dioxide and helium insufflation during laparoscopic radical nephrectomy in a patient with severe pulmonary disease. J Urol 1996; 155:2021.

13. Price HL. Effects of carbon dioxide on the cardiovascular system. Anesthesiology 1960; 21:652.

14. Hardacre JM, Talamini MA. Pulmonary and hemodynamic changes during laparoscopy – Are they important?. Surgery 2000; 127:241.

15. Ortega AE, Richman MF, Hernandez M, et al. Inferior vena caval blood flow and cardiac hemodynamics during carbon dioxide pneumoperitoneum. Surg Endosc 1996; 10:920.

16. Rauh R, Hemmerling TM, Rist M, Jacobi KE. Influence of pneumoperitoneum and patient positioning on respiratory system compliance. J Clin Anesth 2001; 13:361.

17. Sprung J, Whalley DG, Falcone T, et al. The impact of morbid obesity, pneumoperitoneum, and posture on respiratory system mechanics and oxygenation during laparoscopy. Anesth Analg 2000; 94:1345.

18. Fujise K, Shingu K, Matsumoto S, et al. The effects of the lateral position on cardiopulmonary function during laparoscopic urological surgery. Anesth Analg 1998; 87:925.

19. Nord HJ. Complications of laparoscopy. Endoscopy 1992; 24:693.

20. Moncure M, Salem R, Moncure K, et al. Central nervous system metabolic and physiologic effects of laparoscopy. Am Surg 1999; 65:168.

21. Executive summary of the ACC/AHA task force report: guidelines for perioperative cardiovascular evaluation for noncardiac surgery. Anesth Analg 1996; 82:854.

22. American Society of Anesthesiologists: the ASA Directory of Members 1998. Park Ridge, Illinois: American Society of Anesthesiologists, 1998.

23. Gibby GL, Gravenstein JS, Layon AJ, et al. How often does the preoperative interview change anesthetic management? (abstract) Anesthesiology 1992; 77:A1134.

24. Task Force on Preoperative Fasting. Practice guidelines for preoperative fasting and the use of pharmacologic agents to reduce risk of pulmonary aspiration: application to healthy patients undergoing elective procedures. A report by the American Society of Anesthesiologist Task Force on Preoperative Fasting. Anesthesiology 1999; 90:896.

25. Sprung J, O'Hara JF Jr, Gill IS, et al. Anesthetic aspects of laparoscopic and open adrenalectomy for pheochromocytoma. Urology 2000; 55:339.

26. Joris JL, Hamoir EE, Hartstein GM, et al. Hemodynamic changes and catecholamine release during laparoscopic adrenalectomy for pheochromocytoma. Anesth Analg 1999; 88:16.

27. Tauzin-Fin P, Hilbert G, Krol-Houdek M, et al. Mydriasis and acute pulmonary oedema complicating laparoscopic removal of phaeochromocytoma. Anaesth Intensive Care 1999; 27:646.

28. Dhoste K, Lacoste L, Karayan J, et al. Haemodynamic and ventilatory changes during laparoscopic cholecystectomy in elderly ASA III patients. Can J Anaesth 1996; 43:783.

29. Portera CA, Compton RP, Walters DN, Browder IW. Benefits of pulmonary artery catheter and transesophageal echocardiographic monitoring in laparoscopic cholecystectomy patients with cardiac disease. Am J Surg 1995; 169:202.

30. Fahy BG, Hasnain JU, Flowers JL, et al. Transesophageal echocardiographic detection of gas embolism and cardiac valvular dysfunction during laparoscopic nephrectomy. Anesth Analg 1999; 88:500.

31. Collins LM, Vaghadia H. Regional anesthesia for laparoscopy. Anesth Clin N Am 2001; 19:43.

32. Jones SB, Monk TG. Anesthesia and patient monitoring. In: Jones DB, Wu JS, Soper NJ, eds. Laparoscopic surgery. St Louis, 1997:28–36.

33. Chiu AW, Huang WJ, Chen KK, et al. Laparoscopic ligation of bilateral spermatic varices under epidural anesthesia. Urol Int 1996; 57:80.

34. Chiu HH, Ng KH. Complication of laparoscopy under general anaesthesia. Anaesth Intens Care 1977; 5:169.

35. DeGrood PMRM, Harbers JBM, vanEgmond JF, Crul JP. Anaesthesia for laparoscopy: a comparison of five techniques including propofol, etomidate, thiopentone, and isoflurane. Anaesthesia 1987; 42:815.

36. Eger EI, Saidman LJ. Hazards of nitrous oxide anesthesia in bowel obstruction and pneumothorax. Anesthesiology 1965; 26:61.

37. Jones MJ, Mitchell RW, Hindocha N. Effect of increased intra-abdominal pressure during laparoscopy on the lower esophageal sphincter. Anesth Analg 1989; 68:63.

38. Verghese C, Brimacombe JR. Survey of laryngeal mask airway usage in 11,910 patients: safety and efficacy for conventional and nonconventional usage. Anesth Analg 1996; 82:129.

39. Cheney FW, Domino KB, Caplan RA, et al. Nerve injury associated with anesthesia: a closed claims analysis. Anesthesiology 1990; 90(4):1062–9.

40. Johnson RV Lawson NW, Nealon WH. Lower extremity neuropathy after laparoscopic cholecystectomy. Anesthesiology 1992; 77:835.

41. Jorgensen JO, Gilles RB, Lalak NJ, et al. Lower limb venous hemodynamics during laparoscopy: an animal study. Surg Laparosc Endosc 1994; 4:32.

42. Schwenk W, Bohm B, Junghans T, et al. Intermittent sequential compression of the lower limbs prevents venous stasis in laparoscopic and conventional colorectal surgery. Dis Colon Rectum 1997; 40:1056.

43. Harman PK, Kron IL, McLachlan HD, et al. Elevated intra-abdominal pressure and renal function. Ann Surg 1982; 196:594.

44. Richards WO, Scovill W, Shin B, Reed W. Acute renal failure associated with increased intra-abdominal pressure. Ann Surg 1983; 197:183.

45. Derouin M, Couture P, Boudreault D, et al. Detection of gas embolism by transesophageal echocardiography during laparoscopic cholecystectomy. Anesth Analg 1996; 82:119.

46. Yacoub OF, Cardona I Jr, Coveler LA, Dodson MG. Carbon dioxide embolism during laparoscopy. Anesthesiology 1982; 57:533.

47. dePlater RMH, Jones ISC. Nonfatal carbon dioxide embolism during laparoscopy. Anaesth Intens Care 1989; 17:359.

48. Fishburne JI. Anesthesia for laparoscopy: considerations, complications, techniques. J Reprod Med 1978; 21:37.

49. Junghans T, Bohm B, Meyer E. Influence of nitrous oxide anesthesia on venous gas embolism with carbon dioxide and helium during pneumoperitoneum. Surg Endosc 2000; 14:1167.

50. Butler BD, Laine GA, Leman BC, et al. Effect of the Trendelenburg position on the distribution of arterial gas emboli in dogs. Ann Thorac Surg 1988; 45:198.

51. Capelouto CC, Kavoussi LR Complications of laparoscopic surgery. Urology 1993; 42:2.

52. Geissler HJ, Allen SJ, Mehlhorn U, et al. Effect of body repositioning after venous air embolism. An echocardiographic study. Anesthesiology 1997; 86:710.

53. Knos GB, Sung YF, Toledo A. Pneumopericardium associated with laparoscopy. J Clin Anesth 1991; 3:56.

54. Venkatesh R, Kibel AS, Lee D, et al. Rapid resolution of carbon dioxide pneumothorax (capnothorax) resulting from diaphragmatic injury during laparoscopic nephrectomy. J Urol 2002; 167:1387.

55. Gaba DM, Fish KJ, Howard SK. Crisis management in anesthesiology. New York: Churchill Livingstone, 1994:17.

56. Cunningham AJ. Anesthetic implications of laparoscopic surgery. Yale J Biol Med 1998; 71:551–578.

57. Stoelting RK, Dierdorf SF. Anesthesia and co-existing disease, 3rd edn. New York: Churchill Livingstone, 1993:79.

58. Huang SJ, Lee CY, Yeh FC, Chang CL. Hypercarbia is not the determinant factor of systemic arterial hypertension during carboperitoneum in laparoscopy. Ma Zui Xue Za Zhi 1991; 29:592.

59. Ekman LG, Abrahamsson J, Biber B, et al. Hemodynamic changes during laparoscopy with positive end-expiratory pressure ventilation. Acta Anaesthesiol Scand 1988; 32:447.

60. Brown DR, Fishburne JI, Roberson VO, Hulka JF. Ventilatory and blood gas changes during laparoscopy with local anesthesia. Am J Obstet Gynecol 1976; 124:741.

61. Diamant M, Benumof JL, Saidman LJ, et al. Laparoscopic sterilization with local anesthesia: complications and blood-gas changes. Anesth Analg 1977; 56:335–7.

62. Corall IM, Knights K, Potter D, Strunin L. Arterial oxygen tension during laparoscopy with nitrous oxide in the spontaneously breathing patient. Br J Anaesth 1974; 46:925.

63. Dunn MD, McDougall EM. Renal physiology. Laparoscopic considerations. Urol Clin North Am 2000; 27(4):609.

64. Backlund M, Kellokumpu I, Scheinin T, et al. Effect of temperature of insufflated CO_2 during and after prolonged laparoscopic surgery. Surg Endosc 1998; 12:1126.

65. Stoelting RK, Dierdorf SF. Anesthesia and co-existing disease, 3rd edn. New York: Churchill Livingstone, 1993:293.

65. Barry KG, Mazze RI, Schwartz FD. Prevention of surgical oliguria and renal hemodynamic suppression by sustained hydration. N Engl J Med 1964; 270:1371.

66. Green G, Jonsson L. Nausea: the most important factor determining length of stay after ambulatory anaesthesia. A comparative study of isoflurane and/or propofol techniques. Acta Anaesthesiol Scand 1993; 37:742.

67. Gan TJ. Postoperative nausea and vomiting – can it be eliminated? JAMA 2002; 287(10):1233.

68. Apfel CC, Laara E, Koivuranta M, et al. A simplified risk score for predicting post-operative nausea and vomiting: conclusions from cross-validation between two centers. Anesthesiology 1999; 91:693.

69. Collins KM, Docherty PW, Plantevin OM. Postoperative morbidity following gynaecological outpatient laparoscopy. A reappraisal of the service. Anaesthesia 1984; 39:819.

70. Warner DO. Preventing postoperative pulmonary complications. Anesthesiology 2000; 92:1467.

71. Smetana GW. Preoperative pulmonary evaluation. N Engl J Med 1999; 340:937.

72. Joris JL. Anesthesia for laparoscopic surgery. In: Miller RD, ed. Anesthesia. Philadelphia: Churchill Livinstone, 2000:2012.

5

The physiology of laparoscopic genitourinary surgery

J Stuart Wolf Jr

Laparoscopy may be minimally invasive, but in some ways it is more physiologically stressful on the patient than open surgery. During laparoscopy with gas insufflation, the patient is exposed to physiologic derangements that may be unfamiliar to the operating surgeon. Fortunately, there is now available considerable clinical and experimental research directed towards the physiology and pathophysiology of gas insufflation, and the knowledgeable practitioner can successfully manage most of the physiologic effects of laparoscopy. Prior to the development of operative laparoscopy, diagnostic laparoscopy carried a low 0.6 – 2.4% complication rate, and only a third of these could be attributed to physiologic problems.[1] In one large survey of operative laparoscopy (laparoscopic cholecystectomy), one-half of the mortality was due to non-technical ('physiologic') causes.[2] The main purpose of studying this topic is to avoid these physiologic complications.

Most of the work on this topic has concerned intraperitoneal insufflation of gas to produce pneumoperitoneum. Many of the phenomena that have been described likely pertain to gas insufflation into the preperitoneal and retroperitoneal spaces as well; where important differences exist, this will be pointed out, but otherwise the term 'pneumoperitoneum' is used to refer to any gas insufflation for pelvic, abdominal, or retroperitoneal laparoscopy

Hemodynamic considerations

Laparoscopy affects hemodynamics in both stimulatory and inhibitory manners. The mechanical effect of the pneumoperitoneum and the absorption of the carbon dioxide (CO_2) are the primary determinants of hemodynamic changes associated with laparoscopy. Volume shifts due to positioning of the patient for laparoscopy play a role in some situations. These divisions are useful clinically because each component can be varied independently,

allowing the surgeon to alter the patient's hemodynamic response during laparoscopy.

Physiology

Effects of increased intra-abdominal pressure

Insufflation of gas elevates the intra-abdominal pressure, which subsequently increases the systemic vascular resistance. This is a direct compressive phenomenon, primarily affecting the sphlanchnic circulation (Figure 5.1),[3] in both capillaries and capacitance vessels, and in both the venous and arterial systems.[4-9] Blood flow to all abdominal and retroperitoneal viscera except the adrenal gland is diminished at 20 mmHg of intra-abdominal pressure in animal models.[3,10,11]

The volume status of the subject determines the magnitude of the effect of intra-abdominal pressure on systemic vascular resistance. Using an intra-abdominal pressure of 20 mmHg in dogs, Kashtan and associates[7] found that cardiac output fell slightly in the presence of normovolemia, decreased significantly with experimental simulation of hypovolemia, and actually increased with experimental simulation of hypervolemia. Others have confirmed the adverse effects of hypovolemia[12] and the beneficial effect of volume loading[13] in the presence of increased intra-abdominal pressure.

Cardiac output is limited by venous return. At low levels of intra-abdominal pressure (less than 10 mmHg), there is augmentation of venous return (and therefore cardiac output), due to 'autotransfusion' from partially emptied abdominal capacitance vessels.[14,15] As intra-abdominal pressures rise above 20 mmHg, venous return and cardiac output tend to decrease (Figure 5.2).[4-6,16]

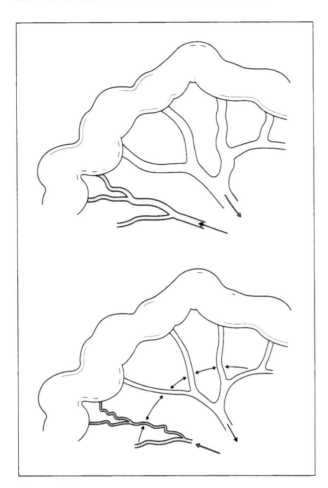

Figure 5.1
Sphlanchnic circulation can be markedly restricted.
(Reproduced with permission from Wolf and Stoller ML.[1])

Mean arterial pressure is the product of cardiac output and arterial resistance. At intra-abdominal pressure ≤ 20 mmHg, there is elevation of mean arterial pressure.[5,8,9,14–18] With intra-abdominal pressure > 40 mmHg, arterial pressure falls as cardiac output decreases more than arterial resistance rises.[6,19] Venous pressure is determined, similarly, by the volume of blood collected from the capillaries and the venous resistance. As noted earlier, the venous resistance rises with insufflation.[4,14] It is, however, more difficult to measure and interpret venous pressures during laparoscopy compared with traditional open urologic surgery. The central venous pressure measured by a catheter within the right atrium is the sum of intracardiac (transmural) and intrathoracic (pleural) pressures. The former reflects venous return and is the effective cardiac filling pressure. Intrathoracic pressure, which impedes venous return, rises during laparoscopy.[5,7] It is the increase in this component that is the primary reason the measured central venous pressure rises during laparoscopy. Consequently, the measured central venous pressure is not necessarily a good indicator of cardiac filling unless intrathoracic pressure is taken into account.

The complex effects of increased intra-abdominal pressure on hemodynamics are best summarized by considering again the role of volume status. In general, a small increase in intra-abdominal pressure will increase venous pressure more than it increases resistance, thereby augmenting venous return and cardiac output. As intra-abdominal pressure rises above a certain point, the increase in resistance exceeds the increase in pressure and venous return falls. This transition point occurs at a low intra-abdominal pressure in the hypovolemic state because

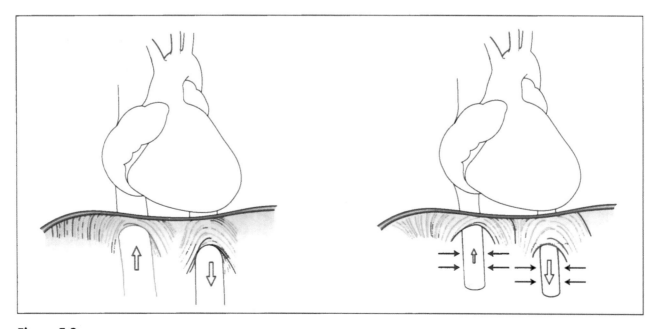

Figure 5.2
Reduction of venous return and cardiac output during laparoscopy. (Reproduced with permission from Wolf and Stoller.[1])

vessels collapse easily. In the hypervolemic state, the transition point occurs at a higher intra-abdominal pressure because the full vessels do not collapse as readily; there is less increase in resistance and the pressure increase remains proportional to the elevation of intra-abdominal pressure. In other words, the balance between resistance and pressure changes that determines venous return – and therefore cardiac output – is dependent upon circulating blood volume. Given the avoidance of hypovolemia, maintaining an intra-abdominal pressure less than 20 mmHg should prevent significant hemodynamic alterations in most patients.

Effects of CO_2

The insufflated gas is another determinant of the hemodynamic effects of laparoscopy. The absorption of CO_2, the most commonly used gas, has contradictory effects at different sites. The direct effects of CO_2 are cardioinhibitory, reducing heart rate, cardiac contractility, and vascular resistance.[20] Stimulation of the sympathetic nervous system by CO_2 counteracts these effects, as sympathetic efferents and circulating catecholamines elevate heart rate, cardiac contractility, and vascular resistance. If acidosis develops, parasympathetic stimulation occurs as well.[20] Overall, moderate hypercapnia elevates cardiac output and blood pressure and decreases systemic vascular resistance. The decrease in systemic vascular resistance counteracts the increase created by the mechanical effects of pneumoperitoneum. Insufflation of gases that lack the chemical activity of carbon dioxide results in a lower cardiac output for a given intra-abdominal pressure.[17,18,21–23]

Effects of positioning

Since laparoscopic retraction can be awkward during laparoscopy, positioning of the patient to use gravity as a retractor is critical. The head-down tilt (Trendelenburg) position during pelvic laparoscopy tends to modestly increase cardiac output.[8,9,24,25] Conversely, the head-up tilt (reverse Trendelenburg) position for upper abdominal laparoscopy is associated with a decrease in cardiac output.[26] The lateral position has minimal effect on hemodynamics unless extreme lateral flexion is applied, which can obstruct the vena cava by impinging on it.[27]

Integrated cardiovascular response

Table 5.1 delineates the hemodynamic effects of an intra-abdominal pressure of 15 mmHg and moderate hypercapnia. The response of any individual patient may differ, however. Measured central venous pressure, systemic vascular resistance, heart rate, and mean arterial pressure all increase when CO_2 is insufflated at 15 mmHg pressure, and the effect on cardiac output in this situation in healthy patients ranges from a decrease of 17–19%,[8,16] to no net change,[4,9] to an increase of 7%.[17] Intra-abdominal pressure less than 5–10 mmHg may increase cardiac output in normovolemic patients by 4–15%,[14,15] while intra-abdominal pressure above 40 mmHg risks marked reduction of cardiac output.[4]

Retroperitoneal insufflation

Although not as extensively studied as intraperitoneal insufflation, findings suggest that the impact of retroperitoneal insufflation on hemodynamics is less. In two different experimental studies in pigs, extraperitoneal insufflation tended to alter venous pressures and cardiac output in the same direction but with less magnitude compared to intraperitoneal insufflation.[28,29] Giebler and associates did not find any change in cardiac output up to retroperitoneal insufflation pressures of 20 mmHg,[30] and subsequently confirmed the distinction between

Table 5.1 *Hemodynamic response to laparoscopy*

	Intra-abdominal pressure of 15 mmHg	Moderate hypercapnia (PaCO$_2$ of 45 mmHg)	Combined
Central venous pressure	Increase	Increase	Increase
Systemic vascular resistance	Increase	Decrease	Increase
Heart rate	Increase	Increase	Increase
Mean arterial pressure	Increase	Increase	Increase
Cardiac output	Decrease	Increase	Variable

PaCO$_2$ = arterial partial pressure of carbon dioxide.

intraperitoneal insufflation (decreased venous return) and retroperitoneal insufflation (slightly augmented venous return) with a clinical study using the same testing methodology in both groups.[31] The smaller volume of gas in the latter group may account for some of the difference.

Physiologic complications

Tension pneumoperitoneum

When intra-abdominal pressure is excessive (> 40 mmHg), the increased vascular resistance becomes overwhelming and tension pneumoperitoneum can occur. Venous return, cardiac output, and blood pressure drop precipitously,[32] which can be fatal.[33] The effect of elevated intra-abdominal pressure is potentiated by hypovolemia,[6,7] so volume status must be optimized before laparoscopy. Parra and associates[34] reported a case of tension pneumoperitoneum during urologic laparoscopy when a malfunctioning insufflator allowed the intra-abdominal pressure to exceed 32 mmHg, resulting in hypotension and bradycardia. Although the procedure was completed following release of the excess pressure and administration of atropine, the patient suffered a cerebrovascular accident that was thought to be due to the intraoperative event. Whenever hemodynamic compromise due to excessive intra-abdominal pressure is suspected, immediate desufflation will quickly improve the situation and the surgeon may be able to complete the procedure at a lower intra-abdominal pressure.[32]

Although brief periods of intra-abdominal pressure above 20 mmHg during laparoscopy are well tolerated by most patients, in general the pressure should be kept below 15–20 mmHg. Even these typically acceptable pressures are no guarantee against problems, as hemodynamic deterioration has been reported at insufflation pressures ≤ 20 mmHg.[35] Moreover, patients with cardiac disease, either ischemic heart disease or with congestive heart failure, are at greater risk for intraoperative cardiac dysfunction and should be monitored even more closely.[36,37] Laparoscopy can be performed safely in patients with cardiac ejection fractions less than 15% with careful preparation.[38]

Cardiac dysrhythmias

Cardiac dysrhythmias have been noted during laparoscopy with a frequency of 17–50%.[39,40] Tachycardia and ventricular extrasystoles due to CO_2 are usually benign, but fatal dysrhythmias can occur with very high arterial partial pressure of CO_2 ($PaCO_2$).[20] Since hypercapnia may also potentiate parasympathetic actions,[20] vagal stimulation

by peritoneal manipulation or distention during CO_2 laparoscopy can occasionally produce bradydysrhythmias; asystolic arrest during CO_2 laparoscopy has been reported.[41,42] Avoidance of hypercapnia will prevent tachydysrhythmias. As vagal reactions may be more profound during laparoscopy under local anesthesia, some recommend premedication with atropine in this setting.[43]

Fluid overload

The need for intravenous fluid administration is much less during laparoscopy than during open surgery. Not only is the insensible loss of fluid less because there is no body cavity open to air but also urine production is decreased.[44] In one study, urine output during laparoscopy was only 0.03 ml/kg/h, compared to 1.70 ml/kg/h immediately postoperatively, despite an average intravenous intraoperative fluid administration of 13.0 ml/kg/h.[45] An intra-abdominal pressure < 10 mmHg caused only mild oliguria, while pressure > 10 mmHg produced a 50–100% decrease in urine output in a rodent model.[46] Increased renal vein resistance (with subsequent decreased renal blood flow) and renal parenchymal compression are potential mechanisms.[44,46–50] Pigs exposed to pneumoperitoneum > 10 mmHg pressure experienced a 65% fall in urine output, compared to a 29% increase with intra-abdominal pressure ≤ 10 mmHg.[51] This combination of decreased insensible losses and decreased urine output predisposes to volume overloading during laparoscopy. In Clayman's nephrectomy series, 2 of the first 10 patients developed transient congestive heart failure, possibly due to administration of excessive intravenous fluid and blood products at a time when the decreased urine output during laparoscopy was not yet appreciated.[52] In an effort to prevent this volume overload, however, patients must not be allowed to become hypovolemic, as this will exacerbate the adverse hemodynamic effect of pneumoperitoneum. The volume status of the patient should be optimized prior to insufflation, and then intraoperative fluid administration should be limited to appropriate replacement for blood loss plus a maintenance rate of 5 ml/kg/h.

Renal failure

Corresponding to the decreased urine output during laparoscopy, there is a reduction in creatinine clearance. During laparoscopic cholecystectomy the creatinine clearance fell in 29 of 48 patients in one study, with the decrease being > 50% in 8 patients.[53] In a porcine study,[51] the creatinine clearance decreased 18% with intra-abdominal pressures ≤ 10 mmHg and 53% with pressures

> 10 mmHg. Encouragingly, all renal indices returned almost to baseline within 2 hours of the release of pneumoperitoneum. Moreover, the temporary renal insult does not potentiate the toxicity of nephrotoxic agents such as aminoglycosides[54] and even experiments in a chronic renal insufficiency model failed to reveal anything but a transient effect of pneumoperitoneum.[55] If postoperative renal failure occurs in a laparoscopy patient, then other etiologies should be evaluated before ascribing the event to the pneumoperitoneum. Nonetheless, there has been a single case report of acute renal failure lasting for 2 weeks following laparoscopy in a 67-year-old man with chronic renal insufficiency, renal tubular acidosis, and hypertension.[56]

Hypertension

Hypertension may accompany hypervolemia during laparoscopy. In addition, hypertension during laparoscopy may be due to hypoxemia, hypercapnia, inadequate anesthesia, or moderately increased intra-abdominal pressure. If hypertension is noted during laparoscopy, the cuff reading should be verified, the intra-abdominal pressure checked, and the adequacy of anesthesia ascertained. If there is doubt as to the accuracy of pulse oximetry and capnography in estimating the arterial partial pressure of oxygen (PaO_2) and $PaCO_2$, arterial blood gases should be obtained to evaluate for hypoxemia and hypercapnia.

Elevated intracranial pressure and cerebral ischemia

In a small animal series, the intracranial pressure rose 5 mmHg in pigs exposed to intra-abdominal pressure of 15 mmHg with CO_2 pneumoperitoneum.[57] In 2 myelomeningocele patients with Arnold–Chiari malformations managed with ventriculoperitoneal shunts, the intracerebral pressure increased more than 15 mmHg above baseline during CO_2 pneumoperitoneum at ≤ 10 mmHg intra-abdominal pressure.[58] In another study of 18 patients with ventriculoperitoneal shunts undergoing 19 laparoscopic procedures, there was no trend toward the combined bradycardia and hypertension that would be expected if this intracerebral pressure increase were clinically significant.[59] Cerebral vascular engorgement secondary to restricted venous outflow is the probable mechanism for the increase in intracranial pressure associated with laparoscopy, although in patients with ventricu-

loperitoneal shunts distal obstruction of the catheter may play a role as well. Patients with head trauma or cerebral mass lesions may suffer from an increase in intra-abdominal pressure during laparoscopy. As the cerebral circulation responds to the increased intracranial volume and pressure with a decrease in blood flow, patients with significant cerebral vascular disease may suffer ischemia.[60]

Venous thrombosis

The increased abdominal pressure during laparoscopy restricts lower extremity venous return. Mechanical pressure forces blood out of the sphlanchnic circulation into the lower extremities.[61] Femoral vein pressures generally parallel intra-abdominal pressures. Lower extremity venous stasis during transperitoneal laparoscopy can be demonstrated with Doppler flow studies.[62,63] One group evaluated femoral vein flow during intraperitoneal and preperitoneal gas insufflation in the same patients, and found flow to decrease with the former but not the latter.[64] Deep vein thromboses and pulmonary emboli have been reported following laparoscopy.[65–67] It is not known if laparoscopy poses a greater or lesser risk for venous thrombosis than open surgery, although in one study of 61 low-risk laparoscopic patients there were no cases of deep venous thrombosis detected with lower limb venous duplex scans.[63] Prophylaxis against deep venous thrombosis with sequential compression devices makes intuitive sense and has been shown to be effective in reversing the pneumoperitoneum-induced reduction of femoral vein flow during laparoscopy,[68] but the optimal method of prophylaxis in laparoscopy has not been determined.

Pulmonary, acid–base, and insufflant-related considerations

Investigations of the pulmonary effects of pneumoperitoneum were first directed toward the use of pneumoperitoneum to treat pulmonary tuberculosis and emphysema.[69] These studies focused on the mechanical aspects of pneumoperitoneum. Subsequently, workers have considered the role of gas absorption from pneumoperitoneum. CO_2, the most commonly used insufflant, is rapidly absorbed during laparoscopy and consideration of the effects of absorbed CO_2 is important in understanding the physiology of laparoscopy.

Physiology

Mechanical effect of pneumoperitoneum

Pneumoperitoneum adversely affects pulmonary function. The increased intra-abdominal pressure and volume elevate the diaphragm,[70] reducing both lung capacity and compliance.[15,71] There is worsening of the ventilation/perfusion mismatch.[70]

Gas absorption

When the peritoneal cavity is filled with gas by insufflation, the total sum of gas movement is directed outwards into the surrounding tissue because the intra-abdominal pressure is above atmospheric pressure.[72] Individual gases move in a direction determined by their partial pressure gradients. The rate of their movement is determined by:

- tissue permeance of the gas
- absorptive capacity of the surrounding tissue
- temperature
- the area of tissue exposed.

The peritoneal cavity is lined by well-vascularized mesothelium with high absorptive capacity. Gases with high tissue permeance are absorbed readily. CO_2 has the highest tissue permeance of the gases used for insufflation during laparoscopy (Table 5.2).[73] Insufflated CO_2 rapidly diffuses into the bloodstream. The baseline production of CO_2 in adults is 150–200 ml/min.[74] The amount of CO_2 absorbed from the peritoneal cavity during intraperitoneal CO_2 laparoscopy has been estimated to range from 14 to 48 ml/min.[67] Increasing minute ventilation can usually eliminate this excess CO_2. When the insufflated gas gains access into the extraperitoneal space or subcutaneous tissues, the surface area exposed for gas absorption increases and a greater amount of CO_2 is absorbed.[67,75,76]

CO_2 metabolism and absorption

When CO_2 is absorbed or produced by tissue metabolism, it is primarily hydrated to carbonic acid, a reaction catalyzed by carbonic anhydrase. Carbonic acid rapidly ionizes to bicarbonate, which represents 90% of the CO_2 in the bloodstream, and hydrogen ions.[74] The hydrogen ions reduce hemoglobin. In the alveolar capillaries the hemoglobin is re-oxidized and the hydrogen ions are released to produce carbonic acid, subsequently forming CO_2 and water for expiration. If CO_2 elimination cannot keep pace with the sum of metabolic production and absorption of CO_2, hypercapnia and respiratory acidosis develop. The absolute rise of $PaCO_2$, which represents the 'rapid' compartment of CO_2 storage, is tempered by storage of CO_2 in the 'medium' (primarily skeletal muscle) and 'slow' (fat) compartments. These storage sites can hold up to 120 liters of CO_2.[74] Therefore, all of the absorbed CO_2 is not immediately available for elimination. The situation exists where hypercapnia can develop or persist after the conclusion of an extended laparoscopic procedure.[77]

Physiologic complications

Hypercapnia

Hypercapnia (excess of CO_2 in the blood) occurs when production and absorption of CO_2 exceed its elimination. While moderate hypercapnia is stimulatory to the cardiovascular system overall, if the level of $PaCO_2$ exceeds 60 mmHg the direct cardiodepressive effects predominate. Cardiovascular collapse, severe acidosis, and fatal

Table 5.2 *Insufflant characteristics*

	Solubility[a]	Diffusibility[a]	Tissue Permeance[a]
Nitrogen	1.0	1.0	1.0
Helium	0.7	2.7	1.3
Oxygen	1.9	0.9	1.8
Argon	2.2	0.9	2.0
Nitrous oxide	33.0	0.9	28.0
Carbon dioxide	47.0	0.9	39.0

Reproduced with permission from Stoller and Wolf.[73]
[a]Value relative to nitrogen.

dysrhythmias can occur. The respiratory acidosis associated with hypercapnia is responsible for most effects of hypercapnia, but CO_2 has direct effects as well. Hypercapnia is related directly to the insufflated CO_2, and not to any change in tissue metabolism or pulmonary function. In 3 studies comparing N_2O insufflation to CO_2 insufflation in patients under general anesthesia with controlled respiration at a fixed minute ventilation, the average increase in $PaCO_2$ was 0.5 mmHg in the N_2O group and 10.7 mmHg in the CO_2 group.[21,78,79] Animal studies have also confirmed that hypercapnia during laparoscopy is due to absorption of CO_2 rather than mechanical effects on pulmonary function.[80] The clinical practice during laparoscopy of increasing ventilation rates and tidal volumes in order to increase CO_2 elimination is usually but not always effective. Wittgen and associates[81] converted 2 of 30 laparoscopic cholecystectomies to open surgery because of hypercapnia, and conversion to open surgery because of hypercapnia during laparoscopic pelvic lymphadenectomy has been reported.[65,73] Others have described severe cardiovascular depression or cardiac arrest due to hypercapnia during CO_2 pneumoperitoneum.[41,42,82]

Clinical studies have suggested that subcutaneous emphysema,[67,76,83] elevated intra-abdominal pressure,[4] extraperitoneal insufflation,[67,75,76] and increased duration of insufflation[22,70,79,84] all increase the rate of CO_2 absorption. Other studies have not found extraperitoneal insufflation to be a risk factor.[28,29,85]

Reduction of intra-abdominal pressure is the first maneuver that should be performed when hypercapnia is detected. It allows more effective CO_2 elimination by reducing the mechanical interference with ventilation by pneumoperitoneum, and it decreases CO_2 absorption. Intra-abdominal pressure should be limited to 20 mmHg. In addition, adjustment of ventilation to keep the partial pressure of end-tidal CO_2 (P(et)CO_2) between 30 and 40 mmHg is recommended. Finally, alternative gases may be employed for insufflation.

Introduced in 1924 by Zollikofer of Switzerland, CO_2 is the most popular gas for insufflation. The advantages of CO_2 are its rapid absorption and its inability to support combustion. The rapid absorption of CO_2 is beneficial if hypercapnia can be maintained at a low level ($PaCO_2 \leq 45$ mmHg), because its cardiovascular stimulation offsets some of the hemodynamic burden of pneumoperitoneum.[17,18,21–23] At excessive levels, however, hypercapnia can produce dysrhythmias and cardiodepressive acidosis. For this reason, workers have searched for alternative gases for insufflation. Following the first formal reports of the physiologic hazards of CO_2 pneumoperitoneum,[86] Alexander and Brown described the use of N_2O for insufflation.[78] N_2O is similar to CO_2 in that it is rapidly absorbed (see Table 5.2), but it has few physiologic effects at the blood concentration achieved with intraperitoneal

insufflation and it is less irritating to the peritoneal membrane.[87,88] Unlike CO_2, it can support combustion in the abdominal cavity (see Intra-abdominal explosion section below). N_2O is a suitable alternative for intra-abdominal insufflation if electrocautery or laser techniques are not being used.

Other alternative gases include helium (He) and argon (Ar).[23,80] Experiments with He have revealed no cardiopulmonary problems.[80,89] Successful clinical series of laparoscopic cholecystectomy have been performed,[22] and in one case report a laparoscopic nephrectomy associated with extreme hypercapnia was continued safely after switching the insufflatory gas to He.[90] Helium and argon have less chemical activity than CO_2 and are absorbed slowly (Table 5.2). Hypercapnia is obviated by the use of He or Ar for insufflation, but the clinical effects of a venous gas embolism may be exacerbated (see Venous gas embolism section below). A practice of switching to He or Ar after initial insufflation with CO_2 might be a safe and effective way of preventing hypercapnia.[84,90]

Capnography is used to monitor the P(et)CO_2 during operation. The P(et)CO_2, being about 3–5 mmHg lower than the $PaCO_2$ during general anesthesia, should be maintained between 30 and 40 mmHg. The difference between $PaCO_2$ and P(et)CO_2, the P(a−et)CO_2 gradient, is not significantly worsened during short laparoscopic procedures in healthy patients.[71,77,91] Normal pulmonary function is adequate to eliminate the small amount of absorbed CO_2 and any increase in $PaCO_2$ is minimal. As $PaCO_2$ rises in patients with pulmonary disease, however, P(a−et)CO_2 increases in an unpredictable manner.[81,92] To monitor accurately the CO_2 elimination in patients with pulmonary disease, arterial blood gases may be necessary.

Acidosis

Laparoscopy with CO_2 insufflation causes a mild respiratory acidosis due to the absorption of CO_2.[6,93] Various investigators have reported coexisting minimal metabolic alkalosis[91] and mild metabolic acidosis.[77,79] Experimentally, the trend towards metabolic acidosis is noted at gas insufflation pressures ≥ 20 mmHg.[51] Since the metabolic acidosis is not associated with an increased anion gap, the cause is not likely to be lactate acidosis from splanchnic hypoperfusion, and may instead be related to retained acids due to the decreased urine output at high intra-abdominal pressures.[51]

Extraperitoneal gas collections

Gases insufflated into the peritoneal cavity may leak into several extraperitoneal tissue planes or spaces.

Subcutaneous emphysema is the most common site of extraperitoneal gas. Its presence is often attributed to technical causes such as incorrect insufflation needle placement, excessive intra-abdominal pressure, a malfunctioning insufflator, or leakage around a laparoscopic port, but in practice it is sometimes inevitable. Since subcutaneous gas is a risk factor for hypercapnia, its presence should prompt an assessment for hypercapnia and its effects. Gas that is insufflated inadvertently into the preperitoneal space or omentum will interfere with visualization during intraperitoneal laparoscopy and might also increase the risk of hypercapnia. Preperitoneal insufflation is a not an uncommon reason for aborting a laparoscopic procedure.[34]

A deliberate extraperitoneal approach is now being advocated for many laparoscopic procedures. Aside from the surgical implications of this approach, there are some physiologic ones. First, extraperitoneal insufflation may be associated with increased gas absorption,[67,75,76] although not all have found this to be the case.[28,29,85] Secondly, extraperitoneal gas can more easily gain access into the subcutaneous space or thoracic cavity. In one study, subcutaneous emphysema was noted in 91% of patients undergoing laparoscopy with extraperitoneal insufflation and in 53% of patients in whom the insufflation was intraperitoneal. Pneumomediastinum or pneumothorax was noted in 36% of patients undergoing extraperitoneal laparoscopy and in 6% of patients after transperitoneal laparoscopy.[67,76]

Pneumomediastinum and pneumothorax can inhibit cardiac filling and limit lung excursion, and can be fatal.[94] Insufflated gas may get into the thorax through many pathways: persistent fetal connections (pleuroperitoneal, pleuropericardial, and pericardioperitoneal), around great vessels in an extrafascial plane, in between fibers of the diaphragm (extraperitoneal or extrapleural), or dissection of subcutaneous gas from the anterior neck directly into the superior mediastinum (Figure 5.3).[1] Pneumothorax may also occur secondary to barotrauma when the peak airway pressure rises with pneumoperitoneum.[71] Pneumomediastinum is more common than pneumothorax, and when the latter occurs it is almost always accompanied by pneumomediastinum and subcutaneous emphysema.[1,67,76] If CO_2 or N_2O has been insufflated, the pneumothorax will usually resolve,[95] but thoracostomy should be performed for a large or symptomatic pneumothorax. Pneumopericardium is occasionally noted after laparoscopy.[96] Subcutaneous gas has been present in all reported cases of pneumopericardium, and in 3 of 4 cases there has been radiographic evidence of pneumomediastinum. The mechanism is most likely entry of mediastinal gas into the pericardial space alongside blood vessels, although persistent embryologic pleuropericardial and pericardioperitoneal connections would also allow gas into the pericardium.

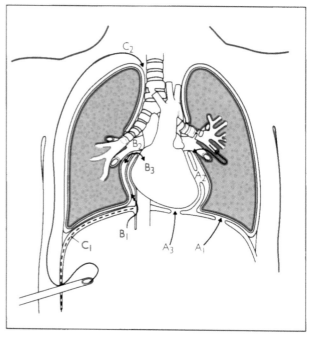

Figure 5.3
Possible routes of gas into mediastinum, pericardial sac, or pleural cavity during laparoscopy include the following: persistent fetal connection at the site of pleuroperitoneal membrane (A1, forme fruste of diaphragmatic hernia), pleuropericardial membrane (A2), and pericardioperitoneal canal (A3); rupture of gas through intact membrane at a weak point such as diaphragmatic hiatus (B1), at pulmonary hilum (B2), and pericardial sac alongside blood vessels (B3); gas outside membrane-bound cavities such as pro- or retroperitoneal gas in between fibers of the diaphragm or alongside great vessels (C1) or subcutaneous gas from the anterior neck (C2); gas from the rupture of an airspace (barotrauma) enters the mediastinum or pleural cavity by dissecting along the pulmonary vasculature (D). (Reproduced with permission from Wolf and Stoller.[1])

Venous gas embolism

A venous gas embolism (VGE) is a gas bubble in the venous system that can pass into the heart and pulmonary circulation. The outflow tract of the right side of the heart can be blocked, producing hypoxemia, hypercapnia, and depressed cardiac output. If the right-heart pressure exceeds that on the left side, a probe patent foramen ovale (present in 20–25% of the population) may open and allow embolization of gas into the arterial system.[5,97,98] The incidence of VGE has been estimated to be between 0.002 and 0.08%,[1] although clinically detectable VGE may occur in as many as 0.59% of laparoscopic cases when careful surveillance is used.[99] Many VGE during laparoscopy have been fatal.[97,98,100] VGE rarely occurs more than a few minutes after initial gas insufflation, but delayed cases have been reported.[97] VGE has been produced experimentally in a bleeding vena cava model, with the riskiest situations appearing to be occlusion of the vena cava distal to the venotomy or following significant blood loss.[101] Clinically, VGE should be suspected when there is hypoxemia, evidence of pulmonary edema, increased airway pressure, hypotension, jugular venous distention, facial plethora, or dysrhythmias. The most useful finding is a sudden fall in $P(et)CO_2$ on capnometry (if the CO_2 embolus is large) and an abrupt but transient increase if it is small.[100,102] The auscultation of a mill-wheel murmur and the appearance of a widened QRS complex with right-heart strain patterns on electrocardiography are less sensitive indicators. When these indicators are noted during initial insufflation, VGE should be suspected. Swift response is required, and includes immediate desufflation, rapid ventilation with 100% oxygen, steep head-down tilt with the right side up, and general resuscitative maneuvers.

The type of the gas comprising the embolus is important. Air (~80% nitrogen) is absorbed very slowly in blood. As Table 5.2 indicates, CO_2 is 47 times more soluble than nitrogen. Graff and associates[103] found the LD_{50} (lethal dose in 50% of subjects) of CO_2 to be 5 times that of air when injected intravenously in dogs. Helium, which has been used as an alternative to CO_2 for insufflation in some series,[22,84,90] is even less soluble than nitrogen. In canine experiments, the intravenous injection of He was lethal on 4 of 6 occasions, whereas the same amount of CO_2 was followed by hemodynamic recovery in all cases (Figure 5.4).[104] Additionally, argon VGE during laparoscopic use of an argon beam coagulator has been reported.[105] These findings argue against the use of He or Ar for initial insuf-

flation, but their use after the pneumoperitoneum has been safely created with CO_2 appears safe.[84]

Hypoxemia

PaO_2 may decrease during laparoscopy because of the decreased cardiac output, increased pulmonary shunt, worsened ventilation/perfusion mismatch, decreased alveolar ventilation, and acidosis associated with laparoscopy.[106] Most clinical studies have suggested a slight but clinically insignificant reduction of PaO_2 during laparoscopy.[6,71,78,81,93] Corall and associates[107] reported that 2 patients with heavy smoking history experienced a drop in PaO_2 to less than 100 mmHg during N_2O laparoscopy, but others have not found PaO_2 during laparoscopy to be affected significantly by preoperative pulmonary status.[81] When severe hypoxemia occurs, other complications such as venous gas embolism, pneumothorax, or ventilator malfunction should be considered.

Hypothermia

Hypothermia may occur during laparoscopy because of the loss of heat to the large volumes of gas exchanged through the patient.[108] Ott found that the core temperature dropped 0.3°C for every 50 liters of CO_2 used, and recommended warming the gas prior to insufflation to prevent hypothermia.[109] Others, however, found that heating the gas made no difference in the slight drop in core temperature.[110] Moreover, another study found the core temperature to increase rather than decrease during

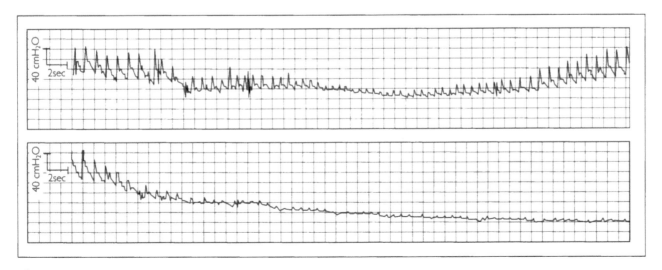

Figure 5.4
Arterial tracing after rapid intravenous injection of 7.5 ml/kg CO_2 (top) and helium (bottom) in a dog. There is recovery within 1 min after the CO_2 injection but complete cardiovascular collapse after helium injection. (Reproduced with permission from Wolf et al.[104])

laparoscopy, even with the use of room temperature gas for insufflation.[111]

Intra-abdominal explosion

In 1933, Fervers[112] reported an intra-abdominal explosion during laparoscopy with oxygen insufflation, and the use of pure oxygen pneumoperitoneum subsequently has been abandoned. N_2O will support combustion[113] and is explosive in the presence of hydrogen or methane.[114] Although the proper conditions for explosion during laparoscopy are rare,[115] death has occurred due to cardiac rupture from an explosion during N_2O pneumoperitoneum.[116] Neuman and associates[117] found that N_2O content in the peritoneal cavity rose to 36% after 30 min duration of CO_2 pneumoperitoneum when the inhaled gas contained 60% N_2O. They also reported that 69% hydrogen (the maximum reported content of hydrogen in bowel gas) was combustible in the presence of 29% N_2O. Therefore, both inhaled and insufflated N_2O should be avoided when electrocautery or laser might be used. Even without N_2O insufflation, electrocautery injury to the colon can be associated with explosion.[118]

Summary

The hemodynamic effects of laparoscopy are determined by the intra-abdominal pressure, the type of gas insufflated, and the position of the patient. Cardiovascular complications of laparoscopy include tension pneumoperitoneum, cardiac dysrhythmias, fluid overload, renal failure, hypertension, elevated intracranial pressure, cerebral ischemia, and venous thrombosis. The intraoperative pulmonary stresses of laparoscopy can also be considerable. Pulmonary, acid–base, and insufflant-related complications include hypercapnia, acidosis, extraperitoneal gas collections, venous gas embolism, hypoxemia, hypothermia, and intra-abdominal explosion.

Most patients tolerate laparoscopy well if the intra-abdominal pressure is limited to 20 mmHg, there is adequate (but not excessive) fluid replacement, and CO_2 levels are monitored appropriately. Nonetheless, it should be remembered that laparoscopy is in many ways associated with more intraoperative physiologic stress than is open surgery. The unique physiologic stresses of laparoscopy require vigilance on the part of the surgeon and anesthesiologist to prevent, monitor for, and treat the potential physiologic complications of laparoscopy.

References

1. Wolf JS Jr, Stoller ML. The physiology of laparoscopy: basic principles, complications, and other considerations. J Urol 1994; 152:294–302.

2. Deziel DJ, Millikan KW, Economou SG, et al. Complications of laparoscopic cholecystomy: a national survey of 4,292 hospitals and an analysis of 77,604 cases. Am J Surg 1993; 165:9–14.

3. Caldwell CB, Ricotta JJ. Changes in visceral blood flow with elevated intraabdominal pressure. J Surg Res 1987; 43:14–20.

4. Motew M, Ivankovich AD, Bieniarz J, et al. Cardiovascular effects and acid-base and blood gas changes during laparoscopy. Am J Obstet Gynecol 1973; 115:1002–12.

5. Ivankovich AD, Miletich DJ, Albrecht RF, et al. Cardiovascular effects of intraperitoneal insufflation with carbon dioxide and nitrous oxide in the dog. Anesthesiology 1975; 42:281–7.

6. Diamant M, Benumof JL, Saidman LJ. Hemodynamics of increased intra-abdominal pressure: interaction with hypovolemia and halothane anesthesia. Anesthesiology 1978; 48:23–7.

7. Kashtan J, Green JF, Parsons EQ, Holcroft JW. Hemodynamic effects of increased abdominal pressure. J Surg Res 1981; 30:249–55.

8. Johannsen G, Andersen M, Juhl B. The effect of general anaesthesia on the haemodynamic events during laparoscopy with CO_2-insufflation. Acta Anaesthesiol Scand 1989; 33:132–6.

9. Torrielli R, Cesarini M, Winnock S, et al. [Hemodynamic changes during celioscopy: a study carried out using thoracic electric bioimpedance]. Can J Anaesth 1992; 37:46–51.

10. Hashikura Y, Kawasaki K, Munakata Y, et al. Effects of peritoneal insufflation on hepatic and renal blood flow. Surg Endosc 1994; 8:759–61.

11. Eleftheriadis E, Kotzampassi K, Botsios D, Tzartinoglou E, Farmakis H, Dadoukis J. Sphlanchnic ischemia during laparoscopic cholecystectomy. Surg Endosc 1996; 10:324–6.

12. Ho HS, Saunders CJ, Corso FA, Wolfe BM. The effects of CO_2 pneumoperitoneum on hemodynamics in hemorrhaged animals. Surgery 1993; 114:381–7.

13. Cullen DJ, Coyle JP, Teplick R, Long MC. Cardiovascular, pulmonary, and renal effects of massively increased intra-abdominal pressure in critically ill patients. Crit Care Med 1989; 17:118–21.

14. Versichelen L, Serreyn R, Rolly G, Vanderkerckhove D. Physiopathologic changes during anesthesia administration for gynecologic laparoscopy. J Reprod Med 1984; 29:697–700.

15. Ekman LG, Abrahamsson J, Biber B, et al. Hemodynamic changes during laparoscopy with positive end-expiratory pressure ventilation. Acta Anaesthesiol Scand 1988; 32:447–53.

16. Lenz RJ, Thomas TA, Wilkins DG. Cardiovascular changes during laparoscopy: studies of stroke volume and cardiac output using impedance cardiography. Anaesthesia 1976; 31:4–12.

17. Marshall RL, Jebson PJR, Davie IT, Scott DB. Circulatory effects of carbon dioxide insufflation of the peritoneal cavity for laparoscopy. Br J Anaesth 1972; 44:680–4.

18. Marshall RL, Jebson PJR, Davie IT, Scott DB. Circulatory effects of peritoneal insufflation with nitrous oxide. Br J Anaesth 1972; 44:1183–7.

19. Richardson JD, Trinkle JK. Hemodynamic and respiratory alterations with increased intra-abdominal pressure. J Surg Res 1976; 20:401–4.

20. Price HL. Effects of carbon dioxide on the cardiovascular system. Anesthesiology 1960; 21:652–63.

21. El-Minawi MF, Wahbi O, El-Bagouri IS, et al. Physiologic changes during CO_2 and N_2O pneumoperitoneum in diagnostic laparoscopy. A comparative study. J Reprod Med 1981; 26:338–46.

22. Bongard FS, Pianim NA, Leighton TA, et al. Helium insufflation for laparoscopic operation. Surg Gynecol Obstet 1993; 177:140–6.

23. Eisenhauer DM, Saunders CJ, Ho HS, Wolfe BM. Hemodynamic effects of argon pneumoperitoneum. Surg Endosc 1994; 8:315–21.

24. Sibbald WJ, Paterson NAM, Holliday RL, Baskerville J. The Trendelenburg position: hemodynamic effects in hypotensive and normotensive patients. Crit Care Med 1979; 7:218–24.

25. Reich DL, Konstadt SN, Raissi S, et al. Trendelenburg position and passive leg raising do not significantly improve cardiopulmonary performance in the anesthetized patient with coronary artery disease. Crit Care Med 1989; 17:313–17.

26. Cunningham AJ, Turner J, Rosenbaum S, Rafferty T. Transoesophageal echocardiographic assessment of haemodynamic function during laparoscopic cholecystectomy. Br J Anaesth 1993; 70:621–5.

27. Lawson NW. The lateral decubitus position. In: Martin JT, ed. Positioning in anesthesia and surgery. Philadelphia: WB Saunders, 1987:155–79.

28. Bannenberg JJ, Rademaker BM, Froeling FM, Meijer DW. Hemodynamics during laparoscopic extra- and intraperitoneal insufflation. An experimental study. Surg Endosc 1997; 11:911–14.

29. Giebler RM, Kabatnik M, Stegen BH et al. Retroperitoneal and intraperitoneal CO_2 insufflation have markedly different cardiovascular effect. J Surg Res 1997; 68:153–60.

30. Giebler RM, Walz MK, Peitgen K, Scherer RU. Hemodynamic changes after retroperitoneal CO_2 insufflation for posterior retroperitoneoscopic adrenalectomy. Anesth Analg 1996; 82:827–31.

31. Giebler RM, Behrends M, Steffens T, et al. Intraperitoneal and retroperitoneal carbon dioxide evoke different effects on caval vein pressure gradients in humans: evidence for the Starling resistor concept of abdominal venous return. Anesthesiology 2000; 92:1568–80.

32. Lee CM. Acute hypotension during laparoscopy: a case report. Anesth Analg 1975; 54:142–3.

33. Arthure H. Laparoscopy hazard. Br Med J 1970; 4:492–3.

34. Parra RO, Hagood PG, Boullier JA, et al. Complications of laparoscopic urological surgery: experience at St. Louis University. J Urol 1994; 151:681–4.

35. Lew JKL, Gin T, Oh TE. Anaesthetic problems during laparoscopic cholecystectomy. Anaesth Intens Care 1992; 20:91–2.

36. Joris JL, Noirot DP, Legrand MJ, et al. Hemodynamic changes during laparoscopic cholecystectomy. Anesthes Analg 1993; 76:1067–71.

37. Safran D, Sgambati S, Orlando R III. Laparoscopy in high-risk cardiac patients. Surg Gynecol Obstetr 1993; 176:548–54.

38. Jones PE, Sayson SC, Koehler DC. Laparoscopic cholecystectomy in a cardiac transplant candidate with an ejection fraction of less than 15%. J Soc Laparoendosc Surg 1998; 2:89–92.

39. Scott DB, Julian DG. Observations on cardiac arrythmias during laparoscopy. Br Med J 1972; 1:411–13.

40. Cimino L, Petitto M, Nardon G, Budillon G. Holter dynamic electrocardiography during laparoscopy. Gastrointest Endosc 1988; 34:72.

41. Shifren JL, Adlestein L, Finkler NJ. Asystolic cardiac arrest: a rare complication of laparoscopy. Obstet Gynecol 1992; 79:840–1.

42. Biswas TK, Pembroke A. Asystolic cardiac arrest during laparoscopic cholecystectomy. Anaesth Intens Care 1994; 22:289–91.

43. Borten M. Choice of anesthesia. In: Laparoscopic complications. Toronto: BC Decker, 1986:173–84.

44. Vukasin A, Lopez M, Shichman S, et al. Oliguria in laparoscopic surgery (abstract #462). J Urol 1994; 151(supplement):343A.

45. Chang DT, Kirsch AJ, Sawczuk IS. Oliguria during laparoscopic surgery. J Endourol 1994; 8:349–52.

46. Kirsch AJ, Hensle TW, Chang DT, et al. Renal effects of CO_2 insufflation: oliguria and acute renal dysfunction in a rat pneumoperitoneum model. Urology 1994; 43:453–9.

47. McDougall EM, Monk TG, Hicks M, et al. Effect of pneumoperitoneum on renal function in an animal model (abstract #938). J Urol 1994; 151(supplement):462A.

48. Chiu AW, Azadzoi KM, Hatzichristou DG, et al. Effects of intra-abdominal pressure on renal tissue perfusion during laparoscopy. J Endourol 1994; 8:99–103.

49. Razvi HA, Fields D, Vargas JC, et al. Oliguria during laparoscopic surgery: evidence for direct parenchymal compression as an etiologic factor. J Endourol 1996; 10:1–4.

50. Guler C, Sade M, Kirkali Z. Renal effect of carbon dioxide insufflation in rabbit pneumoperitoneum model. J Endourol 1998; 12:367–70.

51. McDougall EM, Monk TG, Hicks M, et al. The effect of prolonged pneumoperitoneum on renal function in an animal model. J Am Coll Surg 1996; 182:317–28.

52. Clayman RV, Kavoussi LR, Soper NJ, et al. Laparoscopic nephrectomy: review of the initial 10 cases. J Endourol 1992; 6:127–32.

53. Kubota K, Kajiura N, Teruya M, et al. Alterations in respiratory function and hemodynamics during laparoscopic cholecystectomy under pneumoperitoneum. Surg Endosc 1993; 7:500–4.

54. Beduschi R, Beduschi MC, Williams AL, Wolf JS Jr. Pneumoperitoneum does not potentiate the nephrotoxicity of aminoglycosides in rats. Urology 1999; 53:451–4.

55. Cisek LJ, Gobet RM, Peters CA. Pneumoperitoneum produces reversible renal dysfunction in animals with normal and chronically reduced renal function. J Endourol 1998; 12:95–9.

56. Ben-David B, Croitoru M, Gaitini L. Acute renal failure following laparoscopic cholecystectomy: a case report. J Clin Anesth 1999; 11:486–9.

57. Josephs LG, Este-McDonald JR, Birkett DH, Hirsch EF. Diagnostic laparoscopy increases intracranial pressure. J Trauma 1994; 36:815–19.

58. Poppas DP, Peters CA, Bilsky MH, Sosa RE. Intracranial pressure monitoring during laparoscopic surgery in children with ventriculoperitoneal shunts. J Endourol 1994; 8:S93.

59. Jackman SV, Weingart JD, Kinsman SL, Docimo SG. Laparoscopic surgery in patients with ventriculoperitoneal shunts: safety and monitoring. J Urol 2000; 164:1352–4.

60. Prentice JA, Martin JT. The Trendelenburg position. Anesthesiologic considerations. In: Martin JT, ed. Positioning in anesthesia and surgery. Philadelphia: WB Saunders, 1987:127–45.

61. Borten M. Circulatory changes. In: Laparoscopic complications. Toronto: BC Decker, 1986:185–95.

62. Jorgensen JO, Hanel K, Lalak NJ, et al. Thromboembolic complications of laparoscopic cholecystectomy. BMJ 1993; 306:518–19.

63. Wazz G, Branicki F, Taji H, Chishty I. Influence of pneumoperitoneum on the deep venous system during laparoscopy. J Laparoendosc Surg 2000; 4:291–5.

64. Morrison CA, Schreiber MA, Olsen SB, et al. Femoral venous flow dynamics during intraperitoneal and preperitoneal laparoscopic insufflation. Surg Endosc 1998; 12:1213–16.

65. Kavoussi LR, Sosa E, Chandhoke P, et al. Complications of laparoscopic pelvic lymph node dissection. J Urol 1993; 149:322–5.

66. Mayol J, Vincent HE, Sarmiento JM, et al. Pulmonary embolism following laparoscopic cholecystectomy: report of two cases and review of the literature. Surg Endosc 1994; 8:214–17.

67. Wolf JS JR, Clayman RV, Monk TG, et al. Carbon dioxide absorption during laparoscopic pelvic surgery. J Am Coll Surg 1995; 180:555–60.

68. Schwenk W, Bohm B, Fugener A, Muller JM. Intermittent pneumatic sequential compression (ISC) of the lower extremities prevents venous stasis during laparoscopic cholecystectomy. A prospective randomized study. Surg Endosc 1998; 12:7–11.

69. Wright GW, Place R, Princi F. The physiological effects of pneumoperitoneum upon the respiratory apparatus. Am Rev Tuberc 1949; 60:706–14.

70. Hodgson C, McClelland RMA, Newton JR. Some effects of the peritoneal insufflation of carbon dioxide at laparoscopy. Anaesthesia 1970; 25:382–90.

71. Puri GD, Singh H. Ventilatory effects of laparoscopy under general anaesthesia. Br J Anaesth 1992; 68:211–13.

72. Piiper J. Physiological equilibria of gas cavities in the body. In: Fenn WO, Rahn H, ed. Handbook of physiology, Section 3: Respiration. Washington, DC: American Physiological Society, 1965:1205–18.

73. Stoller ML, Wolf JS Jr. Physiological considerations in laparoscopy. In: Das S, Crawford ED, ed. Urologic laparoscopy. Philadelphia: WB Saunders, 1994:17–34.

74. Nunn JF. Carbon dioxide. In: Applied respiratory physiology. London: Butterworths, 1987:207–34.

75. Mullett CE, Viale JP, Sagnard PE, et al. Pulmonary CO_2 elimination during surgical procedures using intra- or extraperitoneal CO_2 insufflation. Anesth Analg 1993; 76:622–6.

76. Wolf JS Jr, Monk TG, McDougall EM, et al. The extraperitoneal approach and subcutaneous emphysema are associated with greater absorption of carbon dioxide during laparoscopic renal surgery. J Urol 1995; 154:959–64.

77. Liu SY, Leighton T, Davis I, et al. Prospective analysis of cardiopulmonary responses to laparoscopic cholecystectomy. J Laparoendosc Surg 1991; 1:241–6.

78. Alexander GD, Brown EM. Physiologic alterations during laparoscopy. Am J Obstet Gynecol 1969; 105:1078–81.

79. Magno R, Medegård A, Bengtsson R, Tronstad S-E. Acid-base balance during laparoscopy: the effects of intraperitoneal insufflation of carbon dioxide on acid-base balance during controlled ventilation. Acta Obstet Gynecol Scand 1979; 58:81–5.

80. Leighton TA, Liu SY, Bongard FS. Comparative cardiopulmonary effects of carbon dioxide versus helium pneumoperitoneum. Surgery 1993; 113:527–31.

81. Wittgen CM, Andrus CH, Fitzgerald SD, et al. Analysis of the hemodynamic and ventilatory effects of laparoscopic cholecystectomy. Arch Surg 1991; 126:997–1001.

82. Holzman M, Sharp K, Richards W. Hypercarbia during carbon dioxide gas insufflation for therapeutic laparoscopy: a note of caution. Surg Laparosc Endosc 1992; 2:11–14.

83. Sosa RE, Weingram J, Stein B, et al. Hypercarbia in laparoscopic pelvic lymph node dissection. J Urol 1992; 147:A246.

84. Neuberger TJ, Andrus CH, Wittgen CM, et al. Prospective comparison of helium versus carbon dioxide pneumoperitoneum. Gastrointest Endosc 1994; 40:P30.

85. Wright DM, Serpell MG, Baxter JN, et al. Effect of extraperitoneal carbon dioxide insufflation on intra-operative blood gas and hemodynamic changes. Surg Endosc 1995; 9:1169–72.

86. Siegler AM, Berenyi KJ. Laparoscopy in gynecology. Obstet Gynecol 1969; 34:572–7.

87. Sharp JR, Pierson WP, Brady CE III. Comparison of CO_2- and N_2O-induced discomfort during peritoneoscopy under local anesthesia. Gastroenterology 1982; 82:453–6.

88. Minoli G, Terruzzi V, Spinzi GC, et al. The influence of carbon dioxide and nitrous oxide on pain during laparoscopy: a double-blind, controlled trial. Gastrointest Endosc 1982; 28:173–5.

89. Fitzgerald SD, Andrus CH, Baudendistel LJ, et al. Hypercarbia during carbon dioxide pneumoperitoneum. Am J Surg 1992; 163:186–90.

90. Wolf JS Jr, Clayman RV, McDougall EM, et al. Carbon dioxide and helium insufflation during laparoscopic radical nephrectomy in a patient with severe pulmonary disease. J Urol 1996; 155:2021.

91. Verbessem D, Camu F, Devroey P, Steirteghem AV. Pneumoperitoneum induced pH changes in follicular and Douglas fluids during laparoscopic oocyte retrieval in humans. Human Reprod 1988; 3:751–4.

92. Wahba RWM, Mamazza J. Ventilatory requirements during laparoscopic cholecystectomy. Can J Anaesth 1993; 40:206–10.

93. Kenefick JP, Leader A, Maltby JR, Taylor PJ. Laparoscopy: blood-gas values and minor sequelae associated with three techniques based on isoflurane. Br J Anaesth 1987; 59:189–94.

94. Sivak BJ. Surgical emphysema: report of a case and review. Anesth Analg 1964; 43:415–17.

95. Batra MS, Driscoll JJ, Coburn WA, Marks WM. Evanescent nitrous oxide pneumothorax after laparoscopy. Anesth Analg 1983; 62:1121–3.

96. Pascual JB, Baranda MM, Tarrero MT, et al. Subcutaneous emphysema, pneumomediastinum, bilateral pneumothorax and pneumopericardium after laparoscopy. Endoscopy 1990; 22:59.

97. Root B, Levy MN, Pollack S, et al. Gas embolism death after laparoscopy delayed by 'trapping' in portal circulation. Anesth Analg 1978; 57:232–7.

98. Gomar C, Fernandez C, Villalonga A, Nalda MA. Carbon dioxide embolism during laparoscopy and hysteroscopy. Ann Fr Anesth Reanim 1985; 4:380–2.

99. Hynes SR, Marshall RL. Venous gas embolism during gynaecological laparoscopy. Can J Anaesth 1992; 39:748–9.

100. Beck DH, McQuillan PJ. Fatal carbon dioxide embolism and severe haemorrhage during laparoscopic salpingectomy. Br J Anesth 1994; 72:243–5.

101. O'Sullivan DC, Micali S, Averch TD, et al. Factors involved in gas embolism after laparoscopic injury to inferior vena cava. J Endourol 1998; 12:149–54.

102. Shulman D, Aronson HB. Capnography in the early diagnosis of carbon dioxide embolism during laparoscopy. Can Anaesth Soc J 1984; 31:455–9.

103. Graff TD, Arbegast NR, Phillips OC, et al. Gas embolism: a comparative study of air and carbon dioxide as embolic agents in the systemic venous system. Am J Obstet Gynecol 1959; 78:259–65.

104. Wolf JS Jr, Carrier S, Stoller ML. Gas embolism: helium is more lethal than carbon dioxide. J Laparoendosc Surg 1994; 4:173–7.

105. Mastragelopulos N, Sarkar MR, Kaissling G, et al. [Argon gas embolism in laparoscopic cholecystectomy with the Argon Beam One coagulator]. Chirurg 1992; 63:1053–4.

106. Nunn JF. Oxygen. In: Applied respiratory physiology. London: Butterworths, 1987:235–83.

107. Corall IM, Knights K, Potter D, Strunin L. Arterial oxygen tension during laparoscopy with nitrous oxide in the spontaneously breathing patient. Br J Anaesth 1974; 46:925–8.

108. Ott DE. Laparoscopic hypothermia. J Laparoendosc Surg 1991; 1:127–31.

109. Ott DE. Correction of laparoscopic insufflation hypothermia. J Laparoendosc Surg 1991; 1:183–6.

110. Nelskyla K, Yli-Hankala A, Sjoberg J, et al. Warming of insufflation gas during laparoscopic hysterectomy: effect on body temperature and the autonomic nervous system. Acta Anaesth Scand 1999; 43:974–8.

111. Teichman JMH, Floyd M, Hulbert JC. Does laparoscopy induce operative hypothermia? J Endourol 1994; 8:S92.

112. Fervers C. Die Laparoskopie mit dem Cystoskop. Medizinische Klinik 1933; 29:1042–5.

113. Soderstrom RM. Dangers of nitrous oxide pneumoperitoneum. Am J Obstet Gynecol 1976; 124:668–9.

114. Robinson JS, Thompson JM, Wood AW. Laparoscopy explosion hazards with nitrous oxide. Br Med J 1975; 4:760–1.

115. Vickers MD. Fire and explosions in operating theatres. Br J Anaesth 1978; 50:659–64.

116. El-Kady AA, Abd-el-Razek M. Intraperitoneal explosion during female sterilization by laparoscopic electrocoagulation. A case report. Int J Gynaecol Obstet 1976; 14:487–8.

117. Neuman GG, Sidebotham G, Negoiana E, et al. Laparoscopy explosion hazards with nitrous oxide. Anesthesiology 1993; 78:875–9.

118. Altmore DF, Memeo V. Colonic explosion during diathermy colotomy. Dis Colon Rectum 1993; 36:291–3.

6

Laparoscopic access, trocar placement, and exiting the abdomen

Sean P Hedican and Stephen Y Nakada

Introduction

Proper access to the peritoneal cavity or retroperitoneum, including the insertion and positioning of port sites, is as important as the laparoscopic procedure itself for insuring a good surgical outcome. In a recent review, initial access to the peritoneal cavity accounted for anywhere from 6% to 57% of injuries occurring during laparoscopy.[1] In addition, poor trocar planning can result in unnecessary frustration due to crossing of instruments, difficult angles of approach, mirror imaging, and shoulder fatigue. Diligence should also be exercised in exiting the abdomen to prevent inadvertent organ injury and delayed complications (abdominal wall bleeding and/or trocar site hernia formation). This chapter outlines the critical elements involved in safe and effective laparoscopic access, trocar placement, and exiting the abdomen, with emphasis on ways of avoiding potential pitfalls.

Accessing the abdomen
Closed transperitoneal access

Closed laparoscopic access to the peritoneal space is most commonly obtained after initial insufflation via a Veress access needle. The needle is usually inserted at the region of the umbilicus for procedures performed in the supine position. At the umbilicus, the puncture is concealed and there are no intervening layers of muscle encountered, so the Veress needle only has to pass through the fused anterior and posterior rectus sheaths before entering the peritoneum. For flank access, we prefer inserting the Veress needle via the trocar skin incision made for the lower quadrant port of the ipsilateral side of the pathology. Caution should be exercised not to insert the needle too laterally, in close proximity to the superior iliac crest,

because this can result in retroperitoneal insufflation or puncture of the colon (sigmoid on the left and the cecum on the right).

Key steps to insure correct intraperitoneal insertion and avoid injury to underlying viscera or vasculature include insertion of the Veress needle perpendicular to the fascial surface while tenting up the abdominal wall using instruments or manual elevation. Passage through two points of maximum resistance are noted as the needle traverses the fascial layers with less resistance as it passes through muscle and fat. An audible snap of the internal obturator heralds entry into an area of low resistance, which is usually the peritoneal cavity (Figure 6.1), and further advancement of the needle is halted. Intraperitoneal localization is confirmed by:

1. a lack of resistance with gentle side-to-side movements of the needle tip
2. easy injection and drainage of saline through the hub of the Veress needle
3. lack of succus entericus, blood, or air on gentle aspiration with a 10 ml syringe attached to the Veress needle
4. low insufflation pressures (< 10 mmHg) at a low flow rate.

It is important to take into account body habitus when assessing the appropriateness of observed insufflation pressures. Obese patients with a large amount of chest and abdominal wall fat may have a resultant increase in their intraperitoneal pressure. Initial recordings in these patients may be just under 10 mmHg at low insufflation rates and remain stable until the peritoneal cavity nears complete distention.

If all of the localization findings occur as noted above, yet the recorded intraperitoneal pressures appear inappropriately high, or occlusion alarms intermittently sound, then the needle may be entrapped in omentum or bowel mesentery. Gentle incremental withdrawal or angulation

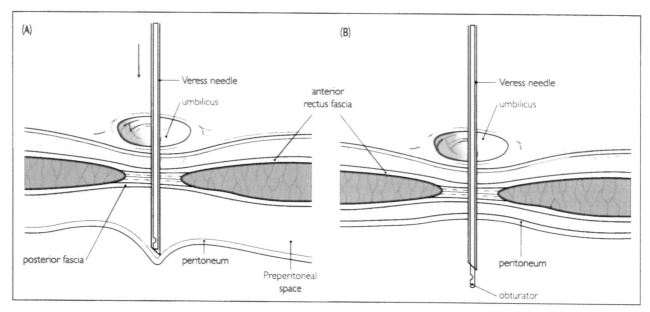

Figure 6.1
(A) Veress needle being inserted with initial retraction of the internal obturator on contact with the skin or fascia. (B) On entry into the peritoneal cavity, the protective obturator snaps forward with an audible engagement to protect the underlying viscera and vasculature.

of the needle is safe to perform with repeat inspection of the pressure after each adjustment. If pressures do not improve, the needle should be removed and reinserted.

After establishment of the pneumoperitoneum at 15–20 mmHg pressure, either a blind or visual trocar technique can be utilized for introduction of the initial port. A blind trocar technique involves insertion of the initial port, utilizing either a fascial cutting or splitting trocar, with entry into the peritoneum determined by both a loss of resistance and audible engagement of the inner protective obturator. Final confirmation is obtained by venting the port or performing a direct camera inspection of the peritoneal contents. The risk of inadvertent injury to underlying viscera or catastrophic vascular injury when utilizing this technique is obviously higher than what is observed using direct vision trocar methods.[1]

Direct vision port introduction utilizes a pistol-shaped introducing obturator with either a fascial splitting clear plastic point (e.g. Optiview, Ethicon Endo-Surgery, Cincinnati, Ohio) (Figure 6.2) or a fascial cutting blade which is activated each time the trigger is pulled (Visiport, U.S. Surgical (USSC) Norwalk, Connecticut) (Figure 6.3). The Optiview comes in both a 10/12 mm pistol as well as a 5 mm size that is shaped like a standard obturator through which a 5 mm laparoscope may be introduced. Once the laparoscope is inserted and focused on the line traversing the plastic tip of the Optiview, it is slowly advanced using a back-and-forth twisting motion through the layers of the abdominal wall. Each layer can usually be identified as it is

traversed. Entry into the peritoneum is recognized initially as a widening dark hole through which the trocar is advanced. Once inside the peritoneum, the visual obturator is removed from the port and taken off of the laparoscope (Figure 6.2). The Optiview, like other non-cutting trocars, splits the fascia along the course of its fibers and, theoretically, has less chance of postoperative hernia formation even without fascial closure.[2] In contrast, the Visiport device has a blade that cuts the fascia and only comes in a 12 mm size. Since it is desirable to cut the fascia along the course of its fibers, the camera of the laparoscope is focused on the blade of the Visiport, which is then oriented in the direction of the fibers by turning the end of the pistol grip handle. As the trigger is depressed and each layer of the abdominal wall is cut, the device is slowly advanced with a twisting motion until it enters the peritoneal cavity. Larger abdominal wall vessels can usually be visualized with this device and avoided by changing the orientation of the blade so it runs parallel and to the side of the vessel.

The use of a visual obturator without prior insufflation has also been described. The theoretic risk for injury to underlying structures is higher due to the lack of separation between the parietal peritoneum and the underlying viscera. In this closed transperitoneal access technique, the visual obturator is utilized in exactly the same fashion as it is with an insufflated abdomen; however, entry into the peritoneum is confirmed by loss of resistance and the visual appearance of bowel or omentum.

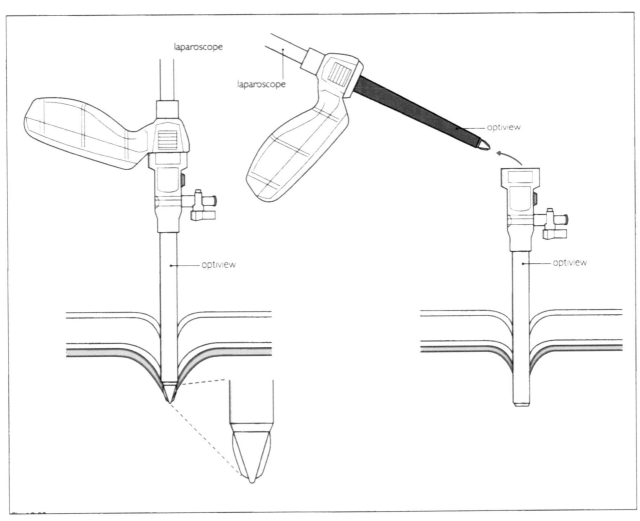

Figure 6.2
(A) 10/12 mm Optiview cannula (Ethicon Endo-Surgery, Cincinnati, Ohio) with its fascial splitting point being introduced. (B) Removal of the pistol-shaped visual obturator and laparoscope from the introduced trocar. The obturator is taken off of the laparoscope, which is then reinserted into the port for initial inspection.

Open transperitoneal access

In cases where standard insertion of an insufflating needle or closed trocar insertion is associated with a significant risk of injury to underlying structures, it may be preferable to perform an open access to the peritoneal cavity. This is often utilized in patients who have had significant prior transperitoneal surgery raising concerns about adhesion formation. Adhesions of omentum, bowel, bowel mesentery, and in some cases solid organs such as the liver to the anterior abdominal wall prevent these structures from falling away from the parietal peritoneum as it is elevated during insertion of the needle or following insufflation. This can result in direct puncture or laceration injuries of these structures with either the Veress needle or the initial trocar. These injuries can even occur utilizing direct vision trocars since it can be difficult to discern the passage of one

of these devices into or through adhered viscera from passage through the preperitoneal layer.

In these circumstances, it is often prudent to use an open access to establish the pneumoperitoneum. This technique is performed by making a 1.5–2 cm incision at the site of desired trocar insertion. The underlying fascia is exposed using deep, narrow retractors and incised. Stay sutures of 0-Vicryl (polyglactin) mounted on a semicircular needle are inserted through the corners of the fascial incision. The underlying muscle fibers are split using a tapered clamp and the posterior fascial layer is incised. The preperitoneal fat is grasped and gentle spreading motions of the Metzenbaum scissors reveal the underlying peritoneal layer. The peritoneum is tented up between grasping, nontoothed forceps and cut (Figure 6.4). Entry into the peritoneum is confirmed by visualization of freely mobile bowel or omentum. A blunt-tipped

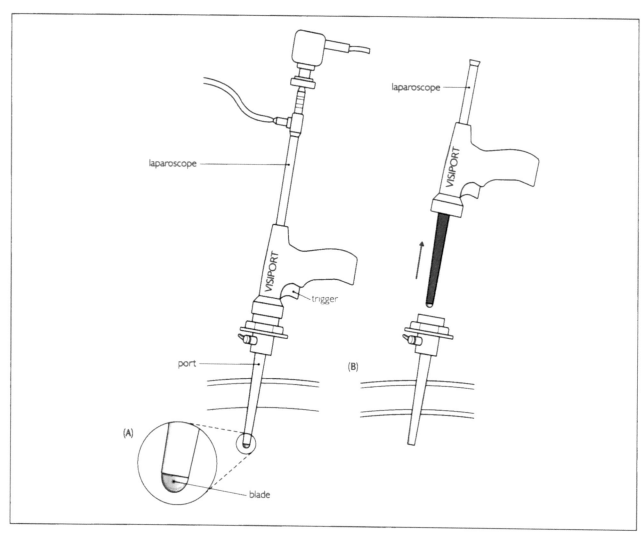

Figure 6.3
(A) Visiport device (USSC, Norwalk, Connecticut) with its cutting blade that is activated each time the trigger is depressed. (B) Removal of the visual obturator and laparoscope from the introduced port.

cannula, such as a Hasson, is inserted through the opening in the peritoneum. The fascial corner stitches are wrapped around the circular suture guides holding the Hasson trocar in place. The cuff is then pushed into the skin incision and locked into position to prevent leakage of the pneumoperitoneum (see Figure 6.4).

One drawback of the open access technique is the larger skin incision required for introduction of the initial cannula than what is necessary using a closed introduction. In addition, a larger fascial incision than the diameter of the port is often made and can result in problematic leakage of the pneumoperitoneum around the cuff of the Hasson cannula. Overall, this approach takes longer to perform than the closed technique and can be extremely difficult in obese patients due to the thickness of the subcutaneous and preperitoneal fat layers.

Hand-assisted access

Early-generation hand-assist devices such as the Pneumo Sleeve (Weck Closure Systems, Research Triangle Park, North Carolina) relied on applied or tape-backed adhesives to secure the device to the skin of the abdominal wall. This required initial insufflation and distention of the abdomen to allow smooth application of the device and to prevent leakage and detachment on creation of the pneumoperitoneum.[3] The latest generation of devices relies on inner and outer abdominal securing rings attached by a wound protector. The pneumoperitoneum is then maintained around the inserted hand via an occlusive gel matrix (GelPort; Applied Medical, Rancho Santo Margarita, California), twisted pneumatic cuff (OmniPort; Weck Closure Systems, Research Triangle Park, North Carolina),

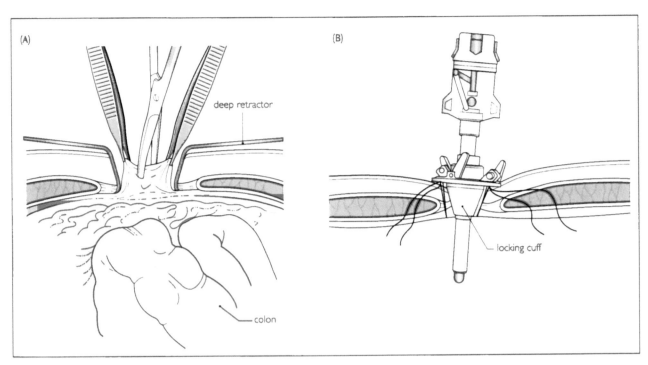

Figure 6.4
(A) Incision of the peritoneum being made for open access port introduction. (B) Insertion of the Hasson port and securing of the locking cuff to prevent leakage of the pneumoperitoneum using the previously placed fascial corner stitches.

or an adjustable iris (Lap Disc; Ethicon Endo-Surgery, Cincinnati, Ohio). With each of these new generation of devices, the incision for the hand-assist port can be made first and the secondary ports inserted under direct inspection or with the aid of an inserted hand in a nonvisualized fashion.

In the method utilizing direct inspection, a 10/12 mm port is inserted via the hand device through the gel matrix (GelPort), aperture of the twisted pneumatic cuff (OmniPort), or adjustable iris (Lap Disc). These devices can be secured around the inserted port in identical fashion to the operating hand and the abdomen insufflated to allow for insertion of the additional trocars under direct vision (Figure 6.5). An alternative to direct inspection is to place the laparoscopic ports with the aid of the inserted hand. The hand is cupped beneath the point of entry of the trocar, palpated as an area of downward-tented peritoneum and transversalis fascia. The inserted hand acts as a backstop to the abdominal wall and shields the peritoneal contents from the entering trocar (Figure 6.6). Non-bladed trocars should be utilized in this method to avoid injury to the surgeon's hand. If any adhesions are felt, it is best to take them down first under direct inspection through the hand-assist port incision prior to inserting additional trocars.

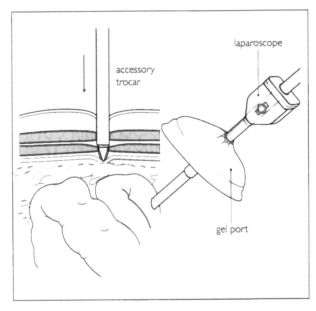

Figure 6.5
A trocar has been inserted through the gel matrix of the GelPort hand-assist device (Applied Medical, Rancho Santo Margarita, California) and direct visual confirmation is being performed of an accessory port as it is introduced into the abdomen.

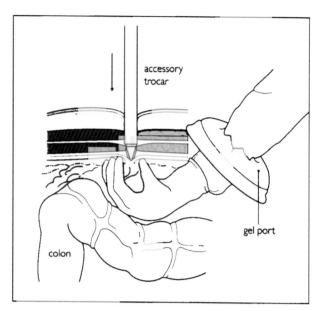

Figure 6.6
Secondary port placement is being performed with the surgeon's hand inserted via the hand-assist device, protecting the abdominal contents as a nonbladed trocar is introduced into the peritoneal cavity.

Closed retroperitoneal access

Depending upon individual surgeon preference or clinical situations in which peritoneal exposure may be limited, access to the retroperitoneum may be desired. Closed access can be obtained via direct retroperitoneal insufflation in the flank position using a Veress needle inserted at the posterior axillary line midway between the 12th rib and the iliac crest. After establishing the pneumoretroperitoneum, a visual or standard cannula can be introduced. An alternative access option is the introduction of a direct vision trocar such as the Optiview or Visiport at the same location without prior insufflation. Regardless of the closed technique utilized, care must be exercised to insert either the needle or direct vision trocar at an angle approximately 10° anterior from vertical.[4] This degree of angulation helps to avoid entry into the psoas and quadratus muscle posteriorly and the bowel and peritoneum anteriorly. Introduction of a visual cannula into the retroperitoneum is performed in exactly the same fashion as it is for transperitoneal surgery; however, the final layer of entry is into the retroperitoneal fat as the cannula traverses the inner muscular fascia. Once this layer is entered, the insufflant is attached and gentle blunt dissection is then performed with the laparoscope to generate adequate space for additional trocars. It is important to sweep the peritoneal envelope medially to prevent transperitoneal placement of the accessory ports, which can result in loss of retroperitoneal distention or inadvertent visceral injury.

Open retroperitoneal/extravesical access

To avoid the risk of colonic injury, open retroperitoneal access is often preferred. In this approach, a several-centimeter incision is made off of the tip of the 12th rib and carried down through the underlying fascia. The muscle fibers are then split along their course using deep, narrow retractors and the retroperitoneum is entered using a tapered clamp. Once the retroperitoneal fat is identified, a finger is inserted via the incision and used to perform blunt dissection to create space for a retroperitoneal dilating balloon. There are several commercially available dilating balloons (e.g. Origin Medsystems, Menlo Park, California) that allow dilation either with or without direct vision. Correct cephalad placement behind Gerota's fascia is critical to maximize the beneficial impact of the balloon on creation of the retroperitoneal space. An alternative and more cost-effective method of balloon dilation utilizes a finger cut from an operative glove and secured to a 16F red rubber catheter with a 2-0 silk suture. The 'finger balloon' is then sequentially inflated using a catheter tip syringe with clamping after each instillation until a total volume of 500 ml of saline is instilled. Once dilation has been performed and the desufflated balloon removed, the surgeon can insert his finger into the retroperitoneum to further sweep the peritoneum medially. Additional trocars can then be introduced directly onto the palpating finger, which is protected using a narrow malleable retractor (Figure 6.7), or under direct vision once the pneumo-retroperitoneum has been established.[5]

Potential pitfalls of accessing the abdomen

Vascular injury

Access-related injuries to the aorta, vena cava, iliac, and epigastric vessels occur in approximately 0.25% of cases.[1] The risk of such injuries can be reduced by using direct vision, open access, or hand-assist techniques for introduction of the initial port. Confirmation of vascular injury is usually the prompt return of a significant quantity of blood via the inserted Veress needle or trocar. Delayed recognition of a major vascular injury until introduction of the laparoscope demonstrates the presence of brisk intraperitoneal or retroperitoneal bleeding is also possible. In such cases the access needle port punctures or lacerates a major vessel prior to being repositioned. Vascular trauma that occurs during establishment of the initial access is often difficult to manage laparoscopically since an adequate number of working ports have not been introduced and the time required for insertion and control is

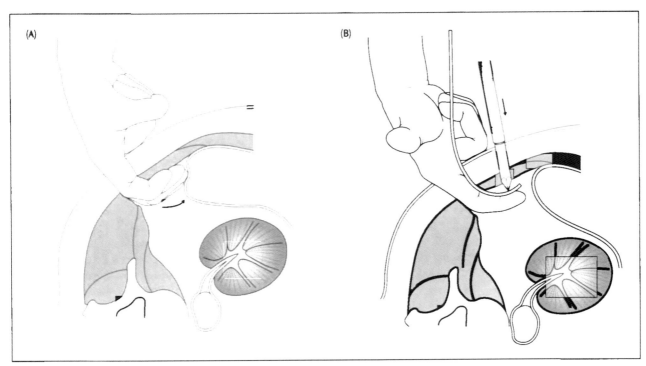

Figure 6.7
(A) Secondary port placement during open retroperitoneal access can be performed after manually sweeping the peritoneal envelope medially off of the abdominal wall. (B) The accessory port is then introduced directly onto the palpating finger, which can be protected with a malleable retractor or use of a nonbladed trocar.

often prohibitive. In the case of such large-vessel entry access injuries, prompt open conversion is usually necessary to avoid catastrophic blood loss.

Venous gas embolism can also occur if insufflation is attempted while the Veress needle is inserted into a large vein. The reported incidence of clinically detectable venous gas embolism is 0.002–0.08% and presents clinically as facial plethora, jugular venous distention, inability to oxygenate, and cardiovascular collapse.[6] A classic mill-wheel murmur is auscultated over the heart and right-heart strain is evidenced on the electrocardiogram. Prompt release of the pneumoperitoneum, head-down with right-side-up positioning, and 100% oxygen administration are critical steps toward reversing this life-threatening situation.[6]

Bowel injury

Inadvertent injury to the bowel during laparoscopy occurs in approximately 0.13% of cases, 32% of which happen during Veress needle or trocar insertion.[7] Selecting an entry point furthest away from areas of scar tissue minimizes the potential for injury. In the flank position, it is often preferable to insert the needle in the lower quadrant of the upside, since the small bowel tends to be displaced medially and injury to the colon, or solid viscera, will be less likely than it would with insertion in the midline or

upper quadrant. Entry into the bowel may be suspected if uneven insufflation of the abdomen is noted, or verified on aspiration of succus entericus or fecal contents. In these cases, leaving the needle in place and performing an open access technique is recommended. If the needle is identified entering the bowel via an isolated puncture site, this can usually be laparoscopically oversewn. Lacerations or thermal injuries of the bowel must be repaired meticulously via the laparoscope or converted to an open exposure if necessary to confirm the quality of the repair. If the needle is not found entering the bowel on initial inspection via the open access, but an injury is still suspected, then the bowel should be run and any suspicious areas oversewn.

It is important to recognize the presenting signs of occult bowel injury following laparoscopy because 70% of these injuries will go unrecognized during the laparoscopic case.[7] Some of the more common presenting signs include focal trocar site pain, leukopenia, and diarrhea.[7] Abdominal–pelvic computed tomography (CT) has been shown to assist in the diagnosis of bowel injuries.[8] Early recognition and intervention is important, as profound sepsis with cardiovascular collapse and death can occur.[7]

Preperitoneal insufflation

Insufflation between the abdominal wall musculature and the peritoneum is usually recognized by a rapid early rise in insufflation pressures. The total volume of infused gas is markedly reduced from what is observed during intraperitoneal insufflation, although it can still be substantial in larger patients. Unfortunately, this condition may not be recognized until introduction of the initial port, when inspection reveals web-like attachments and the confining peritoneum preventing visualization of the bowel. A non-bladed visual cannula can be utilized to advance the lens through this space and into the peritoneal cavity, which is initially collapsed due to the intervening preperitoneal insufflant. The extent of the separation can, however, make this maneuver difficult due to compression of the peritoneal sac and the resultant proximity of the underlying bowel. Once the peritoneum is entered and the line of Toldt is incised, the space rapidly equilibrates. The expansion of introduced gas tracking from the preperitoneal space can actually facilitate the retroperitoneal dissection in some cases.

Omental insufflation

Insertion of the Veress needle into the omentum is usually heralded by intermittent elevations of the intraperitoneal pressures that improve periodically with minor adjustments of the depth of needle penetration. Upon insertion of the initial trocar, a diffuse bubbled appearance of the omentum is noted. The primary detriment of this condition is the negative impact it can have on visualization, which is usually minimal, and the possibility of lacerating an omental vessel.

Trocar placement

The specific trocar arrangements utilized for each operation will be given in their corresponding chapters. These remain a rough guideline that can be altered depending upon the specifics of patient habitus, individualized pathology, instrument preference, and surgeon hand dominance. However, several general principles should be recognized and are outlined in this section.

Trocar introduction

Controlled insertion of laparoscopic trocars of any type is best accomplished by making an epidermal and dermal incision slightly larger than the trocar itself. This prevents 'gripping' of the trocar on introduction that can lead to compression of the abdominal wall and peritoneal envelope with subsequent injury to the underlying viscera or vasculature. An adequate-size incision also prevents excessive pressure at the trocar skin edges during the operation, which can result in tissue necrosis, cellulitis, and larger areas of scarring. The underlying fat is spread down to the level of the fascia using a narrow-tipped clamp. Two-handed introduction of the trocar with the non-dominant hand positioned on the shaft of the trocar, controlling the speed of entry, prevents excessively rapid introduction of accessory ports. An alternative single-handed introduction, with the index finger of the dominant hand extended along the shaft of the trocar to limit the extent of entry, can also be utilized. All ports should be inserted with slight angulation toward the surgical organ of interest. This insures that the anterior and posterior fascial incisions do not line up, thereby reducing the risk of hernia formation. A more perpendicular introduction of the port can also limit excursion toward the surgical organ of interest, causing unnecessary resistance during the dissection.

There are three main types of trocars available on the market: fascial-cutting, fascial-splitting, and radial-dilating trocars. Once initial access has been obtained, these additional ports should always be inserted under direct visual inspection by the laparoscope. Fascial-cutting trocars have an internal obturator with either a mounted pyramidal or single blade that cuts the fascia as it is advanced through it. Once the insufflated peritoneum is entered, the blade retracts within a protective obturator. The port is then advanced until the insufflation side hole is visualized within the peritoneal cavity. It is often best to place a securing suture around the side port of fascial-incising trocars to prevent dislodgment, since there is less resistance to withdrawal during instrument exchanges. The securing suture is tied at the skin level using an air-knot; each end is then wrapped around the side port proximal to the stop-cock, and tied again.

Fascial-splitting trocars require slightly more force to insert than the bladed trocars and are advanced using a back-and-forth twisting motion. Once the fibers of the fascia begin to split, it is important not to release applied pressure to the trocar to prevent the obturator tip from backing out of the fascia and creating a separate fascial opening. The fascia tends to grip these ports more vigorously than the bladed trocars and securing sutures to prevent dislodgment of the port are often unnecessary. Radial-dilating ports (Step System; Weck Closure Systems, Research Triangle Park, North Carolina) also split the fascia, but provide the additional option of increasing the size of the inserted trocar from 5 to 12 mm using a series of stepwise ports with their dilating obturators inserted into a mesh-like sheath. This enables the operating surgeon to minimize port size and enlarge a specific access at any time during a case when necessary (Figure 6.8).

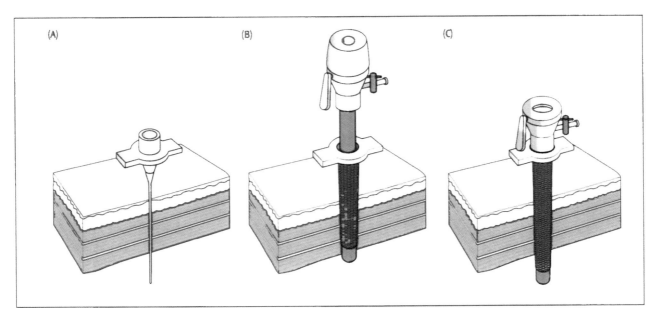

Figure 6.8
(A) The mesh-like expandable sleeve of the Step Access System (Weck Closure Systems, Research Triangle Park, North Carolina) is introduced into the peritoneal cavity over an insufflation needle. (B) The needle is removed and radial dilation is performed to the desired size using a blunt tip obturator and cannula inserted via the mesh sheath. (C) The obturator is removed and the port is ready for use.

Size selection

Port sizes include 2 mm 'needlescopic', 5 mm, 10/12 mm, and 15 mm sizes. Choosing the size of the trocar depends upon the equipment that will be inserted via the specific port. Therefore, each port must be large enough to accommodate the diameter of the largest instrument that will potentially pass through it. For example, one of the largest frequently used pieces of equipment is the Endovascular linear stapling device, which requires a 12 mm port, so a 10/12 mm port should be utilized at all sites where it may be introduced. An alternative to starting with the largest anticipated diameter is to utilize a radial-dilating trocar (e.g. Step System). The mesh-like sleeve allows rapid dilation of the access via a single fascial incision if the port requires upsizing for insertion of a larger instrument than initially anticipated. Separate snap-on flap 'toilet seat' reducers or universal reducer seals allow use of 5 and 10 mm instrumentation via 10/12 mm ports and Versaports (USSC, Norwalk, Connecticut) are produced with universal adapting seals. It is always desirable to utilize the smallest trocars possible to minimize the morbidity of the fascial and muscular puncture and to limit the number of port sites requiring fascial closure. In adult patients, it is not necessary to close 5 mm port sites; however, these should be closed in children due to the risk of omental herniation. Instruments requiring more controlled movements such as the Endovascular stapling or EndoStitch device (AutoSuture, Norwalk, Connecticut) are preferably manipulated using the surgeon's dominant hand at an acceptable angle for application, which dictates location of the appropriate trocar size.

Trocar length

A standard trocar length of 75 mm in pediatric and 100 mm in adult patients of average size adequately penetrates the abdominal wall and provides stable access to the abdominal cavity. In some morbidly obese patients, extra long trocars measuring 120 mm may be required to prevent the trocar from backing out of the peritoneum, which can be time consuming to reintroduce and lead to subcutaneous emphysema. The abdominal pannus is a mobile structure in obese patients and is often hanging medial and inferior to the corresponding fascial entry point for patients in the flank position. More cephalad and lateral introduction of the ports is required in these patients for proper access to retroperitoneal organs when approached in a transperitoneal fashion.[9] This also avoids the excess thickness of the subcutaneous fat contained within the abdominal pannus.

Potential pitfalls of trocar placement

Inadequate trocar spacing

In general, ports should be placed a distance apart corresponding approximately to that between the index and little finger to limit crossing instruments or so-called sword fighting. Instruments may still cross with extreme movements, even with the widest separation of the port sites. Utilizing an angled lens can minimize these interactions, if they are due to the laparoscope. If interactions are due to the instrument of an assistant, the offending device can usually be inserted via a different port site, which results in less interference. Other elements the surgeon should always be aware of when planning port placement include osseous barriers such as the ribs, pelvis, or spine and the edge of any inserted hand-assist device. All of these structures can inhibit deflection of the instruments. The amount of separation required from these areas is fairly minimal when they are close to the fulcrum point of the port. Downward and lateral deflection of instruments should also be inspected prior to insertion of the ports to avoid inadequate tip movements due to contact with the table, padding, or extremities.

Mirror imaging

Any time the angle created between the inserted laparoscope and the operating instrument exceeds 90°, mirror imaging occurs in the primary tower, leading to counter-intuitive movements. In general, positioning the camera port between the operating surgeon's two working ports is preferable. However, as long as the laparoscope is inserted within a 90° array of the two introduced working instruments, the procedure can usually be performed without difficulties due to mirror imaging. It is important to take into consideration the extent of the dissection and to have an appropriate plan for shifting the position of the laparoscope if necessary to avoid counter-intuitive movements. If possible, it is also best to limit the amount of mirror imaging experienced by the assistant surgeon in the secondary tower to expedite the flow of the operation.

Exiting the abdomen

Final inspection

Once the laparoscopic operation has been completed, the areas of the dissection should be thoroughly inspected for any signs of bleeding or occult visceral injury. If questionable biliary or pancreatic injuries are present, a drain may be required for adequate monitoring and drainage. All serosal bowel injuries should be repaired either laparoscopically or via an extended port incision as these can ultimately lead to perforation and fistulization, especially when they are a result of thermal injury.[7]

Once the surrounding structures are determined to be free of injury and hemostasis is deemed adequate, all dissection sites should be reinspected under low insufflation pressures of 5 mmHg pressure. Higher intraperitoneal pressures can tamponade regions of venous bleeding resulting in unnecessary post-insufflation blood loss and possible hematoma formation. Hemostasis of any observed areas of bleeding can then be obtained using the harmonic shears, electrocautery, direct pressure with surgical cellulose (Surgicel, Johnson & Johnson, Inc., Arlington, Texas), hemoclips, laparoscopic suturing, fibrin glue, or other techniques.[10] The entry point of each trocar should also be inspected for bleeding on removal and insertion of the port closure sutures. If vigorous abdominal wall bleeding is noted from any of these sites, it may require placement of a figure-of-eight suture rather than a simple closure stitch, especially in cases of inferior epigastric vessel injury.

Fascial port closure

There are several options available for closure of laparoscopic port sites. In patients with minimal amounts of subcutaneous fat, one option is direct vision closure. This is accomplished using narrow, deep retractors such as the Army–Navy retractors to expose the underlying fascia. Sutures of 0-Vicryl mounted on a semicircular needle are then passed through the cut edges of the fascia, which are then tied together to complete the closure. Subfascial herniations at laparoscopic port sites have been reported, indicating the benefit of including the peritoneal layer in the closure.[11] The peritoneum is not incorporated when a direct vision closure is performed in an adult patient, thereby increasing the risk of this type of herniation.

A more reliable method of closing the port site utilizes a suture-grasping needle such as the Carter–Thomason device (Inlet Medical Inc., Eden Prairie, Minnesota), which includes both the fascia and peritoneum in the closure.[12] One effective technique for obtaining a good fascial closure using the Carter–Thomason device involves removal of the port and insertion of the index finger of the non-dominant hand into the defect. This prevents release of the pneumoperitoneum and allows the surgeon to feel the cut edges of the fascia. The thumb and first two fingers of the dominant hand are inserted into the handle of the device. As the thumb is drawn back in the spring-loaded handle, the jaw opens. The thumb is then squeezed toward the index and middle fingers to close the jaws, which squeeze together to grasp a 0-Vicryl suture approximately 1 cm back from its end.

The grasping needle is inserted below the skin level and through the center portion of the fascial edge until it can be visualized with the laparoscope entering the intraperitoneal space. The speed of entry is controlled by pinching the shaft of the needle between the side of the inserted index finger and the pad of the thumb (Figure 6.9). It is critical to maintain direct vision of the tip of the Carter–Thomason needle as it enters the peritoneum to avoid inadvertent injury to the bowel, solid viscera, or vasculature. The grasping needle is advanced for a distance of 1–2 cm into the peritoneal cavity and is then withdrawn slightly to create slack in the introduced loop of suture. The assistant uses a grasper to grab a portion of the suture within the peritoneal cavity. The handles of the closure device are separated to open the jaws of the grasping needle, which releases the suture as the assistant pulls it from the jaws of the device. The jaws of the Carter–Thomason device are then closed and it is withdrawn. The grasping needle is then reinserted through the fascia on the opposite side of the incision and into the peritoneal cavity. The jaws of the Carter–Thomason device are once again opened, the suture is passed into the jaws, and the end is pulled out through the fascia, completing placement of the simple closure stitch (see Figure 6.9). If the

surgeon does not wish to insert the grasping needle adjacent to his finger, a conical guide with side holes can be utilized or the needle can simply be passed along either side of the port itself.

When a laceration of an abdominal wall vessel occurs at the site of port closure, or a wide gap in the fascial defect exists, the Carter–Thomason device can also be utilized to place a figure-of-eight instead of a simple stitch. Once passage of the suture is complete, the trocar is then reinserted using the blunt obturator and the stitch is tagged until a similar closure suture has been placed at each of the other port sites.

An alternative needle closure device is the EndoClose (AutoSuture, Norwalk, Connecticut), which functions similar to the Carter–Thomason needle but relies on a retractable hook on the internal obturator of the needle to grasp the suture. As the thumb of the dominant hand pushes down on a spring-loaded button on the handle of the device, the obturator advances, releasing the hooked suture, which is then grasped by the assistant. The needle is reinserted through the cut fascia of the opposite side and the button is depressed to once again expose the hook. The suture is wrapped around the needle and slid into the crotch of the hook. As the button is released, the hooked

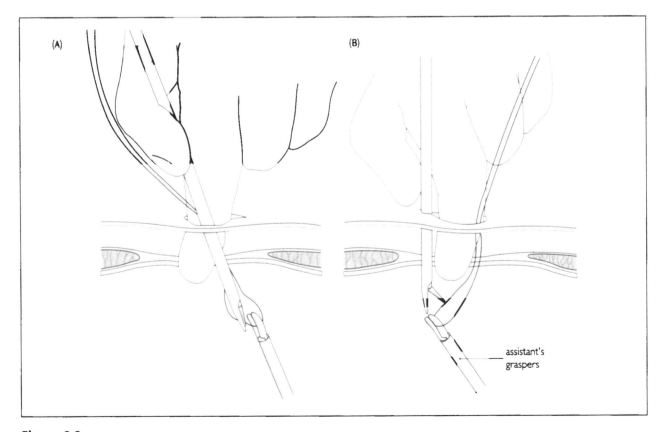

(A)   (B)

assistant's
graspers

Figure 6.9

(A) The Carter–Thomason closure device (Inlet Medical Inc., Eden Prairie, Minnesota) introduces a 0-Vicryl suture through one of the fascial edges, which is then grasped by an assistant. (B) The grasping needle is reinserted through the opposite fascial edge and the assistant transfers the suture back into the jaws of the device, which is then withdrawn to complete the stitch.

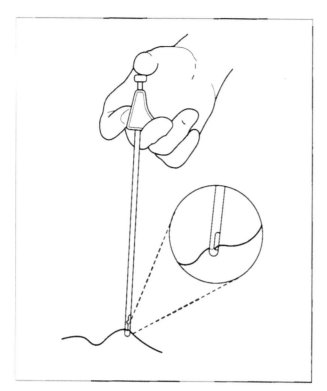

Figure 6.10
The EndoClose (AutoSuture, Norwalk, Connecticut) fascial-suturing needle functions in similar fashion to the Carter–Thomason device, but utilizes a retractable hook instead of grasping jaws to secure and transfer the suture through the fascial edges.

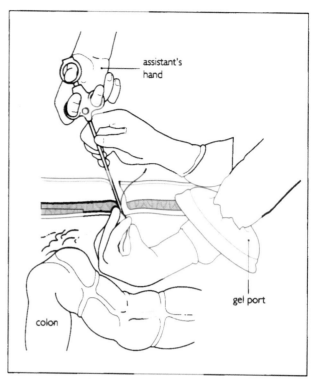

Figure 6.11
Fascial closure being performed using the Carter–Thomason device and a hand inserted via the hand-assist port. The surgical assistant manipulates the handle of the Carter–Thomason device as the primary surgeon grasps the shaft of the needle and controls the speed and location of its insertion. The introduced hand acts like the grasper during a standard laparoscopic closure and performs the suture transfer into and out of the jaws of the fascial closure device.

suture is pulled tight against the edge of the needle by the retracted obturator and the suture is drawn out through the fascia to complete the stitch (Figure 6.10).

Closing the hand-assist port and accessory ports

If a hand-assist port is utilized, the inserted hand is used to grasp the suture and to perform the exchanges between the jaws of the Carter–Thomason or EndoClose device, much like the grasping instrument was utilized during port closure on the standard laparoscopic cases. To control entry of the fascial closure device, the assistant squeezes the handle of the grasper, keeping the jaws closed on the suture, while the operating surgeon advances the grasping needle through the fascia. The inserted hand can be cupped beneath the area of the fascial defect, with the middle finger inserted into the defect to prevent escape of the pneumoperitoneum. Care must be taken to prevent inadvertent injury to the inserted hand. Once the suture enters the abdomen, it is grasped between the thumb and forefinger of the inserted hand and is drawn in further to

facilitate passage to the jaws of the closure device after it has been inserted through the other side of the fascia (Figure 6.11). The trocars are reinserted, as outlined previously, until all closure sutures have been placed, and are then tied down with the inserted hand separating the peritoneal organs from the abdominal wall to prevent entrapment.

Desufflation of the abdomen

The 5 mm trocar sites should be removed prior to tying the fascial closure sutures of the 10/12 mm ports. This allows potential placement of a closure stitch at these sites, while the 10/12 mm ports can still be utilized should port-site bleeding occur. Each of the 10/12 mm ports are removed under visual inspection, leaving the umbilical port (supine case) or the lower quadrant port (flank case) until the end. Once all of the other fascial closure sutures have been tied down, the insufflant is shut off and the side port of the remaining trocar is opened. The patient is positioned so the final exit port is elevated and the laparoscope is directed into all remaining areas of the pneumoperitoneum as a hand is used to compress the abdominal wall, assisting in evacuation of the insufflant. The anesthesiologist is instructed to give the patient several large extended breaths to help in expulsion of any areas of collected pneumoperitoneum beneath the diaphragm. Once desufflation appears complete, the fascial closure suture of the one remaining port is elevated and the trocar is slid out, leaving the laparoscopic lens in place within the peritoneal cavity. The lens is slowly withdrawn in a vertical orientation, taking care to observe the peritoneal contents falling back into the abdominal cavity as the laparoscope passes out through the muscular fascia.

For hand-assisted laparoscopic procedures, desufflation can be performed quite effectively via the hand-assist incision. The omentum should be used to cover the underlying viscera in the base of the incision whenever possible to prevent adhesion formation and reduce the risk of bowel entrapment. The hand-assist incision is then closed using a running #1 polydioxanone surgical (PDS) suture in patients with healthy fascia. If wound healing comorbidities exist, such as steroid use, diabetes, or obesity, interrupted figure-of-eight nonabsorbable permanent sutures should be utilized.

The skin incisions are irrigated with an antibiotic solution and injected with 0.25% bupivacaine. Several interrupted 3-0 Vicryl dermal sutures are placed for hand-assist or organ extraction incisions followed by a running absorbable subcuticular suture and Steri-strips. Band-Aids or small folded gauze dressings are placed at trocar sites and an adhesive island dressing is applied to the hand-assist or organ extraction site.

Potential pitfalls of exiting the abdomen

Inadequate desufflation and shoulder pain

Carbon dioxide insufflant is a peritoneal irritant and residual collections beneath the diaphragm can irritate the muscle, causing referred pain to the region of the shoulder, scapular muscles, and trapezius. Once this condition occurs, the patient can be quite uncomfortable and must await eventual resorption of the pneumoperitoneum. Prevention via careful and complete release of all insufflant is paramount. Methods to reduce the discomfort include periods of supine or head-down positioning to displace the carbon dioxide to regions of the peritoneum away from the diaphragm. Anti-inflammatory pain medication and warm shoulder packs can also provide varying degrees of relief.

Bowel or omental herniation

The incidence of port-site herniation is approximately 1% in most published series and is usually due to a poor fascial closure, but it can result from associated factors such as localized infection, diabetes, coughing, or steroid use.[2,13] Trocar sites where the fascial incision is extended for specimen extraction are also at higher risk for herniation, possibly due to fascial attenuation that can occur from torquing the laparoscopic ports during the procedure and on removal of the specimen.[13] At port sites through which specimen morcellation is performed, it is advisable to place a figure-of-eight or several interrupted sutures as additional tension and stretching of fascial fibers often occurs during the fragmentation process. It has been suggested in the literature and by the manufacturers of fascial-splitting trocars that it is not necessary to close the fascial defects created by these ports due to their low risk of herniation.[2] A case of herniation following use of one of these trocars in a donor nephrectomy patient has recently been reported.[14] As a result, we now recommend closure of the fascia for all 10/12 mm port types.

In pediatric patients, closure of 5 mm ports is also recommended, due to the potential for omental herniation. These ports can usually be closed via the skin incision under direct vision, due to the limited amount of subcutaneous fat in pediatric patients, although fascial closure devices may be more efficient in larger or older children.

Presenting signs of port-site herniation vary depending upon the timing of the occurrence and the presence or absence of bowel ischemia. On occasion, evidence of asymptomatic herniation may be found incidentally during follow-up imaging studies or physical examination. Patients can also present with more subtle signs of intermittent bowel obstruction or, at the other end of the spectrum, with severe acute obstruction manifested by abdominal distention, nausea, and vomiting. If the prolapsed portion of bowel becomes ischemic, focal trocar site pain, diffuse abdominal pain, and eventually signs of bowel necrosis, abdominal wall cellulitis, peritonitis, and sepsis can ensue.

In the acute setting, it may be possible to manage a herniation via laparoscopic reduction. Open exploration, however, is preferable in the acutely ill patient in whom complete bowel inspection and potential resection is required.

Abdominal wall vessel bleeding

Epigastric or abdominal wall vessel lacerations may not become evident until the trocars are removed at the end of the case, since the port can tamponade the point of injury. Placement of a figure-of-eight suture around the bleeding vessel using a grasping needle such as the Carter–Thomason device can be used to obtain hemostasis, which is then confirmed under direct visual inspection. Other methods, such as the use of electrocautery or an inserted Foley catheter whose balloon is inflated and pulled tight against the bleeding point, have also been utilized.[10] On occasion, open exposure and ligation of the lacerated vessel is required. Lack of early recognition of this condition can lead to significant blood loss and large rectus or abdominal wall hematoma formation.

Conclusions

Careful access entry, trocar placement, and exiting the peritoneum or retroperitoneum are critical elements of any laparoscopic operation. These steps require the same degree of forethought and careful execution as the procedure itself to insure success of the operation and avoid potential complications.

References

1. Chandler JG, Corson SL, Way LW. Three spectra of laparoscopic entry access injuries. J Am Coll Surg 2001; 192:478–90.

2. Shalhav AL, Barret E, Lifshitz DA, et al. Transperitoneal laparoscopic renal surgery using blunt 12 mm trocar without fascial closure. J Endourol 2002; 16:43–6.

3. Purohit S, Slakey D, Conerly V, et al. Making hand-assisted laparoscopy easier: preventing CO_2 leak. J Endourol 2001; 15:943–6.

4. Capelouto CC, Moore RG, Silverman SG, Kavoussi LR. Retroperitoneoscopy: an anatomical rationale for direct retroperitoneal access. J Urol 1994; 152:2008–10.

5. Gill IS. Retroperitoneal laparoscopic nephrectomy. Urol Clin N Am 1998; 25:343–60.

6. Wolf JS. Pathophysiologic effects of prolonged laparoscopic operation. Semin Surg Oncol 1996; 12:86–95.

7. Bishoff JT, Allaf ME, Kirkels W, et al. Laparoscopic bowel injury: incidence and clinical presentation. J Urol 1999; 161:887–90.

8. Cadeddu JA, Regan F, Kavoussi LR, Moore RG. The role of computerized tomography in the evaluation of complications after laparoscopic urological surgery. J Urol 1997; 158:1349–52.

9. Nakada SY, Hedican SP, Moon TD. Hand-assisted laparoscopy in the morbidly and profoundly obese. J Endourol 2003; 16 (suppl 1):A113 (abst P21–9).

10. McGinnis DE, Strup SE, Gomella LG. Management of hemorrhage during laparoscopy. J Endourol 2000; 14:915–20.

11. Montz FJ, Holschneider CH, Munro MG. Incisional hernia following laparoscopy: a survey of the American Association of Gynecologic Laparoscopists. Obstet Gynecol 1994; 4:143–8.

12. Carter JE. A new technique of fascial closure for laparoscopic incisions. J Laparoendosc Surg 1994; 4:143–8.

13. Elashry OM, Giusti G, Nadler RB, et al. Incisional hernia after laparoscopic nephrectomy with intact specimen removal: caveat emptor. J Urol 1997; 158:363–9.

14. Lowry PS, Moon TD, D'Alessandro A, Nakada SY. Symptomatic port site hernia associated with a non-bladed trocar following laparoscopic live-donor nephrectomy. J Endourol 2003; 17(7):493–4.

7

Laparoscopic training – basic skills to complex skills

Debora K Moore and Robert G Moore

Over 200 articles have been written dealing with laparoscopic training models, but few are related to urology. In fact, in the last 8 years, <20 articles have been written pertaining to educational aspects of training laparoscopic urological skills![1–13]

Educational principles

To improve our ability as surgical educators, it is helpful to review studies in adult learning theory and the acquisition of technical skills. Research on the acquisition of surgical technical skill has traditionally adopted a theory described by Kopta.[14] He defined three phases of learning a skill – starting with cognitive learning, progressing to integration of knowledge with appropriate motor behavior, and, finally, a phase is reached in which performance is smooth, automatic, and resistant to stress.[15] Later studies question the notion of automaticity. Apparent automaticity observed in expert performance is believed to actually reflect development of a complex cognitive network. This complex network facilitates improved prediction, awareness, and cognitive representation of tasks.[16]

Using the principles of 'learning hierarchies', a concept at the heart of the behavioralist school of thought, an individual must learn basic component skills of a routine before progressing to the full routine ('chunking').[17] More simply put, one breaks a complex task into simple components and then integrates them after successfully mastering each component.

Cognitive theories support the idea that repetitive practice facilitates the subsequent performance of motor activities by permitting more efficient interpretation of proprioceptive, visual, and tactile feedback.[18] Neurophysiologic testing has further illuminated the value of a prior perceptual framework. These are standardized instruments that measure specific components of motor skills, including pure motor ability, imagery, and visuospatial orientation. Schueneman et al conducted neurophysiologic tests on surgical residents, correlating results with

faculty ratings of their surgical skill.[19] They found no correlation between surgical skill and pure motor abilities such as speed and precision. Instead, surgical skill ratings correlated with a complex of activities, including but not limited to visuospatial organization, somatosensory memory, and stress tolerance. 'Visuospatial perceptual skill' is the ability to use landmarks to create a mental picture of relationships in three-dimensional space. 'Somatosensory memory' is the ability to interpret sensory cues based on prior experience. 'Stress tolerance' is the ability to distinguish essential detail from nonessential detail.[20]

Shadmehr and Holcomb looked at neural correlates of motor memory consolidation. They monitored changes in cerebral blood flow, an indirect marker of neural activity, using positron emission tomography to study the acquisition of newly learned motor skills. They concluded that it takes 4–6 hours for the memory of new skills to shift from prefrontal regions of the cortex, a temporary storage site, to the premotor, posterior parietal, and cerebellar cortex structures, which represent permanent storage. Using this information, they felt that allowing for this time passage before teaching a new motor skill should increase functional stability of the previously learned skills.[21]

Current educational theories emphasize the importance of incorporating cognitive learning side by side with skill practice and drills. Frequent feedback is essential and must incorporate both cognitive and technical elements.[22] Lastly, it has been well documented that adult learning is enhanced by a self-directed approach centered on the learner not the teacher, with specific goals identified and in which continued constructive feedback is given.[23]

Using these concepts to train surgeons in laparoscopic surgery requires a program that allows the trainee to enhance proprioceptive and tactile perceptions while developing visuospatial orientation through an operative video camera. Once mastered, this foundation can be used to develop perceptual experience with more difficult surgical skills. Frequent and repetitive practice appears to be important to retention of these skills. If somatosensory memory not pure motor ability is important, tissue models that closely resemble true surgical tissues would be valuable. Improving perceptual skills, providing a thorough knowledge of laparoscopic equipment, including their capabilities and limitations, and adherence to surgical principles, enhances stress tolerance. Finally, in order for an education program to be effective it should honor the principles of adult education, allowing for self-directed learning and continued feedback.

Problems specific to laparoscopic training

Training residents to operate has traditionally been done in the operating room using a system introduced by Halsted more than a century ago.[24, 25]

Customarily, open surgical skills have been acquired by hands-on experience, allowing tactile sensation and direct vision of the tissue under the guidance of an experienced surgeon. Minimally invasive surgery presents significant and unique challenges to the traditional modes of training that need to be addressed in order for it to be performed in a quality fashion.[26]

The first challenge to overcome is working in a three-dimensional field off a two-dimensional image monitor: in simple terms, the operator loses depth perception. Studies have shown that the mind will not accept the lack of depth perception on the video monitor and will subconsciously project depth.[27,28] To compensate for loss in depth perception, visual cues are used to aid in position determination.[29] Motion parallax, the motion of an instrument past the camera while it remains in a fixed position, angulation, the angle of the instruments when introduced into the visual field, and known reference points, all contribute to the estimation of depth on a flat screen. Touching an object in the visual field creates a known reference point and this mentally aids in depth perception during laparoscopic procedures.

Another difficulty encountered in learning to perform laparoscopic surgical skills is that the current trocars and instruments used have restricted degrees of operative movement and many deny any wrist or elbow motion. This problem of restricted degrees of freedom is compounded by the fulcrum or lever effect currently inherent in laparoscopic surgery. Because the trocar, through which the instrument passes, is fixed in the abdominal wall, an upward movement of the instrument handle causes a downward displacement of the end effectors and vice versa. To minimize this restriction, trocar and camera positions should be optimized; ideal positions have been determined by the experts in the field for each individual procedure and approach and can easily be referenced.[30]

Next, when performing laparoscopic surgery, there is a loss of tactile feedback used by surgeons to differentiate tissue types. Using two laparoscopic instruments and frequently touching objects in the visual field provides some sensory input. Again, this maneuver also assists the surgeon in maintaining a three-dimensional orientation to the two-dimensional video image.

Educating surgeons in laparoscopic techniques

Concerns about the adequacy of surgical education have been increasing. Countless problems exist in surgical education, such as increasing constraints imposed on operative time, the changing patient population at teaching hospitals, heightened medicolegal considerations, and the higher cost of running residency programs. With laparoscopy, these problems are amplified and apply not only to surgical residents but also to all surgeons in practice who want to keep up with new techniques. Thus, there is an urgent need to improve on the current quality of residency and post-residency training methods.

In order to progress, educators in urology need to examine the teaching methods being used today critically and to have knowledge about the background literature, as general surgery has been investigating methods to educate surgeons in laparoscopic technique since laparoscopic cholecystectomy appeared on the scene in the mid–late 1980s.[31,32] With the initial high rate of complications with this procedure and even some reported deaths, they have had to re-evaluate how to educate and train surgeons to perform such procedures.[33–35] This literature contains a wealth of information that we can use. Mistakes can be avoided if we are willing to take the time to educate ourselves and apply the information. Dogma needs to be put to rest and we need to base our teaching on scientifically based facts.

Laparoscopic skill development is related to recent and ongoing laparoscopic training and experience

Open surgical skills are based on an ensemble of techniques that can be transferred from one procedure to another. During open surgery training it has been demonstrated that learning basic surgical skills allows surgical residents to build on those skills for more complex or related skills. Transfer of training (TOT) is the term used for this process and it is a necessary process in the development of open surgical technical skills.

Many assumed that TOT from open skills takes place to laparoscopic skills and for years we have heard the comment that 'the best laparoscopic surgeons are the best open surgeons,' but studies by Figert et al refute this.[36] In their study, transference of open surgical skills to laparoscopic skills was specifically examined and it was assumed that more experienced open surgeons have shorter learning curves for new surgical procedures secondary to TOT. No evidence was found for TOT from open surgical experience to newly introduced laparoscopic knot-tying techniques or from one skill training session to a different skill session at least 4 hours later. More notable is that their data suggests that specific laparoscopic skills might not be transferable to acquisition of different laparoscopic surgical skills. These findings may explain why surgical residents and experienced open surgeons do not differ significantly when learning new laparoscopic skills. These findings further support what has been recognized by others but never documented: laparoscopic skill development is related to recent and ongoing laparoscopic training and experience. Collectively, this information supports the concept that specific minimally invasive surgery training is needed to develop laparoscopic surgery skills.[36]

Inherent surgeon characteristics

It has been a commonly held assumption that younger surgeons have a natural advantage in the development of surgical skills. The affects of age, gender, lateral dominance, and prediction of open operative skills among general surgery residents was examined. In one study investigators found that, while age influenced pure motor skills, neither age nor pure motor skills are necessarily important for open operative skills. In fact it was stated that 'contrary to surgical folklore, pure psychomotor skill (manual dexterity) is not the major dimension distinguishing the proficient surgical performance from the mediocre.' It was found that the components necessary for superior open surgical skills included nonverbal, visuospatial problem-solving abilities (i.e. the capacity to rapidly analyze and organize perceptions based on multisensory information) and the ability to distinguish essential from nonessential detail even when the 'signal-to-noise ratio' is high.[18,19]

Rosser et al in the development of the 'Yale Laparoscopic Boot Camp' also found that age and sex did not play a dominant role in skills outcome.[37] All participants who attended the courses, regardless of age, sex, and previous training, learned intracorporeal suturing and performed an anastomosis. The performance of all participants improved in the study. Collectively, the residents took

marginally longer to complete an anastomosis, although their suturing time was not significantly different from that of a trained surgeon. The difference between the residents and trained surgeons was felt to be due to a lack of experience in performing anastomosis rather than in suturing skills. Residents took more time to perform the cup drop drill, which requires considerable depth perception to the two-dimensional environment. However, residents performed significantly better than trained surgeons in the triangle transfer drill, which requires two-hand skills as well as depth and spatial orientation. No difference was noted in the performance of male and female residents in performing either drills or suturing exercises. The finding that trained females took a longer time to complete suturing exercises and rope pass drills was only marginally significant ($p < 0.5$). Rosser et al concluded that age and experience might influence some types of dexterity drills, but overall they do not seem to play a dominant role.[37]

In a related study, Hayward et al compared the abilities of male and female residents in six areas: ethics, judgment, technical skills, knowledge, interpersonal skills, and work habits. Again, no difference was found between female and male residents.[38] Schueneman et al found that left-handed residents were more reactive to stress, more cautious, and more proficient on a neuropsychologic test of tactile-spatial abilities than right-handed counterparts. Although these traits correlated positively with rated open operative skills within the left-handed group, the group received consistently lower ratings than did right-handed residents. They hypothesized that the 'inconvenience' of assisting left-handed residents may overshadow attending surgeon's perceptions of their innate abilities.[19] More recently, Hanna et al re-examined psychomotor skills for endoscopic manipulations for minimally invasive surgery and the differing abilities between right- and left-handed individuals.[39] They found that right-handed subjects performed better with either hand in terms of error rate and first-time accuracy than left-handed individuals. Their findings are consistent with previous reports on psychomotor studies that showed left-handed people have poorer spatial perception than right-handed subjects.[40–43] However, many others have not supported this difference.[44–46] Right-handed subjects also performed tasks in a shorter execution time but with more force on the target than left-handed individuals. The longer execution time by the left-handed subjects with application of less force on the target are in agreement with the reported observations of Schueneman et al and appear to support the concept that left-handed surgical residents are more cautious than right-handed counterparts. These particular findings demonstrate significant, neuropsychologically based differences among surgery residents that pose unique challenges to persons responsible for their education and training.

Teaching surgical skills outside the operating room – the influence of technology, inanimate models, and simulators

Teaching skills in the operating room is inefficient, and expensive, and learning on patients is no longer acceptable. Current curriculums have been designed to train residents outside of the operating room, but no consensus exists as to what type of training is appropriate and how much training is necessary to effectively impact operative performance.[13,47] Rapid acceptance of laparoscopic surgery has resulted in high complications, especially with novice surgeons. It has been consistently reported that surgical complications occur most frequently during the first 10 procedures that the laparoscopic trainee performs.[32,33,35] The importance of adequate education and accruement of appropriate skills before attempting procedures on live patients have been highlighted by this high rate of serious complications.[48]

While it has been proven that texts, lectures, and video are important tools for developing insight into the essentials of an operation, they are of limited value due to their didactic nature. Naturally, laboratories with simple inanimate models or live animals for hands-on training allows each surgeon to practice prior to performing the procedure on a patient and therefore they have been included in the current surgical training models. Inanimate models rather than animal models are popular for training outside the operating room because they are reproducible, offer unlimited practice, are readily available and require no supervision.

In 1997 Martin et al examined the reliability of assessing the technical skills of surgical trainees using live vs bench formats. The bench model simulation gave equivalent results to use of live animals with their testing format.[49] Further studies were conducted and it has been proven that practice in these simulators results in an improvement in the skills practiced and assayed in the same simulator.[50]

These simulators allow for practice at various skill levels and, in addition, since many surgeons may not have access to an animal laboratory facility, it is reasonable to use such inanimate models; however, there are drawbacks. The initial simple box laparoscopic trainer was not designed to simulate a specific surgical procedure and its only function is to serve as a fundamental training device for basic skills used in the majority of surgical operations. Also, the more simple and basic training boxes do not mimic human anatomy and living tissue. Furthermore, Jordon et al argues that the use of a box trainer fails to provide trainees with any clear indications of their level of manual dexterity, their progress in training, or even a comparison with their peers.[51]

Recently, Scott et al showed that skills acquired from dry labs using the Guided Endoscopic Module (GEM, Karl Storz Endoscopy, Culver City, California), a training system, were transferable to the operating room.[52] Until this time, studies in the outcome of dry lab training measured improved skills on the same simulator on which the training took place and not in the operating room, so the true transfer of skills training was unknown.

Once the use of basic simulators was shown to be effective in skill acquisition, the need to make them more sophisticated or lifelike came into play. Use of multimedia interactive computer-based training used in such areas as the military, high-tech industries, and even the business world, was examined. Given the fact that multimedia interactive computer-based training has been shown to decrease the learning curve by 60% and increase retention by 50% when compared to traditional didactic training, its use in laparoscopic surgical training was attractive.[53] Multimedia interactive programs have the advantage that they are self-directed, self-paced, and interactive, which is consistent with the proven methods of adult learning. Since programs can be developed from the experience of many surgeons, the emphasis is placed on correct surgical principles for the performance of a specific procedure. The steps of the procedure and the variety of presentations of complications possible at each step of the procedure become the focus, and the experience of many becomes additive to the teaching process. Multimedia interactivity, input from many experts, and an ability to individualize the pace of the learning experience are unique advantages to these training programs.[22]

Using such a program, the Minimally Invasive Surgical Trainer Virtual Reality system (MIST VR, Mentice, AB, Gothenberg, Sweden), Seymour et al in a randomized, double-blinded study found improvement in the operating room performance of residents.[54] This appears to be the first study demonstrating that it is feasible to train operative skills using virtual reality in surgical trainees without extensive prior minimally invasive experience that transfer to the real environment, i.e. the operating room. Further analysis of virtual reality training for technical error reduction, surgical judgment, or even as a means of certifying surgeons remains to be addressed.

Finally, European physicians have not had the luxury of using animal models for surgical training, and practicing in the patient setting has been frowned upon. Consequently, other methods of surgical education and training have been sought sooner and the European community has undergone a multi-institutional project, named the Minimally Invasive Surgery SIMUlator (MISSIMU), with the joint efforts of clinical European centers and two European Industries.[55] While other projects have utilized three-dimensional reproduction to represent human anatomy, this project is more advanced in that its goal is to provide a virtually 'living' human body, inside which it would be possible to perform laparoscopic surgery with tactile sensations and force feedback.[56,57] We await the outcomes of this project.

What training equipment is necessary?

Training can be obtained with even the most meager budget. Keyser and colleagues compared a simplified mirrored-box simulator (Simuview) to the videolaparoscopic cart system.[58] They found that laparoscopic skills can be measured objectively in a videolaparoscopic cart simulator system and the scores were sufficiently sensitive to distinguish differences in performance between residents at different levels of training. The low-cost mirrored-box simulator also gave a reasonable reflection of relative performance of laparoscopic skills. Therefore, if these skills demonstrate transfer to the operating room, a practical, effective basic laparoscopic skills training and evaluation can be accomplished without the need for costly equipment.

Gallagher et al subjected the MIST VR to a prospective, comparative evaluation with traditional laboratory training methods for psychomotor skill (manual dexterity) acquisition only.[59] They found that participants trained on the MIST VR performed significantly better than case-matched participants trained on a traditional box trainer and a control group who received no training. Although manual dexterity is important for surgical procedures, as recalled from the previous sections, it is only a portion of the skills needed for laparoscopic procedures and, again, the cost vs benefits need to be carefully weighed in this situation. Although the incorporation of new training tools such as multimedia interactive programs into surgical training is exciting, there are still many issues to be resolved. Although presumed, will the increased knowledge and comfort levels afforded its user translate into shortened learning curves and fewer complications? Although this benefit has been shown in other industries, does it also apply to laparoscopic surgery?

Many simulators are appearing on the market but, to date, no comparison studies have been performed. The key question – Is there transfer of training? – has not been addressed for all simulators. Remembering the sage advice that 'a fool and his money are soon parted', one has to examine these simulators critically and look at scientific data, the actual skill transfer to the operating room, and not at advertisements or endorsements from 'laparoscopic superstars'.

Experienced surgeon – another key component for laparoscopic teaching

Once you have embarked on a training model, what else can you do to optimize laparoscopic teaching? The Laparoscopic Education Study Group identified a teacher base skilled in laparoscopy as a key component to establishing a successful education program. Without this, a training program limits preceptorship and tutorial portions of resident laparoscopic education.[60]

To enhance resident training, programs have hired an experienced laparoscopic surgeon. Fowler and Hogle looked at the impact that this had on their program and found that with the addition of an experienced laparoscopic surgeon in a resident training program laparoscopic cases in which residents participate increased by more than 100%.[61] Laparoscopic training sessions and minimally invasive research projects also increased measurably.

More and more residents desire to learn the techniques and acquire the skills needed to perform advanced procedures. Although several fellowships in laparoscopic urology are available, demand for these positions far exceeds their availability and there is no uniformity in the education of these fellows. Numerous residency programs have hired such trained laparoscopic surgeons, often by appointing that surgeon to a position such as 'director of minimally invasive surgery'. The acute goal has been to expose both faculty and residents to more advanced laparoscopic procedures, with the ultimate goal of teaching them to perform the procedures. Our personal communications with other fellowship-trained laparoscopic surgeons acting in this role revealed that this endeavor has received results ranging from enthusiasm, to trepidation, and even animosity in various institutions.

Costs

A final concern is the cost involved with training laparoscopic skills. In 2000, the list price for a video trainer (guided Endoscopic Module) ranged from $215,000–$285,000 depending on the quality of video-imaging equipment installed. At the University of Texas Southwestern Medical Center, a total of 186 residents train in general surgery, urology, and gynecology. The cost of training residents using the video trainer was estimated as $270 per graduating resident.[52] In comparison, Bridges and Diamond,[62] at the University of Tennessee Medical Center–Knoxville, estimated that using operating room time to train residents costs about $48,000 per graduating resident.

Intuitively, training outside of the operating room seems cost-effective, but a comparison with an institution that hires a laparoscopic-trained staff to teach and perform complex laparoscopic cases with simpler methods needs to be made. Staff can generate revenue while the simulator cannot.

How does one measure operative skills?

The teaching model is in effect: now one must answer how does one measure success or progress? A major pitfall of training models is the lack of objective assessment used to document improvement or proficiency. Many studies use time to complete a task as the sole assessment of competency. Time assessment alone does not document the steps taking place between the starting and stopping of the stopwatch. It is believed that using time alone to measure skill level overestimates the true levels of laparoscopic skill. In fact, investigators using a laparoscopic skills assessment device that precisely measures movements of instruments during performance of laparoscopic manipulative skills found that the learning curve for operator speed is shorter than the learning curve for operator accuracy.[63] Therefore, laparoscopic accuracy is a more sensitive indicator of skill acquisition than measurement of laparoscopic speed, suggesting a minimum of both variables needs to be considered in developing teaching modules and proficiency standards. Common sense suggests that the main aspects of evaluation should concentrate on how the task is completed rather than on how fast the task is completed.

Operating room skill assessment

Global assessments of operative performance based on direct observation have been extensively studied in the context of open operations and simulations. Reznick and colleagues have shown that global assessments are superior to checklists in validity and reliability.[23] Global assessments are not procedure-specific but rate skill using general performance criteria. Therefore, such assessments may be used for different operations without modification and appear to be the best tool currently available for evaluating skill level in the operating room. Unfortunately, global assessments are almost as time consuming as the earlier checklists and a dedicated evaluator must be present for enough of the operation to draw conclusions about skill level.[64] Shortcuts using video monitoring have been attempted. Even if the assessment is applied to videotaped footage, so that the evaluator need not be present during the case, the entire operation must be viewed. Further attempts to maximize the efficient use of the reviewer's

time looked at the use of edited videotaping. Skill assessments were made from the edited tapes and compared to direct observation assessments.[26] It was discovered that the videotape evaluations did not demonstrate the difference in skill level between the trained and control groups that the direct observation assessments had detected. Also, correlation between videotape and direct observation scores were poor, and interpreter reliability suffered as a result of the videotape format.

The edited videotape contained only visual information and no audio or visual information from the external operating room environment was recorded. It was believed that this information was crucial to the assessment process. For example, were erratic movements attributable to a lack of resident dexterity or to interruption by the faculty for the purpose of teaching? Equipment problems were not detectable from the videotape and could be misinterpreted as unnecessary delays related to resident skill. Residents were asked to vocalize their operative plan and to identify anatomic landmarks during the evaluation and without sound the videotaping of the operation did not capture this information. Other areas that the evaluators could not assess included 'knowledge of instruments', 'use of assistants', and 'knowledge of specific procedure'. Again, this missing data on the videotape were believed to be the reason that videotape assessments did not correlate with assessments performed in the operating room.[26]

The investigators concluded that the wealth of information in the operating room was important to the evaluation process, including audio or visual information from the external operating room environment.

Role of robotics in education

Robotics represents the current frontier in minimally invasive procedures. Surgeons have recently been sorting through the facts and myriad of misinformation, trying to qualitatively and quantitatively analyze their effects. Sung and Gill compared the da Vinci (Intuitive Surgical, Inc., Mountain View, California) and ZEUS (Computer Motion, Inc., Goleta, California) systems and found that the learning curve and operative times were shorter, yet this may be biased by their being proficient at extremely difficult laparoscopic procedures without the use of robotics.[65] Dr Menon looked at open prostatectomies vs laparoscopic vs robotic prostatectomies.[66] His data are confusing due to the fact that different surgeons were involved at different arms. Experienced laparoscopic surgeons performed the laparoscopic procedures, while Dr Menon – using himself as the only inexperienced laparoscopic surgeon – performed robotic prostatectomies; however, he had previously assisted in over 100 pure laparoscopic procedures and the term 'inexperienced' may be inaccurate. Lee and colleagues have stated that in their experience there is a difference in the learning curve with using robotics but their study uses time for an objective parameter, which when used alone is insufficient. As discussed earlier, performing a procedure quicker does not correlate with better results and, more importantly, failing to consider objective assessments of accuracy may lead to overestimating laparoscopic proficiency.[67]

Turning to our general surgery colleagues, Prasad et al[68] reported that laparoscopic tasks performed with ZEUS robotic assistance allowed for increasing speed and consistency while maintaining precision over multiple repetitions, whereas Dakin and Gagner[69] recently reported that basic laparoscopic task performance was generally faster and as precise using standard instruments when compared to the ZEUS robotic surgical system and the da Vinci Surgical System. In their trial when performing fine tasks neither robotic system was faster than standard instruments. Precision with the robots was enhanced over the standard instruments and in this respect may offer an advantage.

Here, as in other instances, TOT needs to be evaluated; also, inexperienced laparoscopic surgeons are the area of concern and testing in these subjects is paramount. Recent concerns about the availability of the robot and canceling cases because the surgeon does not have the skills necessary to complete the case purely laparoscopically were raised at the World Congress of Endourology 2002. Will complication levels be greater if surgeons who lack the skills to perform conventional lap skills short cut training and use the robot? Which is the correct order to proceed when training for laparoscopic procedures: pure laparoscopic rather than robotic, or vice versa? A better understanding of how robotics affects the learning curves will allow for modifications in the training experience with this new technology. Again, efforts need to be made to examine the appropriate teaching of laparoscopic skills closely to avoid major complications and maximize efficiency in training.

Telepresence surgery

The basic concept of telepresence surgery is that an experienced laparoscopic surgeon at a central site can offer assistance, mentored intervention, or guidance to colleagues less experienced at distant sites or even in nearby operating rooms. This concept became a reality in 1996 when Moore and Kavoussi published one of the first experiences in telepresence surgery.[4] However, although telemedicine mentoring and assistance during the learning curve have been successfully implemented in studies and would provide an acceptable bridge for those at the beginning of the laparoscopic learning curve, the medicolegal issues,

costs, and scheduling constraints continue to hinder its advancement in the United States. Other uses of telepresence surgery have been in teaching medical students.[70] Uses for telepresence surgery will continue to grow and its full potential use is still being determined. Chapter 55 gives a more comprehensive overview of surgical robotics and telepresence surgery.

Courses

Adaptation rates or skills transfer for trained surgeons attending the standard equipment company-sponsored courses remain disappointing. Follow-up surveys on surgeons who participate in these standard courses has revealed a low likelihood of adopting the 'taught' procedure.[2,3,5] These surveys have also shown that if the participants do not seek further training or do not have experienced surgeons to assist or proctor them during their initial cases, complication rates are increased. Furthermore, in advanced laparoscopic procedures, even when the inexperienced surgeon knows the complications that occur during the learning curve phase, the complication is not avoided by this knowledge. Quicker identification may be made from the knowledge but, again, prevention of complications is not reduced.

On the horizon is the use of internet-based 'courses' to educate surgeons. Webcast courses make any location where a computer is installed a classroom and programs without expert faculty can be exposed to minimally invasive techniques via this media. The course may be interactive or a simulation to enhance one's skills. Investigators are moving in this direction and the educational results remain to be seen.[71–73]

Suggestions on what to look for in a laparoscopic training course include:

- What are the course objectives and can they be met in the suggested format?
- What are the basic skill requirements and how may one obtain these skills if they are needed prior to the course?
- Are the principles of adult education being followed?
- What reinforcement material will be included to enable one to practice the skills or review the technique needed to successfully complete the skill being taught at the course?

The course should be used to hone your skills, correct your bad habits, review laparoscopic anatomy, review how the 'experts' handle the problems encountered in the laparoscopic approach, and review the complications and how to remedy or recognize them. Reinforcement material such as an interactive CD-ROM should allow one to 'practice' the procedure at home to ready oneself for performing the procedure independently or a videotape reviewing technique, problems encountered, and troubleshooting for such problems commonly encountered during the procedure also seems appropriate. Edited tapes of the surgical procedure, although highlighting the 'laparoscopic superstar's' talent, really appear to add little to the novice's learning experience, as the editing leaves out any problems that arose during the case and how to deal with them. Another important point to be aware of is that skill transfer from the course to the operative suite is higher when attending the course with a colleague or another person involved with the operating team.[2]

Moore simplified model of laparoscopic training

Currently, laparoscopic intracorporeal suturing is the most difficult exercise to master in the minimally invasive environment. Yet several investigators have shown that with training even the most inexperienced individual can learn to suture. Champion et al taught surgically inexperienced medical students to complete an extracorporeal suture with a 3-throw knot in an average of 3 min 12 s, while Moore et al taught surgically inexperienced first-year medical student intracorporeal laparoscopic suturing in which they had to complete two separate knots.[8,12,74] In this study objective criteria included time to complete the task and knot quality – Was the knot squared? Did it slip? – and each knot's breaking strength was recorded in newtons. The average time to throw two 2-0 silk knots was 7.1 min and 5.2 min for 4-0 silk. These outcomes are excellent when one compares the results of Pattaras et al, who reported that experienced laparoscopic surgeons using 2-0 polyester suture tied knots with 5 half hitches in an averaged 5.08 min/knot.[75]

The fact that training is needed for laparoscopic surgery is not disputed, but today there exists no consensuses on which tasks are suitable, how much training is needed, and who should be trained. Below is an example of our training model. Based on adult educational principles, it provides instant feedback to trainees, which we believe accelerates the laparoscopic learning process, and one-on-one interaction, which we believe avoids the pitfalls of trainees developing bad habits that need to be 'unlearned' if the learning was done entirely on a self-directed individual basis.[76]

In our program we start with didactic lectures with actual dry lab reinforcement to meet cognitive and technical goals. Subject material covered includes but is not limited to:

1. Light sources, video cameras, insufflators.
2. Pneumoperitoneum: physiologic changes and entry to and exit from peritoneal cavity.
3. Energy sources in laparoscopy.
4. Laparoscopic anatomy.
5. Laparoscopic procedures.

Developing basic skills

Drills to increase ambidexterity seem obvious. In our model, subjects are asked to use their non-dominant hand during everyday activities – brushing their teeth, eating, dressing, answering the phone, etc. Next, to overcome what we term 'right/left hand/brain dominance', a series of tracings or patterns are placed on a table in front of a mirror. While looking only into the mirror the pattern is traced right to left and left to right using both the dominant hand and non-dominant hand. The tracings start out very simple and become more and more complex. Instrument use has been previously described and is again demonstrated. Each individual takes time to acclimate to the instruments in a simple video box. The bounce technique (moving the instruments across the field in a stepwise fashion to get to the intended spot) to find one's instruments is taught and the subject practices this until moving the instrument directly to the intended position is not a problem. Subjects are taught to place their trocars in a diamond pattern and reminded that they are to have both hands on an instrument at all times. According to Hanna et al, a combination of a 60° manipulation angle with 60° elevation angle provides the shortest execution time and highest performance score when evaluating optimal port locations for intracorporeal knot tying and this is demonstrated.[77] Appropriate laparoscopic instruments are used to transfer various objects, including but not limited to rope, Penrose drains of various size, washers, needle caps, navy beans, etc. Next, to further laparoscopic spatial orientation, items are placed within other objects or onto a peg of varying sizes using both dominant and non-dominant hands. This is followed by two-handed drills: using two graspers and removing an object from a dish while placing another object into a second dish simultaneously; holding the camera with one hand and moving a washer onto a peg with the other hand; holding an 18-gauge needle in the air with one instrument, uncapping it and placing it down on the surface, picking the pieces up and in midair recapping the needle. Principles of retraction and countertraction are reviewed and demonstrated for cutting objects or various shapes from gauze sponges. A pattern is drawn on a gauze sponge and suspended in the training box at various positions from the 'bull's-eye' position in the working zone and later the pattern is moved to the right or far left of the working area. Next, subjects are asked to try various needle drivers for ease and comfort. A gate made of cloth tape placed between two posts is placed in the training box. Using a needle driver in each hand, a needle is passed from right to left and back again through the gate from left to

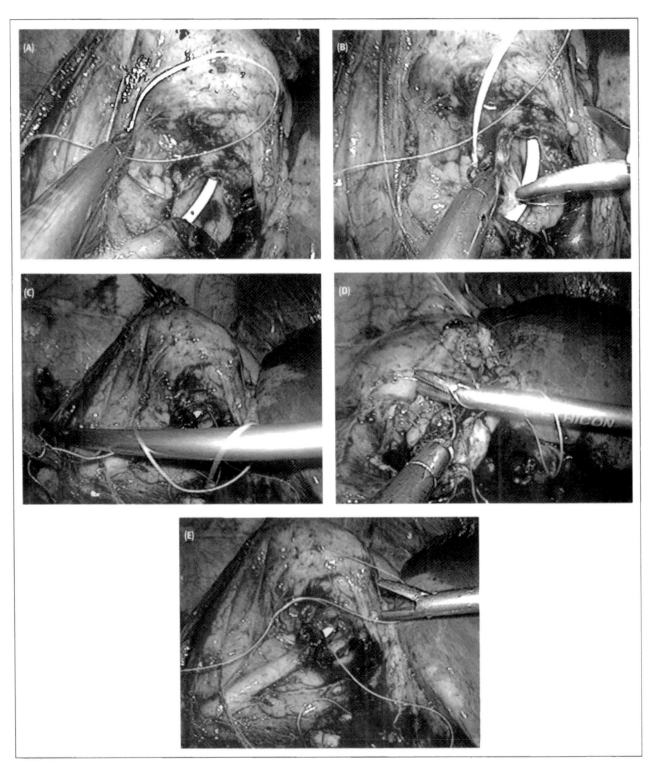

Figure 7.1

Basic steps of intracorporeal knot tying: (A) Using a needle driver the needle is grasped in the middle or proximal third of the shaft of the needle. (B) A second needle driver is used for countertraction on the tissue and the needle is passed from left to right and right to left or vice versa. (C) Typically, we initially employ a surgeon's knot to lock the suture in place. When possible, the memory of the suture is used to our advantage to form the loops around our needle driver. (D) The end of the suture is grasped and drawn through the loops previously thrown around the driver. That the knot is squared is checked and the knot tightened. (E) The above steps are repeated as needed for the number of throws wanted for each specific suture.

right. Appropriate needle angle is discussed and needles of varying sizes are used. At least four positions are used for the gate, with the starting position being the bull's-eye zone with the gate straight up and down. As the subject masters this, the gate is spun to say a right oblique position and the exercise repeated (Figure 7.1).

Complex skills

Once the subject is comfortable with these maneuvers, a demonstration of suturing techniques is reviewed. Several papers exist on laparoscopic suturing.[74,78–80] Correct suture length for tying is discussed, and tricks to aid one in righting the needle, dealing with too short a suture, too long a suture, or what to do if the needle or suture breaks are reviewed and demonstrated. Hints such as gripping the needle in the middle or at the proximal end, holding the needle $> 90°$ to the instrument axis, and inserting the needle between 80° and 100° angle are reinforced, as this aids in improving task accuracy.[81] Under direct supervision, the subjects are allowed to master the conventional suturing and knot. Instant feedback is given to facilitate learning and decrease errors. Notable time-wasting maneuvers are pointed out or obvious need to continue to work on deficits is noted. Drills or further homework are given to compensate for the observed weaknesses by the fellowship-trained surgeon. As evidenced by Emam et al, the subjects are taught that optimal suturing with better quality and reduced execution time is accomplished with vertical suturing toward the surgeon with isoplanar monitor display of the operative field. It was demonstrated in their study that poorer performance was seen with horizontal suturing and was accompanied by more muscle work and fatigue. Also, they found that horizontal suturing did not improve by monitor display of the incision in the vertical plane.[82] Although one cannot always set up the operative field to accommodate vertical suturing, the subjects are made aware of the fact, so that when feasible they can 'help themselves' more easily perform the task which aids in keeping operating room time to a minimum. Once suturing and knot tying is mastered, the subjects are asked to sew together the finger of a latex glove with an ~1–2 inch rent. We have found that the glove is inexpensive and if not handled with care the suture easily rips the latex, reinforcing appropriate tissue handling. Once mastered, more difficult exercises are given such as sewing the finger back on the glove and suturing Penrose tubing of various sizes together at various positions and varying sizes. Maneuvers for hemostasis are reviewed and hypothetical situations are given with a walk through of how one may handle the problem laparoscopically. We believe that rehearsal of such situations decreases anxiety and errors when they appear in the actual operating room.

Subjects become familiar with instruments such as clip applicators, and instructions with stapling devices are also included. Finally, a procedure such as a pyeloplasty followed by a nephrectomy in the animal laboratory is scheduled. Subjects are brought into the animal laboratory and the subject performs the procedure with anatomy review, surgical principle review, and further instruction as it arises. Here, as always prior to starting the procedure, a plan is discussed how the laparoscopic procedure will be safely converted to a hand assist or even an open procedure, what role each individual will play in opening, and who will decide to open; also, appropriate open instruments will be discussed and checked for presence in the operating room. Discussion on how to surgically assist is also given. Here is a chance to also discuss and demonstrate reverse alignment conditions and the maneuvers to improve performance. At times the surgeon has to operate ahead of the camera and, as a result, the image displayed on the monitor will be an inverted mirror image of the operative field, so that the view is upside down and reversed left to right (reverse alignment). While most surgeons will simply transfer the scope to another port, this may result in less optimal angles to work from and adds time to the operative case. Basically, we have found, like Cresswell et al, that the effect on performance produced by reverse alignment of the scope and instruments can be overcome by simply turning the camera through 180° or, if available, digital electronic processing will aid in reducing execution time and execution-time errors.[83] Again, the subjects are given these aids so they may continue operating under optimal conditions in a timely fashion.

Lastly, we believe that videotaping the procedure is a valuable learning tool. Subjects are encouraged to review their performance and look for further areas of improvement, look for wasted movement, review laparoscopic anatomy, review the steps in the procedure while reviewing possible complications at each step and what methods can be performed laparoscopically to remedy the situation. They are asked to make a game plan on how they could improve the overall performance of the procedure.

Conclusion

It has been demonstrated that minimally invasive surgery is safe but only in experienced hands. Being a competent surgeon is more than having psychomotor skills; rather, nonverbal, visuospatial problem-solving abilities and the ability to distinguish essential from nonessential detail even when the signal-to-noise ratio is high appear crucial to superior technique.

Recently, it has been determined that the skills necessary for laparoscopic procedures are unique, and open operative skills often do not transfer. Educational models for open procedures are lacking and not valid for laparoscopic procedures. A critical review of our educational process with the aid of general surgery's own experience in laparoscopic education needs to be done. The need for out-of-the-operating room training is evident, but there is no consensus on which skills need to be taught and how much training is suitable. Realistically, developing an all-inclusive laparoscopic training course may never be done, but we can strive to make our education system better by requiring rigorous scientific validation of the educational interventions used. Application of adult educational principles for adult learning is a must to facilitate learning. Training has to be objectively monitored using proven methods, with documentation of TOT from the educational model to the operating room.

Laparoscopic surgery was once thought of as the future and today, despite several advances with virtually all open procedures being replicated laparoscopically, the final chapter still remains to be written. As always, we must continue to adapt so that we can continue to grow.

References

1. See WA, Cooper CS, and Fisher RJ. Predictors of laparoscopic complications after formal training in laparoscopic surgery. JAMA 1993; 270:2689–92.

2. See WA, Fisher RJ, Winfield HN, Donovan JF. Laparoscopic surgical training: effectiveness and impact on urological surgical practice patterns. J Urol 1993; 149:1054–7.

3. See WA, Cooper CS, Fisher RJ. Urologic laparoscopic practice patterns 1 year after formal training. J Urol 1994; 151:1595–8.

4. Moore RG, Adams JB, Parti AW, et al. Telementoring of laparoscopic procedures: initial clinical experience. Surg Endosc 1996; 10:107–10.

5. Colegrave PM, Winfield HN, Donovan JF, See WA. Laparoscopic practice patterns among North American urologists 5 years after formal training. J Urol 1999; 161:881–6.

6. Cadeddu JA, Wolfe JS Jr, Nakada S, et al. Complications of laparoscopic procedures after concentrated training in urological laparoscopy. J Urol 2001; 166 (6):2109–11.

7. Traxer O, Gettman MT, Napper CA, et al. The impact of intense laparoscopic skills training on the operative performance of urology residents. J Urol 2001; 166(5):1658–61.

8. Moore DK, Riley PL, Smith GS, Moore RG. Saint Louis University laparoscopic conventional knot tying teaching model. J Endourol 2001; D2–P2.

9. Riley PL, Moore DK, Smith GS, et al. Saint Louis University teaching model for basic laparoscopic skills. J Endourol 2001; D2–P3.

10. Shalhav AL, Dabagia MD, Tsien L, Sangi-Haghpeykar H. Training postgraduate urologists in laparoscopic surgery: the current challenge. J Urol 2002; 167(5):2135–7.

11. White MD, Abrahams HM, Kogan BA. Laparoscopic skill training for urology residents: does practice make perfect? J Endourology 2001; D2–P4.

12. Moore DK, Riley PL, Landman J, et al. Objective/subjective evaluation of laparoscopic conventional knot tying using our teaching model. J Endourology 2002; P16–14.

13. Medina M. Formidable challenges to teaching advanced laparoscopic skills. JSLS 2001; 5:153–8.

14. Kopta JA. An approach to the evaluation of operative skills. Surgery 1971; 70:297–303.

15. Ericsson KA. The acquisition of expert performance. In: Ericsson KA, ed. The road to excellence: the acquisition of expert performance in the arts and sciences, sports and games. Mahwah, NJ: Lawrence Erlbaum, 1996.

16. Des Coteaux JG, Leclere H. Learning surgical technical skills. Can J Surg 1995; 38:33–8.

17. Schmidt RA. A schema theory of discrete motor skill learning. Psychol Rev 1975; 82:225–60.

18. Schueneman AL, Pickelman J, Hesslein R, Freeark RJ. Neuropsychologic predictors of operative skill among general surgery residents. Surgery 1984; 96:288–95.

19. Schueneman AL, Pickleman J, Freeark RJ. Age, gender, lateral dominance, and prediction of operative skill among general surgery residents. Surgery 1985; 98:506–15.

20. Cundiff GW. Analysis of the effectiveness of an endoscopy education program in improving residents' laparoscopic skills. Obstet Gynecol 1997; 90:854–9.

21. Schadmehr R, Holcomb H. Neural correlates of motor memory consolidation. Science 1997; 227:88.

22. Rosser JC, Herman B, Risucci DA, Murayama M. Effectiveness of a CD-ROM multimedia tutorial in transferring cognitive knowledge essential for laparoscopic skill training. Am J Surg 2000; 179(4):320–4.

23. Reznick R, Regehr G, MacRae H, et al. Testing technical skill via an innovative 'bench station' examination. Am J Surg 1993; 165:358–61.

24. Halsted WS. The training of the surgeon. Bull Johns Hopkins Hosp 1904; 15:267.

25. Barnes RW, Lang NP, Whitesede MF. Halstedian technique revisited: innovations in teaching surgical skills. Ann Surg 1989; 210:118–21.

26. Scott DJ, Rege RV, Bergen PC, et al. Measuring operative performance after laparoscopic skills training: edited videotape versus direct observation. J Laparoendosc Adv Surg Tech A 2000; 10(4):183–90.

27. Soper NJ, Hunter JG. Suturing and knot tying in laparoscopy. Surg Clin N Am 1992; 72(5):1139–52.

28. Hunter JG, Sakier JM. Minimally invasive surgery. New York: McGraw-Hill, 1993.

29. Overbeeke CJ, Smets GJF, Stratmann MH. Depth on a flat screen II. Percept Mot Skills 1987; 65:120.

30. Moore RG. Secondary trocar placement. In: Smith AD, ed. Smith's textbook of endourology, vol. 2. St Louis: Quality Medical Publishing, 1996:779–86.

31. Sackier JM, Berci G, Paz Partlow M. A new training device for laparoscopic cholecystectomy. Surg Endosc 1991; 5:158–9.

32. Peters JH, Elison EC, Innes JT, et al. Safety and efficacy of laparoscopic cholecystectomy. Ann Surg 1994; 312:3–12.

33. Wherry DC, Rob CG, Marohn MR, et al. An external audit of laparoscopic cholecystectomy performed in the medical treatment facilities of the Department of Defense. Ann Surg 1994; 220:626–34.

34. Giddings T, Gary G, Maran A, et al. Response to the General Medical Council Determination on the Bristol Case. London: The Senate of Surgery, 1998.

35. Fahlenkamp D, Rassweiler J, Fornara P, et al. Complications of laparoscopic procedures in urology: experience with 2,407 procedures at 4 German centers. J Urol 1999; 162:765.

36. Figert PL, Park AE, Witzke DB, Schwartz RW. Transfer of training in acquiring laparoscopic skills. J Am Coll Surg 2001; 193: 533–7.

37. Rosser JC, Rosser LE, Savalgi RS. Objective evaluation of a laparoscopic surgical skill program for residents and senior surgeons. Arch Surg 1998; 133:657–61.

38. Hayward CZ, Sachdeva A, Clarke JR. Is there gender bias in the evaluation of surgical residents? Surgery 1987; 102:297–9.

39. Hanna GB, Drew T, Clinch P, et al. Psychomotor skills for endoscopic manipulations: differing abilities between right and left-handedness individuals. Ann Surg 1997; 225:333–8.

40. Silverman AJ, Adevai G, McGough WE. Some relationships between handedness and perception. J Psychosom Res 1966; 10:151–8.

41. James WE, Mefferd RB, Wieland BA. Repetitive psychometric measures: handedness and performance. Percept Mot Skills 1967; 25:209–12.

42. Miller E. Handedness and the pattern of human ability. Br J Psychol 1971; 62:111–12.

43. McGlone J, Davidson W. The relationship between cerebral speech laterality and spatial ability with special reference to sex and hand preference. Neuropsychologia 1973; 11:105–13.

44. McGee MG. Laterality, hand preference and human spatial ability. Percept Mot Skills 1976; 42:781–2.

45. Newcombe F, Ratcliff G. Handedness, speech lateralization and ability. Neuropsychologia 1973; 11:399–407.

46. Annett M, Turner A. Laterality and the growth of intellectual abilities. Br J Educ Psychol 1974; 44:37–44.

47. Park A, Witzke DB. Training and educational approaches to minimally invasive surgery: state of the art. Semin Laparosc Surg 2002; 9(4):198–205.

48. Coleman J, Nduka CC, Darzi A. Virtual reality and laparoscopic surgery. Br J Surg 1994; 81:1709–11.

49. Martin JA, Regehar G, Reznick R, et al. Objective Structured Assessment of Technical Skills (OSATS) for Surgical Residents. Br J Surg 1997; 84(2):273–8.

50. Derossis AM, Fried GM, Abrahamowicz M, et al. Development of a model for training and evaluation of laparoscopic skills. Am J Surg 1998; 175:482–7.

51. Jordon J, Gallagher AG, McGuigan J, et al. A comparison between randomly alternating imaging, normal laparoscopic imaging, and virtual reality training in laparoscopic psychomotor skill acquisition. Am J Surg 2000; 180:208–11.

52. Scott DJ, Bergen PC, Rege RV, et al. Laparoscopic training on bench models: better and more cost effective than operating room experience? J Am Coll Surg 2000; 191:272–83.

53. Ramshaw BJ, Young D, Garcha I, et al. The role of multimedia interactive programs in training for laparoscopic procedures. Surg Endosc 2001; 15:21–7.

54. Seymour NE, Gallagher AG, Roman SA, et al. Virtual reality training improves operating room performance results of a randomized, double-blinded study. Ann Surg 2002; 236:458–64.

55. Breda G, Nakada SY, Rassweiler JJ. Future developments and perspectives in laparoscopy. Eur Urol 2001; 40:84–91.

56. Hoffman H, Murray M. Anatomic visualize: realizing the vision of a VR-based learning environment. In: Westwood JD, Hoffman HM, Robb RA, Stredney D, eds. Medicine meets virtual reality; the convergence of physical and informational technologies: options for a new era in healthcare. Amsterdam: IOS Press, 1999:134–41.

57. Heinrichs WK, Dev P. Interactive pelvic anatomy. Available at: htpp://summit.stanford.edu/welcome.html and htpp://www.nlm.nih.gov./research/visible/vhp-conf/heinrich/abstract.htm. Accessed 2003.

58. Keyser EJ, Derossis AM, Antoniuk M, et al. A simplified simulator for the training and evaluation of laparoscopic skills. Surg Endosc 2000; 14:149–53.

59. Gallagher AG, Richie K, McClure N, McGuigan J. Objective psychomotor skills assessment of experienced, junior and novice laparoscopic with virtual reality. World J Surg 2001; 25:1478–83.

60. Fung Kee Fung MP, Temple LM, Ash KM. Laparoscopic education study group. What are the components of a successful laparoscopic educational program? J S O G C 1996; 18:859–67.

61. Fowler DL, Hogle N. The impact of a full time director of minimally invasive surgery. Surg Endosc 2000; 14: 444–7.

62. Bridges M, Diamond DL. The financial impact of teaching surgical residents in the operating room. Am J Surg 1999; 177:28–32.

63. Smith CD, Farrell TM, McNatt SS, Metreveli RE. Assessing laparoscopic manipulative skills. Am J Surg 2001; 181:547–50.

64. Streiner DL. Global rating scales. In: Neufeld VR, Norman GR, eds. Assessing clinical competence. New York: Springer, Springer Series on Medical Education 1985; 7:119–41.

65. Sung GT, Gill IS. Robotic laparoscopic surgery: a comparison of the Da Vinci and Zeus systems. Urology 2001; 58(6):893–8.

66. Menon M, Shrivastava A, Tewari A, et al. Laparoscopic and robot assisted radical prostatectomy: establishment of a structured program and preliminary analysis of outcomes. J Urol 2002; 168: 945–9.

67. Yohannes P, Rotariu P Pinto P, et al. Comparison of robotic versus laparoscopic skills: is there a difference in the learning curve? Urology 2002; 60(1):39–45.

68. Prasad SM, Maniar HS, Soper NJ, et al. The effect of robotic assistance on learning curves for basic laparoscopic skills. Am J Surg 2002; 183(6):702–7.

69. Dakin GF, Gagner M. Comparison of laparoscopic skills performance between standard instruments and two surgical robotic systems. Surg Endosc 2002; 17(4):574–9.

70. Kaufmann C, Rhee P, Burris D. Telepresence surgery system enhances medical student surgery training. Stud Health Technol Inform 1999; 62:174–8.

71. El-Khalili N, Brodie K, Kessel D. WebSter: a web-based surgical training system. Stud Health Technol Inform 2000; 70:69–75.

72. Gandsas A, McIntire K, Palli G, Park A. Live streaming video for medical education: a laboratory model. J Laparoendosc Adv Surg Tech A 2002; 12(5):377–82.

73. Riding M, John NW. Force-feedback in Web-based surgical stimulators. Stud Health Technol Inform 2001; 81:404–6.

74. Champion JK, Hunter J, Trus T, Laycock W. Teaching basic video skills as an aid in laparoscopic suturing. Surg Endos 1996; 10:23–5.

75. Pattaras JG, Smith GS, Landman J, Moore RG. Comparison and analysis of laparoscopic intracorporeal suturing devices: preliminary results. J Endourol 2001; 187–92.

76. Bergamaschi R, Dicko A. Instruction versus passive observation: a randomized educational research study on laparo-scopic suture skills. Surg Laparosc Endosc Percutan Tech 2000; 10(5):319–22.

77. Hanna GB, Shimi S, Cuschieri A. Influence of direction of view, target-to-endoscope distance and manipulation angle on endoscopic knot tying. Br J Surg 1997; 84(10):1460–4.

78. Pennings JL, Kenyon T, Swanstrom L. The knit stitch. Surg Endosc 1995; 9:537–40.

79. Frede T, Stock C, Rassweiler JJ, Alken P. Retroperitoneoscopic and laparoscopic suturing: tips and strategies for improving efficiency. J Endourology 2000; 905–14.

80. Park AE. Needle-assisted technique of laparoscopic knot-tying. Contemp Surg 2001; 516–18.

81. Joice P, Hanna GB, Cuschieri A. Ergonomic evaluation of laparoscopic bowel suturing. Am J Surg 1998; 176:373–8.

82. Emam TA, Hanna G, Cuschieri A. Ergonomic principles of task alignment, visual display, and direction of execution of laparoscopic bowel suturing. Surg Endosc 2002; 16:267–71.

83. Cresswell AB, Macmillan AIM, Hanna GB, Cuschieri A. Methods for improving performance under reverse alignment conditions during endoscopic surgery. Surg Endosc 1999; 13:591–4.

8

Renal cystic disease

Chandru P Sundaram

Renal cystic disease includes a variety of cystic anomalies and lesions of the kidneys and can be seen in all age groups. This chapter will include those conditions where minimally invasive options are an accepted treatment modality. A cyst is a sac lined by epithelium within the kidney. The origin for cysts could be from ectopic tubules or collecting ducts. The cysts may be continuous with the nephron or may be isolated despite a communication during pathogenesis. A majority of the cysts arise from the nephron and collecting ducts. Multicystic kidneys, however, are dysplastic kidneys that arise before the formation of the nephron. Classification of renal cystic diseases that are listed in Table 8.1 is based on the system proposed in 1987 by the Committee on Terminology, Nomenclature and Classification of the American Academy of Pediatrics (AAP), Section on Urology.[1]

Table 8.1 *Classification of renal cystic disease*
Genetic
Autosomal recessive (infantile) polycystic kidneys
Autosomal dominant (adult) polycystic kidneys
Juvenile nephronophthisis–medullary cystic disease complex:
Juvenile nephronophthisis
Medullary cystic disease
Congenital nephrosis
Cysts associated with multiple malformation syndromes
Non-genetic
Multicystic kidney (multicystic dysplasia)
Multilocular cyst (multilocular cystic nephroma)
Simple cysts
Medullary sponge kidneys (less than 5% inherited)
Acquired renal cystic disease
Caliceal diverticulum

Simple cysts

A simple renal cyst is an oval-to-round cyst in the kidney, which is lined by a flattened cuboidal epithelium and filled with clear or straw-colored fluid. These are usually acquired lesions and are believed to originate as diverticula of the distal convoluted tubules or the collecting ducts.[2,3] The prevalence of renal cysts as well as the number of cysts in each kidney increases with age. The prevalence in the adult population is about 12–14%.[4,5] In another CT study by Tada et al, the incidence of cysts in patients by the age of 50 was at least 27%.[6] In a longitudinal study, the cysts were seen to increase in size at the mean rate of 2.82 mm or 6.3% per year and cysts in younger patients progressed more rapidly than the older patients.[4] The ratio of men to women with renal cysts was 2 : 1. An autopsy study by Kissane and Smith identified a 50% incidence of simple renal cysts after the age of 50.[7]

Simple cysts are usually asymptomatic and incidentally detected on abdominal imaging. Occasionally, symptoms related to renal cysts include a palpable mass, pain, flank pain, and hematuria. Clinical features related to cysts can be due to infection, hemorrhage, impairment of renal function, and hypertension. Cysts can rupture into the caliceal system and cause hematuria or cause caliceal or ureteral obstruction. Cysts can also cause hypertension secondary to segmental ischemia.

Diagnosis

Ultrasound

Simple cysts can typically be confirmed by a renal ultrasonography. The characteristics of a simple cyst on ultrasonography include a spherical smooth-walled lesion with a thin distinct margin, absence of internal echoes, through transmission of ultrasound waves through the cyst, and acoustic enhancement of the sound waves deep to the cyst. Renal cystic disease should be suspected if two or more cysts are noted in individuals 30 years or younger, or two or more cysts are noted in each kidney in those aged 30–59 years, or four cysts are noted in each kidney in those older than 60 years.[8,9] Other criteria are also helpful: size of the cyst, the location of the cyst, as well as the echogenicity of the cortex can also be determined via ultrasound examination. If all ultrasonographic criteria for the simple cyst are met, no further evaluation is required. However, should there be an equivocal diagnosis on ultrasound, further imaging by computed tomography (CT) or a magnetic resonance imaging (MRI) may be helpful.

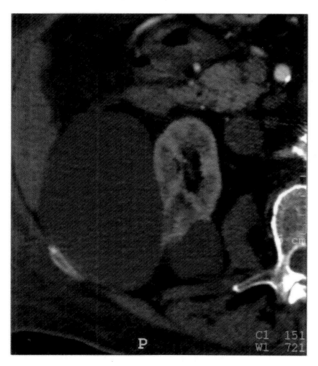

Figure 8.1
Large symptomatic simple cysts treated with aspiration and sclerotherapy. (CT courtesy of Dr Jonas Rydberg.)

Computed tomography

On CT imaging, apart from the distinct smooth spherical or oval thin-walled lesion seen on ultrasound, the CT lesion should be homogenous, with a density of −10 to +20 Hounsfield units, without enhancement following intravenous (IV) contrast injection (Figure 8.1). However, CT imaging is often required in patients with complex lesions. It is important that CT be obtained with and without IV contrast and with thin sections (5 mm or less) through the kidney. When the diagnosis is equivocal, details regarding the CT technique as well as the time of imaging after injection of contrast as well as other details of technique should be determined. A hyperdense cyst can have a density of between 20 and 90 Hounsfield units but will not have enhancement after IV contrast injection. Diagnostic aspiration of the cyst is indicated only in an occasional patient, especially when an infected cyst is suspected. In patients who are poor surgical risks and when cytologic evaluation of the fluid may be helpful, cyst aspiration can be performed. MRI may be helpful, especially in identifying hemorrhagic cysts that are seen on T2 images as extremely bright lesions.

Bosniak classification

In 1986 Bosniak proposed a classification (Table 8.2) for renal cysts to select patients whose cysts are likely to be malignant and who would need close follow-up or surgery due to the risk of malignancy.[10–13] The Bosniak classification was based primarily on CT imaging to evaluate renal masses. Management decisions, however, are made on the basis of patient age and clinical conditions as well as other imaging modalities such as ultrasound and MRI.

Category I consists of simple benign cysts with CT and ultrasound features as previously described in this chapter. Category II are cysts that include one or two thin septations (≤ 1 mm), fine calcification, and hyperdense cysts with homogenously high attenuation with all other features of category I cyst. There can, however, be

Table 8.2 *Renal cyst CT classification based on Bosniak criteria with risk of malignancy*

Type	Wall	Septations	Calcification	Precontrast density on CT (HU)	Enhancement	Risk of malignancy	Require surgical resection
I	Thin	None	None	0–20	None	None	–
II	Thin	None–few	Minimal	0–20	None	Low	+/–
III	Increasing thickness	Multiple	Moderate	0–20	None	Moderate	+/–
IV	Thick	Many	Coarse	> 20	Yes	High	Yes

CT, computed tomography; HU, Hounsfield units.
Parts of table taken from Bosniak MA[10] with permission.

interobserver variation in distinguishing between Bosniak II and Bosniak III lesions. Category III are complicated lesions that have more than minimal calcification and prominent septation with thicker walls or multiple septa (Figure 8.2A,B). Category IV are clearly malignant and are considered cystic renal malignancies with irregular margins and enhancing components. Enhancement is considered significant, with an increase of at least 10 Housefield units with IV contrast.

Category I and II lesions do not require surgery; category III comprises lesions that cannot be definitively distinguished from malignant neoplasms and need to be considered for surgical exploration. Category IIF is a group not clearly defined by Bosniak and consists of lesions that do not clearly fall into the category II and require follow-up. Category IV are clearly considered to be radiologically malignant and require resection.

Occasionally, high-density cysts can be mistaken for enhancing renal tumors if CT imaging is performed after IV contrast alone. In these circumstances a repeated delayed CT imaging may help in differentiating between high-density cysts and solid renal neoplasms. With high-density cysts there is no change in attenuation between the initial post-contrast and the delayed CT, whereas with renal neoplasms there is a decreased attenuation in the delayed CT compared to the post-contrast CT, indicating vascularity.[14]

Nephrotomography, renal angiography, and cyst puncture have been used in the past to differentiate the renal cysts from tumor. However, with advances in sonography, CT, and MRI, invasive procedures are rarely required for diagnostic purposes. Indications for cyst puncture include a possible renal abscess or an infected cyst, when the patient is a high risk for surgery, or when cytologic diagnosis is required for further management for the patient. In the case of an infected cyst or an abscess, percutaneous drainage after cyst puncture may be appropriate.

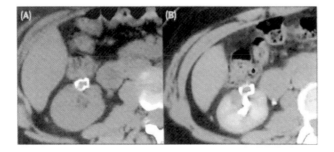

Figure 8.2

(A and B) Bosniak category III cyst with thick calcified wall treated with laparoscopic wedge excision.

Management of simple cysts

Simple cysts rarely require treatment and do not need regular follow-up. Treatment for simple cysts is required if the cyst is symptomatic with pain or causes effects due to compression of the renal parenchyma or the pelvicaliceal system. When simple cysts are to be treated, the options include aspiration, aspiration with sclerotherapy, percutaneous endocytosis, and laparoscopic decortication of cysts.

Percutaneous drainage of simple cysts is minimally invasive, is tolerated well by patients, and can be performed on an outpatient. It is typically performed under ultrasound guidance by the radiologist. However, simple aspiration does not have a high success rate, since in the vast majority of the patients the cyst persists on follow-up imaging. In a study of 156 patients there was no statistically significant difference in change of mean size between the cysts that were aspirated and the cysts that had no intervention.[15] In some patients in whom the symptoms may not be definitively related to the cyst, aspiration may be performed as part of the evaluation, before more invasive options such as decortication are considered if the symptoms resolve with aspiration.

Percutaneous aspiration and sclerotherapy

Indications and contraindications. Sclerotherapy is recommended as an initial treatment of choice for simple renal cysts that are peripheral and symptomatic. Should sclerotherapy not be successful, and in those patients where sclerotherapy is contraindicated, other options should be considered. Sclerotherapy is contraindicated when the following are present or suspected: malignancy, infection, communication with the renal collecting system, and peripelvic location (Figure 8.3A and B).

Technique. The treatment of symptomatic cysts with aspiration and sclerotherapy is more effective and is an effective minimally invasive option with good results. Sclerotherapy has been performed with several agents, including glucose, phenol, iophendylate, and 99% ethanol and bismuth phosphate. Other chemicals for sclerotherapy include 10% povidone-iodine and doxycycline. Ten percent povidone-iodine has also been used in combination with doxycycline.

It has been noted that a repeat injection of 99% ethanol has been more efficacious than a single injection.[16] In a recent study by Paananen et al, 32 patients with simple cysts were treated with ultrasound-guided percutaneous aspiration of the cysts followed by a 99% ethanol sclerotherapy.[17] The procedure was performed under local anesthesia with the patients hospitalized overnight. The cyst was punctured with a 15 cm 18-gauge needle under

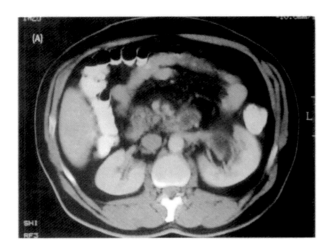
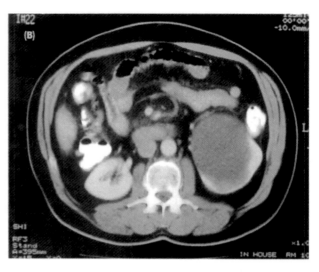

Figure 8.3
(A and B) This large symptomatic simple renal cyst, extending towards the pelvis of the kidney, was treated with laparoscopic decortication.

ultrasound guidance with local anesthesia. Fluid was aspirated from the cyst and sent for cytologic examination. Ten milliliters of contrast was injected under fluoroscopic guidance into the cyst after using the Seldinger technique to insert a 30 cm 5F catheter into the cyst. The fluid from the cyst was aspirated to completion. Contrast was then injected into the cyst to confirm that the cyst walls were smooth and that there was no extravasation. Ninety-nine percent ethanol was then injected into the cysts: one-fourth of the cyst volume but never more than 100 ml. The alcohol was left in the cyst for 20 min and the patient rolled from side to side in different positions at intervals of 5 min. Following this, all the alcohol was aspirated. The cyst was similarly treated once or twice more during the same session. Twenty milliliters of 2% lidocaine hydrochloride has been injected into the cyst for 15 min before the alcohol injection in order to relieve the pain that can sometimes be associated with alcohol sclerotherapy. Other investigators[18] have used 95% alcohol sclerotherapy with three doses at intervals of 24 hours. Alcohol is rarely absorbed through the cyst wall, with detectable levels of alcohol in the urine and blood.

Results: Sclerotherapy with ethanol was successful in the disappearance of the cyst in 22% of cases, and mean size of all cysts decreased from 7.8 cm to 1.7 cm, with a mean follow-up of 55 months. There was no correlation between the size of the cyst and intensity of the pain.[17] Sclerotherapy with bismuth phosphate has also been effective in the treatment of simple renal cysts.[15] Fifty percent acetic acid has also been used for sclerotherapy and in one study was noted to induce faster and more complete regression of the cyst compared with 99% ethanol.[19]

Ureteroscopic approach

Ureteroscopic marsupialization is suitable for small or medium-sized parapelvic and centrally located cysts.[20] This approach can be considered in patients who are poor candidates for more invasive surgery. The flexible ureteroscope can be used to incise the wall of the cyst to allow adequate drainage into the collecting system. Fluoroscopy with retrograde pyelography and ultrasound may be used to assist with localization of the cyst. Electrosurgical energy or a holmium laser can be used to perform a cruciate incision in the cyst wall.

Percutaneous endocystolysis

There have been a few reports of percutaneous decortication of renal cysts.[21–23] This approach involves general anesthesia but is less invasive than the laparoscopic approach.

Indications and results. An ideal patient for this approach is one who has a medium-sized or large solitary posterior cyst, preferably in the mid or lower parts of the kidney. Long-term follow-up of 10 patients who underwent percutaneous resection of renal cysts was reported by Plas and Hubner in 1993.[23] All patients were cured of symptoms without late complications, with a median follow-up of 45.7 months. The cysts had completely resolved in 50% of patients. Cyst recurrence was seen in 30% and there was a 45% decrease in cyst size in 20% of patients. The technique described by Kang and colleagues has been successful in 9 patients with a mean follow-up of 21 months.[21] Eight of 9 patients had complete resolution of pain and 1/9 had significant improvement in pain. Follow-up CT imaging revealed complete or near-complete resolution in 7 patients and small cysts in 2 patients.

Technique. The patient is initially placed in the lithotomy position and a retrograde pyelogram is performed (Figure 8.4). An open-ended ureteral catheter is placed with its tip in the renal pelvis to facilitate injection of indigo carmine solution during the percutaneous procedure.

The patient is then turned to a prone position for the percutaneous cyst decortication. The cyst is localized using fluoroscopy with injection of contrast via the retrograde catheter. Ultrasound may also be used to help localize the cyst accurately and to direct the percutaneous access. A 15 cm 18-gauge needle is used for percutaneous direct access into the cyst. Cyst fluid is aspirated and sent for cytologic examination. An 80 cm J wire is passed through the needle before the needle is removed. The percutaneous

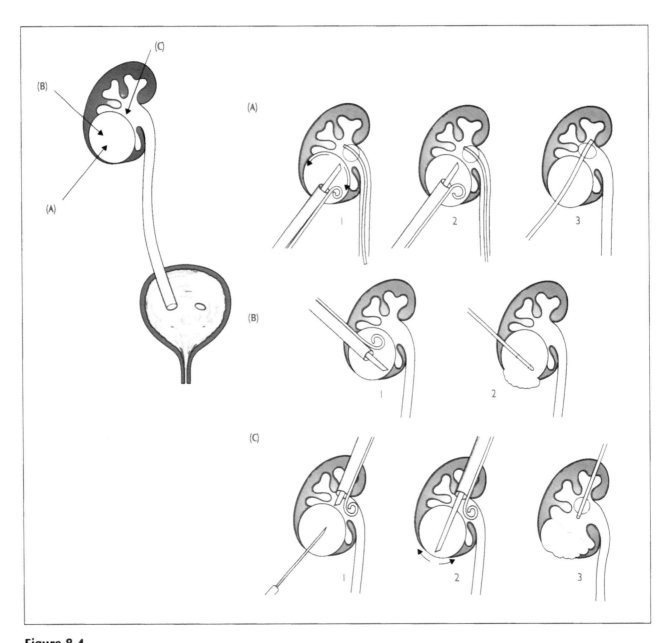

Figure 8.4

Three approaches for percutaneous access for cyst decortication. (A) Direct approach: (1) cyst is punched directly and cyst wall is incised into the pelvis; (2) cyst wall is fulgurated; (3) a nephrostomy tube is placed through the cyst. (B) Direct approach through parenchyma: (1) cyst is punctured through the parenchyma; (2) a nephrostomy tube is placed in the cyst – no communication between the cyst and the collecting system. (C) Indirect approach: (1) collecting system is entered first and cyst is punctured and distended for easy identification; (2) cyst wall is fulgurated; (3) a nephrostomy tube is placed. (from Clayman et al.[24])

tract is dilated over the wire with a balloon dilator to 30F after a second safety guide wire is inserted into the cyst. A 26F rigid nephroscope with an offset lens and a straight working channel is used with glycine irrigant. After initial inspection of the cyst, a 26F resectoscope with a rollerball electrode is used. The lining of the cyst is gently fulgurated with a rollerball electrode. After the cyst wall is fulgurated, a portion of the cyst wall is marsupialized into the retroperitoneum with a grasping forceps. Indigo carmine injected into the collecting system helps identify the cyst wall facing the retroperitoneum. Care is taken to limit the extravasation of glycine into the retroperitoneum to avoid the transurethral resection (TUR) syndrome.

The other percutaneous approach to the cyst is via a direct approach but through adjacent renal parenchyma. The cyst is marsupialized into the retroperitoneum but not into the collecting system. The third approach is an indirect method where percutaneous access is achieved into the collecting system at a site distant to the cyst. After dilation of the tract and insertion of a 30F Amplatz sheath, the cyst is marsupialized into the collecting system. Before the cyst is marsupialized in this manner, an 18 gauge needle is inserted percutaneously into the cyst and saline injected into the cyst to facilitate visualization of the cyst wall to the nephroscopist.[24]

Laparoscopic decortication

Indications. For laparoscopic cyst decortication, indications include:

1. simple cysts that have failed aspiration with sclerotherapy
2. cysts with close proximity to the collecting system (see Figure 8.3A and B) or with a possible communication with the collecting system
3. peripelvic cysts (Figure 8.5)

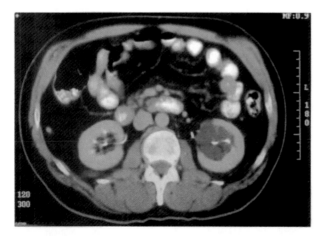

Figure 8.5
Peripelvic cyst is a contraindication for sclerotherapy.

4. cysts that are suspicious for malignancy or where malignancy cannot be definitively be ruled out
5. autosomal dominant polycystic kidney disease.

Laparoscopic cyst decortication can be performed via a transperitoneal or a retroperitoneal approach. For simple cysts, the approach can be dictated by the location of the dominant cyst using a retroperitoneal approach for a more posterior cyst and a transperitoneal approach for a more anteriorly placed cyst.

Preoperative preparation: The patient is placed on a liquid diet and given a Fleets enema the night before the surgery and a bottle of magnesium citrate about 24 hours before surgery. IV cefazolin is administered preoperatively for antibiotic prophylaxis. Should there be suspicion of infected cysts, especially in patients with autosomal dominant polycystic kidney disease, an IV fluoroquinolone such as ciprofloxacin is administered to achieve adequate antibiotic levels within the cyst. Preoperatively, a ureteral catheter is placed in selected patients, such as those with autosomal dominant polycystic kidney disease and with peripelvic cysts. In these patients, access to their retrograde ureteral catheter is maintained to facilitate injection of indigo carmine during the surgery to confirm that no caliceal violation has occurred. In these instances, if a small caliceal injury is noticed the ureteral catheter is used at the end of the procedure to pass a guide wire in a retrograde fashion to insert an indwelling double pigtail ureteral stent under fluoroscopic guidance to drain the collecting system.

Patient positioning: The patient is positioned in a lateral decubitus position with the table flexed. The patient is anchored securely to the table and all bony prominences are well padded to ensure that there is no neuromuscular injury as a result of positioning. Pneumatic compression stockings are applied before the patient is positioned.

Port placement: Pneumoperitoneum is established in the left lower quadrant using the Veress needle or the dilating trocar with the visual obturator (Ethicon Endopath 12 mm trocars). A 2nd 12 mm trocar is inserted at the umbilicus. In obese patients this trocar is inserted at the lateral border of the rectus abdominis muscle. The 3rd trocar is a 5 mm trocar that is inserted in the midline midway between the umbilicus and the xiphisternum. The 4th trocar may occasionally be required if lateral retraction of the kidney is required. This is a 5 mm trocar that is inserted in the subcostal region along the anterior axillary line (Figure 8.6A). If access to the upper pole is required on the right side, an additional 5 mm trocar is inserted medially in the subcostal region to help retract the liver away from the superior pole of the kidney.

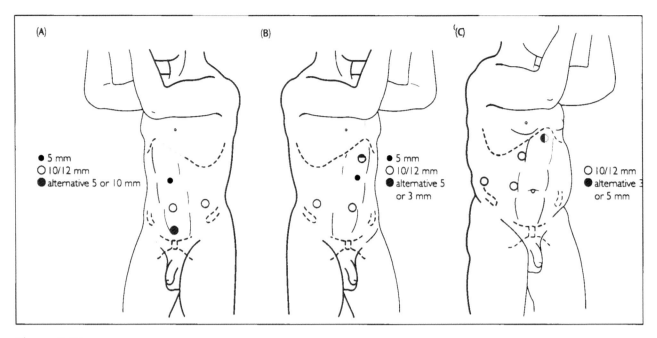

Figure 8.6A
Trocar site placements. Two 10/12 mm trocars are placed: one at umbilicus and one at the level of umbilicus lateral to the edge of rectus muscle. A 5 mm trocar is placed in the midline between umbilicus and the xiphoid process. An additional 5 mm trocar can be inserted medially in the subcostal region. (A) Left-sided procedures. (B) Right-sided procedures. (C) In obese patients, all trocars are shifted laterally.*

Technique: The line of Toldt is incised with a Harmonic Scalpel (Ethicon Endo-Surgery, Inc., Cincinnati, Ohio) and the colon is mobilized medially off the Gerota's fascia (Figure 8.6B). The Gerota's fascia is dissected off the surface of the cyst. The perinephric fat and Gerota's fascia around the cyst is excised in order to expose the entire cyst as well as a normal renal parenchyma surrounding the cyst. Initially, it is preferable not to decompress the cyst in order to dissect the margins completely. However, should the size of the cyst be impeding complete dissection of the cyst, it can be aspirated with a spinal needle to decrease the size. In the case of a simple cyst, the cyst fluid is first aspirated. The wall of the cyst is excised flush with the renal parenchyma and sent for histopathologic examination (Figure 8.6C). The base of the cyst is then inspected and, should there be any suspicion, biopsies of the base are obtained. The biopsy sites would need to be fulgurated in order to obtain adequate hemostasis. The cyst wall that is attached to the renal parenchyma can be fulgurated to prevent recurrence; however, this should be avoided if there is a risk of injury to the collecting system, depending on the preoperative imaging.[25] Once the cyst has been decorticated, perirenal fat can be placed and secured in place to help prevent reaccumulation. Polytetrafluoro-ethylene wick has also been used for a large peripelvic cyst.[26] We do not routinely recommend a drain in patients with a simple cyst (Figure 8.6D).

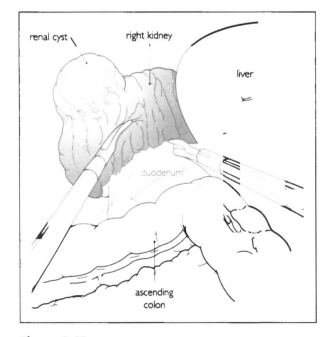

Figure 8.6B
Laparoscopic renal cyst decortication. Mobilization of colon and duodenum to free up Gerota's fascia. Sharp dissection with laparoscopic scissors prevents the possibility of bowel injury. An exophytic cyst can usually be identified or laparoscopic ultrasound can be used. Gerota's fascia is then dissected off the surface of the cyst.*

*(From Fabrizio MD. Laparoscopic evaluation and treatment of symptomatic and indeterminate renal cysts. In: Bishoff JT & Kavoussi LR (eds). Atlas of Laparoscopic Retroperitoneal Surgery. Philadelphia, PA: WB Saunders Company, 2000.)

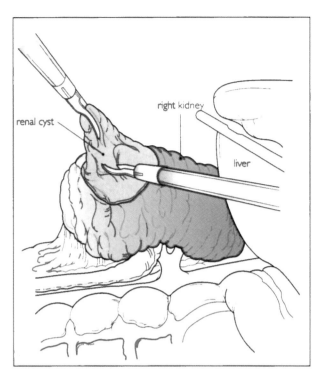

Figure 8.6C
Laparoscopic renal cyst decortication. Cyst fluid is first aspirated. Then the wall of the cyst is excised flush with renal parenchyma and sent for histopathologic examination. The base of the cyst is then inspected and biopsied if indicated. The base of the cyst is then fulgurated.*

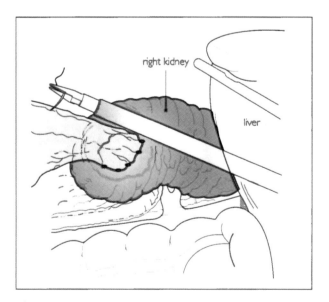

Figure 8.6D
Laparoscopic renal cyst decortication. Decorticated perirenal fat or a piece of omentum can be sutured and secured in place.*

Peripelvic cysts

Peripelvic cysts may be more difficult to treat laparoscopically because of their close relationship to the hilar blood vessels (see Figure 8.5). In these patients, depending on the location of the cysts, it may be necessary to dissect the renal hilar vessels to prevent hemorrhage during cystic cortication. Fluid is aspirated and sent for cytologic analysis. The entire cyst wall may not be accessible for excision. In these circumstances, the cyst wall is excised in those accessible locations between the hilar blood vessels. The cyst wall remnant is not fulgurated because of its proximity to the renal pelvis and hilum. The cyst cavity is then filled with perinephric fat or a polytetrafluoroethylene wick. A 10 mm laparoscopic ultrasound probe (B-K Medical, Copenhagen, Denmark) with a flexible and steerable tip is valuable for peripelvic cysts and other cysts that are not readily visible on the surface of the kidney. The laparoscopic ultrasound probe is inserted through a 12 mm port and has ability to control the angulation of the tip. Should adequate contact between the renal surface and the ultrasound probe not be obtained, irrigation with saline within the abdomen can help with ultrasound visualization.

Indeterminate renal cysts

In the majority of patients with indeterminate cysts where surgical exploration is indicated a laparoscopic partial nephrectomy is feasible and safe. This is especially true with patients with small cysts that are exophytic and peripheral. Rarely it may be necessary to further evaluate the cyst before a decision on excision is made. This is especially true in larger indeterminate cysts where confirmation of malignancy may necessitate a radical nephrectomy. In these rare instances the cyst may be aspirated and the fluid sent for cytology. The cyst wall is also excised and a biopsy of the floor of the cyst performed; further management is based on the results of the frozen section pathology evaluation. If the cyst is confirmed to be benign, the edges of the cyst remnant are fulgurated. Although there is a theoretical risk for dissemination of malignant cells within the abdomen, this has not been reported by the authors.[27,28] If the frozen section pathology confirms malignancy, a radical or partial nephrectomy is performed, depending upon the size and location of the tumor and the patient's renal function and medical condition.

In a recent series of 35 patients with indeterminate renal cysts who were treated with laparoscopic exploration as described, 14% were found to have cystic renal cell carcinoma. There was no evidence of local recurrence or distant metastases with a mean follow-up of 20.2 months.[27]

*(From Fabrizio MD. Laparascopic evaluation and treatment of symptomatic and indeterminate renal cysts. In: Bishoff JT & Kavoussi LR (eds). Atlas of Laparoscopic Retroperitoneal Surgery. Philadelphia, PA: WB Saunders Company, 2000.)

Autosomal dominant polycystic kidney disease

Autosomal dominant polycystic kidney disease (ADPKD) is an inherited disorder which accounts for 10–15% of patients who are on hemodialysis.[29] It is characterized by multiple bilateral renal cysts (Figure 8.7) and can result in progressive renal failure. It is seen in 1 : 500–1000 patients and over 500,000 Americans have been diagnosed with ADPKD.[30] Most patients are diagnosed to have ADPKD between the ages of 30 and 50 years old, although the condition is also diagnosed occasionally in children. Two genes have been implicated with the genesis of ADPKD. These are the PDK genes: PDK-1, which is on the short arm of chromosome 16, and PDK-2, which is on chromosome 4. PDK-3 is also seen in a small percentage of patients who do not have PDK-1 or PDK-2.[31]

Other manifestations of ADPKD include hepatic cysts (Figure 8.8), cerebral aneurysms, mitral valve prolapse, and chronic diverticulosis. Hepatic cysts may be seen in about 60% of patients.[32] However, these cysts rarely are symptomatic. Rarely, they can lead to portal hypertension. Occasionally, large hepatic cysts may need decortication during renal cyst surgery.

Symptoms and signs of the disease typically occur between the ages of 30 and 50 years old.[33] Symptoms include hematuria, flank pain, and gastrointestinal symptoms. Hypertension is also a major presenting sign, while 20–30% of patients with ADPKD can develop renal stones.[34] Pain can be related to cyst size.[35] In a study by Hatfield and Pfister, over 50% of symptomatic patients had cysts over 3 cm in size, but they were present in only 20% of asymptomatic patients.

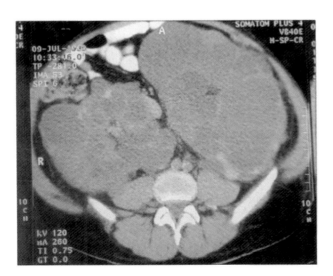

Figure 8.7
Patient with ADPKD (autosomal dominant polycystic kidney disease) and renal pain who underwent laparoscopic left renal cyst decortication.

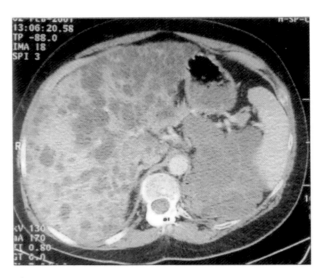

Figure 8.8
Hepatic cysts in this patient required hepatic cyst decortication during laparoscopic renal cyst decortication.

About 64% of patients with ADPKD develop microscopic or gross hematuria.[36] Most episodes of hematuria are due to urinary tract infections or renal cyst rupture and urolithiasis. However, other conditions can coincidentally occur with ADPKD, and therefore hematuria must be investigated in order not to miss other conditions such as upper tract malignancy or bladder carcinoma. Gross hematuria can be seen in as many as about 50% of patients with ADPKD. Hematuria is generally self-limiting and lasts generally for 7 days; it resolves spontaneously with conservative management, such as bed rest, IV hydration, and narcotic analgesics.

Diagnosis

It is usually not difficult to differentiate between localized cystic renal conditions and autosomal dominant polycystic kidney disease. Renal cysts in ADPKD are bilateral and involve both the cortex and medulla. Usually, however, ADPKD can have a symmetric onset, especially in children. In some patients with unilateral nonprogressive localized cystic disease and multiple simple cysts, it may be difficult to differentiate between ADPKD and localized cystic disease. In these patients, long-term follow-up, family history, and imaging of other family members may confirm the diagnosis. ADPKD is often associated with cysts of the liver and pancreas and in a small percentage of patients cerebral aneurysms can also be seen. Localized cystic disease of the kidney comprises multiple cysts in one portion of the kidney, which could be mistaken for a polycystic kidney, multilocular cystic nephroma, or cystic neoplasm. The parenchyma between the cysts have enhancement that is similar to the enhancement in the rest of the renal parenchyma. Also, there is no encapsulation of the cystic mass, as can be seen in neoplasms. In addition, there are often discrete cysts in the rest of the kidney that are not within this cystic lesion.

It is important to obtain a family history of ADPKD when evaluating patients with bilateral renal cysts. If no family history is obtained, a proper diagnosis can still be made in patients with bilateral cysts if two or more of the following symptoms are seen:

1. bilateral renal enlargement
2. three or more hepatic cysts
3. cerebral artery aneurysm
4. solitary cysts of the arachnoid, pineal gland, pancreas, or spleen.[37]

Before laparoscopic decortication, imaging should rule out solid suspicious lesions. Renal ultrasound and CT scan with and without IV contrast is usually adequate. However, in patients with renal impairment, an MRI with IV gadolinium may be required.

Urolithiasis

Urolithiasis occurs in about 20% of patients with ADPKD and is 5–10 times more frequent in those patients compared with the general population (Figure 8.9).[36,38] Uric acid stones constitute the majority of stones seen in patients with ADPKD, although other stones such as calcium oxalate, calcium phosphate, calcium carbonate and struvite are also seen.[36,39] Stone formers amongst ADPKD patients have larger cysts compared with non-stone formers. Increased cyst numbers are also associated with stone formation. It is therefore possible that urinary stasis related to larger cysts and increased number of cysts contributes to stone formation. Causes of stone formation in ADPKD include tubular dilation, urinary stasis, and metabolic abnormalities. High incidences of hypocitraturia and hyperuricosuria have been reported by Torres and associates.[38]

Treatment options for patients with ADPKD are similar to patients without ADPKD, depending on the stone size, location, and caliceal anatomy. Shock wave lithotripsy (SWL), ureteroscopy, and percutaneous nephrolithotomy (PCNL) have therefore been used for ADPKD.[40,41] In a multicenter report of 20 patients from 6 centers, SWL and PCNL were used in 16 and 4 patients, respectively. The stone-free rate was 43% and 80%, respectively, following lithotripsy and percutaneous nephrolithotomy.[42] In another report of 16 renal units, 13 were treated with SWL and 3 with open surgery. The overall stone-free rate was 85% at 3 months, including patients who underwent repeat lithotripsy.[41] Percutaneous nephrolithotomy in patients with ADPKD is performed rarely. However, this approach can be used with larger stones such as stag horn stones. Open surgery is rarely required in the contemporary management of urolithiasis in ADPKD patients.

Management of pain in patients with autosomal dominant polycystic kidney disease

Pain in patients with ADPKD can be multifactorial in etiology. Apart from the pain due to urologic conditions such as urolithiasis, cyst enlargement, cyst rupture, and hydronephrosis, other causes of chronic pain can be a complex problem in these patients. Mechanical back pain can result from increased lumbar lordosis and degenerative changes in the spine.[43] When obvious causes for renal pain are excluded, an MRI of the spine in these patients should be performed in order to rule out disc disease or other spinal abnormalities, such as spinal stenosis and lumbosacral radiculopathy due to disc disease or degenerative spine disease. Appropriate management of the spinal pathology can relieve pain in these patients.

Renal pain in these patients can result from compression of cysts on the surrounding tissues, traction on the pedicle of the kidney, and distention of the capsule. The severity of pain generally correlates with the size and number of the cysts, but there can be exceptions. Often there is a renal and an extrarenal component to the pain. A comprehensive approach to management of pain in these patients should be formulated in conjunction with the nephrologist and the pain clinic. Treatment options for pain in ADPKD patients

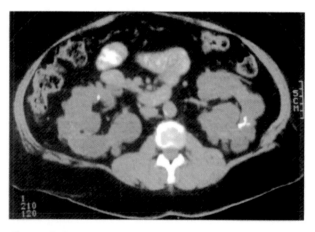

Figure 8.9
CT of a patient who had undergone renal transplantation for renal failure with ADPKD (autosomal dominant polycystic kidney disease) and presented with bilateral urolithiasis and recurrent UTIs (urinary tract infections) from the native kidneys. She was treated with hand-assisted laparoscopic bilateral nephrectomy.

include physical measures, psychobehavioral modifications, systemic analgesics, physical therapy and interventions such as transcutaneous electrical nerve stimulation (TENS), acupuncture, autonomic plexus blockade, neuromodulation by spinal cord stimulation, neuroaxial, opioids, and local anesthetics. Analgesics that have been successfully used include acetaminophen, salsalate, nonsteroidal analgesics, COX-2 (cyclooxygenase 2) inhibitors, tramadol and clonidine, before trying opioids with or without clonidine.[43] After conservative treatments have failed, surgical options must be considered. Aspiration of the cysts is not successful, since this is usually followed by rapid reaccumulation of fluid and recurrence of pain. Bennett et al reported that only 33% of patients who were treated with ultrasound-guided aspiration of cysts were pain-free at 18 months compared with 81% treated with open cyst decortication.[44]

Cyst decortication

Results

The original surgical decortication of renal cysts was performed by Rovsing in 1911.[45] Cyst decompression was performed by other authors who claimed considerable success. However, in 1957, after a report by Bricker and Patton suggested that patients who underwent surgical decompression of polycystic kidneys develop worsening of renal function, this procedure was abandoned for several years.[46] There were also a considerable morbidity and mortality in these patients after surgery during that time.[47] In the 1980s, however, surgical cyst decortication in ADPKD patients was rediscovered with encouraging results.[44,48] In 1992 Elzinga and colleagues reported a group of patients who were prospectively studied after undergoing 32 cyst decompression or decortication operations.[49] They reported up to 80% success 12 months postoperatively and 62% at 24 months following surgery. They also found that among patients following pain relapse the pain was often lessened and fewer patients were taking analgesics in comparison with the preoperative group. More importantly, no deterioration in renal function was observed postoperatively.

With the introduction of urologic laparoscopy in the 1990s there have been several reports of decortication of cysts. In 1995 Teichman and Hulbert reported 6 cases of laparoscopic cyst decortication (LCD) of patients with ADPKD.[50] With a follow-up of 6–40 months, pain relief was achieved in all patients but one, who underwent renal and hepatic cyst decortication. Brown and associates from the Mayo Clinic reported LCD in 13 patients (8 with ADPKD), with 62% of the patients having good pain relief

12–28 months postoperatively.[51] Twenty-nine patients who underwent 35 LCD procedures were meticulously followed prospectively at Washington University with a mean follow-up of 32.3 months.[52] At 12, 24, and 36 months, 73%, 52%, and 81% of patients, respectively, noted a greater than 50% improvement in pain. The mean operating time was 4.9 hours and a mean of 220 cysts (range = 4–692) were treated in each patient. More importantly, the majority of patients had improvement in their hypertension and the procedure was not associated with worsening renal function. LCD in patients with ADPKD is performed primarily for refractory pain caused by enlarged kidneys to multiple cysts. Surgery is also indicated in patients whose renal enlargement causes significant abdominal distention and discomfort. Percutaneous aspiration of cysts has not been successful in the long term. LCD is therefore an acceptable option for patients with enlarging cysts that require surgery.

Preoperative preparation

Patients with renal pain could also have cyst infections. Lipid-soluble antibiotics such as fluoroquinolones are useful in penetrating the cyst wall. Other antibiotics that are also lipid soluble include trimethoprim–sulfamethoxazole and chloramphenicol.[53] Patients receive bowel preparation, and patient positioning and trocar placement are similar to that described for cyst decortication of simple cysts.

Technique

Cyst decortication can be performed laparoscopically via a transperitoneal or retroperitoneal approach. We prefer the transperitoneal approach for laparoscopic surgery in patients with ADPKD because of the greater operating space that is available with this approach. Occasionally, patients with hepatic cysts can also undergo simultaneous hepatic cyst decortication via the laparoscopic approach.

When obtaining pneumoperitoneum with a Veress needle or with dilating trocar, it is important that the CT scan be reviewed in order not to insert the trocar or the Veress needle into the kidney itself. This is an important consideration when dealing with polycystic kidneys that can occupy the entire abdomen and can extend into the lower quadrant. The open approach (Hassan) to obtaining a pneumoperitoneum after insertion of the primary port is an option for the inexperienced laparoscopist and when the entire lateral abdomen is distended with the hugely enlarged kidney.

The line of Toldt is incised and the colon is mobilized off the Gerota's fascia. The plane between the Gerota's fascia and the mesocolon is developed until the colon is mobilized entirely. The colonic mobilization is continued until the hilum of the kidney is exposed in order to access the majority of the cysts. The perinephric fat is usually attenuated in patients with ADPKD. The Gerota's fascia is dissected off the anterior surface of the kidney to expose the majority of the cysts.

The cysts in the lower pole of the kidney are first drained to allow adequate mobilization of the upper pole. The superficial walls of the larger cysts are excised and sent for histopathologic examination. The medium cysts are treated with cruciate incisions on the roof, and the smaller cysts are punctured and drained. The decortication of the cysts is performed with the harmonic scalpel, the hook electrode, or the Endo-shear. Hemostasis is achieved with meticulous cauterization of the edges of the excised cysts with electrocoagulation. Indiscriminate electrocoagulation of the interior of the cyst is avoided to prevent caliceal entry. Incision into the renal parenchyma adjacent to the cyst is avoided to prevent excessive bleeding. The argon beam coagulator is used as required. In this manner the entire anterior wall of the renal cyst is treated. The hilum is dissected in order to be able to treat the cysts in the hilar region without vascular injury. After the superficial cysts have been treated, the retrograde injection of indigo carmine helps to distend and identify the renal collecting system, as previously described in this chapter.

After treating the entire anterior surface of the kidney, the kidney is mobilized in order to expose the posterior surface. The cysts in the posterior surface of the kidney are similarly treated. Complete mobilization of the kidney is essential to decorticate all visible cysts. Incision of the coronary ligament of the liver may be necessary to expose the superior aspect of the right polycystic kidney. A 10 mm flexible ultrasound probe is used to identify the cysts that are not obviously visible and deeper within the kidney parenchyma. Depending on the mobility of the kidney at the end of the procedure, the kidney may need to be fixed to the posterior abdominal wall with 2.0 polyglactin sutures using intracorporeal laparoscopic suturing.[54]

At the end of this procedure it is important that the peritoneum be irrigated with at least 1 liter of saline to ensure that the cyst fluid that has spilled into the peritoneum be evacuated. Certain cyst fluid can cause peritoneal irritation, leading to significant postoperative pain. Peritoneal drainage is not required. Intra-abdominal pressure is decreased to 5 mmHg to ensure that there is no bleeding. The trocars are then removed under vision. When a bladed trocar is used, the 10 and 12 mm trocar sites are closed using 0 polyglactin sutures, utilizing the Carter–Thomason device. The skin at the trocar sites is closed using 2-octly lcyanoacrylate (Dermabond; Ethicon, Inc, Somerville, New Jersey) skin adhesive. After the skin edges are clean and dry, they are held together and the Dermabond is applied with light brush strokes. At least three layers of the adhesive are applied.

Bilateral nephrectomy

Patients who are in end-stage renal failure, on hemodialysis, or who have undergone renal transplantation occasionally require unilateral or bilateral nephrectomy for chronic abdominal pain (see Figure 8.8) or symptoms related to significant abdominal distention. Bilateral nephrectomy for ADPKD can be performed via a transperitoneal or a retroperitoneal approach. We prefer a transperitoneal approach because of the increased space as well as the easier specimen extraction with that approach. It is essential to carefully image these patients preoperatively before cyst decompression is performed, since incidental renal tumors may be seen in these patients and cyst decortication in this situation can cause tumor spillage.

In a recent report by Rehman et al from Washington University, 3 patients underwent bilateral hand-assisted laparoscopic nephrectomy.[55] Bilateral nephrectomy can be performed with a single hand assisted device placed via a periumbilical incision (Figure 8.10). Two additional 12

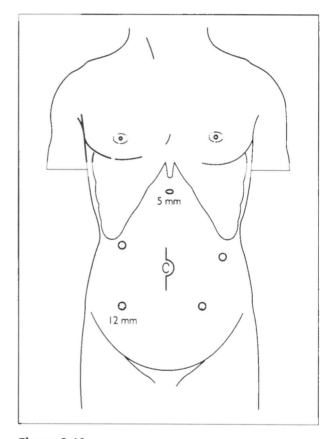

Figure 8.10
Port placement for laparoscopic hand-assisted bilateral nephrectomy for a right-handed surgeon. The lower 12 mm ports are used for the laparoscope and a periumbilical incision is made for the hand-assistance device. An additional 5 mm port may be used in the anterior axillary line for lateral retraction of the kidney during hilar dissection.

mm ports and a 5 mm port are then inserted on each side to perform the bilateral nephrectomy. The patient can be placed in a lateral decubitus position and the position changed after one side is performed. We use the beanbag, which supports the patients laterally on both sides. The patient is then strapped to the table securely with adequate padding at bony prominences. With this arrangement, the patient can be rotated about 40–50° in each direction, in order to elevate the ipsilateral side and perform the operation without having to reposition the patient after the first nephrectomy is performed. Hand assistance in this operation considerably reduces the operating time and is recommended, especially since an incision will have to be made to extract the specimen. The midline incision is adequate for hand assistance on both sides as well as to extract both kidneys.

After initial colonic mobilization, some of the cysts may need to be decompressed in order to facilitate hilar dissection. After the hilar vascular control is obtained, further cyst decortication may be required in order to facilitate the delivery of the specimen to the hand-assist device incision. With a periumbilical incision the left hand can be used for both sides for the right-handed surgeon. Several devices are available for hand assistance. Each device has its own advantages and disadvantages. We have recently used the Lap Disc (Ethicon Endo-Surgery, Cincinnati, Ohio) as well as the GelPort (Applied Medical Resources, Rancho Santa Margarita, California) effectively.

These patients are generally at the higher risk for perioperative complications, since they are typically on dialysis or have had renal transplantation, and are on immunosuppressant medication including steroids. The peritoneum is thoroughly irrigated with saline, since some of the cysts are decompressed before extraction of the specimen. Cyst decortication can cause considerable peritoneal irritation and postoperative pain. To minimize this, some of the cysts can be drained after the lower pole is delivered outside the abdominal incision. With the drainage of cysts outside the abdomen with a partially extracted kidney, peritoneal irritation can be avoided or minimized.

Bilateral nephrectomy has also been performed for ADPKD via a retroperitoneal approach.[56] With the retroperitoneal approach, the patient is placed in the full lateral position and securely strapped to the table. The table is flexed in order to maximize the distance between the costal margin and iliac crest. Access is gained in the retroperitoneal approach using a 1.5 cm incision off the tip of the 12th rib. Balloon dilation is performed with 800–1000 ml of air. Three 12 mm trocars are used: one off the tip of the 12th rib; another 12 mm port at the junction of the lateral erector spinae muscle and the 12th rib; and another 12 mm port 3 cm cephalad to the iliac crest. After the nephrectomy is performed via a standard retroperitoneal approach, a lower midline incision is made 12 cm long. Blunt dissection is performed in a posterolateral

direction, posterior to the rectus abdominus muscle, in order to reach the retroperitoneal space containing the kidney that was previously removed via a retroperitoneal approach. This approach avoids peritoneal violation and the complications associated with it. However, retroperitoneal nephrectomy with a massively enlarged kidney in a limited space can be technically challenging and is recommended only for surgeons with extensive experience with this approach.

Hydatid cyst

Hydatid cysts are parasitic cysts that are associated with echinococcal infestation. Although rare in the continental United States except Alaska, this microorganism is still prevalent in the regions such as the Middle East and Australia. Silber and Moyad[57] described three forms of the disease:

1. a benign sylvatic form of *Echinococcus granulosus* endemic to Alaska, where the renal lesion is a calcified unilocular cyst
2. a pastoral form of *E. granulosus*, where the cyst expands rapidly and can rupture
3. *E. multilocularis*, which, although uncommon, is invasive with a high mortality rate.

The most common symptom is flank pain.[58] Other symptoms are hematuria, malaise, fever, and hydatiduria. Eosinophilia can be present and occasionally daughter cysts can be seen in the urine. The Casoni skin test, the Weinberg (complement fixation) test, and the indirect hemagglutinin test may be helpful in making the diagnosis. Imaging may reveal a calcified cystic renal lesion. CT imaging can detect calcification and the daughter cysts, as well as extrarenal involvement. If the kidney is extensively involved and poorly functioning, a laparoscopic nephrectomy can be performed. Care should be taken during the nephrectomy to avoid spillage of cyst contents into the abdomen, since seeding with daughter cysts can occur.

Partial nephrectomy or total nephrectomy is performed depending upon the size and location of the cyst and the function of the kidney. Intra-operative spillage of cyst contents can be a serious complication. LCD has been described when the cyst is small and the kidney has good function. The retroperitoneal laparoscopic approach is preferred if the cyst is accessible via the retroperitoneal approach. The cyst is exposed and the cyst contents aspirated. The cyst cavity is then filled with dilute povidone-iodine and drained. The cyst is then decorticated, as described for simple cysts. The retroperitoneum is thoroughly irrigated with saline.[59] Other scolecidal agents include 30% saline, 2% formalin, 1% iodine, and 0.5% silver nitrate.

Conclusion

Renal cystic disease can be managed with a variety of minimally invasive options. A thorough evaluation with radiologic imaging is essential to make the initial diagnosis in order to differentiate malignant from the nonmalignant cystic conditions. In the vast majority of patients a definitive diagnosis can be made without the need for invasive interventions such as angiography or aspiration. A few indeterminate complex cysts may require surgical exploration and resection.

Simple cysts rarely require treatment and are often incidental radiologic findings. When simple cysts are symptomatic they can be managed in most cases with aspiration and sclerotherapy. When sclerotherapy fails or is contraindicated, LCD is effective. Other options in selected patients include the ureteroscopic and percutaneous approaches. Laparoscopic decortication is effective in the management of ADPKD. This approach is indicated primarily for renal pain due to cyst enlargement. The procedure has also been found to assist with control of hypertension. This surgery should aim to achieve decortication of all cysts that are accessible without caliceal violation.

References

1. Glassberg KI, Stephens FD, Lebowitz RL, et al. Renal dysgenesis and cystic disease of the kidney: a report of the Committee on Terminology, Nomenclature and Classification, Section on Urology, American Academy of Pediatrics. J Urol 1987; 138(4 Pt 2):1085–92.

2. Baert L, Steg A. On the pathogenesis of simple renal cysts in the adult. A microdissection study. Urol Res 1977; 5(3):103–8.

3. Baert L, Steg A. Is the diverticulum of the distal and collecting tubules a preliminary stage of the simple cyst in the adult? J Urol 1977; 118(5):707–10.

4. Terada N, Ichioka K, Matsuta Y, et al. The natural history of simple renal cysts. J Urol 2002; 167(1):21–3.

5. Yasuda M, Masai M, Shimazaki J. A simple renal cyst. Nippon Hinyokika Gakkai Zasshi – Japanese J Urol 1993; 84(2):251–7.

6. Tada S, Yamagishi J, Kobayashi H, et al. The incidence of simple renal cyst by computed tomography. Clin Radiol 1983; 34(4):437–9.

7. Kissane JM, Smith MG. Pathology of infancy and childhood, 2nd edn. St Louis: CV Mosby, 1975: 587.

8. Ravine D, Gibson RN, Walker RG, et al. Evaluation of ultrasonographic diagnostic criteria for autosomal dominant polycystic kidney disease 1. Lancet 1994; 343:824–7.

9. Nicolau C, Torra R, Badenas C, et al. Autosomal dominant polycystic kidney disease types 1 and 2: assessment of US sensitivity for diagnosis. Radiology 1999; 213:273–6.

10. Bosniak MA. The current radiological approach to renal cysts. Radiology 1986; 158(1):1–10.

11. Bosniak MA. Difficulties in classifying cystic lesions of the kidney. Urol Radiol 1991; 13(2):91–3.

12. Bosniak MA. Problems in the radiologic diagnosis of renal parenchymal tumors. Urol Clin N Am 1993; 20(2):217–30.

13. Bosniak MA. Diagnosis and management of patients with complicated cystic lesions of the kidney. AJR Am J Roentgenol 1997; 169(3):819–21.

14. Macari M, Bosniak MA. Delayed CT to evaluate renal masses incidentally discovered at contrast-enhanced CT: demonstration of vascularity with deenhancement. Radiology 1999; 213(3):674–80.

15. Holmberg G, Hietala SO. Treatment of simple renal cysts by percutaneous puncture and instillation of bismuth-phosphate. Scand J Urol Nephrol 1989; 23(3):207–12.

16. Chung BH, Kim JH, Hong CH, et al. Comparison of single and multiple sessions of percutaneous sclerotherapy for simple renal cyst. BJU Int 2000; 85(6):626–7.

17. Paananen I, Hellstrom P, Leinonen S, et al. Treatment of renal cysts with single-session percutaneous drainage and ethanol sclerotherapy: long-term outcome. Urology 2001; 57(1): 30–3.

18. Fontana D, Porpiglia F, Morra I, Destefanis P. Treatment of simple renal cysts by percutaneous drainage with three repeated alcohol injection. Urology 1999; 53(5):904–7.

19. Seo TS, Oh JH, Yoon Y, et al. Acetic acid as a sclerosing agent for renal cysts: comparison with ethanol in follow-up results. Cardiovasc Intervent Radiol 2000; 23(3):177–81.

20. Kavoussi LR, Clayman RV, Mikkelsen DJ, Meretyk S. Ureteronephroscopic marsupialization of obstructing peripelvic renal cyst. J Urol 1991; 146(2):411–4.

21. Kang Y, Noble C, Gupta M. Percutaneous resection of renal cysts. J Endourol 2001; 15(7):735–8, discussion 738–9.

22. Hulbert JC, Hunter D, Young AT. Castaneda-Zuniga W. Percutaneous intrarenal marsupialization of a perirenal cystic collection – endocystolysis. J Urol 1988; 139(5):1039–41.

23. Plas EG, Hubner WA. Percutaneous resection of renal cysts: a long-term followup. J Urol 1993; 149(4):703–5.

24. Clayman RV, McDougall EM, Nakada SY. Endourology of the uppertract: percutaneous renal and ureteral procedures. In: Walsh PC, Retik AB, Vaughan ED, Wein AJ, eds. Campbell's urology, Philadelphia: WB Saunders, 1998.

25. Hoenig DM, McDougall EM, Shalhav AL, et al. Laparoscopic ablation of peripelvic renal cysts. J Urol 1997; 158(4):1345–8.

26. Rubenstein SC, Hulbert JC, Pharand D, et al. Laparoscopic ablation of symptomatic renal cysts. J Urol 1993; 150(4): 1103–6.

27. Santiago L, Yamaguchi R, Kaswick J, Bellman GC. Laparoscopic management of indeterminate renal cysts. Urology 1998; 52(3):379–83.

28. Bellman GC, Yamaguchi R, Kaswick J. Laparoscopic evaluation of indeterminate renal cysts. Urology 1995; 45(6): 1066–70.

29. Hildebrandt F. Genetic renal diseases in children. Curr Opin in Pediatr 1995; 7(2):182–91.

30. Gabow PA. Autosomal dominant polycystic kidney disease. N Engl J Med 1993; 329(5):332–42.

31. Glassberg KI. Renal dysgenesis and cystic disease of the kidney. In: Walsh PC, Retik AB, Vaughan ED, Wein AJ, eds. Campbell's urology, 7th edn. Philadelphia: WB Saunders, 1998: 1925.

32. Thomsen HS, Thaysen JH. Frequency of hepatic cysts in adult polycystic kidney disease. Acta Medica Scand 1988; 224(4): 381–4.

33. Glassberg KI, Hackett RE, Waterhouse K. Congenital anomalies of the kidney, ureter and bladder. In: Kendall AR, Karafin L, eds. Harry S Goldsmith's practice of surgery: urology. Hagerstown: Harper and Row, 1981: 1.

34. Fick GM, Gabow PA. Hereditary and acquired cystic disease of the kidney. Kidney Int 1994; 46(4):951–64.

35. Hatfield PM, Pfister RC. Adult polycystic disease of the kidneys (Potter type 3). JAMA 1972; 222(12):1527–31.

36. Delaney VB, Adler S, Bruns FJ, et al. Autosomal dominant polycystic kidney disease: presentation, complications, and prognosis. Am J Kidney Dis 1985; 5(2):104–11.

37. Grantham JJ. Polycystic kidney disease: hereditary and acquired. Adv Int Med 1993; 38:409–20.

38. Torres VE, Erickson SB, Smith LH, et al. The association of nephrolithiasis and autosomal dominant polycystic kidney disease. Am J Kidney Dis 1988; 11(4):318–25.

39. Grampsas SA, Chandhoke PS, Fan J, et al. Anatomic and metabolic risk factors for nephrolithiasis in patients with autosomal dominant polycystic kidney disease. Am J Kidney Dis 2000; 36(1):53–7.

40. Ng CS, Yost A, Streem SB. Nephrolithiasis associated with autosomal dominant polycystic kidney disease: contemporary urological management. J Urol 2000; 163(3):726–9.

41. Delakas D, Daskalopoulos G, Cranidis A. Extracorporeal shockwave lithotripsy for urinary calculi in autosomal dominant polycystic kidney disease. J Endourol 1997; 11(3): 167–70.

42. Torres VE, Wilson DM, Hattery RR, Segura JW. Renal stone disease in autosomal dominant polycystic kidney disease. Am J Kidney Dis 1993; 22(4):513–19.

43. Bajwa ZH, Gupta S, Warfield CA, Steinman TI. Pain management in polycystic kidney disease. Kidney Int 2001; 60(5): 1631–44.

44. Bennett WM, Elzinga L, Golper TA, Barry JM. Reduction of cyst volume for symptomatic management of autosomal dominant polycystic kidney disease. J Urol 1987; 137(4): 620–2.

45. Rovsing T. Treatment of multilocular renal cyst with multiple punctures. Hospitalstid 1911; 4: 105–116.

46. Bricker NS, Patton JF. Renal function studies in polycystic disease of the kidneys with observations on the effects of surgical decompression. N Engl J Med 1957; 256: 212.

47. Dalgaard OZ: Bilateral polycystic disease of the kidneys. A follow-up of 284 patients and their families. Acta Med Scand Suppl 1957; 328; 1–255.

48. He SZ, An SY, Jiang HM, et al. Cyst decapitating decompression operation in polycystic kidney: preliminary report of 52 cases. Chinese Med J 1980; 93(11):773–8.

49. Elzinga LW, Barry JM, Torres VE, et al. Cyst decompression surgery for autosomal dominant polycystic kidney disease. J Am Soc Nephrol 1992; 2(7):1219–26.

50. Teichman JM, Hulbert JC. Laparoscopic marsupialization of the painful polycystic kidney. J Urol 1995; 153(4):1105–7.

51. Brown JA, Torres VE, King BF, Segura JW. Laparoscopic marsupialization of symptomatic polycystic kidney disease. J Urol 1996; 156(1):22–7.

52. Lee D, Andreoni CR, Rehman J, et al. Laparoscopic cyst decortication in autosomal dominant polycystic kidney disease: impact on pain, hypertension, and renal function. J Endourol 2003; 17(6):345–54.

53. Bennett WM, Elzinga LW, Barry JM. Management of cystic kidney disease. In: Gardner KD Jr, Brnstein J, eds. The cystic kidney. Boston: Kluwer Academic, 1990: 247–75.

54. Dunn MD, Portis AJ, Naughton C, et al. Laparoscopic cyst marsupialization in patients with autosomal dominant polycystic kidney disease. J Urol 2001; 165(6 Pt1):1888–92.

55. Rehman J, Landman J, Andreoni C, et al. Laparoscopic bilateral hand assisted nephrectomy for autosomal dominant polycystic kidney disease: initial experience. J Urol 2001; 166(1):42–7.

56. Gill IS, Kaouk JH, Hobart MG, et al. Laparoscopic bilateral synchronous nephrectomy for autosomal dominant polycystic kidney disease: the initial experience. J Urol 2001; 165(4):1093–8.

57. Silber SJ, Moyad RA. Renal echinococcus. J Urol 1972; 108(5):669–72.

58. Gogus C, Safak M, Baltaci S, Turkolmez K. Isolated renal hydatidosis: experience with 20 cases. J Urol 2003; 169(1): 186–9.

59. Hemal AK. Laparoscopic management of renal cystic disease. Urol Clin N Am 2001; 28(1):115–26.

9

Laparoscopic/retroperitoneoscopic radical nephrectomy for renal cell cancer

Jens J Rassweiler, Dogu Teber, Yoram Dekel, Michael Schulze, Tibet Erdogru and Thomas Frede

Pathological aspects of renal cell carcinoma

Incidence and etiology

Renal cell carcinoma accounts for 3% of all adult malignancies. Annual incidence in the industrialized countries is reported at between 9 and 11 per 100,000 inhabitants,[1] whereas the global figures show an incidence of 2.4–4.3 cases per 100,000 inhabitants.[2] At the time of diagnosis, 20% of the patients have disseminated disease and another 25% will have locally advanced tumors.[3] Around 60% of the patients who are clinically diagnosed will die due to the disease because of progression and metastatic spread.[4]

Renal cell cancer occurs primarily in the 5th to 6th decade. Men are twice as often afflicted as women. There is some evidence that renal cell carcinoma is more common in the urban population, due to the exposition to carcinogenic industrial agents and tobacco abuse.

Renal cell carcinoma is the most common renal tumor, accounting for 85% of all renal malignancies. The origin of the tumor is reported by a number of investigations[5–7] as being mainly from the proximal tubular cells (clear cell and chromophile carcinoma), followed by the distal tubular system (chromophobe carcinoma), and the collecting system (Bellini duct carcinoma).

The identification of specific genetic alterations has led to the classification of different genetic subtypes beyond the morphology of the cells, such as that described by Kovacs et al.[8] The main interest in this classification is that different genetic subtypes (Table 9.1) have significant different clinical behaviors as regards the course of the disease and the response to therapy. Conventional renal cell carcinomas have a poorer prognosis than papillary renal cell carcinoma.[9,10] Patients with chromophobe renal cell carcinoma survive longer and have less advanced disease than patients with conventional or papillary renal cell carcinoma.[11,12] Tumor progression and more malignant behavior has been associated with various genetic and subtype specific alterations such as duplication of chromosome 5q22 for conventional renal cell carcinoma and trisomy of chromosome 3/3q or loss of chromosome Xp in papillary renal cell types. DNA flow cytometry data also suggest that both prognosis and tumor progression rate may correlate with nondiploid tumor patterns in all subtypes.[13–15] The knowledge of these genetic variabilities is an important step in understanding the different responses of renal cell carcinoma to immunotherapy or other treatment modalities.

Table 9.1 *Heidelberg classification of renal cell carcinoma*

Subtypes of renal cell carcinoma (incidence)	Genetic alterations
Conventional renal cell carcinoma (clear cell) (75–80%)	Allelic loss of chromosomes 3p, 6q, 8p, 9p, 14q; duplication of 5q; mutation in VHL gene
Papillary renal cell carcinoma (10–15%)	Trisomies of chromosomes 3q, 7, 8p, 12q, 16q, 17q, 20; loss of Y chromosome in male
Chromophobe renal cell carcinoma (1–3%)	Monosomy of chromosomes 1, 2, 6, 10, 13, 17, 21
Bellini duct carcinoma (1–2%)	No specific alterations established; loss of DNA sequences in chromosomes 1, 2, 9, 11 and 18 is discussed
Nonclassified renal cell carcinoma (3–5%)	No specific alterations established

Pathologic factors

The TNM (tumor–node–metastasis) classification of the UICC (The International Union against Cancer) is today the worldwide established clinical staging system that demonstrates the anatomic extent of the malignancy; it has taken over from other classification systems (i.e. Robson stage I–IV). The TNM classification takes into account tumor size, invasion beyond the Gerota's fascia, local spread into veins, lymph node and/or adrenal metastasis, and distant metastasis (Table 9.2). All these factors are significant in predicting the clinical outcome of the disease. Patients with tumors limited to the kidney have 85–95% 5-year survival rates, whereas those with distant metastases have a poor prognosis with a 5-year survival rate of < 5%.[16–20] In organ-confined renal cell carcinoma, the microscopic invasion of the renal vein significantly influences the course of the disease, with a poorer 5-year survival rate of 77%.[16] Patients with tumor invasion of the perirenal fat or Gerota's fascia have worse prognosis, with about 50% 5-year survival compared to those with organ-confined disease.

The importance of renal vein invasion as an independent predictor of prognosis is controversially discussed in the literature; the frequency is reported at between 5 and 36%.[21,22] There is some evidence that renal vein invasion alone does not adversely affect survival when the tumor is organ-confined.[23] Similarly, the involvement of the vena cava inferior has no significant impact on survival; 5-year survival rates of 47–69% were published for both

patterns.[24,25] Therefore, an aggressive surgical approach is accepted in cases of vein invasion.

Lymph node involvement implicates a survival rate from 5 to 30% at 5 years.[23] Johnsen and Hellsten reported from autopsy studies that all cases with lymphatic spread also had distant metastases.[26] Therefore, the benefit from an extensive lymphadenectomy is controversial. Incidental detection of unsuspected lymph node metastasis has been reported only in the range of 3%.[27]

Similarly, patients with adrenal gland metastasis also have distant or lymph node metastases, so that only 0.5–2% of them benefit from an adrenalectomy.[28] Some authors therefore recommend that ipsilateral adrenalectomy should only be performed if a lesion is detected preoperatively on a computed tomography (CT) scan or if the renal cell carcinoma is located at the upper pole region of the kidney.[29]

Studies of patients with metastatic disease have shown a prognosis with 5-year survival rates of between 2 and 10%.[17,30] The synchronous presentation of the metastatic disease is associated with a longer survival time compared to patients with asynchronous diagnosis of metastasis; in particular, patients with resectable solitary metastasis are reported to have a 5-year survival rate of 23%.[31]

Apart from the pathologic stage of the tumor (TNM) a number of histopathologic grading systems with regard to cell type, necrosis rate, and nuclear shape have been established. The nuclear grade is the most important independent factor correlating with survival for all stages of renal cell carcinoma.[32] Nevertheless, its application in clinical practice is difficult, due to the high inter-observer variation. Techniques such as nuclear morphometry are promising more objective and reproducible results in grading renal cell carcinoma, but only a few results with this method have been published regarding its prognostic significance.[33]

Stage	Description
Table 9.2 *TNM classification of renal cell carcinoma (UICC 1997)*	
T1	Tumor limited to the kidney, 7 cm or less in diameter
T2	Tumor limited to the kidney, more than 7 cm in diameter
T3a	Invasion of the adrenal gland or perirenal fat
T3b	Invasion of renal vein or infradiaphragmal vena cava
T3c	Invasion of supradiaphragmal vena cava
T4	Tumor infiltration beyond Gerota's fascia
N1	One lymph node metastasis
N2	More than one lymph node metastasis
M1	Distant metastasis

Surgical treatment of renal cell carcinoma

The reported worldwide steady increase of incidence might undoubtedly be a result of the increasing availability of ultrasonography or CT. Because more incidental renal tumors are being diagnosed, the profile of patients seeking treatment for renal carcinoma has changed. Therefore, treatment strategies with different approaches (i.e. high-intensity focus ultrasound, radiofrequency ablation, cryotherapy, radical and partial surgery, laparoscopy) reflect this situation in current reports. Nevertheless, surgical removal is still considered to be the dominant procedure in the management of renal cell carcinoma. During the last 10 years, however, open surgery has increasingly been replaced by the laparoscopic approaches.

History of laparoscopic radical nephrectomy

Clayman et al pioneered laparoscopic nephrectomy, when removing a renal oncocytoma in 1990.[34] Almost 1 year later Coptcoat et al used the same technique for a radical extirpation of a T2 renal cell carcinoma.[35] In 1992, Chiu et al reported on a laparoscopic nephroureterectomy for malignant disease.[36] This technique has become one of the most innovative challenges to the conventional and traditional gold standard of the open approach. Currently, this option is preferred over surgery in many uro-oncologic centers all over the world, particularly focused towards T1 tumors.[37]

Numerous experiences worldwide have demonstrated very good surgical results and low perioperative morbidity, at least comparable to or better in many aspects than open surgery.[38] Additionally, a few published series with long-term follow-up now show a similar oncologic result to the open counterpart.[38] The technique, however, is still demanding, as it requires adequate skills in laparoscopic surgery. The further refinement of the laparoscopic technique is accompanied by a growing number of urologists being adequately trained in this area.

The basic oncologic surgical principles applied to laparoscopic surgery are exactly the same as for open surgery. Moreover, the criteria used for diagnosis, staging, follow-up, and general management are identical as well. Thus, the objective of this chapter is to focus more on the technical aspects of the procedure rather than on those aspects of the disease. Additionally, we review the current state of the art of laparoscopic radical nephrectomy, including a review of long-term follow-up data based on own experience and on the literature.

Technique of laparoscopic radical nephrectomy

Principally, there are two approaches for laparoscopic radical nephrectomy: the transperitoneal and retroperitoneal technique.

Transperitoneal approach

Patient preparation

All patients receive similar preoperative preparation as performed prior to open surgery (including informed consent and bowel preparation). Prior to the procedure, a nasogastric tube and a urinary catheter are inserted. Under general anesthesia, the patient is placed in the lateral tradi-tional flank position, with the table flexed to extend the uppermost flank; the table is then turned to a more oblique position (Figure 34.1).

Trocar placement

After a pneumoperitoneum is attained with the inserted Veress needle, placed lateral to the rectus abdominis muscle on the line with the umbilicus, trocars are inserted through the ventral abdominal wall. Port I (10 mm) is located periumbilically at the lateral edge of the rectus abdominis muscle; Port II (5 mm for the left, 12 mm for the right side) is located subcostally on the mammillary line. Port III (12 mm for the left, 5 mm for the right side) is located above the superior iliac spine on the mammillary line (see Figure 9.1). The laparoscope is passed through Port I and used for endoscopic control of secondary trocar insertion. The ports are fixed with a sterile adhesive tape and sutured to the skin (no grips preferred). After complete inspection of the abdomen, either the descending (left kidney) or ascending (right kidney) colon is mobilized through a laterocolic incision of the peritoneum along the line of Toldt. Since the respective colon is free to fall off medially (Figure 9.2), one or two further 5 mm ports can be inserted through the newly exposed retroperitoneum (Ports IV, V). These two ports are mainly used to grasp the kidney during dissection and for kidney retrieval.[37,39]

Clipping the ureter

The gonadal vein is identified in proximity to the sacral promontory, and clipped and dissected, as is the ureter

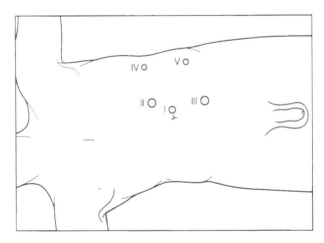

Figure 9.1
Transperitoneal laparoscopic radical nephrectomy – patient positioning and trocar placement for left renal tumor. Positions of ports I–V are indicated.

thereafter (Figures 9.2 and 39.3). Retraction of the ureter can be established with an ENDO BOWEL clamp inserted through Port IV or V and may be helpful during dissection of the renal hilum. The lower pole of the kidney is isolated, including the fatty capsule.

Renal vessel control

Once the vessels are identified and dissected, the clipping and transection is performed, following the principles of open surgery and starting with the artery. There are a number of different ligating systems, including the Lapro-Clip® (Tyco-Braun), an absorbable single ligating clip; the Challenger® titanium clip (Aesculap); the nonabsorbable lockable plastic Hemo-lock-clips® (Weck); or the Endo-GIA® endoscopic stapling device (Tyco), particularly used for the vein. On most occasions, we prefer titanium clips for the artery (three clips on the stay side) and the

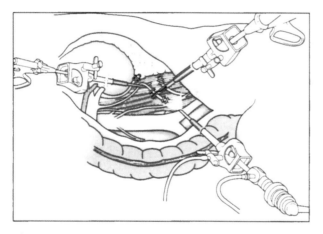

Figure 9.2
Transperitoneal laparoscopic radical nephrectomy – dissection and clipping of the ureter.

Lapro-Clip for the renal vein. Only for larger renal veins, do we prefer an endoscopic stapler (Figure 9.4). Dissection of the renal vessels is carried out bimanually with EndoShears, endodissector, and right-angle-clamp, quite similar to open surgery.

Organ retrieval

Now the upper pole of the kidney, including the fatty capsule, is dissected free of the respective adrenal gland and the relevant peritoneum. Next, the organ is grasped in the hilar region and moved down into the pelvic area, preventing any interference with insertion of the organ bag. In selected cases (i.e. upper pole renal cell carcinoma) we have additionally taken out the adrenal gland by use of clips or the Endo-GIA stapler. For retrieval of the specimen we strongly recommend the LapSac, because of the strength and rigidity of the organ bag, particularly when further morcellation of the specimen is planned (Figure 9.5). The LapSac is twirled around a 4.5 mm converter-reduced Endo Grasp and passed through Port III. The organ bag unfolds intra-abdominally and is held open by three Endoclamps (via Port II, IV, and V) while the kidney is maneuvered into the LapSac.[40]

Digital fragmentation

After the endodissector pulls the drawstring, thereby closing the bag, the trocar sleeve is removed and the neck of the bag is pulled out over the surface of the abdomen (via Port II for the right kidney and Port III for the left side). The port site is further incised (20 mm) and covered

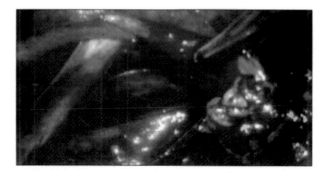

Figure 9.3
Transperitoneal laparoscopic radical nephrectomy – dissection and clipping of the ureter (endoscopic view).

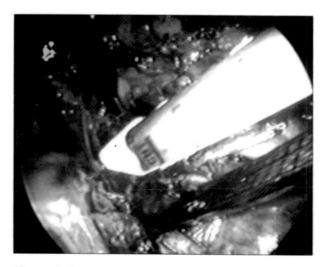

Figure 9.4
Transperitoneal laparoscopic radical nephrectomy – clipping and transsection of a large renal vein with the endoscopic stapler (Endo-GIA, Tyco).

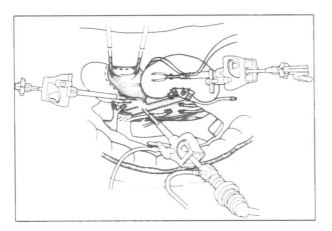

Figure 9.5
Transperitoneal laparoscopic radical nephrectomy –
Entrapment of the specimen in the organ bag (LapSac).

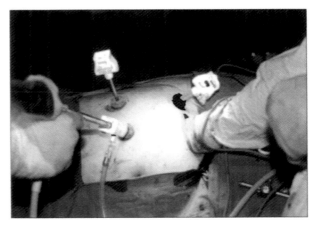

Figure 9.7
Transperitoneal laparoscopic radical nephrectomy – removal of
the complete specimen via a muscle-splitting incision in the
lower abdomen. This incision can also be used for a hand-
assisted technique.

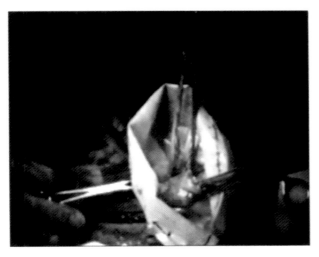

Figure 9.6
Transperitoneal laparoscopic radical nephrectomy – digital
fragmentation and stepwise removal of specimen with ring
forceps.

with an adhesive drape, making forceps removal of
fatty tissue and digital fragmentation of the kidney into
3–5 pieces possible (Figure 9.6). This is done very carefully
to distinguish between fatty capsule, normal renal tissue,
and renal tumor, which is sent separately for histopathologic analysis. We never used a mechanical liquidizer, aspirator, or morcellator device.[34,41]

Complete organ removal

In some cases we have used a 8–10 cm muscle-splitting
lower abdominal incision for complete organ removal.[42,43]
This access can also be used for a *hand-assisted laparoscopic*

approach, particularly towards the end of the procedure
(Figure 9.7).

Before all trocar sleeves are removed under direct vision,
the renal fossa has to be inspected to rule out any active
bleeding. This permits drainage of blood and irrigation
fluid and may reveal postoperative bleeding. The enlarged
incision (for organ removal) is closed with fascia and skin
suture. All other port incisions are sutured sub- and intra-
cutaneously or covered with adhesive strips.

Retroperitoneal approach

Patient preparation

All patients receive similar preoperative preparation as
performed prior to open surgery or transperitoneal
laparoscopic nephrectomy.

Access to the retroperitoneum

Under general anesthesia, the patient is placed in the
typical kidney position. The Trendelenburg position is not
necessary. A 15–18 mm incision is made in the 'muscle-
free' triangle between the lateral edges of the M. latissimus
dorsi and M. obliquus externus (Figure 9.8). A canal down
to the retroperitoneal space is then created by blunt dissection with Overhold forceps. The canal is then dilated with
the index finger, which dissects the plane between the
lumbodorsal aponeurosis and Gerota's fascia, pushing the
peritoneum medially, and thus creating a retroperitoneal
cavity for correct placement of the secondary trocars
(Figure 9.9).

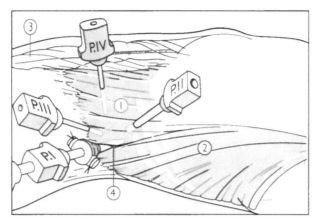

Figure 9.8
Retroperitoneal laparoscopic radical nephrectomy – patient positioning and trocar placement. 1 = M. obliquus externus, 2 = M. latissimus dorsi, 3 = M. rectus abdominis, 4 = muscle-free triangle. Positions of Ports P.I–P.IV are indicated.

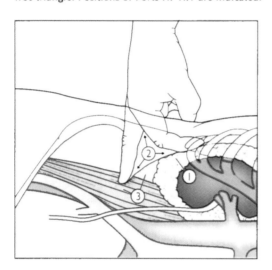

Figure 9.9
Retroperitoneal laparoscopic radical nephrectomy – finger dissection of the retroperitoneal space between the lumbodorsal aponeurosis and Gerota's fascia. 1 = perirenal fat, 2 = retroperitoneal space, 3 = Gerota's fascia.

Placement of secondary trocars

We then place the next two secondary trocars directly under palpation lateral to the index finger introduced via the primary access.[44] To avoid any injury to the surgeon's finger, the canal needs to be dilated using forceps (Figure 9.10): Port II (10/11 mm) for the right hand of the surgeon (use of EndoShears and Endoclip applicator); Port III (5 mm) for the left hand of the surgeon (use of endodissector). Then, the trocar site of Port I is closed with a matress suture around the sheath to avoid gas leakage and the trocar is connected to the CO_2 insufflator to establish a pneumoretroperitoneum (12 mmHg, 3.5 l/min), and retroperitoneoscopy is performed.

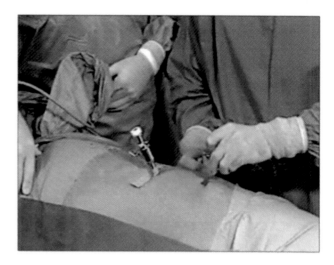

Figure 9.10
Retroperitoneal laparoscopic radical nephrectomy – placement of secondary trocars under palpatory control.

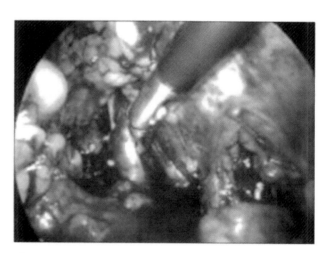

Figure 9.11
Retroperitoneal laparoscopic radical nephrectomy – dissection of the renal artery with right-angle forceps.

Finally, if necessary, medially to the edge of the peritoneum, another 5 mm trocar (Port IV) is inserted under endoscopic view, serving for retraction of the kidney during the dissection. As with the open procedure, the surgeon and the camera assistant stand on the dorsal side of the patient.

Early control of the renal artery

The first step in the retroperitoneal approach is the horizontal incision of Gerota's fascia to expose the psoas muscle. Thereafter, the renal hilum can be accessed easily followed by dissection of the renal artery using right-angle forceps (Figure 9.11). Subsequently, the renal artery is clipped and transected, followed by isolation of the renal vein. Early control of the renal hilum is one of the main advantages of the retroperitoneal approach.

Dissection of the kidney and ureter

After early control of the hilar vessels, the lower pole of the kidney and the ureter are dissected, identifying and transecting the gonadal vein (Figure 9.12). Finally, the upper

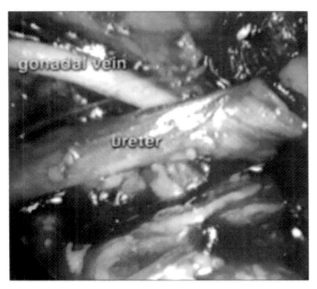

Figure 9.12
Retroperitoneal laparoscopic radical nephrectomy – dissection of the ureter and gonadal vein.

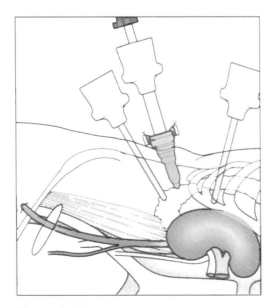

Figure 9.13
Retroperitoneal laparoscopic radical nephrectomy – en bloc removal of the specimen via a muscle-splitting retroperitoneal incision in the lower abdomen.

pole and the medial part of the kidney are dissected, which includes the perirenal fat. When indicated, the adrenal gland is taken en bloc with the specimen, requiring clipping of the adrenal vessels.

Organ entrapment

For adequate retrieval of the specimen, an adequate organ bag (i.e. LapSac) has to be inserted. The organ bag is pulled out on the skin surface via Port I. For morcellation of the specimen, the initial incision is enlarged to 25–30 mm. En bloc removal of the specimen can also be performed via a muscle-splitting retroperitoneal incision in the lower abdomen (Figure 9.13).

Heilbronn experience with laparoscopic radical nephrectomy

Patients

Since 1992, we have performed in the Department of Urology at the SLK-Klinikum in Heilbronn 80 laparoscopic radical nephrectomies in 78 patients (48 male, 30 female) with localized renal cell carcinoma. Stage and grade are listed in Table 9.3; the majority were pT1 tumors, and there had been two bilateral renal cell carcinomas in patients under dialysis. All relevant perioperative data were recorded, concerning operative time, complications, conversion, and reintervention rate, as well as hospital stay (Table 9.4). The follow-up time averaged 80 (7–144) months. Outcomes were determined by local recurrence, regional progression, development of metastases, and disease-specific survival.

Table 9.3 *Heilbronn experience with laparoscopic radical nephrectomy – pathological classification*

Tumor	Stage	n
Renal cell carcinoma	pT1	38
	PT2	10
	pT3a	3
	pT3b	2
Oncocytoma		2
Total		55

Table 9.4 *Heilbronn experience with laparoscopic radical nephrectomy – perioperative data*

Criteria	Nephrectomy (RCC)
Total number	80
Access:	
• Transperitoneal	18
• Retroperitoneal	62
Specimen retrieval:	
• Morcellation	25
• By incision	55
Mean operating time	141 min
Mean blood loss	135 ml
Conversion to open surgery	0
Complications:	5.0%
• Bleeding	1
• Pulmonary embolism	1
• Ileal stenosis	1
Reintervention	1
Hospital stay	7 days
Back to normal activity	21 days

RCC = renal cell carcinoma.

Results

Perioperative data

The operating time averaged 141 (90–410) min; there was no difference whether a transperitoneal (n = 18) or retroperitoneal (n = 62) approach was used (see Table 34.3). In 25 cases the specimen was entrapped in an organ bag (LapSac®, Cook Urological, Spencer, Indiana) and retrieved after digital morcellation, whereas in 55 instances the intact organ was removed via a 6–8 cm incision in the lower abdomen (see Figures 9.7 and 9.13). In 5 cases, this incision was also used for manual assistance during the procedure. The mean estimated blood loss was 135 (100–700) ml. There was no conversion to open surgery.

We observed one bleeding from the surface of the spleen, which could be managed by laparoscopic tamponating using a hemostatic gauze (Tachotamp®, Ethicon, Norderstedt, Germany). Another patient developed bleeding from one of the trocar sites (Port III) 6 hours after a right radical nephrectomy, which was controlled by a transcutaneous suture. Two months later the same patient suffered from ileus due to a stenosis of the terminal ileum, most probably induced by the aforementioned suture. The patient was successfully treated by a segmental ileal resec-

tion. One patient had a pulmonary embolism which could be managed conservatively. The mean postoperative hospital stay was 7 (4–16) days (see Table 9.4).

Pathology

The tumor was right sided in 33 (41%) patients, left sided in 43 (54%), and bilateral in 2 (5%) patients. The tumor was located at the upper pole in 21 (26%), at the central area in 40 (50%), and at the lower pole in 19 (24%) of the cases. Mean tumor size was 4.1 cm (range 0.5–8). The pathologic examination revealed renal cell carcinoma in 78 (97.5%) and an oncocytoma in 2 (2.5%) specimens. In the renal cell carcinoma group, the tumor stage was pT1 in 61 (76%), pT2 in 12 (15%), pT3a in 3 (45%) and pT3b in 2 (2.5%) of the specimens. Since we did not use any morcellator (i.e. Cook morcellator), the pathologist was able to define the exact pathologic staging in all cases. The surgical margins were negative in all cases.

Follow-up data

The mean observation time was 65 months (36–85 months). There was no port-site metastasis. One patient with a pT2G2 tumor developed a local recurrence and bone metastases 4 years after laparoscopic radical nephrectomy. He died 56 months after the procedure. Another 3 patients with pT1G3, pT2G3 and T3a tumor developed pulmonary and bony metastases 12, 18 and 31 months after the procedure and died 34 months after surgery. The cumulative overall disease-free survival rate after 5 years is 91%, revealing 96% for pT1/pT2 and 82% for pT3 tumors (Table 9.5).

Table 9.5 *Heilbronn experience with laparoscopic radical nephrectomy – follow-up data*

Criteria	Radical nephrectomy (RCC)
Total	55
Mean observation time	65 months
Dead of disease	4
Dead of other causes	–
Overall survival	91%
Disease-free survival (5 years)	
• Overall	91%
• pT1/pT2	96%
• pT3	80%

RCC = renal cell carcinoma.

Worldwide experience with laparoscopic radical nephrectomy

Laparoscopic radical nephrectomy has largely overtaken traditional surgery in many centers all over the world (Table 9.6). Beyond the discussion of access (retroperitoneal or transperitoneal), the contempory review of the literature documents the perioperative benefits of laparoscopy compared to the open approach.

In a multicenter study, Ono et al[45] compared 103 patients operated on by laparoscopy (85 transperitoneal and 18 retroperitoneal) with 46 operated on by the classic open procedure. The mean blood loss was documented as 254 ml vs 465 ml and the mean of the patients requiring transfusion were 5% vs 9% respectively for the two groups (see Table 9.6).

Gill et al[46] compared, retrospectively, 34 patients operated on laparoscopically using a retroperitoneal approach with 34 patients who underwent traditional open methods. They found a mean blood loss of 97.4 ml vs 295.1 ml and a complication rate of 13% vs 24% for comparable cases (see Table 9.6).

The meta-analysis of minor complications is reported in the current literature between 3 and 15% and major complications between 3 and 10% (Table 9.7). In open cases a complication rate between 10 and 20% was described for similar tumor stages.[47] The complication rate of 34% published by Dunn et al[48] rather reflects the learning curve of the pioneer and the benefit other centers gained from this experience.

Table 9.6 *Laparoscopic vs open radical nephrectomy – review of the literature*

Criteria	Abbou et al[37]		Ono et al[45]		Gill et al[46]		Jeschke et al[66]	
	Lap	Op	Lap	Op	Lap	Op	Lap	Op
Patients (*n*)	29	29	103	46	34	34	31	34
Tumor size (cm)	4.1	5.7	3.1	3.3	5.0	6.1	3.8	5.7
OR time (min)	145	121	282	198	186	174	125	145
Blood loss (ml)	100	285	254	465	98	370	na	na
Complication (%)	7	27	na	na	13	24	na	na
Hospital stay (days)	4.8	9.7	na	na	1.4	5.8	6.8	11.5
Follow-up (months)	15	13	29	39	10	29	na	na

Lap = operated on by laparoscopy, Op = operated on by the classic open procedure, OR = operating room, na = not available.

Table 9.7 *Worldwide experience of laparoscopic radical nephrectomy – perioperative data*

Main author	Patients (*n*)	Operating time (h)	Blood loss (ml)	Complication rate		Conversion	Hospital stay (days)
				Minor	Major		
Barret[59]	72	2.9	–	3%	8%	8%	4.4
Abbou[37]	29	2.4	100	8%		3.4%	4.8
Dunn[64]	60	5.5	172	34%	3%	1.6%	3.4
Ono[45]	103	4.7	254	3%	10%	3.4%	–
Chan[64]	67	4.2	289	15%		1.5%	3.8
Gill[62]	100	2.8	212	11%	3%	2%	1.6
Janetschek[58]	121	2.4	154	5%	4%	0%	6.1
Rassweiler*	80	2.5	135	5.0%			7

* Present series.

The mean operating time, initially reported in the range of 240 min, decreased in recent publications to 150 min (see Tables 9.6 and 9.7). We made the same observation (see Table 9.4), underlining the importance of the learning curve in achieving comparable or better operating times than the open approach.[46,48,49] A major key to that problem is that the same experienced laparoscopic team treats all cases. Dunn et al reported a decrease of the operating time by nearly half comparing the first 10 and the last 10 patients who underwent a laparoscopic radical nephrectomy in the same institution.[48]

As far as the duration of the hospital stay was concerned, different authors described a significant advantage of laparoscopy: Gill et al[46] 1.4 vs 5.8 days; Abbou et al[37] 4.8 vs 9.7 days.

The comparison of complication rate, length of hospital stay, blood loss, and a decreasing operating time confirms significant lower perioperative morbidity (see Table 9.7).

Much more important than the technical feasibility of laparoscopic radical nephrectomy is the long-term outcome. In the meantime, studies are available with longer follow-up, including our own experience (Table 9.8). It has to be noted that, at the beginning all authors limited their range of indications to small-sized renal tumors (3–6 cm) according to clinical stage T1. However, like in our series, histopathology also evidenced pT3 tumors among the treated cases.[50–52] This has to be taken into consideration when looking at the long-term results. The overall 5-year disease-free survival rates are excellent, ranging between 89 and 96% (see Table 9.8). Portis et al recently published the long-term follow-up of a multi-institutional study with a mean follow-up of 5 years. The authors observed equivalent overall survival (81 vs 89%), cancer-specific survival (98 vs 92%), as well as recurrence-free survival (92 vs 92%) rates compared to the traditional open technique in these centers.[38] Our own 5-year experience at Heilbronn confirms these results (see Tables 9.5 and 9.8).

Discussion

Since the first laparoscopic nephrectomy reported by Clayman et al in 1991,[34] experience with laparoscopy in urology, especially in laparoscopic nephrectomy, has increased continuously. The role of laparoscopic radical nephrectomy for malignancies of the kidney and ureter is still under debate. Primary concerns are focused on the safety of the procedure, the reproducibility of the technique compared with open surgery, and the risk of tumor cell spillage leading to port-site metastases. Further concerns have been related to cost-effectiveness and the steep learning curve of the procedure.

In the meantime, more than 10 years after one of the authors had the honor of assisting Malcolm Coptcoat with the first radical nephrectomy for renal cell cancer,[35] the technique of transperitoneal laparoscopic radical nephrectomy has been standardized, fulfilling all principles of uro-oncological surgery. During the last decade, various authors, including ourselves, have proposed a retroperitoneal approach (Tables 9.7 and 9.8), advocating the

Table 9.8 *Worldwide experience with laparoscopic radical nephrectomy – oncologic aspects*

Main author	Patient (n)	Specimen removal	pT stage	Surgical margin	Follow-up months	Recurrence port site/local/distant (%)	5-year survival
Janetschek[49]	73	Intact	T1–T3a	Negative	13.3	0 / 0 / 0	na
Abbou[63]	41	Intact	T1–T3b	Negative	24.7	0 / 2 / 0	na
Ono[45]	103	Morcellated and intact	–	–	29	0 / 1 / 3	92%
Chan[64]	67	Morcellated and intact	T1–T3b	Negative	35.7	0 / 0 / 3	na
Gill[65]	100	Intact	T1–T3b	Negative	16.1	0 / 0 / 2	na
Portis[38]	64	Morcellated and intact	T1–T3b	Negative	54	0 / 1 / 2	
Rassweiler*	80	Morcellated and intact	T1–T3b	Negative	65	0 / 2 / 4	91%

na = not applicable; * = present series.

advantage of earlier control of the renal artery and the reduced need for dissection (i.e. deflection of the colon). However, we feel that, like in open surgery, the access should be of secondary interest. The reproducibility of the procedure has been documented in multicenter studies,[46,47] as well as in a review of the literature. The complication rate is acceptable and still decreasing; with increasing experience, even the operative time does not exceed that of open surgery (see Tables 9.3, 9.6, and 9.7). The retrieval of the specimen is accomplished mostly by a small incision after entrapment in an organ bag rather than by morcellation.

Some authors have used this incision earlier during the procedure to perform hand-assisted laparoscopy (see Figure 9.7). They emphasize that this would speed up the procedure and reduce the learning curve.[39,42,43,48] According to our own early experience, we could reduce the operative time by about 60 min.[42,43] However, standardization of the use of the hand has proved to be very difficult, particularly because the surgeon has to insert different hands for left- and right-sided radical nephrectomies. Particularly, with regards to a standard training program of laparoscopy and retroperitoneoscopy in urology, we feel that hand-assistance should be limited to managing problematic situations. By contrast, the increasing expertise of first-generation laparoscopists has offered a variety of dissecting techniques and retraction standards for the following generations. This enables them to perform the operations much easier and with less complications than the pioneers.[53,44] Subsequently our own operating room times have dropped significantly, and are now in the same range as for open surgery (see Tables 9.4 and 9.7).

Concerning the cost-benefit analysis of laparoscopic radical nephrectomy, the situation in the United States differs significantly from that in Europe: the operating times reported by the different groups are mostly longer, the charges for the operating room are higher, and the postoperative hospital stay is shorter for both open and laparoscopic surgery than in Europe.[39,50,52] Therefore, the higher perioperative costs of laparoscopy cannot be completely compensated by the reduction of hospital stay. At our center, we have exchanged almost all of our disposable instruments by reusable armamentarium (i.e. metaltrocars, endo-shears, endo-graspers, clip-appliers). Even if the operating time in some centers may still be 60 min longer for laparoscopy, these costs can mostly be compensated by the reduced postoperative hospital stay. Consequently, a significant benefit for the social security system can be obtained by the shorter convalescence of about 2–3 weeks compared with open surgery.[50,52,55]

In summary, despite some technical modifications by the different groups, laparoscopic radical nephrectomy can be regarded as a standardized and safe procedure that allows the transmission and reproduction of the surgical principles of the open procedure. Additionally, the perioperative morbidity of the patients can be reduced significantly by use of laparoscopy.

Much more important, however, is the long-term oncologic outcome of the procedure. The overall 5-year disease-free survival rates are excellent, ranging between 89 and 96%, and do not differ from contemporary series of open surgery (see Table 9.6). Additionally, the recently published comparative study with long-term follow-up by Portis et al[38] was able to document almost identical results for laparoscopic and open surgery.

Even after open surgery of clinical T1 tumors, local recurrence as well as distant metastases have been observed.[47,56–58] It must be mentioned that, until now, among more than 2000 reported cases of laparoscopic radical nephrectomy, 3 port-site metastases have been documented.[59,60] However, 2 of them occurred at the same institution during the first 20 cases.[68] In all cases, the specimen was morcellated. Thus, the role of intact specimen removal is still controversial, although there is no difference in morbidity and oncologic outcome as reported recently.[61] Despite the risk of understaging the tumor on a preoperative CT scan, morcellation can be safely performed without compromising survival.[62] According to our own experience, with fragmentation rather than complete morcellation of the kidney, adequate tumor staging had never been a problem.

In conclusion, despite some technical modifications concerning access, laparoscopic radical nephrectomy has become a well standardized and thus reproducible, but technically demanding procedure. Laparoscopic radical nephrectomy has met all oncologic standards in comparison to open surgery. Ideal indications are for small tumors (T1) that are not candidates for nephron-sparing surgery. The complication rates are acceptable and still decreasing. The long-term results are excellent and correspond to the results of open surgery.

References

1. Boeckmann W, Jakse G. Nierenzellkarzinom. In: Rübben H, ed. Uro-Onkologie. Berlin: Springer, 1997:25–55.

2. Parkin DM, Pisani P, Ferlay J. Global cancer statistic. CA Cancer J Clin 1999; 49:33–64.

3. Mickisch GHJ. Lymphnode dissection for renal cell carcinoma – the value of operation and adjuvant therapy. Urologe(A) 1999; 38:326–31.

4. Thrasher JB, Paulson DF. Prognostic factors in renal cancer. Urol Clin North Am 1993; 20:247–62.

5. Tannenbaum M. Ultrastructural pathology of human renal cell carcinoma. Pathol Ann 1971; 6:249–77.

6. Fisher ER, Hovart B. Comparative ultrastructural study of so-called renal adenoma and carcinoma. J Urol 1972; 108:382–6.

7. Thoenes W, Störkel S, Rumpelt HJ. Histopathology and classification of renal cell tumors (adenomas, oncocytomas and carcinomas). Pathol Res Pract 1986; 181:125–43.

8. Kovacs G, Akhtar M, Beckwith BJ, et al. The Heidelberg classification of renal cell tumours. J Pathol 1997; 183:131–3.

9. Sene AP, Hunt L, McMahon RF, et al. Renal cell carcinoma in patient undergoing nephrectomy: analysis of survival and prognostic factors. Br J Urol 1992; 70:125–34.

10. Amin MB, Corles CL, Renshaw AA, et al. Papillary (chromophil) renal cell carcinoma: histomorphologic characteristics and evaluation of conventional pathologic prognostic parameters in 62 cases. Am J Surg Pathol 1997; 21:621–35.

11. Ljungberg B, Iranparvar Alamdari F, Stenling R, et al. Prognostic significance of the Heidelberg classification of renal cell carcinoma. Eur Urol 1999; 36:565–9.

12. Crotty TB, Farrow GM, Lieber MM. Chromophobe renal cell carcinoma: clinicopathological features of 50 cases. J Urol 1995; 154:964–7.

13. Schullerus D, Herbes J, Chundek J, et al. Loss of heterocygosity at chromosomes 8p, 9p and 14q is associated with stage and grade of non-papillary renal cell carcinomas. J Pathol 1997; 183:151–5.

14. Jiang F, Richter J, Schrami P, et al. Chromosomal imbalances in papillary renal cell carcinoma differences between histological subtypes. Am J Pathol 1998; 153:1467–73.

15. Kovacs G, Fuzesi L, Emanual A, et al. Cytogenetics of papillary renal cell tumors. Genes Chromosomes Cancer 1991; 3:249–55.

16. Hermanek P, Schrott KM. Evaluation of the new tumor, nodes and metastases classification of renal cell carcinoma. J Urol 1990; 144:238–42.

17. Hatcher PA, Anderson EE, Paulson DF, et al. Surgical management and prognosis of renal cell carcinoma invading the vena cava. J Urol 1991; 145:20–3, discussion 23–4.

18. Ljungberg B, Larsson P, Stenling R, et al. Flow cytometric deoxyribonucleic acid analysis in stage I renal cell carcinoma. J Urol 1991; 146: 697–9.

19. Ljungberg B, Landberg G, Alamdari FI. Factors of importance for prediction of survival in patients with metastatic renal cell carcinoma treated with or without nephrectomy. Scand J Urol Nephrol 2000; 34:246–51.

20. Minervini R, Minervini A, Fontana N, et al. Evaluation of the 1997 tumor, nodes and metastases classification of renal cell carcinoma: experience in 172 patients. Br J Urol 2000; 86:199–202.

21. Skinner DG, Colvin RB, Vermillion CD, et al. Diagnosis and management of renal cell carcinoma. A clinical and pathological study of 309 cases. Cancer 1971; 74:1165–77.

22. Ljungberg B, Stenling R, Österdahl B, et al. Vein invasion in renal cell carcinoma: impact on metastatic behavior and survival. J Urol 1995; 154:1681–4.

23. Golimbu M, Joshi P, Sperber A, et al. Renal cell carcinoma survival and prognostic factors. Urology 1986, 27:291–301.

24. Skinner DG, Rand Pritchett T, Lieskovsky G et al. Venal caval involvement by renal cell carcinoma: surgical resection provides meaningful long-term survival. Ann Surg 1989; 210:387–92.

25. Swierzewski DJ, Swierzewski MJ, Libertino JA, et al. Radical nephrectomy in patients with renal cell carcinoma with venous, vena cava and atrial extension. Am J Surg 1994; 168:205–9.

26. Johnsen JA, Hellsten S. Lymphatogenous spread of renal cell carcinoma: an autopsy study. J Urol 1997; 157:450–3.

27. Blom JH, van Poppel H, Marechal JM, et al. Radical nephrectomy with or without lymph node dissection: preliminary results of the EORTC randomized phase III protocol 30881. EORTC Genitourinary Group. Eur Urol 1999, 36:570–5.

28. Wunderlich H, Schlichter A, Reichelt O, et al. Real indications for adrenalectomy in renal cell carcinoma. Eur Urol 1999, 35:272–6.

29. Gill IS, McClennan BL, Kerbl K, et al. Adrenal involvement from renal cell carcinoma: predictive value of computerized tomography. J Urol 1994; 152:1082–5.

30. Ljungberg B, Mehle C, Stenling R, et al. Heterogeneity in renal cell carcinoma and its impact on prognosis – a flow cytometric study. Br J Cancer 1996; 74:123–7.

31. O'Dea MJ, Zincke H, Utz DC, et al. The treatment of renal cell carcinoma with solitary metastasis. J Urol 1978; 120:540–2.

32. Fuhrman SA, Lasky LC, Limas C. Prognostic significance of morphologic parameters in renal cell carcinoma. Am J Surg Pathol 1982; 6:655–63.

33. Carducci MA, Piantadosi S, Pound CR, et al. Nuclear morphometry adds significant prognostic information to stage and grade for renal cell carcinoma. Urology 1999: 53:44–9.

34. Clayman RV, Kavoussi LR, Soper NJ, et al. Laparoscopic nephrectomy: initial case report. J Urol 1991; 146:278–82.

35. Coptcoat MJ, Rassweiler J, Wickham JEA, Joyce A. Laparoscopic nephrectomy for renal cell carcinoma. Proc. Third International Congress for Minimal Invasive Therapy, Boston, 10–12 November 1991 (abstract No. D-66).

36. Chiu AW, Chen MT, Huang WJS, et al. Laparoscopic nephroureterectomy and endoscopic incision of bladder cuff. Min Inv Ther 1992; 1:299–303.

37. Abbou CC, Cicco A, Gasman D, et al. Retroperitoeal laparoscopic versus open radical nephrectomy. J Urol 1999; 161:1776–80.

38. Portis AJ, Yan Y, Landman J, et al. Long-term follow-up after laparoscopic radical nephrectomy. J Urol 2002; 167:1257–62.

39. Wolf S, Moon TD, Madisom WI, Nakada SY. Hand-assisted laparoscopic nephrectomy: comparison to standard laparoscopic nephrectomy. J Urol 1998; 160:22–7.

40. Rassweiler J, Stock C, Frede T, et al. Organ retrieval systems for endoscopic nephrectomy: a comparative study. J Endourol 1998; 12:325–33.

41. Coptcoat MJ, Ison KT, Wickham JEA. Endoscopic tissue liquidization and surgical aspiration. J Endourol 1988; 2:321–9.

42. Tschada RK, Henkel TO, Seemann O, et al. First experiences with laparoscopic radical nephrectomy. J Endourol 1994; 8:S80 (abstract No. P1-68).

43. Tschada RK, Rassweiler JJ, Schmeller N, Theodorakis J. Laparoscopic radical nephrectomy – the German experience. J Urol 1995; 153:479 A (abstract 1003).

44. Rassweiler JJ, Seemann O, Frede T, et al. Retroperitoneoscopy: Experience with 200 cases. J Urol 1999; 160:1265–9.

45. Ono Y, Kinukawa T, Hattori R, et al. The long-term outcome of laparoscopic radical nephrectomy for small renal cell carcinoma. J Urol 2001; 165:1867–70.

46. Gill IS, Schweizer D, Hobart MG, et al. Retroperitoneal laparoscopic radical nephrectomy: the Clevland Clinic experience. J Urol 2000; 163:1665–70.

47. Swanson DA, Borges PM. Complications of transabdominal radical nephrectomy for renal cell carcinoma. J Urol 1983; 129:704–7.

48. Dunn MD, Portis AJ, Shalhav AL, et al. Laparoscopic versus open radical nephrectomy: a 9-year experience. J Urol 2000; 164:1153–9.

49. Janetschek G, Jeschke K, Pechel R, et al. Laparoscopic surgery for stage T1 renal cell carcinoma: radical nephrectomy and wedge resection. Eur Urol 2000; 38:131–8.

50. McDougall EM, Clayman RV, Elashry OM. Laparoscopic nephroureterectomy for upper tract transitional cell cancer: Washington University experience. J Urol 1995; 154:975–80.

51. Cadeddu JA, Moore RG, Nelson JB, et al. Laparoscopic nephrectomy for renal cell cancer: a multi-center evaluation of efficacy. J Urol 1998; 159:147 A (abstract No. 557).

52. McDougall EM, Clayman RV, Elashry OM. Laparoscopic radical nephrectomy for renal tumor: The Washington University experience. J Urol 1996; 155:1180–5.

53. Rassweiler J, Fornara P, Weber M, et al. Laparoscopic nephrectomy: the experience of the laparoscopic working group of the German Urological Association. J Urol 1998; 160:18–21.

54. Barrett PH, Fentie DD, Taranger LA, et al. Laparoscopic assisted nephroureterectomy (TCC). J Endourol 1998; 12:S103 (abstract No. F 1–3).

55. Rassweiler J, Coptcoat MJ. Laparoscopic surgery of the kidney and adrenal gland. In: Janetschek G, Rassweiler J, Griffith D, eds. Laparoscopic surgery in urology. New York: Thieme Stuttgart, 1996; 139–55.

56. Levy DA, Slaton JW, Swanson DA, Dinney CPN. Stage specific guidelines for survival after radical nephrectomy for local renal cell carcinoma. J Urol 1998; 159:1163–7.

57. Mickisch G, Tschada R, Rassweiler J, et al. Das lokale Rezidiv nach Nierentumoroperation. Akt Urol 1990; 21:77–81.

58. Moch H, Gasser TC, Urrejola C, et al. Metastatic behavior of renal cell cancer: an analysis of 871 autopsies. J Urol 1997; 157:66 A (abstract No. 254).

59. Barrett PH, Fentie DD, Taranger L. Laparoscopic radical nephrectomy with morcellation for renal cell carcinoma: the Saskatoon experience. Urology 1998; 52:23–8.

60. Castilho LN, Fugita OEH, Mitre AI, Arap S. Port site tumor recurrences of renal cell carcinoma after videolaparoscopic radical nephrectomy. J Urol 2001; 165:519.

61. Landman J, Lento P, Hassen W, et al. Feasibility of pathological evalution of morcellated kidneys after radical nephrectomy. J Urol 2001; 164:2086–9.

62. Gettman MT, Napper C, Corwin TS, Cadeddu J. Laparoscopic radical nephrectomy: prospective assessment of impact of intact versus fragmented specimen removal on postoperative quality of life. J Endourol 2002; 16:23–5.

63. Cicco A, Salomon L, Hoznek H, et al. Carcinological risks and retroperitoneal laparoscopy. Eur Urol 2000; 38:606–12.

64. Chan DY, Cadeddu JA, Jarret TW, et al. Laparoscopic radical nephrectomy: cancer control for renal cell carcinoma. J Urol 2001; 166:2095–100.

65. Gill IS, Meraney AM, Schweizer DK et al. Laparoscopic radical nephrectomy in 100 patients: a single center experience from the United States. Cancer 2001; 92:1843–55.

66. Jeschke K, Wakonig J, Winzely M, Henning K. Laparoscopic radical nephrectomy: overcoming the main problems. BJU Int 2000; 85:163–5.

10

Nephron-sparing minimally invasive surgery for renal malignancy*

Yair Lotan, Jeffrey A Cadeddu, and Jay T Bishoff

Introduction

The increase in incidentally found small renal tumors has served as an impetus to develop less-invasive parenchymal-sparing techniques for tumor treatment[1] (Figure 10.1). Recent studies have shown that renal parenchymal-sparing procedures yield comparable outcomes with regard to tumor control compared with radical nephrectomy for small tumors.[2–5] The indications for partial nephrectomy include resection of nonfunctioning moieties of duplicated systems, urolithiasis in calyceal diverticula, and excision of small tumors or tumors in solitary kidneys. To reduce the morbidity of partial nephrectomy, newer minimally invasive approaches have been developed: laparoscopic partial nephrectomy (LPN) and ablative technologies. While laparoscopic techniques aim to reproduce open tumor resection with negative margins, ablative techniques aim to destroy renal tumors without the need for resection. In this chapter, we will explore the current experience with laparoscopic partial nephrectomy with a focus on the various hemostatic modalities. We will also discuss the current ablative techniques and possible future areas of development.

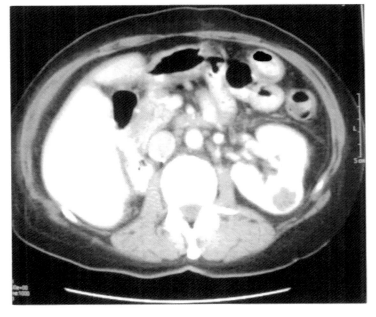

Figure 10.1
X-ray. A 3 cm left renal lesion consistent with renal cell carcinoma. (Courtesy of Tung Shu.)

*The views expressed in this article are those of the authors and do not reflect the official policy of the Department of Defense, or other Departments of the U.S. Government.

Laparoscopic partial nephrectomy

With the emergence of laparoscopy as a less-morbid approach to various urologic procedures, efforts have been made to apply this technique to small renal tumors.

Technical aspects

The goal of LPN is to successfully reproduce the oncologic surgical principles of open partial nephrectomy, which include:

1. complete survey of the renal unit to exclude the presence of synchronous lesions missed by preoperative imaging

2. wide, en bloc tumor excision with a normal parenchymal margin and without tumor spillage
3. vascular control and hemostasis
4. water-tight closure of the collecting system

Approach

Both transperitoneal and retroperitoneal approaches have been used for LPN (see Table 10.1). While some authors have used the transperitoneal approach exclusively[6] (Figure 10.2), because of its larger working space, several authors have used a retroperitoneal approach for posterior and lateral tumors[7,8] (Figure 10.3). The benefit of a retroperitoneal approach may be decreased bowel irritation and lower risk of bowel injury, although this complication is uncommon. Most patients have been discharged early regardless of approach, and the main consideration should be the surgeon's preference.

Special equipment

Intraoperative laparoscopic ultrasound (Figure 10.4) permits the surgeon to identify multifocal tumors, to determine an adequate surgical margin, and to assess the

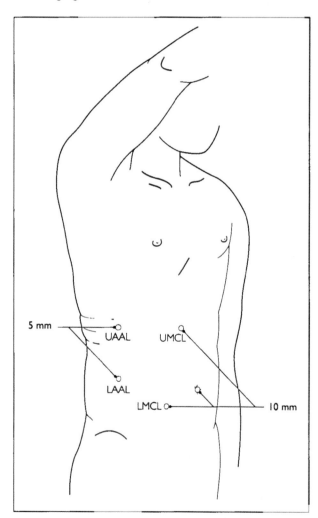

Figure 10.2
Transperitoneal access for laparoscopic nephron-sparing renal surgery. Five trocars are used with three 12 mm trocars: one umbilicus and two mid-clavicular with upper (UMCL) and lower (LMCL) trocars and two 5 mm trocars: one in the anterior axillary line upper (UAAL) and lower (LAAL).

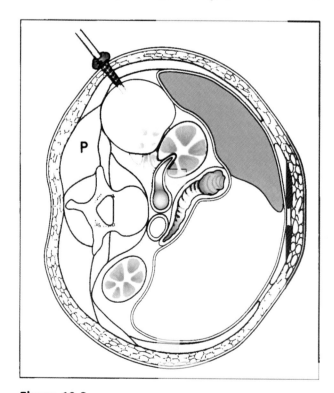

Figure 10.3
Retroperitoneal access for laparoscopic nephron-sparing surgery. A balloon is placed between the psoas muscle (P) and Gerota's fascia. As the balloon is inflated, the kidney is mobilized anteriorly. As the working space is created, renal helium can be accessed directly.

Table 10.1 *LPN series: operative data and complications*

Year	Author	n	Approach (No.)	Hilar control	Hemostasis	EBL (ml) (range)	Mean OR time (min)	Mean hospital stay (days)	No. of urine leaks (%)	No. of complica- tions (%)	Conversion
2002	Gill et al[8]	50	Transperitoneal (28) Retroperitoneal (22)	Yes	Suture over bolsters	270 (40–1500)	180	2.2	1 (2)	6 (12)	0
2000	Janetschek et al[9]	25	Transperitoneal (15) Retroperitoneal (10)	No	Bipolar, argon beam, fibrin glue	287 (20–800)	163.5	5.8	2 (4)	3 (12)	0
2001	Stifelman et al[11]	11	Transperitoneal	No	Hand assistance, harmonic scalpel, argon beam, Surgicel	319	274	3.3	0	2 (18)	1
2000	Harmon et al[10]	15	Transperitoneal (7) Retroperitoneal (8)	No	Laparoscopic coagulating shears, argon beam, Surgicel	368 (75–1000)	170	2.6	0	0	0
2001	Gettman et al[34]	10	Transperitoneal (9) Retroperitoneal (1)	No	Radiofrequency ablation	198 (50–700)	193	NA	0	0	0
2001	Yoshimura et al[14]	6	Transperitoneal	No	Microwave tissue coagulator	< 50	186	NA	0	2 (33)	0
1999	Hoznek et al[7]	7	Retropertioneal	Yes (5)	Bipolar, harmonic scalpel, glue	129 (0–400)	133	7.3	1 (14)	1 (14)	0
2000	Wolf et al[6]	10	Transperitoneal	No	Hand assistance (8), argon beam, gelatin sponge with fibrin glue	460	199	2	0	3 (30)	0

EBL = estimated blood loss, OR = operating room, NA = not available.

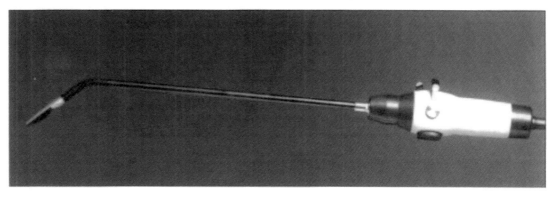

Figure 10.4
Laparoscopic ultrasound probe (B-K Medical, Copenhagen, Denmark). Laparoscopic flexible tipped ultrasound probe is used to image renal lesions to guide for nephron-sparing therapy.

tumor(s) position relative to the collecting system and renal vasculature. Endoscopic retrieval devices like the Endocatch bag allow removal of the tumor specimen without tumor spillage, peritoneal implantation, or trochar site seeding.

Hemostasis

The main challenge that has limited the widespread use of laparoscopy in the management of small renal tumors has been unreliable parenchymal hemostasis. While Gill et al achieved good results with duplication of open techniques,[8] the difficulty of suturing and concerns with warm ischemia have led to the development of innovative means of achieving hemostasis without the need for hilar control or suturing. These techniques to decrease blood loss have ranged from the use of various energy sources, such as bipolar electrocautery,[9] ultrasonic scalpel,[7,10,11] argon beam,[6,9–11] laser,[12,13] and microwave,[14] to the use of tamponading devices, such as cable ties,[15–18] loops,[19] electrosurgical snare electrodes,[20] and hand assistance.[6,11] Table 10.1 provides details concerning the operative course and hemostatic control methods for various series for LPN. However, a brief discussion of each technique is warranted.

Duplication of open techniques: suturing and hilar control. In an effort to duplicate open surgical techniques, Gill and colleagues performed LPN in 50 patients.[8] Initially only the renal artery was clamped but persistent venous oozing hampered tumor excision. Subsequently, both the vein and artery were clamped using a laparoscopic Satinsky clamp with a mean warm ischemia time of 23 min (Figure 10.5). Hemostasis was achieved with intracorporeal suturing and bolsters (Figure 10.6). While this group had good results, this technique is challenging because of the advanced skills necessary to complete intracorporeal suturing in less than 30 min.

Hoznek et al also clamped the hilum for bleeding that was not controlled with bipolar coagulation. Warm ischemia never exceeded 10 min. After resection, the lesion was covered with oxidized regenerated cellulose mesh with gelatin resorcinol formaldehyde glue.[7]

Hand assistance. Hand-assisted laparoscopy has been used to decrease morbidity during radical and donor nephrectomy. Recently it has been applied to nephron-sparing surgery as well. Wolf and colleagues performed LPN in 10 patients and used the Pneumosleeve (Dexterity, Atlanta, Georgia) to facilitate this procedure in 8 patients.[6] The approach was transperitoneal in all cases. Use of hand assistance allowed for 'pinching' of the tumor base to tamponade bleeding. A gelatin sponge soaked with fibrin glue was applied with pressure to achieve hemostasis. In addition, the argon beam was used to seal the edges of the fibrin glue. The

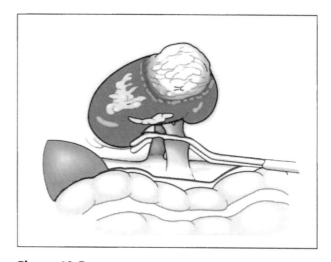

Figure 10.5
Laparoscopic partial nephrectomy. To facilitate resection of the renal tumor during laparoscopic partial nephrectomy, a laparoscopic Satinsky clamp (AESCULAP) is used to obtain control of both the renal artery and vein.

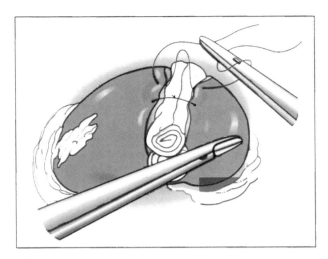

Figure 10.6
Laparoscopic partial nephrectomy. After the resection of the renal tumor is completed, hemostasis is obtained via intra-corporeal suturing of the renal parenchyma over bolsters with No. 1 polydioxanone suture.

argon beam coagulator is frequently used as a hemostatic adjunct.[21] There was one major complication involving an arteriovenous (AV) fistula and one of the patients who was undergoing standard laparoscopy required conversion to hand assistance to control hemorrhage.

Stifelman and colleagues performed LPN in 11 patients, 9 of whom had < 4 cm renal lesions.[11] They used three different devices: the Intromit (Applied Medical, Rancho Santa Margarita, California), Hand Port (Smith Nephew, Andover, Massachusetts), and Pneumosleeve. The renal artery was identified and isolated but not clamped. A combination of the harmonic scalpel and argon beam was used for resection and hemostasis. Subsequently, the intra-abdominal hand was used to compress the parenchyma and Surgicel (Johnson & Johnson, Summerville, New Jersey) was pressed manually into the defect. Three or four pledget sutures were then placed to reapproximate the renal capsule. The results of this technique were good with no positive margins, no transfusion requirement, and two minor complications (18%). One patient was converted to an open procedure to ensure negative margins because of deep invasion of the tumor. There were no recurrences in a mean of 8 months follow-up.

Laser energy. Laser partial nephrectomy has been described using the CO_2,[22,23] Nd:YAG,[12,24,25] and holmium laser.[13,26] Lasers have different energy levels and tissue penetration according to their wavelength. The CO_2 laser wavelength of 10.6 μm provides sharp cutting with minimal tissue penetration. Compared with the CO_2 laser, the Nd:YAG laser (1064 nm) has a deeper thermal effect and thus improved tissue coagulation. Because of the shallow tissue penetration of the CO_2 laser, adequate hemostasis of

larger vessels is problematic even with hilar occlusion.[22,23] Benderev et al. performed open lower pole laser partial nephrectomy in six dogs following hilar occlusion.[25] While there was minimal blood loss, two large urinomas occurred, suggesting that the laser may not adequately seal the collecting system.

The holmium:YAG laser operates in the near infrared region of the electromagnetic spectrum (2100 nm) and is effective in cutting through soft tissue. Lotan et al developed a successful technique of laparoscopic Ho:YAG laser partial nephrectomy without the necessity of hilar occlusion in the porcine model and subsequently applied it successfully to 3 patients.[13,26] Settings of 0.2 J at 60 pulses/s provided an almost continuous delivery of energy, but higher energy of 0.8 J at 40 pulses/s was also utilized to assist with hemostasis. Importantly, with the addition of fibrin glue to the cut surface of the remaining parenchyma, the collecting system was closed. While the Ho:YAG laser provides adequate hemostasis without hilar occlusion for patients with peripheral tumors during LPN, blood splattering and smoke generation during resection can obscure the operating field and diminish its clinical value.

Cable ties/loops. While initial efforts using a porcine model demonstrated the potential of tourniquets for stabilization of the kidney and vascular tamponade,[15] the initial attempt at using a plastic tie band to control bleeding was unsuccessful in clinical practice.[16] Cadeddu et al later refined this technique in the laboratory[18] and then used it clinically.[17] In a porcine model, a ¼-inch wide, 10-inch long standard commercial plastic cable tie was engaged in a loop and laparoscopically positioned around the lower pole, and 8 large amputations involving the collecting system and 8 smaller amputations excluding the collecting system were performed using laparoscopic scissors. Fibrin glue was applied to seal the cut surface prior to cable-tie removal. Median cable tie ischemia time was 15 min (range 7–48) and median blood loss was 30 ml (range 10–300). In each case, hemostasis was attained with fibrin glue. One animal died from urinary extravasation on postoperative day 4. This technique was utilized in a patient with a 3 cm upper pole renal cell carcinoma.[17] Bleeding was kept to minimal ooze by the cable tie: estimated blood loss (EBL) < 100 ml. The argon beam coagulator along with two layers of fibrin glue and oxidized cellulose, was then used to seal the parenchymal surface prior to removal of the cable tie. Two additional patients have undergone successful LPN using this technique (JA Cadeddu, pers comm).

Following a similar concept, a double-loop apparatus has also been used to stabilize the kidney and provide polar compression to allow for a retroperitoneal LPN.[19] The advantage of a cable tie or tourniquet technique is that it allows normal parenchyma in the remaining kidney to maintain perfusion. The obvious disadvantages are that a necessary margin of normal parenchyma between the tumor and hilum restricts the technique to polar lesions, and slippage of the cable tie off the kidney is possible.

Endosnare. With the aim of providing both a tourniquet effect and simultaneous hemostasis, Elashry et al have developed a unique electrosurgical snare electrode (Cook Urological Inc., Spencer, Indiana) in combination with an electrosurgical generator (ERBE USA, Inc., Marietta, Georgia) for LPN.[20] The endosnare device generator provides both cutting and coagulation energy. The device is positioned around the pole of the kidney and the wire is pulled through the kidney until the pole is completely transected.

This device was compared with two different ultrasonic dissectors, the Cavitron Ultrasonic Surgical Aspirator (CUSA) and the ultrasonic shears, in a porcine LPN. The electrosurgical snare was found to be significantly faster and associated with less intraoperative bleeding. However, the argon beam electrocoagulator was necessary in certain cases to control persistent oozing from the cut parenchymal surface. There was no evidence of extravasation at 6 weeks. Unfortunately, there has been no human application at this time. As with other tourniquet devices, this technique is limited to polar lesions.

Radiofrequency ablation assisted LPN. While most technologic innovations focus on instruments that cut and coagulate simultaneously, radiofrequency ablation (RFA) has been used to coagulate the renal lesion prior to excision in order to prevent bleeding. Several investigators have demonstrated parenchymal thrombosis and coagulation as a result of RFA. Corwin and Cadeddu were the first to describe the use of RFA to facilitate LPN in this manner.[27] A 15-gauge RITA Starburst XL probe (RITA Medical Systems, Inc., Mountain View, California) was used for

RFA and was deployed approximately 0.5–1.0 cm beyond the computed tomography (CT)-measured tumor diameter (Figures 10.7 and 10. 8). After ablation for 2 cycles, the tumor is resected. Experience suggests that this technique should be limited to peripheral exophytic tumors.[28]

Microwave tissue coagulator. A microwave tissue coagulator has also been used to provide hemostasis prior to resection in patients with peripheral exophytic masses.[14,29–31] Yoshimura et al used the Microtaze OT-110M (Azwell Inc., Osaka, Japan) microwave generator with 4 probes ranging in length from 1 to 3 cm and 0.6 cm in diameter.[14] After laparoscopic exposure in 6 patients, the renal parenchyma was punctured with a needle-type monopolar probe along the resection line at 5–8 mm intervals. There were 5–23 coagulations performed at 70–75 W for 40–45 s per session. The tumor was subsequently

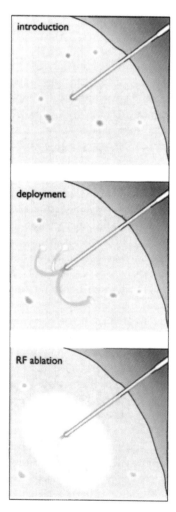

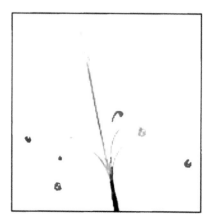

Figure 10.7
Radiofrequency ablation probe. Radiofrequency ablations of small renal lesions are carried out with a RITA Starburst XL probe (RITA Medical Systems, Inc., Mountain View, California).

Figure 10.8
Radiofrequency ablation. The RITA probe is placed directly into the renal lesion under ultrasound monitoring. Prongs are deployed approximately 0.5 – 1.0 cm beyond the measured tumor diameter to completely ablate the tumor.

resected with the endoscissors along the coagulation zone without the need for renal pedicle occlusion.

Collecting system transection

As in open surgery, a drain should be placed after LPN to detect and drain urine leaks. Preoperative ureteral catheterization can be used to help identify calyceal injuries, and intracorporeal suture repair has been performed by some investigators[8] (Figure 10.9). However, materials such as oxidized cellulose mesh,[10,11] gelatin resorcinol formaldehyde glue,[7] and fibrin glue[6,9] have also been used successfully to seal the transected parenchyma and collecting system.

Clinical outcomes

Winfield et al performed the first LPN in 1992 on a patient with a lower pole diverticulum.[32] Subsequently, McDougall et al described their experience with 12 patients who underwent wedge resection or polar partial nephrectomy and reported a high complication rate (50%) and open conversion rate (33%) associated with LPN.[33]

Table 10.2 summarizes the oncologic outcomes for series of LPN. In a commendable effort to duplicate open surgical techniques, Gill and colleagues performed LPN in 50 patients.[8] Of these, 24 (48%) had either compromised contralateral kidney function (20) or a solitary kidney (4). The mean tumor size was 3.0 cm. The mean operative time was 3.0 hours and hospital stay was 2.2 days. Renal cell carcinoma was confirmed in 34 patients (68%), and all patients had negative margins. There were few complications (12%) with 1 case of intraoperative hemorrhage, 1 case of delayed hemorrhage, and one urine leak.

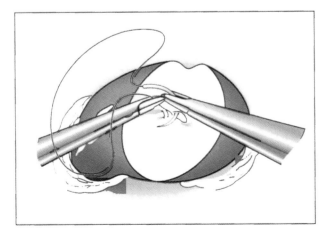

Figure 10.9
Laparoscopic partial nephrectomy. Intracorporeal laparoscopic suture repair of the violated urinary collecting system is completed using 4-0 polydioxanone suture.

Janetschek et al treated 98 patients with renal masses diagnosed by computed tomography (CT) scans that were T1 based on the 1997 TNM (tumor, node, metastasis) staging system.[9] The laparoscopic approach was used for all the patients with radical versus wedge resection determined by the tumor location, size, health, and age of patient and status of contralateral kidney. A wedge resection was performed in 25 patients with no conversions required. Both the transperitoneal (15) and retroperitoneal (10) approaches were used, depending on tumor location. No hilar control was obtained and hemostasis was achieved primarily with use of bipolar coagulation, argon beam, and fibrin glue as adjunctive measures. There were 3 complications, 2 of which involved a urine leak that required intervention. No tumors recurred over 22 months.

Harmon et al used laparoscopic coagulating shears for extended wedge resection in 15 patients.[10] Mean tumor size was 2.3 cm and both the transperitoneal (7) and retroperitoneal (8) approaches were used. The renal vessels were dissected but not clamped. The argon beam coagulator (Birtcher Medical Systems, Ervin, California) was used to demarcate the renal capsule 1 cm beyond the tumor margin, and then the tumor was resected using the laparoscopic coagulating shears. The argon beam and oxidized cellulose gauze (Surgicel) were used for hemostasis. There were no complications associated with this procedure but blood loss was 500 ml or greater in 33% of the patients.

The clinical experiences and outcomes using coagulative techniques (RFA and microwave) are less mature. Gettman et al published a multicenter experience using RFA-assisted LPN. Ten patients underwent laparoscopically guided RFA with subsequent tumor excision.[34] The RITA or Radiotherapeutics device (RITA Medical Systems, Inc., Mountain View, CA) was employed (Figures 10.7 and 10.8). Mean tumor size was 2.1 cm. Median operative time was 193 min, and EBL was 198 ml (50–700). There were no perioperative complications, and negative margins were obtained in all cases.

Jacomides et al recently reported their experience with laparoscopic RFA followed by excision of tumor in 6 patients.[28] Mean tumor size was 1.8 cm. Mean operative time was 203 min and mean EBL was 80 ml. There were no perioperative complications and no urinary extravasation. A patient with the multiple treatments had a transient increase in creatinine from 1.3 to 1.8 mg/dl but this normalized within 2 weeks. Mean hospital stay was 2.5 days. Of the 6 patients, 1 patient had a focal positive margin that was felt to result from a technical error during excision. The patient had RFA 1 cm beyond the level of excision and was not re-explored. At 1-year follow-up, the patient remains recurrence free. Likewise, at a mean follow-up of 9.8 months there was no enhancement on CT scan in any of the patients.

Table 10.2 *LPN oncologic outcomes*

Year	Author	Patients	Mean tumor size (cm)	Pathology	Positive margin	Tumor recurrence	Mean follow-up (months)
2002	Gill et al[8]	50	3	RCC (68%), AML (16%), oncocytoma (10%), other (6%)	0	0	7.2
2000	Janetschek et al[9]	25	1.9	RCC (76%), AML (4%), oncocytoma (4%), multilocular cyst (16%)	0	0	22.2
2001	Stifelman et al[11]	11	1.9	RCC (44%), AML (22%), benign cysts (33%)	0	0	8
2000	Harmon et al[10]	15	2.3	RCC (80%), oncocytoma (20%)	0	0	8
2001	Gettman et al[34]	10	2.1	RCC (90%), AML (10%)	0	NA	NA
2001	Yoshimura et al[14]	6	1.8	NA	1 (17%)	0	3
2000	Rassweiler et al[110]	53	2.4	NA	NA	0	36
1999	Hoznek et al[7]	7	NA	RCC (43%), AML (29%), other (29%)	0	0	22
2000	Wolf et al[6]	10	2.4	RCC (73%), benign (27%)	0	0	NA

AML = angiomyolipoma, RCC = renal cell carcinoma, NA = not available.

Yoshimura et al used the Microtaze OT-110M microwave generator in 6 patients.[14] The mean tumor size was 1.8 cm. Mean operative time was 186 min (range 131–239) and blood loss was minimal in all cases (less than 50 ml). There were no major complications. One patient had a positive margin on frozen sections that was subsequently treated with further laparoscopic resection. Limited follow-up of 3–4 months has detected no recurrences or metastatic disease. While hemostasis was effective, multiple needle placements may increase the error rates and lead to incomplete margin ablation.

New approaches

Several new approaches have been presented recently that may simplify the performance of LPN.

Water jet

Basting et al recently reported their clinical experience and the histologic effects of a new water jet resection device on kidney tissue[35,36] (Figure 10.10A and 10.10B). A series of 24 patients underwent open surgery for renal cell carcinoma, nephrolithiasis, complicated cysts, or oncocytoma. The renal pedicle was exposed and controlled prior to resection. The renal capsule was incised and then the water jet was used to cut the parenchyma. A high-pressure pump is used to generate pressure between 16 and 22 bar that 'jets' water through a 0.12 mm pinhole. The high pressure allows the water jet to create a corridor in the desired dissection line without interfering with the intrarenal vessels and pelvicalyceal system. Resection took between 14 and 40 min with minimal intraoperative blood loss. The intrarenal vessels remained undamaged and could be ligated selectively. No significant postoperative complications occurred. Histologic evaluation demonstrated a sharp dissection line without thermal alterations or deep necrosis. Only a small disruption zone could be seen at the margins of the dissection.

Fibrin sealant powder

Fibrin sealant powder (FSP) is a lyophilized human fibrinogen and thrombin preparation that can be applied as a dry spray through a gas-propelled device. Perahia et al randomized farm pigs to laparoscopic heminephrectomy using:

1. Conventional-bolstering sutures placed intracorporeally with vascular control using a pedicle clamp ($n=13$); or
2. FSP application with regional ischemia using a laparoscopic kidney clamp ($n=13$).[37]

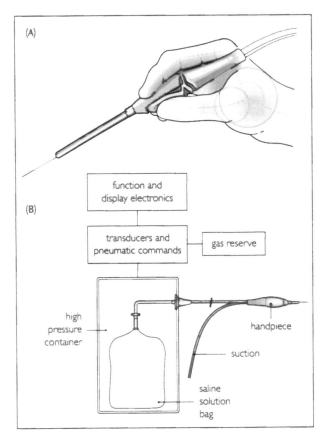

Figure 10.10
(A and B) Water Jet (Saphir Medical S.A., Dardilly, France). The water jet resection devise is a hand-held instrument used to cut through the renal parenchyma to resect renal lesions. A high-pressure pump generates high pressure that 'jets' through a 0.12 mm pinhole to slice through the renal parenchyma.

There were no differences in operating room (OR) time or blood loss between the groups. Urine extravasation was greater at 2 days in the FSP group but was nonexistent at 6 weeks. The authors found FSP application provides good hemostasis and eliminates the need for placing sutures. This application is awaiting clinical trials.

Photopolymerized polyethylene glycol-lactide hydrogels

Photopolymerized polyethylene glycol (PEG)-lactide hydrogels have recently been evaluated for use as hemostatic barriers to limit parenchymal bleeding after LPN. Ramakumar and colleagues used a porcine model to perform wedge excision with vascular control and compare a 'conventional' strategy of 'clamp and wait' with application of hydrogels.[38] For the hydrogel group, primer and macromer were applied through laparoscopic ports. The hydrogel was polymerized on the cut surface of the kidney using a green xenon light source, and the vascular pedicle clamp was released. The polymer gels remained adherent to the cut surface of the kidney with significantly less blood loss than the control group (2.5 ml vs 52.5 ml, $p < 0.001$). No leakage or peeling of the hydrogel was observed at pressures up to 200 and 100 mmHg for ex-vivo vascular and retrograde ureteral perfusion, respectively. This application also awaits clinical trial.

Summary

LPN is both safe and feasible for small renal tumors < 4 cm. Exophytic tumors are ideal for resection using current technologies. While Gill et al have been successful in attaining vascular control and parenchymal suturing,[8] most other authors have attempted to simplify the operative technique by utilizing alternative means of hemostatic control. The use of the argon beam coagulator along with some form of gauze buttress to apply pressure is common and usually effective. Radiofrequency ablation followed by excision is a promising adjunct.

In general, tumor control has been good but awaits long-term follow-up to establish its equivalence with open techniques. However, morbidity is low overall, with short hospital stays for most series (see Tables 10.1 and 10.2).

Ablation

In an attempt to decrease morbidity of surgical intervention for small renal tumors, tumor ablation has been evaluated for both laparoscopic and percutaneous approaches. For ablation to be effective, several factors must be addressed:

1. complete tumor destruction
2. safe, focused treatment
3. reproducible lesions
4. real-time monitoring of lesion formation
5. ability to determine treatment success.

While several energy modalities have been explored, cryotherapy and radiofrequency ablation have been the most extensively evaluated in both experimental and clinical settings. Other technologies such as high-intensity focused ultrasound, interstitial photon radiation energy, and ferromagnetic self-regulating reheatable thermal rod implants have also been evaluated.

Cryoablation

Cryoablation is the most extensively utilized ablation technology. Multiple animal studies have evaluated the effects

of cryoinjury on renal tissues[39–50] (Figure 10.11). The principle of cryoablation, as with any ablative technique, is precise localization of the renal tumor and complete destruction of the lesion without injury to adjacent structures.

Technical aspects

Temperature

Temperature plays a pivotal role in cell destruction during cryoablation. A temperature below $-20°C$ has been found to be important for cell death. Uchida et al evaluated renal cell lines by phase microscopy 24 hours after subjecting them to 60 min of tempertures of -5, -10, -20 and $-30°C$.[51] About 95% of renal cancer cells survived after cooling for 60 min at a temperature of about $-10°C$ but only 15% survived at a temperature of $-20°C$. These findings were confirmed in a porcine model by Chosy et al, who demonstrated complete ablation of tumor at a temperature of $-19.4°C$,[48] and by Schmidlin and colleagues, who found the threshold temperature for complete tissue ablation to be $-16.1°C$.[45]

Ice ball size

In order to guarantee complete ablation, it is important to extend the ice ball a sufficient distance beyond the tumor borders. The margin of cell death beyond the probe is an important consideration in deciding the depth of probe deployment. Campbell and coauthors demonstrated that a temperature less than $-20°C$ was achieved 3.1 mm behind

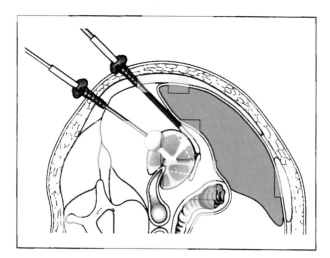

Figure 10.11
Laparoscopic renal cryosurgery. Laparoscopic renal cryosurgery is performed with a retroperitoneal access and laparoscopic intraoperative ultrasonic guidance.

the leading edge of the ice ball.[39] The fact that temperatures sufficient for cell death were found in close proximity to the probe suggests that the cryoprobe does not need to be inserted far beyond the tumor edge to obtain a negative margin.

Freeze–thaw cycle

Initial researchers used a single freeze–thaw cycle[48] to destroy tumor cells. However,[45,51,52] most current clinical series have utilized double freeze–thaw cycles[53] to ensure greater tumor destruction.[54–56]

While there is concern that vascular flow to the kidney may affect the freezing of tissue, renal artery occlusion does not significantly alter the freezing process and provided no practical advantage in an animal model.[39]

Monitoring

Imaging

Due to the destructive nature of the ice ball, it is important to monitor the extent of the lesion as it develops. Direct vision is not a sufficient predictor of tissue destruction, with incomplete ablation noted in 11% of samples taken within the visible margins of the iceball.[48] Real-time ultrasound, including intraoperative laparoscopic ultrasound, has been utilized to monitor the ice ball[46,53–57] (Figures 10.12 and 10.13). The evolving renal ice ball is visualized as a hyperechoic, crescentic advancing edge with posterior acoustic shadowing.[47] On the other hand, renal tumors are mildly hyperechoic or of mixed echogenicity and the renal sinus fat is hyperechoic. The ultrasound probe is placed

opposite the tumor, allowing precise placement of the cryoprobe up to the deep margin of the tumor. Zegel et al found that intraoperative ultrasonography accurately delineated tumor size, cryoprobe placement, and depth of freezing.[58] An echogenic interface was generated by the marked differences at the junction of the normal renal parenchyma and frozen tissue.

Open magnetic resonance imaging (MRI) has also been used to monitor iceball formation during percutaneous cryoablation.[44,59,60] The advantages of MRI include a three dimensional view with good soft tissue imaging. The iceball is seen as a signal void on T1-weighted images. MRI has the advantage of allowing imaging distal to the iceball, achieved secondary to the iceball acoustic shadowing effect.[46,56,57]

Outcome

Histology

Multiple animal studies have evaluated histologic changes as a result of cryoinjury. Acutely, cryoinjury results in sharply demarcated lesions with minimal inflammation[41] (Figure 10.14). At 1 week, four distinct zones are seen: central necrosis, inflammatory infiltrate, hemorrhage, and fibrosis with regeneration. At 13 weeks, the necrotic tissue is replaced with a circumscribed area of fibrosis.[46,49] These findings have been confirmed in human renal tumors.[52]

Radiology

Both CT and MRI have been used to follow-up patients after cryoablation. Gill and Novick use MRI for follow-up

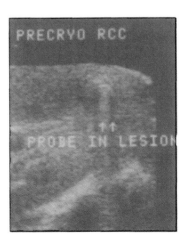

Figure 10.12
Laparoscopic renal cryosurgery. An ultrasound image of a cryoablation probe being placed into a renal lesion. (Courtesy of Tung Shu.)

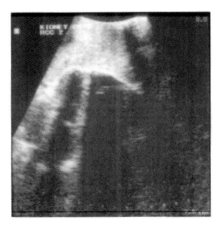

Figure 10.13
Laparoscopic renal cryosurgery. An ultrasound image of an 'ice ball'; a hypoechoic lesion created by cryosurgical ablation of a renal lesion. (Courtesy of Tung Shu.)

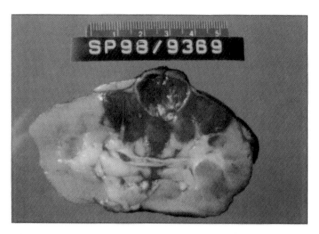

Figure 10.14
Laparoscopic renal cryosurgery. Gross pathologic renal
specimen demonstrates acute post-surgical changes of a renal
lesion and surrounding parenchyma. (Courtesy of Tung Shu.)

and noted that the primary criterion for successful cryoablation is nonenhancement of lesions after gadolinium
administration.[61] All cryolesions are isointense to the adjacent normal parenchyma on T1-weighted images and
hypointense on T2-weighted images. On day 1, half the
cases may have a hyperintense peripheral rim at the border
of the cryolesion and normal kidney. On day 30, the
cryolesions demonstrate an increase in signal intensity on
both T1- and T2-weighted images but no enhancement.[56]
MRI also demonstrates sequential contraction of the
cryolesion.[55] The disadvantage of radiologic follow-up,
however, is that most cryolesions do not resolve
completely.[57,62]

Clinical series

There have been multiple clinical series evaluating
cryotherapy. These series, however, have been limited by
relatively short follow-up (< 3 years) and small numbers
of patients. The patients have for the most part been
selected carefully to include small (< 4 cm), peripheral
lesions. Most have been approached laparoscopically but
the percutaneous[51] and open approaches have also been
utilized. Table 10.3 summarizes the results of these trials.

Rukstalis performed open renal cryoablation on 29
patients with a median preoperative lesion size of 2.2 cm.[63]
Five serious adverse events occurred in 5 patients, with
only 1 event directly related to the procedure. One patient
experienced a biopsy-proven local recurrence, and 91.3%
of patients (median follow-up 16 months) demonstrated a
complete radiographic response with only a residual scar
or small, nonenhancing cyst.

Bishoff et al treated 8 patients with small (average 2 cm)
exophytic renal masses.[46] They underwent laparoscopic
biopsy and cryosurgical ablation using a 3 or 4.8 mm

probe (Cryomedical Sciences Inc., Rockville, Maryland)
for one 15 min or two 5 min freeze cycles to a temperature
of −180°C; the ice ball was extended at least 7 mm beyond
the tumor margin.[46] There were no intraoperative or postoperative complications in the 8 patients. The estimated
blood loss was 140 ml, and the mean hospital stay was
3.5 days. At a mean clinical follow-up of 7.7 (range 1–18)
months and radiographic follow-up of 5 months, there
have been no tumor recurrences or significant changes in
the serum creatinine concentration.

The Cleveland Clinic group have one of the larger experiences with cryoablation and have published their series
with initial and intermediate results.[55,56,64] Sung et al
reported the intermediate follow-up results of laparoscopic renal cryoablation in 50 patients (34 tumors) with a
mean tumor size of 2.1 cm.[64] As dictated by the tumor
location, cryoablation was performed by either the
retroperitoneal ($n = 38$) or the transperitoneal ($n = 12$)
laparoscopic approach using real-time ultrasound monitoring. A double freeze–thaw cycle was routinely
performed. The mean surgical time was 2.6 hours, cryoablation time 20.5 min, and blood loss 50.6 ml. For a mean
intraoperative ultrasonographic tumor size of 2.1 cm, the
mean cryolesion size was 3.5 cm. Sequential MRI demonstrated a gradual contraction in the mean diameter of the
cryolesions with complete resolution in 9 patients with
2-year follow-up. Of 31 patients who underwent CT-
guided biopsy at 3–6 months, 30 had negative biopsies.
One patient had a 1.3 cm heterogeneous enhancing nodule
on 18-month MRI and underwent a nephrectomy based
on a positive needle biopsy.

Shingleton and Sewell have reported in several studies
on the feasibility and safety of performing percutaneous
cryoablation of renal tumors using open MRI.[49,59,60] They
recently reported their 1-year follow-up with a total of 35
patients with mean tumor size of 3.7 cm. Patients were
hospitalized overnight for observation. Follow-up imaging
with MRI or CT and physical examinations were done at
1 week, and at 1, 3, 6, and 12 months. Complications
occurred in 5 patients: a superficial wound abscess in 1,
self-limiting gross hematuria in 4. At mean follow-up of 12
months, all patients were alive with no evidence of residual
or new tumors. Five patients underwent retreatment for
residual enhancing mass.

Harada et al also evaluated the feasibility of performing
percutaneous cryosurgery, treating 4 patients with renal
tumors with local anesthesia using a horizontal open MRI
system (AIRIS II, Hitachi Medical Corp., Tokyo, Japan).[65]
Mass size was radiographically documented as 4 cm or less
in diameter. A 2 or 3 mm cryoprobe was advanced into the
renal mass under real-time MR monitoring. Follow-up
dynamic CT and physical examination were done after 2
weeks and 6 weeks. Cryoablated tumors resolved, and there
were no serious complications and no clinically significant
changes during the procedures and follow-up study.

Table 10.3 *Ablation series*

Technique	Year	Author	Patients (tumors)	Mean tumor size (cm)	Successful ablation[a]	Mean follow-up (months)	Major complication	Minor complication	LOS (days)	Histology
Laparoscopic cryoablation	2001	Sung et al[64]	50	2.1	30/31 (97%)[c]	18.8	NA	NA	NA	NA
Laparoscopic cryoablation	1999	Bishoff et al[46]	8	2	8/8 (100%)	7.7	0	0	3.5	NA
Laparoscopic cryoablation	2002	Kmi et al[111]	12	2.2	10/12 (83%)	10	NA	NA	3.25	8/12 RCC
Laparoscopic (*n* = 3)/ Open (*n* = 4) cryoablation	2000	Rodriguez et al[57]	7	2.2	6/7 studied with partial resolution (no growth)	14	0	Pelvic vein thrombosis, worsening of CVA symptoms (resolved)	4.4	5/7 RCC, 2/7 indeterminate
Percutaneous cryoablation	2001	Shingleton and Sewell[49]	35	3.7	30/35 (86%)	12	0	Gross hematuria (*n* = 4), wound infection (*n* = 1)	NA	NA
Percutaneous cryoablation	2001	Harada et al[65]	4	< 4	4/4 (100%)	1.5	0	NA	NA	NA
Percutaneous RF ablation	2001	McGovern et al[91]	17 (19)	1–5.5	15/18 (84%)	6–36	No	Ureteral obstruction requiring stent (*n* = 2) and gross hematuria/perinephric bleeding (*n* = 1)	15/18 outpatient, 3 admissions	RCC
Percutaneous RF ablation	2000	Gervais et al[90]	8 (9)	3.3	7/9 (78%)	10.3	Large perinephric hematoma and anuria	Reaction to fentanyl	12/14 outpatient, 2 admissions	RCC (*n* = 7)
Percutaneous RF ablation	2002	Pavlovich et al[89]	21 (24)	2.4	19/24 (79%)	2	No	Pain on hip flexion (*n* = 2), flank numbness (*n* = 2)	1	Known VHL (*n* = 19) or hereditary papillary renal cancer (*n* = 2)
Percutaneous RF ablation	2002	Ogan et al[81]	13	2.4	12/13 (93%)	2.9	No	Perinephric hematoma (*n* = 1)	0.9	Biopsy in 5 patients: RCC (40%) oncocytoma (40%) AML (20%)
Percutaneous RF ablation	2002	de Baere et al[112]	5	3.3	5/5 (100%)	9[b]	NA	Hematuria (*n* = 2), subcapsular hematoma (*n* = 1)	1.8	RCC (biopsy proven prior to treatment)
Laparoscopic RF ablation	2002	Jacomides et al[28]	8 (11)	2.1	8/8 (100%)	9.8	No	No	1.5	RCC (75%), AML (12.5%), oncocytoma (12.5%)

[a] Successful ablation defined as no contrast enhancement on follow-up CT imaging.
[b] Median.
[c] Negative CT-directed biopsy at 3–6 months.
AML = angiomyolipoma, RCC = renal cell carcinoma, NA = not available, LOS = length of stay, RF = radiofrequency, CT = computed tomography, CVA = cerebrovascular accident, VHL = Von Hippel–Lindau disease.

Complications

Bleeding. A concern with cryoablation is bleeding at the probe site and from cracks in the parenchyma during thawing. In an animal study, Nakada et al noted a crack in the renal parenchyma of one kidney during the thaw phase; at harvest that animal was found to have an intraperitoneal hemorrhage.[43] Rodriguez and coauthors routinely packed the probe site with microfibrillar collagen hemostat and applied pressure for 2–3 min in addition to using the argon beam coagulation as necessary to control bleeding.[57]

Injury to collecting system. Campbell et al. observed an obstructive stricture of the ureteropelvic junction in 1 animal after cryotherapy.[39] Barone and Rodgers performed cryoinjury on white rabbits with solitary kidneys using a liquid nitrogen probe.[40] Transient gross hematuria was noted in 25% of the animals and microscopic hematuria in 50%. In an interesting study presented by Sung, cryolesions were intentionally extended to the collecting system and unless the cryoprobe physically penetrated the calyces, the collecting system healed in a water tight fashion.[66]

Effect on renal function. Barone and Rodgers performed cryoinjury on white rabbits with solitary kidneys.[40] Serum blood urea nitrogen and creatinine levels reached maximum levels at 72 hours and gradually returned toward normal thereafter. Carvalhal et al. followed 22 patients after laparoscopic renal cryoablation for a minimum of 6 months.[67] No significant differences were found between the preoperative and latest postoperative serum creatinine (sCr) levels (1.13 and 0.91 mg/dl, respectively), systolic and diastolic blood pressure values (135.6 vs 131.2 mmHg and 78 vs 72.7 mmHg, respectively), or in the estimated creatinine clearance. The number or dose of antihypertensive medications did not change during the follow-up period for any patient. In 3 patients with a solitary kidney, the blood pressure and sCr values remained unchanged (mean preoperative sCr 1.43 mg/dl, and mean postoperative sCr after a minimum of 6 months 1.33 mg/dl). Laparoscopic renal cryoablation did not have a deleterious impact on renal function or blood pressure during a mean follow-up of 20.6 months.

Summary

Cryoablation has shown good results, with relatively few complications and low morbidity. Long-term follow-up is necessary to demonstrate oncologic control. At this time, percutaneous cryoablation is limited by the availability of open MRI.

Radiofrequency ablation

RFA has been shown to be an effective and safe method for destroying living tissues (see Figures 10.7 and 10.8). Energy generated by the RF probes creates temperature to >100°C and induces coagulative necrosis in tissues. This technology has been used in multiple organs, including liver,[68] nerves,[69,70] bone,[71] prostate,[72–75] and heart.[76–79]

Zlotta and colleagues were the first to evaluate this technology for renal tumors.[80] They used a RITA generator and measured power delivery, impedance, and total energy delivered. Initially, 4 ex-vivo kidneys were treated. Then, 2 patients with localized renal cancer were treated immediately prior to nephrectomy and 1 patient received percutaneous treatment 1 week prior to nephrectomy. In the patient with the RITA treatment 1 week prior to nephrectomy, the kidney demonstrated extensive coagulative necrosis with no residual tumor cells. No damage was seen beyond the target lesion. The CT scan after 1 week of treatment demonstrated absence of contrast in the targeted lesion. Importantly, several parameters concerning RF were established:

1. the lesions observed were similar to lesions that were forecast
2. the dimensions of thermal lesions created by RF could be monitored by tissue impedance, power delivery, time of application, and total energy delivered to the tissues
3. the treatment is safe and reproducibly destroyed renal tissue
4. the CT scan is an effective modality for following lesions after treatment
5. ultrasound is not effective in assessing lesions during ablation.

Indications

As with most nephron-sparing procedures, RFA is limited to small lesions and is best for exophytic lesions. Endophytic lesions raise concerns about injury to the collecting system and hilar structures, whereas large lesions (> 4 cm) are difficult to ablate completely with the current technology.

Techniques

Approach

The surgeon's preference should always be the primary decision-making tool in determining the approach for RFA. Anterior lesions are easier to approach transperitoneally, but posterior and lateral lesions can be treated from either a retroperitoneal or transperitoneal approach. For percutaneous ablation, it is important to determine if the bowel or lung will limit percutaneous access. Whereas the morbidity of percutaneous approaches is less than for the laparoscopic approach, tumor position in relation to adjacent organs is critical in determining the safety of percutaneous RFA. Ogan et al had to change the management of 3 patients initially scheduled for percutaneous RFA to a laparoscopic approach due to inability to safely guide the needle using a CT scanner.[81]

Radiofrequency generators

There are temperature- and impedance-based RF generators. The RITA system is a temperature-based system and delivers energy at 150 W until the average temperature at the various prongs averages at over 100°C. The Radiotherapeutics device delivers energy up to 200 W. Typically, an ablation cycle starts at 50 W, with an increase of 10 W each minute to a maximum of 90 W. This setting is maintained until impedance has reached 200 ohms, at which time power passively decreases to less than 10 W. Both manufacturers recommend repeating the treatment cycle. Conceptually, temperature-based probes generate a temperature above that necessary to destroy the tumor cells and monitor this temperature level. Impedance-based probes generate energy that enters the tissues and the impedance rises when the tissue is charred and no more energy can be transferred, which signals successful treatment.

In a porcine model, when the 2 probes were compared using manufacturer recommendations, they generated similar-sized lesions with no viable cells.[82]

'Wet' radiofrequency ablation

During RFA, desiccation of tissue causes a rise in impedance, which limits the amount of energy that is delivered to tissues. Infusion of saline into the treatment area can limit early desiccation of tissue around the needle tip and allow greater delivery of energy.

Polascik and colleagues studied the use of an RF electrode (RFT system; United States Surgical Corp., Norwalk, Connecticut) with a continuous 14.6% saline infusion (2 ml/min).[83] A VX-2 tumor was implanted in 14 rabbit kidneys and treatments of 30 or 45 s were applied prior to sacrifice. Mean lesion sizes increased from 1.4 cm × 1.0 cm to 1.8 cm × 1.5 for the 30 s and 45 s treatment groups. No acute complications were noted.

In another study of 'wet' RFA, Patel and colleagues infused 14.6% saline at 10 ml/min for 15 s into normal renal parenchyma of New Zealand white rabbits prior to

ablation.[84] Fifty watts of energy were delivered at 475 kHz for 1 or 2 min. There were no complications in 48 treated animals with no fistula/urinoma and no perinephric hematomas. Treatments for 1 min and 2 min created average lesions of 7 cm^3 and 10 cm^3, respectively. Impedance did not limit the delivery of energy during the treatments.

Although 'wet' RFA may allow larger lesion formation, most current studies have used 'dry' RFA.

Histology

Zlotta et al evaluated acute and 1-week histologic changes after RFA.[80] Macroscopic discoloration was noted in all specimens treated. Microscopic lesions were consistent with intense stromal and epithelial edema as well as hypereosinophilia and pyknosis. In a patient with the RITA treatment 1 week prior to nephrectomy, the kidney demonstrated extensive coagulative necrosis with no residual tumor cells.

Rendon et al also noted significant acute cellular effects, including cytoplasmic vacuolization, chromatic condensation, and cellular shape changes after RFA.[85]

Corwin et al performed laparoscopic RFA in 11 farm pigs,[86] and acute hematoxylin and eosin (H&E) staining revealed preserved renal parenchymal architecture with only minimal cellular changes. However, nicotinamide adenine dinucleotide staining (NADH) for metabolic activity demonstrated complete cell death.

To assess the chronic histologic changes of RFA, Hsu et al performed RFA on 11 pigs, with 5 survival animals.[87] Initially, lesions show intense inflammation and coagulative necrosis. Subsequently, there was near total resorption of the necrotic foci by day 90.

Radiologic monitoring

Unlike cryoablation, real-time monitoring of RFA is not possible. Several investigators have noted that ultrasound was useful for needle placement but could not accurately demonstrate the region of treatment.[80,86,88] For percutaneous RFA, ultrasound and CT scan can be used for localization. Ogan et al have noted the importance of deploying the probe approximately 0.5–1.0 cm beyond the CT-measured tumor diameter for effective cancer control.[81]

Post-procedure, CT scan and MRI are effective in evaluating lesions for follow-up. Loss of lesion enhancement is the key to evaluating for successful treatment.[80,81,88] CT scanning often reveals either spherical lesions or wedge-shaped regions, suggesting intrarenal vascular injury leading to segmental infarction.[88,89]

Hilar occlusion

With the goal of evaluating the effects of hilar occlusion on the extent of RFA, Corwin et al performed laparoscopic RFA in 11 farm pigs.[86] They used the RITA probe and delivered 50 W with average temperature of 100°C for 8 min. There were no perioperative complications or urinoma formations. Lesions formed were symmetrical with a rounded, spherical contour. The lesion dimensions were larger in the hilar occlusion group, but this was not statistically significant.

Outcomes

Clinical series

Table 10.3 summarizes the outcome of treatment with RFA. Tumor sizes mostly range from 2–3 cm and follow-up was less than 2 years for most series. Success was primarily defined as no enhancement on surveillance imaging and ranged from 78 to 100%.

Gervais and colleagues performed percutaneous RFA in 8 patients.[90] This preliminary experience was limited to patients with life expectancy shorter than 10 years, significant comorbidities, and/or a solitary kidney. A total of 9 tumors were treated in these 8 patients, with diagnosis based on needle biopsy ($n = 7$), enlarged enhancing renal mass with 2 nondiagnostic biopsies ($n = 1$), and enlarged enhancing mass on MRI ($n = 1$). All procedures were performed with intravenous (IV) sedation (RF generator: Cosman Coagulator CC-1; Radionics, Burlington, Massachusetts). Follow-up was performed using CT and MRI at 1, 3, and 6 months. Four patients were treated in one ablation session and 4 required more than one session because of imaging evidence of a residual tumor. All 5 exophytic and all 3 small tumors (< 3 cm) were free of enhancement at 6 months. Only 1 of the 3 central tumors was free of enhancement. No patients developed metastases or renal insufficiency. The authors found that centrally located and larger tumors were more difficult to treat and, in fact, the 2 failures occurred in tumors the size of 4.4 and 5 cm despite several repeat treatments.

Pavlovich et al recently published their initial experience with RFA in 21 patients with known VHL (Von Hippel–Lindau disease) or hereditary papillary renal cancer and < 3 cm solid renal masses.[89] Twenty-four tumors were treated percutaneously using conscious sedation. The RITA Starburst XL probe was used to deliver 50 W with temperature set to 100°C for a minimum of two 10–12 min cycles. A third cycle was applied for deep medullary tumors and those close to 3 cm. Of the 24 treatments, 19 were considered satisfactory, based on accurate targeting and maintenance of $> 70°C$ temperature at all probe electrodes during therapy. Results were based on a follow-up CT scan at 2 months. Of the 24 lesions, 5 had focal areas of persistent growth enhancement. While 4 of the 5 were believed to have been insufficiently treated, 1 lesion fulfilled the criteria for a satisfactory treatment.

McGovern et al also performed percutaneous RITA for 19 RCC in a total of 17 patients.[91] These were done in an outpatient setting using IV sedation with an internally cooled RF electrode. Tumor sizes ranged from 1 to 5.5 cm, with follow-up ranging from 6 months to 3 years. There was complete response in 15 of 18 patients and partial response in 3 patients.

Ogan et al recently reported on 12 patients with 13 tumors who underwent percutaneous RFA.[81] To qualify for treatment, lesions were < 4 cm, posterior or lateral in location, and enhancing on imaging studies. Mean tumor size was 2.4 cm. A RITA Starburst XL probe was deployed approximately 0.5–1.0 cm beyond the CT-measured tumor diameter. Target temperature was 105°C and tumors were treated for one or two 5–8 min cycles based on surgeon preference. There were no major complications and 1 patient developed a small perinephric hematoma. Mean length of stay was 0.9 days. Twelve of the 13 patients demonstrated complete ablation on the most recent CT scan, with mean follow-up of 4.9 months.

Despite 2 case reports of laparoscopic RFA, experience lags behind that with percutaneous treatment. Jacomides et al recently reported the only series of laparoscopic RFA on 8 patients.[28] A RITA Starburst XL probe was deployed to ablate a volume approximately 0.5–1.0 cm beyond the CT-measured tumor diameter. Eleven tumors were treated with mean size of 2.1 cm. Mean operative time was 140 min. There were no perioperative complications and no urinary extravasation. Mean hospital stay was 1.5 days. With a mean follow-up of 9.8 months there was no enhancement on CT scan in any of the patients.

Effect on renal function

Gill and colleagues used a porcine model to evaluate acute and chronic changes that resulted from performing bilateral RFA of kidneys.[92] Serum creatinine remained stable at 90 days despite bilateral RFA.

No series published at this time has found significant changes in serum creatinine.[81,89,90]

Injury to adjacent structures

RFA can cause thermal injury to adjacent structures, such as the psoas muscle[88,93] and bowel.[93] In an effort to evaluate ways to protect surrounding structures from thermal injury during RFA, Rendon et al studied the use of hydro- and gas-dissection in the perirenal space.[93] In 3 pigs, a 13-gauge cannula was inserted percutaneously under ultrasound guidance and positioned under Gerota's fascia with a total of 30–60 ml of sterile saline injected to create a fluid space. In 2 pigs, a 22-gauge venous access catheter was used to infuse 500 ml of CO_2 under Gerota's fascia. These techniques prevented injury to adjacent structures. A disadvantage of the CO_2, however, was interference with ultrasound. These techniques have important clinical implications since the threat of injuring anterior structures such as bowel is an important consideration in planning appropriate treatment of renal lesions.

Pavlovich et al noted pain on hip flexion ($n = 2$) and cutaneous flank numbness ($n = 2$) after percutaneous RFA. The pain on flexion resolved within 2 weeks but the numbness persisted at 2 months.[89]

Injury to the collecting system can result in hematuria.[89,91] Fortunately, this can usually be managed conservatively. Perinephric bleeding is not uncommon and has been noted in several series.[81,90,91] Rarely, patients may need a blood transfusion.[90]

Incomplete treatment

Despite the promising results, one of the criticisms of ablation technology is the uncertainty of complete tumor destruction. In a related study, Rendon and coauthors evaluated nephrectomy specimens after RFA.[85] Ten patients with < 3.5 cm renal masses underwent RFA using a LeVeen electrode (Radiotherapeutics Corp., Sunnyvale, California) prior to a partial nephrectomy or with ultrasound/CT guidance in a group treated 7 days prior to open surgery. In several cases it was concluded that viable tumor persisted in 5–10% of the volume. In 2 of these patients, a CT scan did not demonstrate enhancement at 7 days post-treatment. All the areas of tumor positivity occurred at the margins of the lesions and not the center. Several important points are noted from this study. First, RFA depends on appropriate probe placement and ablation of a margin of normal renal parenchyma around the tumor. It is possible that variability in blood flow may allow tissue at the margins to remain viable so the RF probe needs to be deployed > 0.5 cm beyond the tumor margin. Secondly, the CT scan may not be accurate at 1 week post-treatment and may take longer to demonstrate enhancement with residual tumor. Finally, H&E staining is not sufficient to assess viability, whereas NADH staining has been shown to more accurately establish metabolic activity in tissues.

Large tumors and centrally located tumors increase the risk of inadequate treatment with RFA because of technical problems with appropriate positioning of the probes to provide adequate treatment to the periphery of the tumors. McGovern et al had an incomplete response in 3 patients with tumors greater than 3.5 cm.[91] Gervais et al found that only 1 of the 3 patients with central tumors was

free of enhancement. These tumors were 4.4 and 5 cm in size and were unresponsive despite several repeat treatments.[90]

Conclusion

RFA offers a promising modality for managing small renal tumors laparoscopically or percutaneously. Initial results are favorable but long-term results are necessary to evaluate oncologic control.

High-intensity focused ultrasound

High-intensity focused ultrasound (HIFU) uses focused ultrasound waves that are generated by a cylindrical piezo-electric element to create heat in tissues (Figure 10.15). A parabolic reflector focuses the ultrasound waves, and the ultrasound is coupled by degassed water between the source and the patient's skin. In a manner similar to extracorporeal shock wave lithotripsy, the sound waves penetrate the skin, with only slight absorption, prior to converging on the focus point. A high power density, exceeding 100 W/cm², can achieve temperatures above 65°C within a pulse duration of less than 5 s.[94] The size of the ablated tissue is similar to the focal zone but can be controlled by the power and duration of ultrasound pulses.[94] Tissue destruction occurs as a result of both thermal and mechanical (cavitation) effects.

HIFU has been utilized for various clinical applications, from treatment of glaucoma[95] to liver[96] and prostate tissue ablation.[97] Experimental applications in animals have been performed to evaluate HIFU effects on renal tissues.[28,98–102] Chapelon and colleagues used a 1 and 2.25 MHz transducer to perform in-vivo tissue destruction on 124 rat and 16 canine kidneys.[98] The rat experiments were used to define the constants necessary to produce a localized tissue lesion at the focus of the transducer. Subsequently, in the canine experiments, extracorporeal HIFU was performed and kidney lesions were achieved in 10 animals (63%). These lesions were histologically determined to be coagulation necrosis.

Watkin et al performed HIFU in 18 porcine kidneys.[103] No macroscopic lesions were detected in 5 kidneys. In 13 kidneys, 67% of total shots fired were detected within the target area. Lesion sizes ranged from 4 to 17 mm in length and 0.5 to 2.5 mm in width. Individual lesions were well circumscribed with a pale central area surrounded by a hemorrhagic rim. Histologically, in the central zone, tubules were obliterated and nuclei were pyknotic and hyperchromatic. In the periphery, the tubules were

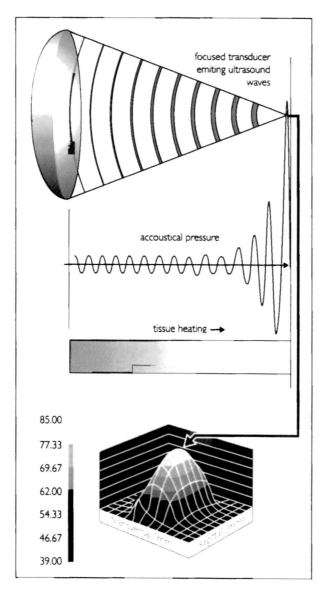

Figure 10.15
High-intensity focused ultrasound (HIFU). Focused ultrasound
waves generated by a piezoelectric element create heat in
tissues. A parabolic reflector focuses the ultrasound waves, and
the ultrasound is coupled by degassed water between the
source and the patient's skin. The sound waves penetrate
the skin with only slight absorption, prior to converging on the
focus point tumor. Tissue destruction occurs as a result of both
thermal and mechanical effects.

distended and filled with amorphous material, and the
nuclei were hyperchromatic but not significantly pyknotic.
Due to anatomic constraints such as rib interference, only
the lower pole could be treated. There was an acute skin
burn in 1 animal and skin changes with red discoloration
in 9 other treatments.

Paterson and colleagues developed a probe that allows
for HIFU application laparoscopically.[104] They directly

applied HIFU to renal tissue in a porcine model ($n = 13$)
and created lesions in 12 of 13 kidneys. There were no
significant complications, and they achieved homogenous
lesions with complete tissue necrosis throughout the entire
volume.

There have been few human applications of HIFU for
renal tissue. Susani et al performed HIFU in 2 patients
prior to radical nephrectomy.[105] Hemorrhagic necrosis was
found in the specimens but the amount of tumor necrosis
did not allow recognition of the treatment zone.[105]
Vallancien et al. performed phase I and II studies in
patients with renal tumors.[28,101,102] Four patients with T2
and T3 kidney tumors were treated 2, 6, 8, and 15 days
prior to nephrectomy. The final pathology revealed coagulative necrosis in the targeted areas. There was a second-
degree skin burn in 1 patient due to an error in dosimetry.

Kohrmann et al presented the first report on a patient
with renal cell carcinoma who underwent HIFU with curative intent.[94] HIFU was applied to 3 tumors in 3 sessions
with the patient under general anesthesia or sedation analgesia, followed by MRI for 6 months. General anesthesia
was required to apply high-energy levels of focused ultrasound. After treatment, MRI showed necrosis in the 2
tumors in the lower kidney pole within 17 and 48 days,
respectively. The necrotic tumor area shrank thereafter but
at 6 months did not completely disappear. The tumor in
the upper pole was not affected by treatment because the
ultrasound energy was absorbed by the interposed ribs.
Successful HIFU application depended on optimum
energy coupling, a sufficiently high ultrasound energy
level, and general anesthesia.

HIFU is still an experimental modality with little clinical
history. A better method for focusing energy is needed to
avoid skin burns and other complications. Furthermore,
studies need to prove that HIFU provides complete tissue
destruction before it is used for cancer control.

Interstitial photon radiation energy

Interstitial photon radiation energy uses a probe to deliver
controllable local radiation therapy without exposing
intervening layers of tissue. A miniature X-ray generator
device produces low-energy X-ray photons, which attenuate rapidly in tissues, resulting in sharply defined bound-
aries. This technology was evaluated in 12 dogs and 11
renal lesions were generated.[106] The lesions were well
demarcated and demonstrated coagulative necrosis that
organized into fibrosis over time. There were no
hematomas or urinomas. A single 10 min treatment
(15 Gy at a radius of 1.3 cm) resulted in a 2.5 cm lesion.
Further studies are necessary to evaluate this technology's
potential.

Interstital laser thermoablation

Laser ablation of target tissue using one or several laser fibers has been described in the treatment of head and neck, liver, brain, and kidney tumors as well as the treatment of benign prostate hyperplasia and uterine fibroids.

Using MR-guided interstitial laser thermoablation (ILT), de Jode et al treated kidney tumors in 3 patients. Laser energy from a neodymium : YAG source was percutaneously delivered to the tumors under real-time MR guidance in an open access scanner. Follow-up gadolinium-enhanced MRI confirmed necrosis in the target tissue. One patient showed areas of enhancement consistent with viable tumor and underwent an additional ablation of the enhancing areas.[107]

In a porcine model, Gettman et al studied the size and histology of lesions created with interstitial laser coagulation (ILC) via a laparoscopic approach with and without hilar occlusion in the porcine model.[108] For each kidney, a 600 μm bare-tip silicon laser fiber was attached to a diode laser (wavelength=805 nm) and inserted 0.5 cm into the lower pole for 15 min at 6 W. Histology revealed cellular inflammation in acute lesions; chronic lesions demonstrated coagulative necrosis with progressive fibrosis. NADH staining showed viable cells within the treatment zone of surviving animals.

The histologic evidence of viable cells within the treatment zone suggests that additional refinement of the ILC technique in the animal model is warranted before further application in humans.

Ferromagnetic thermal rod implants

Rehman and colleagues evaluated the use of ferromagnetic self-regulating reheatable thermal rod implants for in-situ tissue ablation.[109] Ferromagnetic compounds, when placed in a magnetic field, develop an electric current. In tissue, the ferromagnetic compounds meet resistance to transmission of the current, leading to heat generation. The goal of the study was to evaluate the effect of permanently implanting palladium and cobalt rods that self-regulate to 70°C in solid abdominal organs. In 16 pigs, renal, hepatic, uterine, and pancreatic rods were placed in 1 cm parallel rows to ablate 7 g of tissue. The animals were treated in an extracorporeal magnetic field of 50 gauss rms at a frequency of 50 kHz. The tissue surrounding the rods exceeded 50°C and confluent tissue necrosis was noted in 7 of 9 (78%) kidneys. Necrosis extended 2 mm beyond the periphery of the rods and there were no 'skip areas' of viable tissue. This application is awaiting human trials.

Conclusions

There have been tremendous strides in the management of small renal tumors. Progress has been made in decreasing the morbidity of procedures and improving the safety and feasibility of minimally invasive approaches. Ablative technologies currently offer the promise of outpatient, low-morbidity procedures to manage small tumors without the need for open or laparoscopic surgery. Technologies such as HIFU possess the potential to allow for management of renal tumors without any incision.

At this time, the most extensive experience has been with cryoablation, but is limited primarily to laparoscopic applications. On the other hand, although RFA is increasingly popular and allows percutaneous treatment, physicians have less experience in its use. Long-term cancer control by these modalities has not yet been established, but early results are promising.

References

1. Smith SJ, Bosniak MA, Megibow AJ, et al. Renal cell carcinoma: earlier discovery and increased detection. Radiology 1989; 170:699–703.

2. Licht MR, Novick AC. Nephron sparing surgery for renal cell carcinoma. J Urol 1993; 149:1–7.

3. Thrasher JB, Robertson JE, Paulson DF. Expanding indications for conservative renal surgery in renal cell carcinoma. Urology 1994; 43:160–8.

4. Duque JL, Loughlin KR, O'Leary MP, et al. Partial nephrectomy: alternative treatment for selected patients with renal cell carcinoma. Urology 1998; 52:584–90.

5. Fergany AF, Hafez KS, Novick AC. Long-term results of nephron sparing surgery for localized renal cell carcinoma: 10-year followup. J Urol 2000; 163:442–5.

6. Wolf JS Jr, Seifman BD, Montie JE. Nephron sparing surgery for suspected malignancy: open surgery compared to laparoscopy with selective use of hand assistance. J Urol 2000; 163:1659–64.

7. Hoznek A, Salomon L, Antiphon P, et al. Partial nephrectomy with retroperitoneal laparoscopy. J Urol 1999; 162:1922–6.

8. Gill IS, Desai MM, Kaouk JH, et al. Laparoscopic partial nephrectomy for renal tumor: duplicating open surgical techniques. J Urol 2002; 167:469–7; discussion 475–6.

9. Janetschek G, Jeschke K, Peschel R, et al. Laparoscopic surgery for stage T1 renal cell carcinoma: radical nephrectomy and wedge resection. Eur Urol 2000; 38:131–8.

10. Harmon WJ, Kavoussi LR, Bishoff JT. Laparoscopic nephron-sparing surgery for solid renal masses using the ultrasonic shears. Urology 2000; 56:754–9.

11. Stifelman MD, Sosa RE, Nakada SY, Shichman SJ. Hand-assisted laparoscopic partial nephrectomy. J Endourol 2001; 15:161–4.

12. Janetschek G, Daffner P, Peschel R, Bartsch G. Laparoscopic nephron sparing surgery for small renal cell carcinoma. J Urol 1998; 159:1152–5.

13. Lotan Y, Gettman MT, Ogan K, et al. Clinical use of the Holmium:Yag laser in laparoscopic partial nephrectomy. J Endourol 2002; 16(5):289–92.

14. Yoshimura K, Okubo K, Ichioka K, et al. Laparoscopic partial nephrectomy with a microwave tissue coagulator for small renal tumor. J Urol 2001; 165:1893–6.

15. McDougall EM, Clayman RV, Chandhoke PS, et al. Laparoscopic partial nephrectomy in the pig model. J Urol 1993; 149:1633–6.

16. Winfield HN, Donovan JF, Lund GO, et al. Laparoscopic partial nephrectomy: initial experience and comparison to the open surgical approach. J Urol 1995; 153:1409–14.

17. Cadeddu JA, Corwin TS. Cable tie compression to facilitate laparoscopic partial nephrectomy. J Urol 2001; 165:177–8.

18. Cadeddu JA, Corwin TS, Traxer O, et al. Hemostatic laparoscopic partial nephrectomy: cable-tie compression. Urology 2001; 57:562–6.

19. Gill IS, Delworth MG, Munch LC. Laparoscopic retroperitoneal partial nephrectomy. J Urol 1994; 152:1539–42.

20. Elashry OM, Wolf JS Jr, Rayala HJ, et al. Recent advances in laparoscopic partial nephrectomy: comparative study of electrosurgical snare electrode and ultrasound dissection. J Endourol 1997; 11:15–22.

21. Quinlan DM, Naslund MJ, Brendler CB. Application of argon beam coagulation in urological surgery. J Urol 1992; 147:410–12.

22. Meiraz D, Peled I, Gassner S, et al. The use of the CO_2 laser for partial nephrectomy: an experimental study. Invest Urol 1977; 15:262–4.

23. Hughes BF, Scott WW. Preliminary report on the use of a CO_2 laser surgical unit in animals. Invest Urol 1972; 9:353–7.

24. Landau ST, Wood TW, Smith JA Jr. Evaluation of sapphire tip Nd:YAG laser fibers in partial nephrectomy. Lasers Surg Med 1987; 7:426–8.

25. Benderev TV, Schaeffer AJ. Efficacy and safety of the Nd:YAG laser in canine partial nephrectomy. J Urol 1985; 133:1108–11.

26. Lotan Y, Gettman MT, Lindberg G, et al. Video of laparoscopic partial nephrectomy using holmium laser. J Endourol 2001 15(S1).

27. Corwin TS, Cadeddu JA. Radio frequency coagulation to facilitate laparoscopic partial nephrectomy. J Urol 2001; 165:175–6.

28. Jacomides L, Ogan K, Watumull L, Cadeddu JA. Laparoscopic application of radio frequency energy enables in-situ renal tumor ablation and partial nephrectomy. J Urol 2003; 169:49–53; discussion 53.

29. Hirao Y, Fujimoto K, Yoshii M, et al. Non-ischemic nephron-sparing surgery for small renal cell carcinoma: complete tumor enucleation using a microwave tissue coagulator. Jpn J Clin Oncol 2002; 32:95–102.

30. Tanaka M, Kai N, Naito S. Retroperitoneal laparoscopic wedge resection for small renal tumor using microwave tissue coagulator. J Endourol 2000; 14:569–72.

31. Murota T, Kawakita M, Oguchi N, et al. Retroperitoneoscopic partial nephrectomy using microwave coagulation for small renal tumors. Eur Urol 2002; 41:540–5.

32. Winfield HN, Donovan JF, Godet AS, Clayman RV. Laparoscopic partial nephrectomy: initial case report for benign disease. J Endourol 1993; 7:521–6.

33. McDougall EM, Elbahnasy AM, Clayman RV. Laparoscopic wedge resection and partial nephrectomy – the Washington University experience and review of the literature. JSLS 1998; 2:15–23.

34. Gettman MT, Bishoff JT, Su LM, et al. Hemostatic laparoscopic partial nephrectomy: initial experience with the radiofrequency coagulation-assisted technique. Urology 2001; 58:8–11.

35. Basting RF, Djakovic N, Widmann P. Use of water jet resection in organ-sparing kidney surgery. J Endourol 2000; 14:501–5.

36. Basting RF, Corvin S, Antwerpen C, et al. Use of water jet resection in renal surgery: early clinical experiences. Eur Urol 2000; 38:104–7.

37. Perahia B, Bishoff JT, Cornum RL, et al. The laparoscopic heminephrectomy: made easy by the new fibrin sealant powder. J Urol 2002; 167 (S):2.

38. Ramakumar S, Colegrove PM, Nelson JR, Slepian MJ. Photopolymerized PEG-lactide hydrogels: an effective means for hemostasis during laparoscopic partial nephrectomy. J Urol 2002; 167 (S):2.

39. Campbell SC, Krishnamurthi V, Chow G, et al. Renal cryosurgery: experimental evaluation of treatment parameters. Urology 1998; 52:29–33; discussion 33–4.

40. Barone GW, Rodgers BM. Morphologic and functional effects of renal cryoinjury. Cryobiology 1988; 25:363–71.

41. Sindelar WF, Javadpour N, Bagley DH. Histological and ultrastructural changes in rat kidney after cryosurgery. J Surg Oncol 1981; 18:363–79.

42. Nakada SY, Lee FT Jr, Warner TF, et al. Laparoscopic renal cryotherapy in swine: comparison of puncture cryotherapy preceded by arterial embolization and contact cryotherapy. J Endourol 1998; 12:567–73.

43. Nakada SY, Lee FT Jr, Warner T, et al. Laparoscopic cryosurgery of the kidney in the porcine model: an acute histological study. Urology 1998; 51:161–6.

44. Shingleton WB, Farabaugh P, Hughson M, Sewell PE Jr. Percutaneous cryoablation of porcine kidneys with magnetic resonance imaging monitoring. J Urol 2001; 166:289–91.

45. Schmidlin FR, Rupp CC, Hoffmann NE, et al. Measurement and prediction of thermal behavior and acute assessment of injury in a pig model of renal cryosurgery. J Endourol 2001; 15:193–7.

46. Bishoff JT, Chen RB, Lee BR, et al. Laparoscopic renal cryoablation: acute and long-term clinical, radiographic, and pathologic effects in an animal model and application in a clinical trial. J Endourol 1999; 13:233–9.

47. Onik GM, Reyes G, Cohen JK, Porterfield B. Ultrasound characteristics of renal cryosurgery. Urology 1993; 42:212–15.

48. Chosy SG, Nakada SY, Lee FT Jr, Warner TF. Monitoring renal cryosurgery: predictors of tissue necrosis in swine. J Urol 1998; 159:1370–4.

49. Shingleton WB, Sewell PE Jr. Percutaneous renal cryoablation for renal tumors: one-year follow-up. J Urol 2001; 165(S):186.

50. Cozzi PJ, Lynch WJ, Collins S, et al. Renal cryotherapy in a sheep model; a feasibility study. J Urol 1997; 157:710–2.

51. Uchida M, Imaide Y, Sugimoto K, et al. Percutaneous cryosurgery for renal tumours. Br J Urol 1995; 75:132–6; discussion 136–7.

52. Edmunds TB Jr, Schulsinger DA, Durand DB, Waltzer WC. Acute histologic changes in human renal tumors after cryoablation. J Endourol 2000; 14:139–43.

53. Johnson DB, Nakada SY. Laparoscopic cryoablation for renal-cell cancer. J Endourol 2000; 14:873–8; discussion 878–9.

54. Johnson DB, Nakada SY. Cryosurgery and needle ablation of renal lesions. J Endourol 2001; 15:361–8; discussion 375–6.

55. Gill IS, Novick AC, Soble JJ, et al. Laparoscopic renal cryoablation: initial clinical series. Urology 1998; 52:543–51.

56. Gill IS, Novick AC, Meraney AM, et al. Laparoscopic renal cryoablation in 32 patients. Urology 2000; 56:748–53.

57. Rodriguez R, Chan DY, Bishoff JT, et al. Renal ablative cryosurgery in selected patients with peripheral renal masses. Urology 2000; 55:25–30.

58. Zegel HG, Holland GA, Jennings SB, et al. Intraoperative ultrasonographically guided cryoablation of renal masses: initial experience. J Ultrasound Med 1998; 17:571–6.

59. Shingleton WB, Sewell PE Jr. Percutaneous renal tumor cryoablation with magnetic resonance imaging guidance. J Urol 2001; 165:773–6.

60. Shingleton WB, Sewell PE Jr. Percutaneous renal cryoablation of renal tumors in patients with von Hippel–Lindau disease. J Urol 2002; 167:1268–70.

61. Gill IS, Novick AC. Renal cryosurgery. Urology 1999; 54:215–19.

62. Chan DY, Rodriguez R, Kavoussi LR. Laparoscopic renal ablation. Urology 2001; 58:132.

63. Rukstalis DB, Khorsandi M, Garcia FU, et al. Clinical experience with open renal cryoablation. Urology 2001; 57:34–9.

64. Sung GT, Meraney AM, Schweizer DK, et al. Laparoscopic renal cryoablation in 50 patients: intermediate follow-up. J Urol 2001; 165 (S):158.

65. Harada J, Dohi M, Mogami T, et al. Initial experience of percutaneous renal cryosurgery under the guidance of a horizontal open MRI system. Radiat Med 2001; 19:291–6.

66. Sung GT, Gill IS, Hsu TH, et al. Effect of intentional cryo-injury to the renal collecting system. J Urol 2003; 170:619–22.

67. Carvalhal EF, Gill IS, Meraney AM, et al. Laparoscopic renal cryoablation: impact on renal function and blood pressure. Urology 2001; 58:357–61.

68. Rossi S, Di Stasi M, Buscarini E, et al. Percutaneous radiofrequency interstitial thermal ablation in the treatment of small hepatocellular carcinoma. Cancer J Sci Am 1995; 1:73.

69. Lord SM, Barnsley L, Wallis BJ, et al. Percutaneous radiofrequency neurotomy for chronic cervical zygapophyseal-joint pain. N Engl J Med 1996; 335:1721–6.

70. Lord SM, Barnsley L, Bogduk N. Percutaneous radiofrequency neurotomy in the treatment of cervical zygapophysial joint pain: a caution. Neurosurgery 1995; 36:732–9.

71. de Berg JC, Pattynama PM, Obermann WR, et al. Percutaneous computed-tomography-guided thermocoagulation for osteoid osteomas. Lancet 1995; 346:350–1.

72. Zlotta AR, Djavan B, Matos C, et al. Percutaneous transperineal radiofrequency ablation of prostate tumour: safety, feasibility and pathological effects on human prostate cancer. Br J Urol 1998; 81:265–75.

73. Schulman CC, Zlotta AR, Rasor JS, et al. Transurethral needle ablation (TUNA): safety, feasibility, and tolerance of a new office procedure for treatment of benign prostatic hyperplasia. Eur Urol 1993; 24:415–23.

74. Schulman C, Zlotta A. Transurethral needle ablation of the prostate (TUNA): pathological, radiological and clinical study of a new office procedure for treatment of benign prostatic hyperplasia using low-level radiofrequency energy. Arch Esp Urol 1994; 47:895–901.

75. Zlotta AR, Raviv G, Peny MO, et al. Possible mechanisms of action of transurethral needle ablation of the prostate on benign prostatic hyperplasia symptoms: a neurohistochemical study. J Urol 1997; 157:894–9.

76. Calkins H, Langberg J, Sousa J, et al. Radiofrequency catheter ablation of accessory atrioventricular connections in 250 patients. Abbreviated therapeutic approach to Wolff–Parkinson–White syndrome. Circulation 1992; 85:1337–46.

77. Calkins H, Mann C, Kalbfleisch S, et al. Site of accessory pathway block after radiofrequency catheter ablation in patients with the Wolff–Parkinson–White syndrome. J Cardiovasc Electrophysiol 1994; 5:20–7.

78. Calkins H, Leon AR, Deam AG, et al. Catheter ablation of atrial flutter using radiofrequency energy. Am J Cardiol 1994; 73:353–6.

79. Calkins H. Radiofrequency catheter ablation of supraventricular arrhythmias. Heart 2001; 85:594–600.

80. Zlotta AR, Wildschutz T, Raviv G, et al. Radiofrequency interstitial tumor ablation (RITA) is a possible new modality for treatment of renal cancer: ex vivo and in vivo experience. J Endourol 1997; 11:251–8.

81. Ogan K, Jacomides L, Dolmatch BL, et al. Percutaneous radiofrequency ablation of renal tumors: technique, limitations, and morbidity. Urology 2002; 60:954–8.

82. Gettman MT, Lotan Y, Corwin TS, et al. Radiofrequency coagulation of renal parenchyma: comparison of effects of energy generators on treatment efficacy. J Endourol 2002; 16:83–8.

83. Polascik TJ, Hamper U, Lee BR, et al. Ablation of renal tumors in a rabbit model with interstitial saline-augmented radiofrequency energy: preliminary report of a new technology. Urology 1999; 53:465–72; discussion 470–2.

84. Patel VR, Leveillee RJ, Hoey MF, et al. Radiofrequency ablation of rabbit kidney using liquid electrode: acute and chronic observations. J Endourol 2000; 14:155–9.

85. Rendon RA, Kachura JR, Sweet JM, et al. The uncertainty of radio frequency treatment of renal cell carcinoma: findings at immediate and delayed nephrectomy. J Urol 2002; 167:1587–92.

86. Corwin TS, Lindberg G, Traxer O, et al. Laparoscopic radiofrequency thermal ablation of renal tissue with and without hilar occlusion. J Urol 2001; 166:281–4.

87. Hsu TH, Fidler ME, Gill IS. Radiofrequency ablation of the kidney: acute and chronic histology in porcine model. Urology 2000; 56:872–5.

88. Crowley JD, Shelton J, Iverson AJ, et al. Laparoscopic and computed tomography-guided percutaneous radiofrequency ablation of renal tissue: acute and chronic effects in an animal model. Urology 2001; 57:976–80.

89. Pavlovich CP, Walther MM, Choyke PL, et al. Percutaneous radio frequency ablation of small renal tumors: initial results. J Urol 2002; 167:10–15.

90. Gervais DA, McGovern FJ, Wood BJ, et al. Radio-frequency ablation of renal cell carcinoma: early clinical experience. Radiology 2000; 217:665–72.

91. McGovern FJ, McDougal WS, Gervais DA, Mueller PR. Percutaneous radiofrequency ablation of human renal cell carcinoma. J Urol 2001; 165(5):157.

92. Gill IS, Hsu TH, Fox RL, et al. Laparoscopic and percutaneous radiofrequency ablation of the kidney: acute and chronic porcine study. Urology 2000; 56:197–200.

93. Rendon RA, Gertner MR, Sherar MD, et al. Development of a radiofrequency based thermal therapy technique in an in vivo porcine model for the treatment of small renal masses. J Urol 2001; 166:292–8.

94. Kohrmann KU, Michel MS, Gaa J, et al. High intensity focused ultrasound as noninvasive therapy for multilocal renal cell carcinoma: case study and review of the literature. J Urol 2002; 167:2397–403.

95. Silverman RH, Vogelsang B, Rondeau MJ, Coleman DJ. Therapeutic ultrasound for the treatment of glaucoma. Am J Ophthalmol 1991; 111:327–37.

96. ter Haar GR, Robertson D. Tissue destruction with focused ultrasound in vivo. Eur Urol 1993; 23 (Suppl 1):8–11.

97. Madersbacher S, Kratzik C, Susani M, Marberger M. Tissue ablation in benign prostatic hyperplasia with high intensity focused ultrasound. J Urol 1994; 152:1956–60; discussion 1960–1.

98. Chapelon JY, Margonari J, Theillere Y, et al. Effects of high-energy focused ultrasound on kidney tissue in the rat and the dog. Eur Urol 1992; 22:147–52.

99. Kohrmann KU, Back W, Bensemann J, et al. The isolated perfused kidney of the pig: new model to evaluate shock wave-induced lesions. J Endourol 1994; 8:105–10.

100. Back W, Kohrmann KU, Bensemann J, et al. Histo-morphologic and ultrastructural findings of shockwave-induced lesions in the isolated perfused kidney of the pig. J Endourol 1994; 8:257–61.

101. Vallancien G, Chopin D, Davila C, et al. [Focused extracorporeal pyrotherapy. Initial experimental results]. Prog Urol 1991; 1:149–53.

102. Bataille N, Vallancien G, Chopin D. Antitumoral local effect and metastatic risk of focused extracorporeal pyrotherapy on Dunning R-3327 tumors. Eur Urol 1996; 29:72–7.

103. Watkin NA, Morris SB, Rivens IH, ter Haar GR. High-intensity focused ultrasound ablation of the kidney in a large animal model. J Endourol 1997; 11:191–6.

104. Paterson RF, Shalhav AL, Lingeman JE, et al. Laparoscopic partial kidney ablation with high intensity focused ultrasound. J Urol 2002; 167(S):2

105. Susani M, Madersbacher S, Kratzik C, et al. Morphology of tissue destruction induced by focused ultrasound. Eur Urol 1993; 23 (Suppl 1):34–8.

106. Chan DY, Koniaris L, Magee C, et al. Feasibility of ablating normal renal parenchyma by interstitial photon radiation energy: study in a canine model. J Endourol 2000; 14:111–16.

107. de Jode MG, Vale JA, Gedroyc WM. MR-guided laser thermoablation of inoperable renal tumors in an open-configuration interventional MR scanner: preliminary clinical experience in three cases. J Magn Reson Imaging 1999; 10:545–9.

108. Gettman MT, Lotan Y, Lindberg G, et al. Laparoscopic interstitial laser coagulation of renal tissue with and without hilar occlusion in the porcine model. J Endourol 2002; 16:565–70.

109. Rehman J, Landman J, Lee D, et al. Ferromagnetic self-regulating reheatable thermal rod implants for in situ tissue ablation. J Urol 2002; 167(S):1.

110. Rassweiler JJ, Abbou C, Janetschek G, Jeschke K. Laparoscopic partial nephrectomy. The European experience. Urol Clin North Am 2000; 27:721–36.

111. Kim SC, Rubenstein J, Yap RL, et al. Laparoscopic renal cryosurgery: the Northwestern experience. J Urol 2002; 167 (S):1.

112. de Baere T, Kuoch V, Smayra T, et al. Radio frequency ablation of renal cell carcinoma: preliminary clinical experience. J Urol 2002; 167:1961–4.

11

Novel therapies of advanced renal cell cancer-coupling immunotherapy with minimally invasive technique

Stephen E Pautler, Jan Roigas and McClellan M Walther

Introduction

The incidence of kidney cancer is increasing in the United States,[1,2] with an estimated incidence of 30,800 cases in 2001 with 12,100 deaths.[3] Approximately, one-third of patients presenting with kidney cancer have metastatic disease at presentation,[2] which greatly reduces the ability to cure patients. Surgical resection of the primary tumor and solitary metastases offers a potential cure for only about 20% of patients. Systemic therapies for metastatic kidney cancer have a poor response rate, although a great effort worldwide to improve these outcomes is ongoing. This chapter will discuss the role of cytoreductive laparoscopic radical nephrectomy (LRN) and we will briefly discuss recent advances of systemic therapies in the context of metastatic kidney cancer.

Diagnosis

The classically described presentation of kidney cancer with gross hematuria, flank pain, and a palpable mass occurs infrequently. Currently, an increasing number of patients are presenting with incidentally discovered renal masses.[4] With a larger use of computer tomography (CT) imaging, a stage migration toward more localized disease has occurred, but 40% of patients still present with metastatic disease. Symptoms attributed to metastatic renal cell carcinoma (RCC) include gross hematuria, flank pain, weight loss, and a variety of paraneoplastic syndromes.

Patients presenting with a solid renal mass suspicious for RCC should undergo a complete history and physical examination. Ancillary investigations include a contrast CT scan of the abdomen/pelvis (Figure 11.1), chest radiograph, blood work (Table 11.1) and urinalysis with urine cytology and/or cystoscopy reserved for cases of possible transitional cell carcinoma. Bone scans are recommended

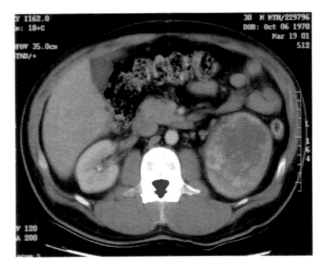

Figure 11.1
Computed tomography of left renal tumor. A 30-year-old male underwent cytoreductive laparoscopic radical nephrectomy with morcellation for an 8 cm × 8 cm left-sided renal tumor that proved to be renal cell carcinoma. The patient had small volume lung metastases and was placed on a randomized trial of systemic interleukin-2 immunotherapy.

for patients with symptomatic bone pain or elevations in the serum calcium or alkaline phosphatase levels. Chest CT can be performed to better characterize abnormalities on the plain film.[5] Magnetic resonance imaging (MRI) is an excellent modality to delineate renal vein or vena cava involvement with tumor thrombus[6] and is recommended in any questionable cases.

Treatment options

Treatment options are limited for patients with metastatic RCC. Based on the biological and clinical observations in

Table 11.1 *The basic work-up for a renal mass that is suspicious for renal cell carcinoma*

Blood work:
    Complete blood count
    Coagulation profile
    Serum electrolytes
    Alkaline phosphatase
    Serum calcium
    Transaminases (ALT and AST)

Urine:
    Urinalysis
    Urinary cytology[a]

Radiographic work-up:
    Pre- and post-contrast CT of the abdomen
    Chest radiograph

Bone scan[b]

Percutaneous biopsy of renal mass[c]

Cystoscopy[d]

[a]Urine cytology is reserved for instances where transitional cell carcinoma is suspected and all cases of presenting with hematuria.
[b]Bone scan is recommended for patients with elevated serum calcium or symptoms of bone pain.
[c]Percutaneous biopsy of the renal mass is limited to cases where the origin of the tumor is in question, such as multifocal renal tumors, renal lymphoma, or possible metastatic disease from another source.
[d]Cystoscopy is reserved for patients who present with hematuria.
ALT = alanine transaminase, AST = aspartate transaminase, CT = computed tomography.

the past, a wide variety of chemotherapeutic, hormonal and immunotherapies have been assessed. Currently, the only Food and Drug Administration (FDA) approved therapy is systemic administration of interleukin-2 (IL-2). Objective responses ranging from 10% to 20% have been seen in various clinical trials.[7,8] A small cohort of patients with advanced RCC at an isolated site of disease is amenable to surgical treatment. In select patients with resection of pulmonary metastases from RCC, for example, a 5-year survival of 35–39% has been found.[9,10]

With respect to novel therapies for advanced RCC, a recent innovation was the concept of laparoscopic cytoreduction prior to administration of systemic immunotherapy. The role of cytoreductive nephrectomy remains somewhat controversial. Clear indications for cytoreductive nephrectomy include the palliation of unmanageable pain attributed to the primary tumor or gross hematuria. Surgery as treatment of paraneoplastic syndromes such as hypercalcemia has had mixed utility in the short term.[11] At the present time, we perform cytoreductive nephrectomy for palliative reasons when indicated. Additionally, we limit elective cytoreductive nephrectomy to patients being

treated with systemic immunotherapies in the context of prospective trials.

Other minimally invasive procedures have a limited role in the treatment of advanced kidney cancer. Two techniques that do merit attention are percutaneous embolization and percutaneous radiofrequency ablation (RFA). One of the most widely studied minimally invasive modalities in metastatic RCC is embolization.[12–16] Palliative percutaneous, transvenous embolization is effective for the control of hemorrhage or gross hematuria caused by large renal tumors.[17] With respect to cancer control, embolization with or without surgery has limited success.[12–16] Initial reports of this strategy had encouraging results[15,16] but several other studies revealed less impressive responses and survival rates.[12,13] Embolization in combination with radioactive iodine has been reported with some moderate success.[18] The current role of embolization in advanced kidney cancer appears to be limited to palliative indications. Further study of the role of embolization of the renal primary will probably occur in the context of the study of other systemic adjuvant therapies.

RFA techniques are currently being developed and studied for the treatment of small primary renal tumors.[19–21] RFA causes coagulative necrosis through molecular friction and heating of the targeted tissue. Short-term outcomes of RFA for small renal tumors have been encouraging, with a 79% success rate.[20] Experience with renal RFA has been limited to smaller tumors (< 5 cm) and, thus far, long-term outcomes have not been reported.[19,21] Experience with RFA for renal tumors in advanced RCC is extremely limited. RFA has been utilized after failure of embolization for the control of gross hematuria due to a renal tumor in the setting of metastatic disease and a solitary kidney.[22] The technique was considered a success, although complete tumor ablation has not been attempted. Additionally, RFA has been applied to the treatment of a splenic metastasis of RCC.[23] The role of RFA in this context remains to be defined.

Indications and contraindications for cytoreductive laparoscopic radical nephrectomy

Palliative indications for cytoreductive nephrectomy include gross hematuria causing shock or requiring repeated blood transfusions, irretractable pain due to local invasion or compression by the primary tumor, and paraneoplastic syndromes in selected patients.[24] Cytoreductive nephrectomy prior to the administration of systemic immunotherapies is a relative indication. Results of immunotherapy trials in which cytoreduction was not performed are extremely poor, with rare responses seen in the primary renal tumor.[25]

Specific contraindications to cytoreductive LRN include level III vena cava tumor thrombus, extensive contiguous organ extension precluding laparoscopic resection and poor performance status of the patient. Relative contraindications include pregnancy, uncorrected coagulopathies, brain metastases, and extreme obesity. With increasing laparoscopic experience, vascular techniques have evolved to the point where level I–II vena caval thrombi have been resected successfully.[26,27] Additionally, diaphragm invasion, splenic and distal pancreatic involvement do not contraindicate a laparoscopic approach if the surgeon is experienced with the advanced laparoscopic techniques required to complete these procedures.[28] Difficult LRN are demanding procedures and should be performed by experienced urologic laparoscopists.

Patient and preoperative preparation

Preoperatively, patients undergo a mechanical/antibiotic bowel prep and are hydrated overnight with intravenous fluids. Generally, a first-generation cephalosporin antibiotic is administered prophylactically. For deep venous thrombosis prophylaxis, patients receive subcutaneous heparin and pneumatic stockings are utilized during the operation. Central venous and arterial line monitoring are essential, as the blood loss encountered during cytoreductive LRN can exceed LRN for localized kidney cancer. A Foley catheter is placed. We utilize an orogastric tube for stomach decompression and inhaled nitrous anesthesia is avoided. Patients are positioned with the ipsilateral flank up, the ipsilateral arm supported by a Kraske arm board, and all pressure points are padded (Figure 11.2).

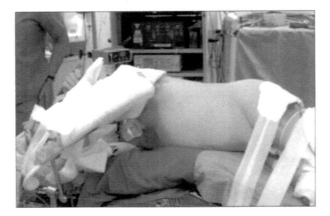

Figure 11.2
Patient positioning for a left laparoscopic radical nephrectomy. Careful padding of all pressure points is mandatory to prevent postoperative complications.

Recommended equipment and instruments

Standard laparoscopic equipment is used for cytoreductive LRN (Table 11.2). Particularly useful tools include the harmonic scalpel and endoshears. An endovascular stapling device is used for control of the renal artery and vein in separate firings of the instrument. For cytoreductive LRN, specimen removal by morcellation is an attractive option to decrease the morbidity associated with intact extraction. The risk of port-site recurrence in this patient population is unknown but such an event is not likely to have a profound impact on patient survival. In cases where morcellation is performed, an impermeable sac such as the LapSac (Cook Urological, Spencer, Indiana) is recommended. Metastases related to tumor morcellation are extremely rare. Laparoscopic ultrasonography is a useful adjunct for the intraoperative assessment of the renal vein and should be available.

Approach and tips

The transperitoneal approach is recommended for the majority of cytoreductive LRN with access achieved by

Table 311.2 *Instruments recommended for use in a cytoreductive laparoscopic radical nephrectomy*

Necessary equipment:
  Hasson cannula
  0° laparoscope
  30° laparoscope
  12 mm trocar (×3)
  5 mm trocar (×2)
  10 mm right-angle dissector
  Maryland dissector
  Endoshears
  5 mm harmonic scalpel
  10 mm clip applier
  Endovascular stapler
  Suction-irrigator
  10 mm fan retractor
  10 mm spoon forceps

Optional equipment:
  5 mm 0° laparoscope
  Laparoscopic ultrasound probe
  5 mm clip applier
  LapSac[a]
  Tissue morcellator
  Sponge forceps
  5 mm atraumatic locking grasping forceps (×3)
  Carter–Thomason port closure kit

[a]Lapsac (Cook Urological, Spencer, Indiana).

Hasson technique. In many patients, the primary renal tumor for cytoreduction is quite bulky (> 10 cm), leading to possible distortion of the normal anatomic landmarks. The open access technique allows controlled access to the abdomen without the possibility of a Veress needle injury to the primary tumor or displaced intra-abdominal viscera. As previously reported, no difference in bowel injuries was seen between the open (Hasson) or closed (Veress) techniques in several studies,[29-31] although these access techniques have not been studied prospectively in the cytoreductive LRN patient population. The transperitoneal approach yields the largest working area and allows the surgeon to identify familiar structures. We have reserved the retroperitoneal approach for a subset of patients with small renal primaries and no evidence of lymphadenopathy or local invasion as seen on preoperative imaging.

The steps of the procedure follow those of a standard LRN for localized disease, as made popular by Clayman and colleagues.[32] Briefly, the bowel is mobilized off the retroperitoneum and kidney (Figures 11.3 and 11.4). For right-sided tumors, liver retraction is important to give access to the upper pole and adrenal gland (Figures 11.5–11.7). Dissection onto the vena cava is performed and the renal vein is identified. Subsequent dissection of the upper pole and ligation of the adrenal vein is performed. Next, the ureter is identified and the lower pole mobilized and elevated to facilitate access to the hilum. With

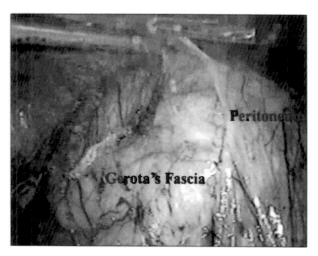

Figure 11.3
The peritoneal attachments of the colon are incised at the 'white' line of Toldt to expose Gerota's fascia.

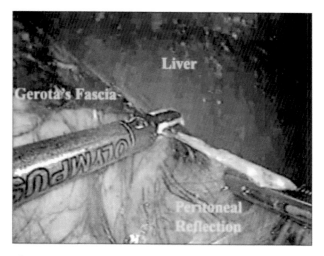

Figure 11.5
The peritoneal reflection is incised under the liver.

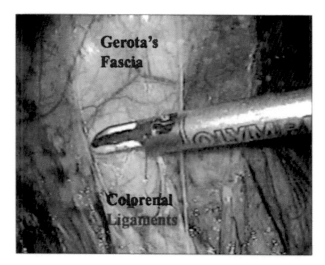

Figure 11.4
To further expose Gerota's fascia and the tumor, the colon mesentery is separated from Gerota's fascia by incising the colorenal ligament.

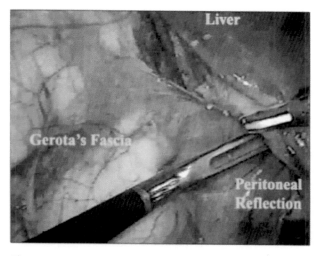

Figure 11.6
The peritoneal reflection is incised under the liver.

particularly large tumors, retraction using 5 mm instruments is difficult and in these situations a spoon forceps allows enough purchase to effectively retract the kidney. The renal artery is controlled with clips or an endovascular stapler. We advocate close inspection of the renal vein to ensure that it collapses, suggesting no secondary arterial blood flow (Figure 11.8). The renal vein is routinely ligated using an endovascular stapler (Figure 11.9). Following ligation of the ureter, the remainder of the kidney is mobilized and the specimen removed by morcellation or intact extraction (Figure 11.10). For left-sided tumors, the bowel is mobilized; the gonadal vein is identified and followed to the hilum. Other important differences include the ligation

of the adrenal and lumbar veins and gentle handling of the tail of the pancreas if it is encountered during dissection. Mobilization of the lateral attachments of the spleen to the abdominal wall allows the spleen to fall medially and out of the dissection field, similar to the dissection performed during laparoscopic adrenalectomy.[33]

Recently, Moore et al described operative techniques to assist in controlling parasitic tumor blood vessels for primary renal lesions greater than 8 cm in size.[34] With this approach, the renal unit is mobilized before securing the renal vessels. A vascular Endo-GIA stapler (US Surgical, Norwalk, Connecticut) is used to control all attachments to Gerota's fascia (Figure 11.11). This technique has

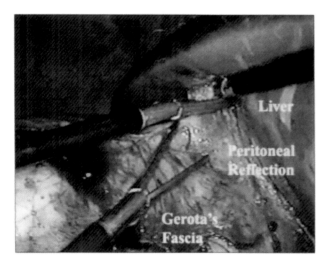

Figure 11.7
The peritoneal reflection is dissected away from the upper pole of Gerota's fascia.

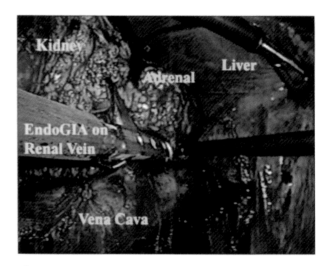

Figure 11.9
The right renal vein (RV) is ligated using an endovascular stapler. During cytoreductive LRN, bulky lymph nodes can obscure the renal hilum, mandating meticulous dissection of the vessels prior to ligation.

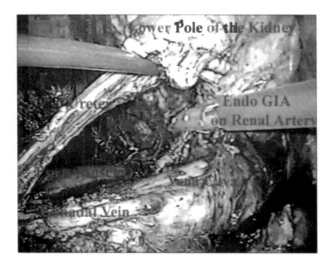

Figure 11.8
The renal vessels are exposed by upward retraction of the ureter at the lower pole. The renal artery is secured first with a vascular GIA stapler.

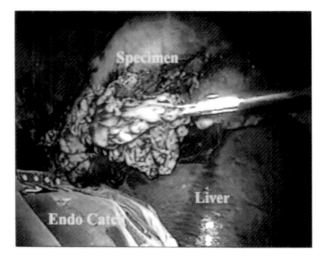

Figure 11.10
The tumor specimen is entrapped with an Endo Catch II device and extracted through an extended umbilical incision.

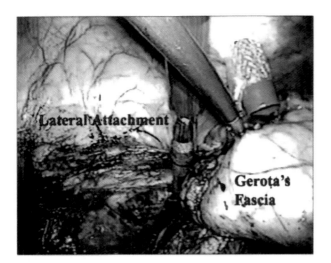

Figure 11.11
All parasitic vessels and attachments to Gerota's fascia are secured by vascular GIA staplers.

demonstrated a decrease in blood loss compared with open cytoreductive nephrectomy series and other laparoscopic series.[35–45]

In cases in which a level I renal vein thrombus is known or suspected, laparoscopic sonography can be employed to confirm the distal extent of the thrombus and the blood flow. In situations where the renal artery has been secured and flow in the renal vein has not decreased, the laparoscopic ultrasound probe in Doppler mode can be used to identify secondary arteries or aberrant vessels.

Extensive dissection of intra-abdominal disease is possible through a laparoscopic approach. Ipsilateral lymphadenectomy is routinely performed for visible disease. Careful hemostasis and judicious use of clips is recommended to prevent unnecessary bleeding or postoperative lymphocele formation. For tumors that are invasive into the diaphragm, resection is possible with the use of the harmonic scalpel. Defects in the diaphragm generally require suture repair, and chest tube placement is recommended at the completion of the operation to prevent hemothorax.[28] The patient must be monitored for hypercarbia or other signs of cardiorespiratory compromise during a diaphragm resection. In unstable patients, urgent chest tube placement or conversion to open is performed. Laparoscopic resection of the spleen and/or the tail of the pancreas can be performed when indicated. The endovascular-stapling device is useful for controlling the splenic hilum, short gastric vessels, and for coming across the pancreatic parenchyma. There are reports of misfiring staplers and urgent control of hemorrhage is mandatory.[35] Urologists must be aware of this possibility and should be prepared in the event that this occurs. If conversion is required, the two subcostal working ports are connected using a scalpel. Rapid control of the hilum is obtained using this approach.

Complications

Open cytoreductive nephrectomy is associated with significant complication rates, ranging from 13 to 50%.[36–40] Laparoscopic cytoreduction appears comparable with respect to the incidence and type of complications. The complications of cytoreductive LRN are similar to those of LRN for localized disease. Several important differences require discussion. First, due to the advanced nature of the kidney cancer, the average blood loss during cytoreductive LRN is greater than that encountered during procedures for localized cancers. Bulky lymphadenopathy and parasitic tumor vessels can contribute to the increased bleeding observed. Cytoreductive LRN can lead to skin blistering and contralateral psoas necrosis due to the prolonged operating times with the patients in the flank position. Preventive measures such as not using a beanbag or kidney rest during patient positioning reduces these problems. Unresectability of a kidney tumor can occur with extensive involvement of the duodenum, head of the pancreas, common bile duct, or great vessels. These situations are not always predicted by preoperative imaging.

Results

The current treatment of metastatic RCC is changing with advances in the fields of immunotherapy, gene therapy, and chemotherapy. The role of cytoreductive surgery in the treatment algorithm is also evolving. Several issues surrounding debulking surgery for kidney cancer merit discussion. Historically, a large percentage of patients who underwent cytoreduction were unfit to receive systemic immunotherapy postoperatively for various reasons, such as progressive disease, postoperative complications, and declining performance status.[39,40] In the recent experience of the National Cancer Institute, 38% of patients who underwent open cytoreduction did not receive systemic high-dose IL-2.[7] The mortality rate from open cytoreductive nephrectomy ranges up to 4%.[24] The rationale for cytoreduction has been based on several observations. First, primary tumors rarely respond to systemic immunotherapy and, with removal, the greatest chance of response is afforded to the patient and the major source of further metastases is eliminated. Additionally, patients may have less pulmonary toxicity as a result of IL-2 administration postoperatively.[40,41] Two recently published prospective randomized trials identified a survival advantage of 3–10 months for patients who underwent open cytoreduction followed by interferon-alpha 2b (IFN-α2) administration in comparison to those who received IFN-α2 alone.[42,43] The reason for the survival advantage is not obvious, as both arms had the same response rate to the systemic therapy and the nephrectomy arm had a slight performance status advantage relative to the control arm.[44] Although the clinical significance of the observed survival advantage is unclear, these studies provide the basis for further investigation into the role of cytoreductive nephrectomy in randomized prospective controlled trials.

To date, limited results are available for cytoreductive LRN. In a pilot study, Walther et al demonstrated the feasibility of the procedure.[45] The goal of minimally invasive surgery is the reduction of morbidity while providing similar surgical outcomes as open surgery. The results of the cytoreductive LRN pilot project support this concept. Advantages were seen for the pure laparoscopic approach with specimen morcellation. Patients required less postoperative narcotics, a shorter hospital stay, and had a shorter recovery time to be fit for the administration of systemic IL-2 therapy. In this initial experience, blood loss was higher than reported for LRN in localized disease,[45,46] probably reflecting the difficulty of the procedure with findings such as bulky lymphadenopathy, local invasion, and large tumors. Operative times for cytoreductive LRN were significantly longer when compared to open cytoreduction.

Specimen removal during LRN remains a somewhat controversial subject. The arguments against morcellation include the risk of port-site seeding and the lack of accurate pathologic staging. Port-site metastases have rarely been reported with localized kidney cancer[47,48] but not in the cytoreductive setting. Additionally, patients with advanced RCC have other documented metastases that require the administration of systemic therapy and portsite seeding would not be a catastrophic event. Histologic confirmation of RCC in advanced disease is important prior to pursuing systemic immunotherapy, whereas staging information does not alter patient management. Evidence exists that accurate histologic diagnosis is possible from morcellated kidney tumors in both the localized[26,49–51] and cytoreductive setting.[52]

Conclusion

Early experience with cytoreductive LRN for advanced RCC has been encouraging. These cases can be difficult and can require a broad range of ablative laparoscopic techniques. Further prospective multi-institutional studies of laparoscopic cytoreduction are required to define the role of this procedure in the care of this devastating disease.

Treatment of advanced renal cell carcinoma

About one-third of patients diagnosed with RRC have metastatic disease at the time of first presentation and

another 20–30% will develop metastases during further follow-up. For these patients therapeutic options are limited and cure from cancer is a rarity. It is a common observation that metastatic RCC does not respond to conventional therapies such as chemotherapy, hormonal therapy, or radiation therapy. However, since the clinical implementation of immunotherapy, progress has been made and, together with malignant melanoma, metastatic RCC is a classic example of a disease which can at least, partially, be managed with immunomodulatory treatment strategies.

Several recent studies have provided evidence for a treatment approach in patients with metastatic RCC that combines the operation on the primary tumor and the subsequent immunotherapy for treatment of unresectable metastases.[42,43] Currently, there is no therapeutic standard defined for the immunomodulatory treatment of metastatic RCC. Therapeutic strategies are still in the experimental phase and include the unspecific activation of the immune system on the basis of cytokines such as IL-2 or IFN-α2, specific vaccination approaches, and adoptive immunotherapeutic concepts. Thus, treatment of metastatic RCC is often performed in phase I or II studies. There is only limited clinical experience from phase III studies, providing information on the efficacy of different treatment schedules and long-term survival data. Also, the performance of studies with a 'no treatment' arm remains unacceptable from the ethical point of view. Thus, to date, the treatment of metastatic RCC is still an experimental approach but it offers the great chance of identifying new, innovative, and effective therapeutic strategies.

Cytokine treatment

The cytokines IL-2 and IFN-α2 play an important role in the treatment of metastastic RCC. IL-2 was clinically introduced by Rosenberg in 1985 and has been approved by the FDA.[52] With the intravenous application of IL-2, response rates of 15% have been reported, with an estimated longterm survival of 10–20% after 5 and 10 years.[53] One of the problems of high-dose intravenous application of IL-2 is the degree of side-effects, which require hospitalization of the patients.

The combination of IL-2 and IFN-α2 has been prospectively analyzed in the CRECY study (Cancer du Rein Ètude Cytokine) in 1996 on 425 patients.[54] Although the combination of the cytokines resulted in a significantly enhanced response rate and duration of the progression-free survival, mean survival was not significantly different (IFN-α2, 13 months; IL-2, 12 months; and IFN-α2 + IL-2, 17 months; $p = 0.55$).

Considering the side-effects of intravenous IL-2, efforts have been made to reduce toxicity by subcutaneous application of IL-2. In a multi-institutional trial on 152 patients, Atzpodien and coworkers reported a 25% response rate with subcutaneous IL-2 in combination with IFN-α2.[55]

On the basis of preclinical data, the cytokines IL-2 and IFN-α2 have been further combined with the pyrimidine antagonist 5-fluorouracil (5-FU). Recently, Atzpodien and coworkers have published their results of a prospective randomized trial comparing immunochemotherapy using subcutaneous IL-2, subcutaneous IFN-α2 and intravenous 5-FU with tamoxifen. Here, in 41 patients treated with immunochemotherapy, median survival was 24 months with a 5-year survival rate of 24.8% compared with 13 months and 13.5% in the tamoxifen-treated control group.[56] The results of the immunochemotherapeutic regimen discussed are controversial. In the studies of Negrier et al[57] and Ravaud et al[58] low rates of objective remissions were observed. In a multicenter phase III study with 131 patients, the effects of 5-FU were tested by comparing IL-2 and IFN-α vs IL-2, IFN-α, and 5-FU. No complete responses were observed and only 5 partial responses in the triple drug arm.[56] In the multicenter phase II study of Ravaud on 105 assessable patients, objective remissions occurred in only 1.8%.[58] However, it has to be considered that, in both trials, a treatment protocol was used with a lower cumulative dose of the cytokines combined with a higher cumulative dose of 5-FU compared with the original subcutaneous treatment schedule.

Another treatment option for patients specifically suffering from pulmonary metastases of RCC is the inhalative application of IL-2, which was first reported by Huland and coworkers. With the inhalative approach, response rates of up to 15% and stabilizations of another 55% of patients, with the advantage of a reduced toxicity compared with intravenous IL-2, have been reported.[59,60] However, a prospective randomized trial comparing the inhalative treatment with intravenous or subcutaneous application of IL-2 has not yet been performed. The inhalative IL-2 approach is cost-intensive and requires a high patient compliance.

Recent efforts focus on the further clinical improvement of immunotherapy. The rationale of a combination of immunotherapy and local radiation has been tested in vitro using the RENCA murine renal carcinoma model.[61,62] Taken together, these studies have demonstrated an enhanced therapeutic efficacy of the combined treatment, resulting in a reduced number of pulmonary metastases, the reduction of primary tumor size, and an increased survival. Brinkmann and coworkers have demonstrated in an initial report that the simultaneous application of radiation therapy and immunochemotherapy might result in a high rate of objective remissions in patients suffering from symptomatic bone or lymph node metastases or local recurrences.[63] Of 12 patients, 9 with bone metastases and 3 with local recurrences were locally irradiated. Complete remissions were reached in 4 patients (33%) and partial remissions in another patient (8%), which was a high rate when compared to results with immunotherapy alone. Only 4 patients (33%) remained progressive under combined therapy. After a median follow-up of 28 months, 75% of the patients were still alive. All patients had subjective pain relief after 2 weeks of treatment. Figure 11.12A and B are CT scans of a 35-year-old female patient with a

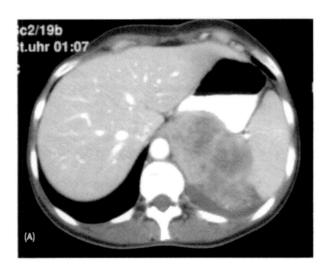 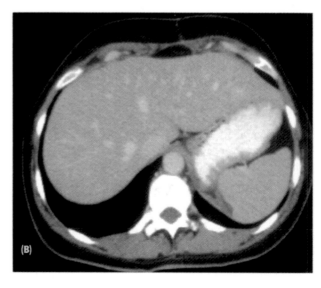

Figure 11.12

(A and B) A 35 year old female patient with a left clear cell renal carcinoma following R2 resection (pT3a pN2 G2) and subsequent progression of retroperitoneal lymph node metastases. The patient received 3 cycles of immunochemotherapy combined with local radiation therapy of the left retroperitoneal masses. A complete response was achieved. The patient has NED after a follow-up of 34 months (left side: CT scan prior to therapy, right side: CT scan after 3 cycles of imunochemotherapy and radiation therapy).

left clear cell renal carcinoma following cytoreductive nephrectomy resection (pT3a pN2 G2) and subsequent progression of retroperitoneal lymph node metastases. After 3 cycles of immunochemotherapy combined with local radiotherapy, complete remission was achieved.

Vaccination therapy

In contrast to the cytokine treatment, most vaccination approaches aim at the development of a specific antitumor immune response. Principally, the lysis of tumor cells depends on the binding of immunologic effector cells (such as CD8+ cytolytic T lymphocytes) on tumor-associated antigens which are presented on the surface of the tumor cell. Vaccines contain the information of specific known or unknown tumor-associated antigens which can be mediated via native or modified intact tumor cells, tumor cell lysates, or defined fragments from tumor cells (peptides). The development of an immune response further depends on the presentation of antigens via professional antigen-presenting cells such as dendritic cells and costimulatory signals which are antigen independent and serve for the activation of immune effector cells.

Therefore, current vaccination strategies include the use of native or modified tumor cells, tumor cell lysates, isolated immunogenic peptides, or in-vitro pulsed dendritic cells. Although there are a large variety of different vaccination concepts, only a limited number of phase I/II trials have shown clinical efficacy of vaccines in the treatment of metastatic RCC.

Kugler and coworkers reported on 17 patients treated with a hybrid cell vaccine generated via electrofusion of allogenous tumor cells and autologous dendritic cells.[64] Fused cells represented tumor-associated antigens as well as costimulating capabilities of dendritic cells. After a mean follow-up of 13 months, 4 complete remissions (23.5%) and 2 partial remissions (11.8%) were observed. This study provided evidence for the clinical efficacy of an individualized immune therapeutic approach based on the induction of cytolytic T lymphocytes against multiple and different tumor-associated antigens.

In another study, 37 patients were treated with pulsed dendritic cells either loaded with autologous tumor cell lysate or with the lysate of the renal cancer cell line A-498 and with the addition of keyhole limpet hemocyanin.[65] After a mean follow-up of 24.6 months and 29 evaluable patients, 2 complete and 1 partial remissions were seen. Remissions occurred only in patients treated with dendritic cells pulsed with autologous tumor cell lysate. Both studies mentioned refer to the potential capabilitiy of dendritic cell-based vaccines for inducing a specific immune response leading to tumor regression in metastatic RCC.

Another concept for vaccination is the use of heat shock proteins associated with tumor-derived peptides eliciting antigen-specific cytolytic T lymphocytes. Heat shock proteins serve as molecular chaperones for tightly bound cellular peptides that are believed to represent a cellular repertoire of immunogens. Using an autologous heat shock protein-peptide vaccine 1 complete and 3 partial remissions were observed in 29 patients with metastatic RCC.[66] Heat shock protein-based vaccines will be further investigated, either in combination with a variety of known immunogenic peptides, cytokines, or dendritic cells.

Adoptive immunotherapy

Because of the immunogenic properties of RCC and its susceptibility to immunotherapy, an innovative therapeutic approach is nonmyeloablative allogeneic stem cell transplantation, first reported for metastastic RCC by Childs and coworkers in 2000.[67] This therapeutic strategy aims, in the same way as observed in hematologic cancers, at the development of a graft-vs-tumor effect, which can lead to the regression of metastases. In the above-mentioned study only stem cell allografts from an HLA-identical sibling or a sibling with one mismatch of an antigen were transplanted. The graft-vs-tumor effect strongly correlated with the occurrence of a complete donor-T-cell chimerism and the development of a graft-vs-host disease. After a median follow-up of 402 days in 19 treated patients, 10 objective remissions (53%) were observed, with regression occurring in different metastatic sites such as lymph nodes, subcutaneous metastases, or liver and bone metastases. However, stem cell transplantation was associated with a 12% mortality rate (2 patients died due to severe graft-vs-host disease or bacterial sepsis).

Taken together, the stem cell transplantation technique offers an interesting therapeutic concept for selected patients which needs to be further evaluated in multicenter clinical trials.

References

1. Chow WH, Devesa SS, Warren JL, Fraumeni JF Jr. Rising incidence of renal cell cancer in the United States. JAMA 1999; 281:1628–31.

2. Hock LM, Lynch J, Balaji KC. Increasing incidence of kidney cancer in the last 2 decades in the United States: an analysis of surveillance, epidemiology and end results program data. J Urol 2002; 167:57–60.

3. American Cancer Society. Cancer Facts and Figures, 2001.

4. Jayson M, Sanders H. Increased incidence of serendipitously discovered renal cell carcinoma. Urology 1998; 51:203–5.

5. Lim DJ, Carter MF. Computerized tomography in the pre-operative staging for pulmonary metastases in patients with renal cell carcinoma. J Urol 1993; 150:1112–14.

6. Sohaib SAA, Teh J, Nargund VH, et al. Assessment of tumor invasion of the vena caval wall in renal cell carcinoma cases by magnetic resonance imaging. J Urol 2002; 167:1271–5.

7. Walther MM, Yang JC, Pass HI et al. Cytoreductive surgery before high dose interleukin-2 based therapy in patients with metastatic renal cell carcinoma. J Urol 1997; 158:1675–8.

8. Fyfe G, Fisher RI, Rosenberg SA, et al. Results of treatment of 255 patients with metastastic renal cell carcinoma who received high-dose recombinant interleukin-2 therapy. J Clin Oncol 1995; 13:688–96.

9. Cerfolio RJ, Allen MS, Deschamps C, et al. Pulmonary resection of metastatic renal cell carcinoma. Ann Thorac Surg 1994; 57:339–44.

10. Friedel G, Hürtgen M, Penzenstadler M, et al. Resection of pulmonary metastases from renal cell carcinoma. Anticancer Res 1999; 19:1593–6.

11. Walther MM, Patel B, Choyke PL, et al. Hypercalcemia in patients with metastatic renal cell carcinoma: effect of nephrectomy and metabolic evaluation. J Urol 1997; 158:733–9.

12. Gottesman JE, Scardino P, Crawford ED, et al. Infarction-nephrectomy for metastatic renal carcinoma. Urology 1985; 25:248–50.

13. Kurth KH, Debruyne FMJ, Hall RR, et al. Embolization and postinfarction nephrectomy in patients with primary metastatic renal adenocarcinoma. Eur Urol 1987; 13:251–5.

14. Flanigan RC. The failure of infarction and/or nephrectomy in stage IV renal cell cancer to influence survival or metastatic regression. Urol Clin North Amer 1987; 14:757–62.

15. Swanson DA, Wallace S. Surgery of metastatic renal cell carcinoma and use of renal infarction. Sem Surg Oncol 1988; 4:124–8.

16. Kauffmann GW, Richter GM, Rohrbach R, Wenz W. Prolonged survival following palliative renal tumor embolization by capillary occlusion. Cardiovasc Intervent Radiol 1989; 12:22–8.

17. Wolff JM, Brehmer B Jr, Adam G, Jakse G. Management of haematuria due to secondary renal tumour with selective arterial embolization. Int Urol Nephrol 1998; 30:15–17.

18. Lang EK, Sullivan J. Management of primary and metastatic renal cell carcinoma by transcatheter embolization with iodine 125. Cancer 1988; 62:274–82.

19. Gervais DA, McGovern FJ, Wood BJ, et al. Radio-frequency ablation of renal cell carcinoma: early clinical experience. Radiology 2000; 217:665–72.

20. Pavlovich CP, Walther MM, Choyke PL, et al. Percutaneous radio frequency ablation of small renal tumors: initial results. J Urol 2002; 167:10–15.

21. de Baere T, Kuock V, Smayra T, et al. Radio frequency ablation of renal cell carcinoma: preliminary clinical experience. J Urol 2002; 167: 1961–4.

22. Wood BJ, Grippo J, Pavlovich CP. Percutaneous radio frequency ablation for hematuria. J Urol 2001; 166:2303–4.

23. Wood BJ, Bates S. Radiofrequency thermal ablation of a splenic metastasis. J Vasc Interv Radiol 2001; 12:261–3.

24. Flanigan RC, Yonover PM. The role of radical nephrectomy in metastatic renal cell carcinoma. Sem Urol Oncol 2001; 19:98–102.

25. Wagner JR, Walther MM, Linehan WM, et al. Interleukin-2 based immunotherapy for metastatic renal cell carcinoma with the kidney in place. J Urol 1999; 162:43–5.

26. Dunn MD, Portis AJ, Shalhav AL, et al. Laparoscopic versus open radical nephrectomy: a 9-year experience. J Urol 2000; 164:1153–9.

27. Gill IS, Schweizer D, Hobart MG, et al. Retroperitoneal laparoscopic radical nephrectomy: the Cleveland Clinic experience. J Urol 2000; 163:1665–70.

28. Pautler SE, Richards C, Libutti SK, et al. Intentional resection of the diaphragm during cytoreductive laparoscopic radical nephrectomy. J Urol 2002; 167:48–50.

29. Chandler JG, Corson SL, Way LW. Three spectra of laparoscopic entry access injuries. J Am Coll Surg 2001; 192:478–90.

30. Penfield AJ. How to prevent complications of open laparoscopy. J Reprod Med 1985; 30:660–3.

31. McKernan JB, Champion JK. Access techniques: Veress needle – initial blind trocar insertion versus open laparoscopy with the Hasson trocar. Endosc Surg Allied Technol 1995; 3:35–8.

32. Dunn MD, McDougall EM, Clayman RV. Laparoscopic radical nephrectomy. J Endourol 2000; 14:849–55.

33. Gagner M, Pomp A, Heniford BT, et al. Laparoscopic adrenalectomy: lessons learned from 100 consecutive procedures. Ann Surg 1997; 226:238–46.

34. Moore DK, Shu T, Amato RJ, Moore RG. Laparoscopic cytoreductive nephrectomy for metastatic renal cell carcinoma prior to thaladimide based immunotherapy. Urology (submitted)

35. Fentie DD, Barrett PH. Laparoscopic radical nephrectomy: Editorial comment. J Endourol 2000; 14:855–6.

36. Rackley R, Novick A, Klein E, et al. The impact of adjuvant nephrectomy on multimodality treatment of metastatic renal cell carcinoma. J Urol 1994; 152:1399–403.

37. Bennett RT, Lerner SE, Taub HC, et al. Cytoreductive surgery for stage IV renal cell carcinoma. J Urol 1995; 154:32–4.

38. Franklin JR, Figlin R, Rauch J, et al. Cytoreductive surgery in the management of metastatic renal cell carcinoma: the UCLA experience. Sem Urol Oncol 1996; 14:230–6.

39. Levy DA, Swanson DA, Slaton JW, et al. Timely delivery of biological therapy after cytoreductive nephrectomy in carefully selected patients with metastatic renal cell carcinoma. J Urol 1998; 159:1168–73.

40. Walther MM, Alexander RB, Wiess GH, et al. Cytoreductive surgery prior to interleukin-2-based therapy in patients with metastatic renal cell carcinoma. Urology 1993; 42:250–7.

41. Wagner JR, Walther MM, Linehan WM, et al. Interleukin-2 based immunotherapy for metastatic renal cell carcinoma with the kidney in place. J Urol 1999; 162:43–5.

42. Flanigan RC, Salmon SE, Blumenstein BA, et al. Nephrectomy followed by interferon alfa-2b compared with interferon alfa-2b alone for metastatic renal-cell cancer. N Engl J Med 2001; 345:1655–9.

43. Mickisch GH, Garin A, van Poppel H, et al. Radical nephrectomy plus interferon-alfa-based immunotherapy compared with interferon alfa alone in metastatic renal-cell carcinoma: a randomised trial. Lancet 2001; 358:966–70.

44. Tannock IF. Removing the primary tumor after the cancer has spread. N Engl J Med 2001; 345:1699–700.

45. Walther MM, Lyne JC, Libutti SK, Linehan WM. Laparoscopic cytoreductive nephrectomy as preparation for administration of systemic interleukin-2 in the treatment of metastatic renal cell carcinoma: a pilot study. Urology 1999; 53:496–501.

46. Gill IS, Kavoussi LR, Clayman RV, et al. Complications of laparoscopic nephrectomy in 185 patients: a multi-institutional review. J Urol 1995; 154:479–83.

47. Fentie DD, Barrett PH, Taranger LA. Metastatic renal cell cancer after laparoscopic radical nephrectomy: long-term follow-up. J Endourol 2000; 14:407–11.

48. Castilho LN, Fugita OE, Mitre AI, et al. Port site tumor recurrences of renal cell carcinoma after videolaparoscopic radical nephrectomy. J Urol 2001; 165:519.

49. Barrett PH, Fentie DD, Taranger LA. Laparoscopic radical nephrectomy with morcellation for renal cell carcinoma: the Saskatoon experience. Urology 1998; 52:23–8.

50. Landman J, Lento P, Hassen W, et al. Feasibility of pathology evaluation of morcellated kidneys after radical nephrectomy. J Urol 2000; 164:2086–9.

51. Pautler SE, Hewitt SM, Linehan WM, Walther MM. Specimen morcellation after laparoscopic radical nephrectomy: confirmation of histological diagnosis using needle biopsy. J Endourol 2002; 16:89–92.

52. Rosenberg SA, Lotze MT, Muul LM, et al. Observations on the systemic administration of autologous lymphokine-activated killer cells and recombinant interleukin-2 to patients with metastatic cancer. N Engl J Med 1985; 313:1485–92.

53. Fisher RI, Rosenberg SA, Fyfe G. Long-term survival update for high-dose recombinant interleukin-2 in patients with renal cell carcinoma. Cancer J Sci Am 2000; 6:55–7.

54. Negrier S, Escudier B, Lasset C, et al. Recombinant human interleukin-2, recombinant human interferon alfa-2a, or both in metastatic renal cell carcinoma. N Engl J Med 1998; 338:1272–8.

55. Atzpodien J, Lopez-Hanninen E, Kirchner H, et al. Multi-institutional home-therapy trial of recombinant human interleukin-2 and interferon alpha-2 in patients with metastatic renal cell carcinoma. J Clin Oncol 1995; 13:497–501.

56. Atzpodien J, Kirchner H, Illiger HJ, et al. IL-2 in combination with IFN-alpha and 5-FU versus tamoxifen in metastatic renal cell carcinoma: long-term results of a controlled randomized clinical trial. Br J Cancer 2001; 85:1130–6.

57. Negrier S, Caty A, Lesimple T, et al. Treatment of patients with metastatic renal carcinoma with a combination of subcutaneous interleukin-2 and interferon alfa with or without fluorouracil. J Clin Oncol 2000; 18(24):4009–15.

58. Ravaud A, Audhuy B, Gomez F, et al. Subcutaneous interleukin-2, interferon alpha-2a, and continuous infusion of fluorouracil in metastatic renal cell carcinoma: a multicenter phase II trail. J Clin Oncol 1998; 16:2728–32.

59. Huland E, Heinzer H, Mir TS, Huland H. Inhaled interleukin-2 therapy in pulmonary metastatic renal cell carcinoma: six years of experience. Cancer J Sci Am 1997; 3:98–105.

60. Heinzer H, Mir TS, Huland E, Huland H. Subjective and objective prospective, long-term analysis of quality of life during inhaled interleukin-2 immunotherapy. J Clin Oncol 1999; 17:3612–20.

61. Dybal EJ, Haas GP, Maughan RL, et al. Synergy of radiation therapy and immunotherapy in murine renal cell carcinoma. J Urol 1992; 148:1331–7.

62. Younes E, Haas GP, Dezso B, et al. Local tumor irradiation augments the response to IL-2 therapy in a murine renal adenocarcinoma. Cell Immunol 1995; 165:243–51.

63. Brinkmann OA, Bruns F, Prott FJ, Hertle L. Possible synergy of radiotherapy and chemo-immunotherapy in metastatic renal cell carcinoma (RCC). Anticancer Res 1999; 19:1583–7.

64. Kugler A, Stuhler G, Walden P, et al. Regression of human metastatic renal cell carcinoma after vaccination with tumor cell-dendritic cell hybrids. Nature Med 2000; 6:332–6.

65. Holtl L, Zelle-Rieser C, Gander H, et al. Dendritic cell-based immunotherapy for metastatic renal cell cancer. Eur Urol 2002; 1(Suppl 1):110.

66. Amato RJ, Murray L, Wood L, et al. Active specific immunotherapy in patients with renal cell carcinoma (RCC) using autologous tumor derived heat shock protein–peptide complex–96 (HSPP-96) vaccine. ASCO, Program/ Proceedings 1999; 18: #1278.

67. Childs R, Chernoff A, Contentin N, et al. Regression of metastatic renal-cell carcinoma after nonmyeloablative allogeneic peripheral-blood stem-cell transplantation. N Engl J Med 2000; 343:750–8.

12

Minimally invasive techniques to treat urothelial tumors of the renal pelvis and ureter

Peter A Pinto and Thomas W Jarrett

Incidence/epidemiology/etiology

Transitional cell carcinoma (TCC) involving the renal pelvis accounts for approximately 10% of all renal tumors and 5% of all urothelial tumors.[1] Tumors involving the ureter are even less common. Upper tract urothelial tumors most commonly affect patients in their sixth to seventh decade of life.[2] Occurrence of these tumours is approximately twice as common in males as in females[3] and they are more commonly seen in whites.[4]

The preceding statistical information is different for cases involving Balkan nephropathy: this is degenerative interstitial nephropathy, which is endemic to rural areas of Balkan countries, and is believed to be related to increased exposure to radon and minerals in the water.[5] These cases have a much higher incidence of upper tract urothelial cancers.

Approximately 2–4% of bladder cancer cases develop upper tract disease, although this could be as high as 25% in cases of bladder carcinoma-in-situ.[6] Patients with initial upper tract TCC develop bladder cancer in 25–75% of cases.[7]

Multiple factors can contribute to the development of upper tract TCC, and they are most likely similar to the causes of urothelial carcinoma involving the bladder. The most important causes are cigarette smoking, exposure to occupational carcinogens, analgesics, coffee, cyclophosphamide, and chronic infections and stones.

Presentation

Gross hematuria is the most common presenting symptom, accounting for approximately 75% of cases.[8] Those patients who develop renal colic can experience dull pain as the tumor grows and obstructs, or acute pain from clot colic. Other presenting symptoms are similar to those found with lower tract urothelial carcinoma.

Diagnosis

Imaging studies such as intravenous pyelography (IVP), computed tomography (CT), ultrasonography, and magnetic resonance imaging (MRI) are usually the first diagnostic procedures undertaken when one suspects upper tract urothelial carcinoma.

IVP has been the most commonly performed study revealing a radiolucent filling defect in approximately 50–75% of cases.[8] High-grade ureteral tumors can cause nonvisualization of the renal unit or severe hydronephrosis.

Recently, there has been debate over the ideal imaging study for hematuria. Contrast CT scans are arguably as good or better for detecting urologic pathology.[9] This imaging modality also provides staging information along with unveiling pathology outside the urinary tract.

Not all filling defects can be attributed to malignant processes. Benign conditions such as calculi, blood clots, sloughed papillae, fungal balls, endometriosis, tuberculosis, ureteritis or pyelitis cystica, and vascular phenomena can present in a similar fashion.[10] In addition, before determining if a patient is a candidate for endourologic management, one needs to know the grade and location of the urothelial carcinoma. Therefore, before planning definitive treatment, retrograde pyelography and ureteropyeloscopy may be necessary. Selective urine cytology, brush cytology, or biopsy of the lesion can be obtained at the same setting to confirm the diagnosis and determine the grade of the lesion.

Pathology

More than 90% of upper tract urothelial tumors are TCC.[11] Less than 10% are attributed to squamous cell carcinoma and less than 1% to adenocarcinoma. These are both usually associated with stones and inflammation.[12,13] Although rare, inverted papillomas, sarcomas, fibroepithelial polyps, and metastatic lesions can involve the upper tract.

Endoscopic treatment and results

The propensity of upper tract TCC towards ipsilateral recurrence and the limitations of upper tract endoscopy have led to radical nephroureterectomy as the gold standard treatment.[14] Even though the cancer-related risks are greater for any alternative treatment, in some select patients the risk of major open surgery or chronic renal failure outweighs the risks of cancer.[15] In other patients with small volume of low-grade disease, the risk of progression is minimal.[16] Thus, the removal of the entire renal unit may not be warranted in a situation where the tumor can be safely removed endoscopically. Recent advances in technology and techniques have permitted the effective endourologic management of upper tract TCC, thus allowing renal-sparing therapy. Still the gold standard is radical nephroureterectomy. Although traditionally performed open, advances in laparoscopic techniques have allowed minimally invasive surgery to play a role. The history, techniques, and results of endoscopic management of upper tract TCC will now be discussed.

In 1912, Hugh Hampton Young described the first endoscopic evaluation of the upper urinary tract.[17] Subsequent advances in techniques and technology allow us to reach all parts of the urinary tract with minimal morbidity via antegrade and retrograde approaches. Diagnosis and treatment of upper tract TCC have become possible with these improvements, as tumor biopsy and ablation using various energy sources is possible even through the smallest of instruments. In addition, miniaturization has made follow-up surveillance of the upper tract more practical with the use of smaller ureteroscopes, which usually do not require previous stenting, or active dilation of the distal ureter.

Tumors of the upper urinary tract can be approached in a retrograde or antegrade fashion. The approach chosen depends largely on the tumor location and volume. In general, a retrograde ureteroscopic approach is used for low-volume ureteral and renal tumors. An antegrade percutaneous approach is preferred for larger tumors of the upper ureter or kidney, or those which cannot be adequately manipulated in a retrograde approach due to location (i.e. lower pole calyx) or previous urinary diversion. In cases with multifocal involvement, a combined antegrade/retrograde approach can be considered.

The basic principles for treating TCC of the upper urinary tract are similar to those of the bladder counterpart. The tumor is biopsied and ablated using electrocautery or laser energy sources. A staged procedure should be considered for high-volume disease or disease that is thought to represent high pathologic grade and/or stage. In such cases where subsequent nephroureterectomy will be most likely to be necessary for cure, biopsy and partial ablation is done to minimize the risks of perforation or major complications. Endoscopic management is completed only after the pathology shows the patient is an acceptable candidate for continued minimally invasive endoscopic management. If the pathology is unresectable, high grade, or invasive, the patient should proceed immediately to nephroureterectomy provided he is medically fit. In addition, patients accepting renal sparing therapy must be committed to a lifetime of follow-up with radiographs and endoscopy.

Retrograde approach

The ureteroscopic approach to tumors was first described by Goodman in 1981 and is generally favored for ureteral and smaller renal tumors. With the advent of small-diameter rigid and flexible ureteroscopes, tumor location is not as much of a limiting factor as previously thought. The advantages of a ureteroscopic approach are mainly low morbidity when compared to the percutaneous and open surgical counterparts and the maintenance of a closed system. With a closed system, nonurothelial surfaces are not exposed to the possibility of tumor seeding.

The major disadvantages of a retrograde approach are related to the smaller instruments required. The smaller endoscopes have a smaller field of view and working channel. This limits the size of tumor that can be approached in a retrograde fashion. In addition, all portions of the upper urinary tract, such as the lower pole calyces, cannot be reliably reached with working instruments. The smaller instruments limit the ability to remove large volumes of tumor and obtain deep specimens for reliable tumor staging. Retrograde ureteroscopy is difficult in patients with prior urinary diversion.

Technique and instrumentation

A wide variety of ureteroscopic instruments are available, each with its own distinct advantages and disadvantages. In general, rigid ureteroscopes are used primarily for the distal and midureter. Access to the upper ureter and kidney with rigid endoscopy is unreliable, especially in the male patient. Larger, rigid ureteroscopes provide better visualization because of their larger field of view and better irrigation. Smaller rigid ureteroscopes (8F) are generally preferred, as they do not require active dilation of the ureteral orifice.

Newer-generation flexible ureteropyeloscopes are now available in sizes less than 8F, which facilitates simple and reliable passage to all portions of the urinary tract.[18,19] These are generally preferred in the upper ureter and kidney, where the rigid ureteroscope cannot be reliably passed. Flexible ureteroscopes, however, have technical limitations such as a small working channel, which limits irrigant flow and the diameter of working instruments. Further limitations of flexible ureteroscopy include access to certain areas of the kidney, such as the lower pole, where the infundibulopelvic angle may limit passage of the scope or prior urinary diversion.

Endoscopic evaluation and collection of urinary cytology. Cystoscopy is performed and the bladder inspected for concomitant bladder pathology. The ureteral orifice is identified and inspected for lateralizing hematuria. A retrograde pyelogram is performed to show upper tract anatomy and possible filling defects. A small-diameter ureteroscope is passed directly (6.9 or 7.5F) into the ureteral orifice and the distal ureter inspected prior to any trauma from a previously placed guide wire or dilation. A guide wire is then placed through the ureteroscope and up the ureter to the level of the renal pelvis under fluoroscopic guidance. The flexible ureteroscope is used to visualize the remaining urothelium. When a lesion or suspicious area is seen, a normal saline washing of the area is performed before biopsy or intervention.[20] If the ureter will not accept the smaller ureteroscope, acute dilation of the ureter will be necessary.

Special circumstances include patients with prior urinary diversion and tumor confined to the intramural ureter. With cases of prior urinary diversion, identification of the ureteroenteric anastomosis is difficult and may require antegrade percutaneous passage of a guide wire down the ureter prior to endoscopy. The wire can be retrieved from the diversion and the ureteroscope can be passed in a retrograde fashion. The nephrostomy tract need not be fully dilated in this setting. A second situation is a tumor confined to the intramural tumor. In such cases where tumor is seen protruding from the ureteral orifice, aggressive transurethral resection of the entire most distal ureter can be done with acceptable results.[21]

Biopsy and definitive treatment. The following three general approaches can be used for tumor ablation:

- bulk excision with ablation of the base
- resection of the tumor to its base
- diagnostic biopsy followed by ablation with electrocautery or laser energy sources.

Regardless of the technique used, special attention to biopsy specimens will be necessary. Specimens are frequently minute in size, should be placed at once in fixative, and specifically labeled for either histologic or cytologic evaluation.[22] The pathologist is asked to review the specimen to evaluate the adequacy of the tissue submitted and to coordinate the method of its pathologic processing.

Ureteroscopic techniques. The tumor is debulked using either grasping forceps (Figure 12.1A-1) or a flat wire basket (Figure 12.1A-2) engaged adjacent to the tumor. The tumor base is then treated with either electrocautery or laser energy sources. This technique is especially useful for low-grade papillary tumors with a narrow stalk. The specimen is sent for pathologic evaluation.

A ureteroscopic resectoscope is used to electrosurgically remove the tumor (Figure 12.1B). Only the intraluminal tumor is resected and no attempt is made to resect deep (beyond lamina propria) as one would with a bladder tumor due to the high risk of perforation. Extra care is necessary in the mid and upper ureter where the wall is quite thin and prone to perforation. Ureteral resectoscopes tend to be larger (12F) and require active dilation of the ureteral orifice. With larger-volume disease of the distal ureter, Jarrett and associates described extensive dilation of the ureter followed by resection with a long standard resectoscope.[23]

The tumor is adequately biopsied and sent to pathology for diagnostic evaluation. The tumor bulk is then ablated to its base using laser or electrosurgical energy (Figure 12.1C). Multiple biopsy specimens are usually required, especially when using the small flexible 3F biopsy forceps. Electrosurgery delivered via a small Bugbee electrode (2 or 3F) can be used to fulgurate tumors. The variable depth of penetration can make use in the ureter quite dangerous. Thus, fulguration circumferentially or of a large area should be avoided due to the high risk of stricture formation. More recently, laser energy with either neodymium:YAG[24-26] or holmium:YAG[27,28] sources has been popular. Each has characteristic advantages and can be delivered through a small flexible fiber (200 or 365 µm), allowing for delivery of energy even through small flexible ureteroscopes without significantly altering irrigant flow or scope defection.

The holmium:YAG laser is well suited for use especially in the ureter. With a tissue penetration less than 0.5 mm, it can safely ablate tumor with excellent hemostasis and minimal risk of full-thickness injury to the urothelium. However, its shallow depth of penetration may make its use cumbersome with larger tumors, especially in the renal pelvis. Settings most commonly used are an energy of 0.6–1.0 J with a frequency of 10 Hz. The neodymium:YAG laser has a tissue penetration of up to 5–6 mm, depending on laser settings and duration of treatment. Unlike the holmium laser, which ablates tumor, the neodymium:YAG laser works by coagulative necrosis, with subsequent sloughing of the necrotic tumor. The safety margin is significantly lower and can limit its safe use in the ureter where the ureteral wall is quite thin. Settings most commonly used for the neodymium:YAG laser are 15 W for 2 s duration for ablating tumor and 5–10 W for 2 s for coagulation. A ureteral stent is placed for a variable duration to aid with the healing process. Large tumors usually require multiple treatment sessions over several months.

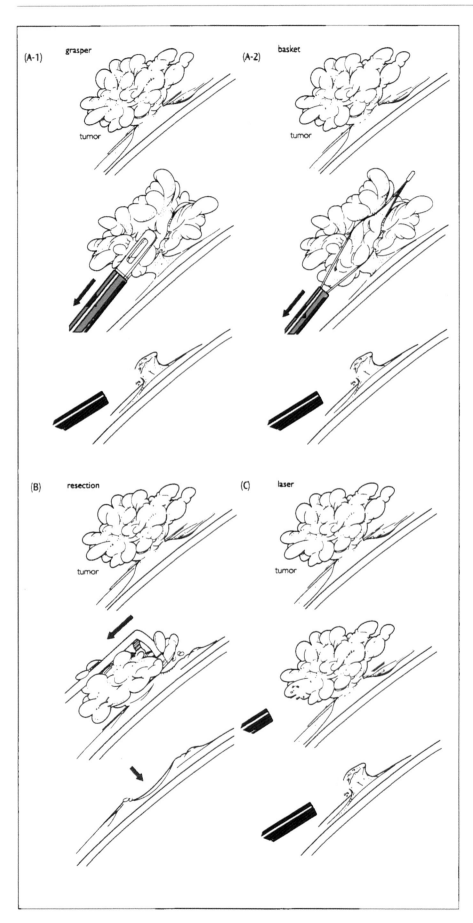

Figure 12.1
Techniques for ureteroscopic treatment of ureteral and renal tumors. (A-1) The tumor is identified and removed piecemeal using grasping forceps to its base. (A-2) Alternatively, a flat wire basket can be deployed alongside the tumor. The tumor is engaged and removed with care not to avulse the adjacent ureter. With either of these techniques, the base is treated with electrocautery or a laser energy source. (B) The tumor is identified and removed using a ureteroscopic resectoscope. The technique differs from the technique for bladder tumors in that only intraluminal tumor is resected. No attempt is made to resect deep, as with a bladder tumor. The scope is not arching deep into the tissue. (C) The tumor is biopsied for diagnostic purposes. The bulk of the tumor is then ablated using electrosurgical or laser energy. Laser energy is generally preferred because it has more reliable delivery of energy and depth of penetration. The two most commonly used energy sources are holmium:YAG and neodymium:YAG (Reproduced with permission of Elsevier Science from Sagalowsky AI, Jarrett TW. Management of urothelial tumors of the renal pelvis and ureter. In: Walsh PC, Retik AB, Vaughan ED Jr, Wein AJ, eds. Campbells urology, 8th edn, Vol. 4. Philadelphia: WB Saunders, 2002: 2845–75.)

Results of retrograde approach

Multiple series have shown the safety and efficacy of ureteroscopic treatment of upper tract TCC.[29–31] In a literature review of 205 patients, the overall recurrence rate for ureteral and renal pelvic lesions was 33% and 31.2%, respectively, and the risk of bladder recurrence was 43%.[32] In the two largest series there was a single cancer death directly attributed to recurrent upper tract disease.[31] As with any TCC, the most important prognostic indicator for tumor recurrence was grade. Keeley and associates showed a recurrence rate of 26% for grade 1 tumors and 44% for grade 2, which roughly correlates with previously established recurrence rates for open conservative surgery.[33]

Procedure complications were uncommon and usually related to patient comorbidities. Complications specific to ureteroscopic therapy included ureteral perforation, which can be managed with indwelling ureteral stent and ureteral stricture. Stricture formation ranged from 5 to 13%.[29–31] The complication rates have dropped in more contemporary series, most probably related to smaller endoscopes, improved laser energy sources, and refinements in endoscopic techniques.

Two major concerns of the ureteroscopic approach are the accuracy of ureteroscopic biopsies and the limitations of biopsies, especially with regard to staging.[34] Retrospective reviews of patients who underwent ureteroscopic biopsy followed by nephroureterectomy found the accuracy of ureteroscopic diagnosis to be 89–94% and the pathologic grading to match the open surgical technique in 78%–92%.[31,35] From prior studies we know that there is an excellent correlation between grade of the lesion and stage.[36,37] This holds true for the ureteroscopic approach, because 87% of patients with grade 1 or 2 tumors had noninvasive disease (Ta or T1), whereas 67% of patients with grade 3 tumors had invasive disease (T2 or T3).[33] This information supports the notion that tumor grade is the most important prognostic factor and, although stage cannot be directly assessed, noninvasive disease can be expected in most cases of low-grade tumor.

A final concern is whether the ureteroscopic approach promoted progression of local disease to other urothelial surfaces or metastatic disease. There have been reports of increased tumor appearance in refluxing ureters of patients with bladder tumors[38] and in the ipsilateral urinary tract and bladder following ureteroscopic treatment. However Kulp and Bagley reported on 13 patients who underwent multiple ureteroscopic treatments followed by nephroureterectomy and found no unusual propagation of TCC in the specimens.[39] Concerns that ureteroscopy may promote metastatic spread were raised by Lim and associates, who found tumor cells in renal lymphatics after ureteroscopy.[40] However, Hendin and associates showed no increased risk of metastatic disease in a group of patients who underwent ureteroscopy prior to nephroureterectomy when compared to those undergoing nephroureterectomy alone.[41]

Antegrade approach

The percutaneous approach was first described by Tomera et al in 1982 and is generally favored for larger tumors located proximally in the renal collecting system and/or proximal ureter.[42]

The main advantage of the percutaneous approach is the ability to use larger instruments, which can remove a large volume of tumor in any portion of the renal collecting system. Since deeper biopsies are obtained, tumor staging as well as grading is possible. In addition, a percutaneous approach may avoid the limitations of flexible ureteroscopy, especially when working in a complicated calyceal system or difficult areas to access such as the lower pole calyx or the upper urinary tract of patients with urinary diversion. With a percutaneous approach, the established nephrostomy tract can be maintained for immediate postoperative nephroscopy and administration of topical adjuvant therapy.

The main disadvantages are the increased morbidity compared with ureteroscopy and the potential for tumor seeding outside the urinary tract. Establishment of the nephrostomy tract has inherent risks and usually cannot be done as an ambulatory procedure. Distinct risks related to percutaneous removal are loss of urothelial integrity and exposure of nonurothelial surfaces to tumor cells. This open system provides the possibility of tumor implantation in the nephrostomy tract.

Technique and instrumentation

Establishment of the nephrostomy tract. Under a single general anesthesia, cystoscopy is performed and an open-ended ureteral catheter is positioned in the pelvis. Contrast is injected through the ureteral catheter to define the calyceal anatomy, and a percutaneous nephrostomy tract is established through the desired calyx (Figure 12.2). Tumors in peripheral calyces are best approached with direct puncture distal to the tumor. Disease in the renal pelvis and upper ureter is best approached through an upper or middle pole access so as to allow scope maneuvering through the collecting system and down the ureteropelvic junction. The tract is dilated using either sequential (Amplatz) or balloon dilation so as to accommodate a large 30F sheath. Correct positioning of the nephrostomy tract is crucial to the success of the procedure and should be performed by the urologist or by the radiologist after direct consultation with the operating surgeon.

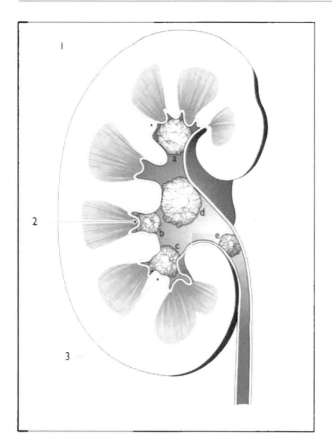

Figure 12.2
Nephrostomy tract puncture site. The position of the
nephrostomy is imperative for successful percutaneous
resection of transitional cell carcinoma of the renal collecting
system and upper ureter and requires careful preoperative
evaluation of radiographs for tumor location. Tumors located
in peripheral calyces (A–C) are best approached by direct
puncture as far distally in the calyx as possible. Tumors located
in the renal pelvis (D) and upper ureter (E) are best approached
by puncture to an upper (1) or middle (2) calyx, which allows
the scope to be maneuvered in the renal pelvis and down the
ureter. Lower calyx puncture (3) for tumor in the lower calyx.
(Reproduced with permission of Elsevier Science from
Sagalowsky AI, Jarrett TW. Management of urothelial tumors of
the renal pelvis and ureter. In: Walsh PC, Retik AB, Vaughan ED
Jr, Wein AJ, eds. Campbells urology, 8th edn, Vol. 4.
Philadelphia: WB Saunders, 2002: 2845–75.)

A nephroscope is inserted and the previously placed
ureteral catheter is grasped, brought out of the tract, and
exchanged for a stiff guide wire, thus providing both antegrade and retrograde control and ensuring that access is
not compromised with nephroscopy. Complete nephroscopy is performed using rigid and flexible endoscopes
when necessary. Any suspicion of upper ureteral involvement
warrants flexible antegrade ureteroscopy.

Biopsy and definitive therapy. Following identification, the tumors need to be removed using one of three
following techniques (Figure 12.3). In the first technique,
which uses a cold-cup biopsy forceps through a standard
nephroscope, the bulk of the tumor is grasped using
forceps and removed in piecemeal fashion until the base is
reached (Figure 12.3A). A separate biopsy of the base is
performed for staging purposes and the base is cauterized
using a Bugbee electrode and cautery. Low-grade papillary
lesions on a thin stalk are easily treated in this manner with
minimal bleeding.

Alternatively, a cutting loop from a standard resectoscope is used to remove the tumor to its base (Figure
12.3B). Once again the base should be resected and sent
separately for staging purposes. This approach is more
effective for larger broad-based tumors where simple
debulking to a stalk is not possible.

For the third technique, which uses flexible or rigid
endoscopes, the tumor is biopsied and treated with
holmium:YAG or neodymium:YAG laser at 25–30 W
(Figure 12.3B, C, and D).

Regardless of technique, a nephrostomy tube is left
in place. This access can be used for second-look follow-
up nephroscopy to ensure complete tumor removal.
Nephroureterectomy is indicated if the pathology shows
high-grade or invasive disease.

Second-look nephroscopy. Follow-up nephroscopy is
performed 4–14 days later to allow for adequate healing. At
second-look nephroscopy, the tumor resection site is identified and any residual tumor is removed. If no tumor is
identified, then the base should be biopsied, and treated
using cautery or the neodymium:YAG laser (15–20 W and
3 s exposures). The nephrostomy tube can be removed
several days later if all tumors have been removed. If the
patient is being considered for adjuvant topical therapy,
then a small 8F nephrostomy tube is left to provide access
for instillations. Some authors have advocated a third-look
nephroscopy prior to final nephrostomy tube removal.[43]

Results of antegrade approach

Owing to the rarity of the disease, there are only several
retrospective series with adequate numbers and follow-up
to draw reasonable conclusions.[43–45] In a literature review
of 84 patients, Okada and associates found an overall
recurrence rate of 27%.[46] Tumor grade strongly predicted
outcomes, as Jarrett et al[43] showed the recurrence rate for
grades 1, 2, and 3 lesions to be 18, 33, and 50%, respectively. The only cancer-related mortalities in this series
were in patients with high-grade disease. Lee et al reviewed
their 13-year experience with percutaneous management,
comparing 50 patients who underwent percutaneous
management to 60 who underwent nephroureterectomy

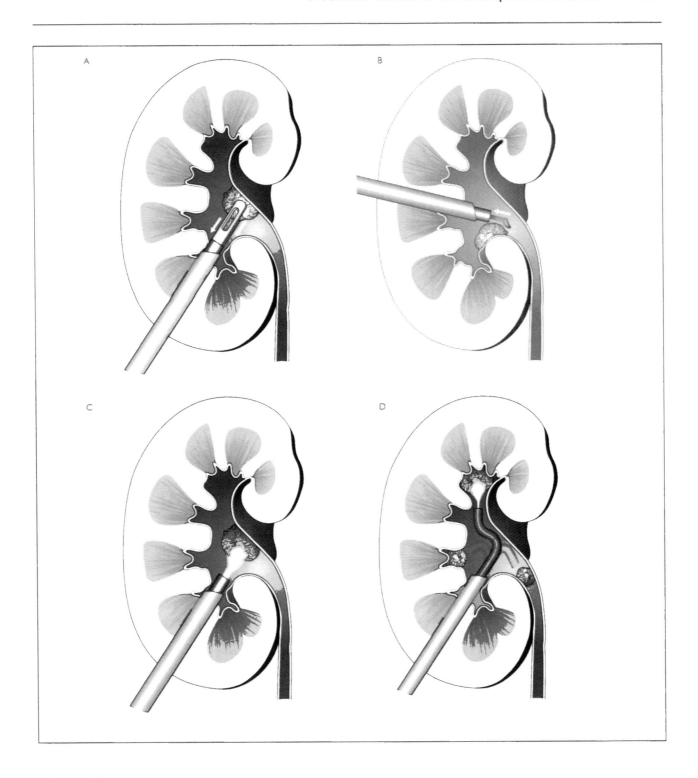

Figure 12.3

Techniques for percutaneous removal of transitional cell carcinoma of the renal collecting system. (A) The tumor is identified and debulked using forceps to its base. The base is biopsied and sent separately for evaluation. This technique works well for papillary tumors on a narrow stalk. Broad-based tumors may cause excessive bleeding and are best approached with resection or laser therapy. (B) Using a standard resectoscope, the tumor is identified and resected to its base. Special care should be taken to avoid resection into major renal vasculature. The tumor is identified, biopsied for diagnostic purposes, and treated using holmium or neodymium laser sources. This can be done via a standard nephroscope (C) or using a flexible cystoscope (D). (Reproduced with permission of Elsevier Science from Sagalowsky AI, Jarrett TW. Management of urothelial tumors of the renal pelvis and ureter. In: Walsh PC, Retik AB, Vaughan ED Jr, Wein AJ, eds. Campbells urology, 8th edn, Vol. 4. Philadelphia: WB Saunders, 2002: 2845–75.)

and found no significant difference in overall survival.[47] As expected, patients with low-grade disease did well, regardless of modality chosen, and patients with high-grade disease did poorly, regardless of treatment option.

Most would agree from the literature that percutaneous management is acceptable in patients with low-grade (grade 1) disease, regardless of the status of the contralateral kidney, provided the patient is committed to lifelong follow-up. Patients with grade 3 disease do poorly, regardless of modality chosen, but should probably have the gold standard nephroureterectomy to maximize cancer therapy (provided they are medically fit). The largest area of controversy surrounds the use of percutaneous management for patients with grade 2 disease and a normal contralateral kidney. Jabbour et al retrospectively evaluated 24 patients and found a disease-specific survival of 95% overall, and 100 and 80% for stage Ta and T1 lesions, respectively.[48] This study shows an acceptable result with noninvasive grade 2 disease. With more invasive lesions, the potential for disease progression and metastatic disease are not insignificant and nephroureterectomy should be strongly considered.

Complications from percutaneous management of tumors are similar to those for benign renal processes and include bleeding, perforation of the collecting system, or secondary ureteropelvic junction obstruction. Complications increased in number and severity with higher tumor grade.[43] This finding is probably due to the more extensive pathology and treatments necessary to eradicate the tumor. Unlike ureteroscopic resection, the percutaneous method was able to adequately stage tumors and, as expected, stage increased with tumor grade.

A major concern of the percutaneous approach is the potential seeding of nonurothelial surface with tumor cells. Although there have been several reported cases of nephrostomy tract infiltration with high-grade tumors,[42,49,50] there were no occurrences in the three largest series.[43–45] Tract seeding is a possibility but appears to be an uncommon event.

Adjuvant therapy

Any procedure short of nephroureterectomy will have a higher local recurrence due to the established risk of ipsilateral recurrence. Several approaches are available to minimize these risks. These fall into two basic categories: instillation of immunotherapeutic or chemotherapeutic agents and brachytherapy of the nephrostomy tract.

Instillation therapy

Instillation therapy can be performed in several acceptable fashions. Accepted techniques include antegrade instillation via a nephrostomy tube (Figure 12.4), or retrograde via direct instillation into a ureteral catheter or by reflux in a patient with an indwelling ureteral stent or iatrogenically created vesicoureteral reflux. Patel and Fuchs described a convenient technique of outpatient instillation via a ureteral catheter placed suprapubically. Regardless of the technique chosen, administration to the upper urinary tract should be performed under low pressure and in the absence of active infection to minimize the risk of bacterial sepsis and/or systemic absorption of the agent.

Results

It makes clinical sense that the same agents used to treat urothelial carcinoma of the bladder would be effective in the upper urinary tract. Many studies have described small retrospective series of patients undergoing therapy with thiotepa,[29,44] mitomycin,[30,31,51,52] and bacille Calmette-Guérin BCG.[43,51,53–55] Although the cumulative experience appears convincing, no individual study has shown statistical improvement with relation to survival and recurrence rates. Possible reasons for this include:

1. insufficient numbers to show clinical significance owing to the relative rarity of the disease
2. tumors of the upper urinary tract have a different tumor biology than their bladder counterparts or
3. the delivery system is inadequate and, unlike the bladder, does not allow for uniform delivery of the agent with adequate dwell time to enable a clinical response.

No doubt further studies are required to settle this issue.

The most common complication of treatment is bacterial sepsis. In order to minimize this risk, patients must be evaluated for active infection prior to treatment and a low-pressure delivery system should be used. Agent-specific complications of the various therapies include ramification of systemic absorption of the agent. Specific to the upper urinary tract, Bellman et al described the complications of BCG following percutaneous management.[56] Most commonly seen was granulomatous involvement of the kidney in the absence of systemic signs of BCG infection. Mukamel et al saw an inordinate decrease in renal function among patients receiving BCG who had vesicoureteral reflux.[57]

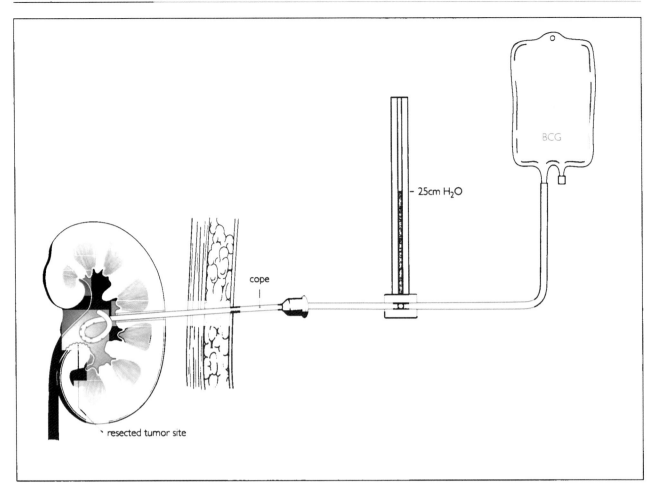

Figure 12.4
Set-up for administration of topical immunotherapy or chemotherapy to the upper urinary tract via a previously placed nephrostomy tube. Therapy is instilled via gravity with a mechanism that prevents excessive intrarenal pressures. High pressures have been linked to complications of systemic absorption and bacterial sepsis. (Reproduced with permission of Elsevier Science from Sagalowsky AI, Jarrett TW. Management of urothelial tumors of the renal pelvis and ureter. In: Walsh PC, Retik AB, Vaughan ED Jr, Wein AJ, eds. Campbells urology, 8th edn, Vol. 4. Philadelphia: WB Saunders, 2002: 2845–75.)

Brachytherapy

Brachytherapy to the nephrostomy tract via iridium wire or delivery system has been described by Patel et al[44] and Nurse et al.[58] There were no instances of tract recurrences in this series, although the authors acknowledge the rarity of the event. The only major complication that has been attributed to brachytherapy is fistula formation requiring nephroureterectomy.

Oral immunotherapy

Bropirimine is an oral agent which induces an interferon response in the urinary tract and thus is an immunotherapeutic agent. Early studies have shown some promise in the bladder and upper urinary tract but significant drop out due to drug-related toxicity.[59]

Follow-up

The propensity of upper tract tumors towards multifocal recurrence and metastatic spread with more dysplastic lesions makes follow-up complicated. Postoperative evaluation must routinely include evaluation of the bladder, ipsilateral (if organ-sparing therapy was chosen), and contralateral urinary tracts, and of extraurinary sites for local and metastatic spread. A follow-up regimen is thus dependent on the time from surgery, the approach chosen (organ-sparing vs radical), and the potential for metastatic spread.

All patients should be assessed at regular 3-month intervals, the first year after being rendered tumor free, by endoscopic or open surgical approaches.[31] This is largely based on work with bladder TCC which shows that most tumor recurrences following bladder resection are in the first year.[60,61] The upper urinary tract is more difficult to monitor, and delayed recognition of upper tract tumor recurrence may lead to rapid disease progression and poor results.[62] Evaluation should include history, physical examination, urinalysis, urine cytology (for high-grade lesions), and office cystoscopy due to the high risk of bladder recurrences in patients treated both conservatively and with nephroureterectomy.[62,63] This is performed every 3 months for the first year, every 6 months for the next 2 years, and yearly thereafter. If the patient's primary pathology was high grade, a urine cytology may be helpful in assessing for tumor recurrence.[63] Its utility, however, is decreased with less dysplastic tumors.[64–66]

Bilateral disease, either synchronous or metachronous, is seen in 1–4% of patients,[63,67,68] and thus imaging of the contralateral kidney by intravenous urogram or retrograde pyelogram is required on a yearly basis. Retrograde pyelography may be necessary if the patient is not a candidate for contrast injection or if the intravenous urogram is not of adequate quality. In addition, CT or sonography may be helpful in distinguishing stones from soft tissue densities. Further evaluation of filling defects on imaging studies usually requires ureteroscopic evaluation. If the patient requires endoscopic evaluation of the upper urinary tract, cystoscopy can be performed in conjunction with that procedure.

If an organ-sparing approach is chosen, the ipsilateral urinary tract must be assessed as well as the remainder of the urinary tract. The frequency and duration of the follow-up depends largely on the grade and stage of the lesion but is usually every 6 months for the first several years and yearly thereafter. Radiographic evaluation of the upper tracts alone is not adequate, as Keeley and associates showed that 75% of early tumor recurrences were visible endoscopically and not radiographically.[31] With tumors approached in a percutaneous fashion, immediate follow-up nephroscopy can be performed through the established nephrostomy tract.

The burden of repeated endoscopic evaluation of the upper urinary tracts used to be a major deterrent to conservative therapy in the past. The use of smaller 7.5F flexible ureteroscopes has greatly eased the burden of follow-up, as ureteroscopes can be reliably passed up the ureter without the need for dilation of the ureteral orifice or prior stenting. Others have advocated resection of the ureteral orifice to facilitate subsequent surveillance ureteroscopy in the office setting.[69] Even though technology has somewhat facilitated follow-up, both physician and patient must be committed to organ-sparing treatment.

Metastatic restaging is required in all patients at significant risk for disease progression to local or distant sites. This group encompasses patients with high-grade and/or high-stage disease. Metastatic restaging is generally not necessary for low-grade disease, where the risks of invasive and subsequent metastatic disease are negligible. There have been several approaches in the literature for

bladder cancer which dictate follow-up based on tumor staging.[70,71] Since there are no established protocols for the upper urinary tract, we can adapt follow-up based on those findings. Physical examination, chest X-ray, and comprehensive metabolic panel with liver enzymes should be performed every 3 months for the first year, every 6 months for years 2 through 3, and annually for years 4 through 5. Subsequent years necessitate evaluation of the urothelium only. CT or MRI of the abdomen and pelvis should be performed every 6 months for the first 2 years and annually for years 3 through 5. Bone scans need only to be performed for elevated alkaline phosphatase or symptoms of bone pain.

Laparoscopic nephroureterectomy

The gold standard therapy for people not at risk for renal failure and the risks of dialysis remains nephroureterectomy. Laparoscopy has greatly minimized the morbidity of the procedure with the avoidance of a multiple incisions or a single large incision to approach the entire urinary tract.

Laparoscopic nephroureterectomy has two distinct portions: removal of the kidney and complete ureterectomy with a cuff of bladder. The nephrectomy portion of the procedure can be confined to the kidney for low-grade noninvasive lesions. Inclusion of Gerota's fascia with or without the adrenal should be considered for parenchymal invasive lesions. Multiple approaches to the nephrectomy portion of the procedure have been described, including transabdominal and retroperitoneal laparoscopic approaches and hand-assisted techniques. All these techniques are equally effective in cancer control and in minimizing morbidity, provided that the principles of surgical oncology are applied. The choice of approach depends on patient factors as well as surgeon comfort. For hand-assisted techniques, one must consider placing the hand incision in a location that can be used for both specimen extraction and dissection of the distal ureter if necessary.

Multiple techniques for complete ureterectomy have been described to decrease morbidity. Such variations include transurethral resection of the distal ureter, total laparoscopic excision, and open removal via extravesical, transvesical, or combined approaches. Regardless of approach, an incision for intact extraction is always required for accurate pathologic staging.

An important factor with regards to TCC when performing distal ureterectomy is distal recurrence and the possibility of tumor seeding. Unlike renal cell carcinoma, where tumor implantation at extrarenal sites is a relatively uncommon event, there are multiple reports of seeding from TCC. Any approach that violates this closed system places the patient at risk for tumor seeding, especially with high-grade lesions. In addition, the propensity toward distal recurrence makes anything short of complete ureterectomy with a bladder cuff unacceptable, with the exception of rare, unusual circumstances. One should avoid approaches which involve removal of the distal ureter, leaving an 'open system' prior to control of the proximal ureter.

The authors' preference is to perform a standard laparoscopic radical nephrectomy with a dissection of the distal ureter as far distally as can safely be done. The incision for extractions is then placed strategically to complete removal of the distal ureter and bladder cuff. A low midline or Pfannenstiel incision is usually adequate if the ureteral dissection was carried out below the iliac vessels. In some cases where there is marked fibrosis of the periureteral tissue (prior surgery or multiple ureteroscopies), dissection below the iliac vessels is quite difficult. In such cases, a Gibson's incision provides exposure of the distal and mid ureter and can be used for specimen extraction. This approach allows flexibility in placing the incision and provides the patient with a procedure which is oncologically sound.

Results

The first laparoscopic nephroureterectomy was performed in 1991 by Clayman and associates.[72] Since that time, the technical aspects and safety of laparoscopic procedures have been well established. There are multiple published series of laparoscopic nephroureterectomy.[73–77] Each varies with regard to approach (transperitoneal vs retroperitoneal), management of the distal ureter by open removal, transurethral resection 'pluck technique', and total laparoscopic management. As with other laparoscopic renal procedures, there is no clear-cut benefit of any one approach with regard to morbidity, cosmesis, or return to activity.

Hard and fast conclusions regarding cancer-related outcomes cannot be determined because there is only a single study with follow-up beyond 2 years.[77] The overall bladder recurrence rate of the combined studies is 16%, which is comparable to that of open nephroureterectomy. In the largest series, Shalhav and colleagues found that although the procedure took much longer than open nephroureterectomy, patients had a much shorter recovery time and equivalent outcomes with regard to bladder recurrence, metastatic disease, and cancer-specific survival.[77] There were no reports of foreign bodies eroding into the bladder when the stapling device was used.

Local recurrence and port-site seeding are major concerns. There have been three reported instances of port-site seeding involving TCC of the upper urinary tract. Two of these cases were discovered after simple nephrectomy for presumed benign disease in which the principles of surgical oncology were inadvertently not followed.[78,79]

In the third case, the proximal coil of a ureteral stent was seen protruding from the collecting system in the area of the tumor.[80] Another case was in an intended nephroureterectomy for high-grade disease (Barrett, pers comm). Although the potential for seeding exists, it does not appear any higher than that for the open surgical counterpart as long as good surgical principles are followed.

References

1. Fraley EE. Cancer of the renal pelvis. In: Skinner DG, DeKernion JB, eds. Genitourinary cancer. Philadelphia: WB Saunders, 1978; 134.

2. Anderstrom C, Johansson SL, Pettersson S, Wahlqvist L. Carcinoma of the ureter: a clinicopathologic study of 49 cases. J Urol 1989; 142:280.

3. Jemal A, Taylor M, Samuels A, et al. Cancer Statistics, 2003. Ca Cancer J Clin 2003; 53:5–26.

4. Say CS, Hori JM. Transitional cell carcinoma of the renal pelvis: experience from 1940–1972 and literature review. J Urol 1974; 112:438–42.

5. Petkovic SD. Epidemiology and treatment of renal pelvic and ureteral tumors. J Urol 1975; 114:858–65.

6. Solsona E, Iborra I, Ricos JV, et al. Upper urinary tract involvement in patients with bladder carcinoma in situ (Tis): its impact on management. Urology 1997; 49(3):347–52.

7. Messing EM. Urothelial tumors of the urinary tract. In: Walsh PC, Retik AB, Vaughan ED Jr, Wein AJ, eds. Campbell's urology, 8th edn. Philadelphia: WB Saunders. 2002; 2767.

8. Murphy DM, Zincke H, Furlow WL. Management of high grade transitional cell cancer of the upper urinary tract. J Urol 1981; 135:25.

9. Gray Sears CL, Ward JF, Sears ST, et al. Prospective comparison of computerized tomography and excretory urography in the initial evaluation of asymptomatic microhematuria. J Urol 2002; 168(6):2457–60.

10. Malek RS, Aquilo JJ, Hattery RR. Radiolucent filling defects of the renal pelvis: classification and report of unusual cases. J Urol 1975; 114(4):508–13.

11. Huffman JL. Management of upper tract transitional cell carcinomas. In: Vogelzang, NJ, Scardino PT, Shipley WU, et al. eds. Comprehensive textbook of genitourinary oncology 2nd edn. Philadelphia: Lippincott, Williams and Wilkins 2000; 367.

12. Babaian RJ, Johnson DE. Primary carcinoma of the ureter. J Urol 1980; 123:357.

13. Spires SE, Banks ER, Cibull ML, et al. Adenocarcinoma of renal pelvis. Arch Pathol Lab Med 1993; 117:1156.

14. Cummings KB. Nephroureterectomy: rationale in the management of transitional cell carcinoma of the upper urinary tract. Urol Clin North Am 1980; 7:569–78.

15. Held PJ, Brunner F, Okada M, et al. Five year survival found for end-stage renal disease patients in the United States, Europe and Japan, 1982–1987. Am J Kidney Dis 1990; 15:451–7.

16. Murphy DM, Zincke H, Furlow WL. Primary grade 1 transitional cell carcinoma of the renal pelvis and ureter. J Urol 1980; 123:629–31.

17. Young HH, McKay RW. Congenital valvular obstruction of the prostatic urethra. Surg Gyn Obst 1929; 48:509.

18. Abdel-Razzak O, Bagley DH. The 6.9 F semirigid ureteroscope in clinical use. Urology 1993; 41:45–8.

19. Grasso M, Bagley A. 7.5/8.2 F actively deflectable, flexible ureteroscope: a new device for both diagnostic and therapeutic upper urinary tract endoscopy. Urology 1994; 43:435–41.

20. Bian Y, Ehya H, Bagley DH. Cytologic diagnosis of upper urinary tract neoplasms by ureteroscopic sampling. Acta Cytol 1995; 39:733–40.

21. Palou J, Salvador J, Millan F, et al. Management of superficial transitional cell carcinoma in the intramural ureter: What to do? J Urol 2000; 163:744–7.

22. Tawfiek ER, Bibbo M, Bagley D. Ureteroscopic biopsy: technique and specimen preparation. Urology 1997; 50:117–19.

23. Jarrett TW, Lee CK, Pardalidis NP, Smith AD. Extensive dilation of distal ureter for endoscopic treatment of large volume ureteral disease. J Urol 1995; 153:1214–17.

24. Smith JA Jr, Lee RG, Dixon JA. Tissue effects of neodymium:YAG laser photoradiation of canine ureters. J Surg Oncol 1984; 27:168–71.

25. Schmeller NT, Hofstetter AG. Laser treatment of ureteral tumors. J Urol 1989; 141:840–3.

26. Carson CC. Endoscopic treatment of upper and lower urinary tract lesions using lasers. Semin Urol 1991; 9:185–91.

27. Bagley D, Erhard M. Use of the holmium laser in the upper urinary tract. Tech Urol 1995; 1:25–30.

28. Razvi HA, Chun SS, Denstedt JD, Sales JL. Soft-tissue applications of the holmium:YAG laser in urology. J Endourol 1995; 9:387–90.

29. Elliott DS, Blute ML, Patterson DE, et al. Long-term follow-up of endoscopically treated upper urinary tract transitional cell carcinoma. Urology 1996; 47:819–25.

30. Martinez-Pineiro JA, Garcia Matres MJ, Martinez-Pineiro L. Endourological treatment of upper tract urothelial carcinomas: analysis of a series of 59 tumors. J Urol 1996; 156:377–85.

31. Keeley FX, Bibbo M, Bagley DM. Ureteroscopic treatment and evaluation of the upper tract TCC. J Urol 1997; 157:1560.

32. Tawfiek ER, Bagley D. Upper-tract transitional cell carcinoma. Urology 1997; 50:321–9.

33. Keeley FX, Kulp DA, Bibbo M, et al. Diagnostic accuracy of ureteroscopic biopsy in upper tract transitional cell carcinoma. J Urol 1997; 157:33–7.

34. Huffman JL. Ureteroscopic management of transitional cell carcinoma of the upper urinary tract. Urol Clin North Am 1988; 15:419–24.

35. Guarnizo E, Pavlovich CP, Seiba M, et al. Ureteroscopic biopsy of upper tract urothelial carcinoma: Improved diagnostic accuracy and histopathological considerations using a multi-biopsy approach. J Urol 2000; 163:52–5.

36. Chasko SB, Gray GF, McCarron JP Jr. Urothelial neoplasia of the upper urinary tract. Pathol Annu 1981; 16(pt 2):127–53.

37. Heney N, Nocks B, Daly J, et al. Prognostic factors in carcinoma of the ureter. J Urol 1981; 125:632–6.

38. De Torres Mateos JA, Banus Gassol JM, Palou Redota J, Morote Robles J. Vesicorenal reflux and upper urinary tract transitional cell carcinoma after transurethral resection of recurrent superficial bladder carcinoma. J Urol 1987; 138:49–51.

39. Kulp DA, Bagley DH. Does flexible uretero-pyeloscopy promote local recurrence of transitional cell carcinoma? J Endourol 1994; 8:111–13.

40. Lim DJ, Shattuck MC, Cook WA. Pyelovenous lymphatic migration of transitional cell carcinoma following flexible ureterorenoscopy. J Urol 1993; 149:109–11.

41. Hendin BN, Streem SB, Levin HS, et al. Impact of diagnostic ureteroscopy on long-term survival in patients with upper tract transitional cell carcinoma. J Urol 1999; 161:783–5.

42. Tomera KM, Leary FJ, Kinke H. Pyeloscopy in urothelial tumors. J Urol 1982; 127:1088–9.

43. Jarrett TW, Sweetser PM, Weiss GH, Smith AD. Percutaneous management of transitional cell carcinoma of the renal collecting system: 9-year experience. J Urol 1995; 154:1629–35.

44. Patel A, Soonawalla P, Shepherd SF, et al. Long-term outcome after percutaneous treatment of transitional cell carcinoma of the renal pelvis. J Urol 1996; 155:868–74.

45. Clark PC, Streem SB, Geisinger MA. 13 year experience with percutaneous management of upper tract transitional cell carcinoma. J Urol 1999; 161:772–5.

46. Okada H, Eto H, Hara I, et al. Percutaneous treatment of transitional cell carcinoma of the upper urinary tract. Int J Urol 1997; 4:130–3.

47. Lee BR, Jabbour ME, Marshall FF, et al. 13-year survival comparison of percutaneous and open nephroureterectomy approaches for management of transitional cell carcinoma of renal collecting system: equivalent outcomes. J Endourol 1999;13(4):289–94.

48. Jabbour ME, Desgrandchamps F, Cazin S, et al. Percutaneous management of grade II upper urinary tract transitional cell carcinoma: the long-term outcome. J Urol 2000; 163:1105–7.

49. Slywotzky C, Maya M. Needle tract seeding of transitional cell carcinoma following fine-needle aspiration of a renal mass. Abdom Imaging 1994; 19:174–6.

50. Huang A, Low RK, DeVere WR. Nephrostomy tract tumor seeding following percutaneous manipulation of a ureteral carcinoma. J Urol 1995; 153:1041–2.

51. Eastham JA, Huffman JL. Technique of mitomycin C instillation in the treatment of upper urinary tract urothelial tumors. J Urol 1993; 150(2 pt 1):324–5.

52. Weston PM, Greenland JE, Wallace DM. Role of topical mitomycin C in upper urinary tract transitional cell carcinoma. Br J Urol 1993; 71:624–5.

53. Smith AY, Vitale PJ, Lowe BA, Woodside JR. Treatment of superficial papillary transitional cell carcinoma of the ureter by vesicoureteral reflux of mitomycin C. J Urol 1987; 138:1231–3.

54. Studer UE, Casanova G, Kraft R. Percutaneous bacillus Calmette-Guerin perfusion of the upper urinary tract for carcinoma in situ. J Urol 1989; 142:975–7.

55. Sharpe JR, Duffy G, Chin JL. Intrarenal bacillus Calmette-Guerin therapy for upper urinary tract carcinoma in situ. J Urol 1993; 149:457–60.

56. Bellman GC, Sweetser P, Smith AD. Complications of intracavitary bacillus Calmette-Guerin after percutaneous resection of upper tract transitional cell carcinoma. J Urol 1994; 51:13–15.

57. Mukamel E, Vilkovsky E, Hadar H, et al. The effect of intravesical bacillus Calmette-Guerin therapy on the upper urinary tract. J Urol 1991; 146:980–1.

58. Nurse DE, Woodhouse CR, Kellett MJ, Dearnley DP. Percutaneous removal of upper tract tumors. World J Urol 1989; 7:131.

59. Sarosdy MF. A review of clinical studies of bropirimine immunotherapy of carcinoma in situ of the bladder and upper urinary tract. Eur Urol 1997; 31 (Suppl) 1:20–6.

60. Varkarakis MJ, Gaeta J, Moore RH, Murphy GP. Superficial bladder tumor: aspects of clinical progression. Urology 1974; 4:414–20.

61. Loening S, Narayana A, Yoder L, et al. Factors influencing the recurrence rate of bladder cancer. J Urol 1980; 123:29–31.

62. Mazeman E. Tumors of the upper respiratory tract calyces, renal pelvis, and ureter. Eur Urol 1976; 2:120–6.

63. Murphy DM, Zincke H, Furlow WL. Management of high grade transitional cell cancer of the upper urinary tract. J Urol 1981; 125:25–9.

64. Grace DA, Taylor WN, Taylor JN, Winter CC. Carcinoma of the renal pelvis: a 15-year review. J Urol 1967; 98:566–9.

65. Sarnacki CT, McCormack LJ, Kiser WS, et al. Urinary cytology and the clinical diagnosis of urinary tract malignancy: a clinicopathologic study of 1400 patients. J Urol 1971; 106:761–4.

66. Zincke H, Aguilo JJ, Farrow GM, et al. Significance of urinary cytology in the early detection of transitional cell cancer of the upper urinary tract. J Urol 1976; 116:781–3.

67. Babaian RJ, Johnson DE. Primary carcinoma of the ureter. J Urol 1980; 123:357–9.

68. Petkovic SD. Epidemiology and treatment of renal pelvic and ureteral tumors. J Urol 1975; 114:858–65.

69. Kerbl K, Clayman RV. Incision of the ureterovesical junction for endoscopic surveillance of transitional cell cancer of the upper urinary tract. J Urol 1993; 150:1440–3.

70. Korman HJ, Watson R, Soloway MS. Bladder cancer: Clinical aspects and management. Monogr Urol 1996; 16:83–110.

71. Slaton JW, Swanson DA, Grossman HB, Dinney CPN. A stage specific approach to surveillance after radical cystectomy for transitional cell carcinoma of the bladder. J Urol 1999; 162:710–14.

72. Clayman RV, Kavoussi LR, Figenshau RS, et al. Laparoscopic nephroureterectomy: initial case report. J Laparoendosc Surg 1991; 1:343.

73. Chung HJ, Chiu AW, Chen KK, et al. Retroperitoneoscopy-assisted nephroureterectomy for the management of upper urinary urothelial cancer. Min Invas Ther and Allied Technol 1996; 5:266–71.

74. Keeley FX, Tolley DA. Laparoscopic nephroureterectomy: making management of upper tract transitional cell carcinoma entirely minimally invasive. J Endourol 1998; 12:139.

75. Salomon L, Hoznek A, Cicco A, et al. Retroperitoneoscopic nephroureterectomy for renal pelvic tumors with a single iliac incision. J Urol 1999; 161: 541–4.

76. Jarrett TW, Chan DY, Cadeddu JA, et al. Laparoscopic nephroureterectomy for the treatment of transitional cell carcinoma of the upper urinary tract. Urology 2001; 57(3):448–53.

77. Shalhav AL, Dunn MD, Portis AJ, et al. Laparoscopic nephroureterectomy for upper tract transitional cell cancer: the Washington University experience. J Urol 2000; 163:1100.

78. Ahmed I, Shaikh NA, Kapadia CR. Track recurrence of renal pelvic transitional cell carcinoma after laparoscopic nephrectomy. Br J Urol 1998; 81(2):319.

79. Otani M, Irie S, Tsuji Y. Port site metastasis after laparoscopic nephrectomy: unsuspected transitional cell carcinoma within a tuberculous atrophic kidney. J Urol 1999; 162(2):486–7.

80. Ong Am, Bhayani SB, Pavlovich CP. Trocar site recurrence after laparoscopic nephroureterectomy. J Urol 2003; 170(4 Pt 1):1301.

13

Minimally invasive hand-assisted nephrectomy for the treatment of renal cancer

Steven J Shichman and Joseph R Wagner

Hand-assisted laparoscopic nephrectomy (HALN) was introduced in 1996 when Bannenberg et al performed the first nephrectomy in the pig.[1] They reported that the HALN technique was quick and easy to perform and, compared with conventional laparoscopic nephrectomy, operative times were shorter (30–45 min versus 90 to 120 min). In 1997 Nakada and colleagues reported the first HALN in a human for removal of a chronically infected kidney from stone disease.[2] Since 1997, numerous publications have reported the use of hand-assisted techniques for radical nephrectomies, nephroureterectomies, donor nephrectomies, partial nephrectomies, and dismembered pyeloplasties.[3–7] Since 1998, we have performed over 500 hand-assisted laparoscopic renal procedures using hand-assisted techniques.

Hand-assisted techniques utilize all the principles of standard laparoscopy, but offer surgeons the advantage of using their most versatile instrument – their hands. The hand aids in dissection, exposure, retraction, and maintaining hemostasis. The hand may also assist in more advanced techniques, such as intracorporeal suturing and knot tying. Furthermore, by maintaining tactile sensation, the surgeon is able to palpate vessels and organs that he may not be able to discern by visualization alone, thereby potentially minimizing the risk of injury to vital structures, particularly during difficult dissections. In essence, hand-assisted laparoscopy combines the advantages of laparoscopic and open surgery. As said by Dr RV Clayman, 'one hand is worth a thousand trocars'.[8]

Indications

Indications for HALN can include almost any scenario in which an open nephrectomy is warranted. The most common indications include nephrectomy for functional renal masses (renal cell carcinoma being the most common pathology), nonfunctioning kidneys, and renovascular hypertension. Hand-assisted techniques can also be applied to nephroureterectomy (hand-assisted laparo-

scopic nephroureterectomy, HALNU) for live donor renal transplants and upper tract transitional cell carcinoma.

Care must be taken in evaluating whether a patient is appropriate for HALN (Table 13.1). The most favorable patients, especially during the initial learning phase, include those who are relatively thin and have left-sided tumors. Patients with virgin abdominal cavities and small, lower pole tumors located away from the renal hilum are ideal candidates.

Several conditions make a patient less than ideal for initial attempts at hand-assisted cases. Obese patients can be a significant challenge, since excessive adipose tissue can make dissection tedious and difficult. Multiple prior abdominal surgeries predispose to intraperitoneal adhesions, which are time consuming to lyse and increase the risk of visceral injury. Patients with extremely muscular abdominal walls have reduced abdominal wall compliance, which reduces the working space and thereby restricts the use of the hand. Relative contraindications to hand-assisted techniques also include extremely large tumors, extensive renal vein or inferior vena cava (IVC) thrombus, history of severe perirenal and/or intra-abdominal inflammatory conditions, ipsilateral abdominal wall stomas, and pregnancy. As the surgeon's experience grows, patients with relative contraindications become more amenable to the hand-assisted technique. Absolute contraindications include caval thrombus extending above the hepatic veins, large tumors with direct extension into the body wall or adjacent viscera, and uncorrectable bleeding disorders.

Hand-access devices

The purpose of the hand-access device is to enable the surgeon to comfortably insert his nondominant hand into the abdominal cavity through a small incision without the loss of the pneumoperitoneum.

There is no perfect hand-access device. Each device has its advantages and disadvantages. Factors determining the ideal choice of a hand-access device for a specific case

Table 13.1 *Favorable aspects, relative contraindications, and absolute contraindications to performing hand-assisted laparascopic nephrectomy*

Favorable aspects	Relative contraindications	Absolute contraindications
Thin body habitus	Morbid obesity	Caval thrombus extending above
Small tumors	Severe intraperitoneal adhesions	hepatic veins
Left-sided tumors	Severe perirenal and perihilar adhesions	Direct extension of tumor into body
Lower pole tumors	Muscular abdominal wall	wall or adjacent viscera
Tumors located away from the	Extremely large tumors (> 15 cm)	Uncorrectable bleeding disorder
renal hilum	Extensive renal vein or IVC thrombus	
Minimal or no previous	Ipsilateral abdominal wall stoma	
abdominal surgery	Pregnancy	

IVC, inferior vena cava.

include the patient's body habitus and pathology, and the surgeon's experience and preference using each individual device. All devices require a similar size incision (3–4 inches) in the abdominal wall, but vary widely on how they maintain a seal around the surgeon's arm and wrist. Unlike the first-generation devices, none of the new products adheres to the body wall using adhesive seals. These adhesive seals were tedious and difficult to apply and were very prone to leakage.

Devices, which are currently on the market, include the following:

1. GelPort – Applied Medical Resources Corporation, Rancho Santa Margarita, California.
2. Lap Disc – Ethicon Endosurgery, Inc., Cincinnati, Ohio.
3. OmniPort – InterMed, Selling, Nevada
4. HandPort – Smith & Nephew, Largo, Florida, recently acquired by Ethicon Endosurgery, Inc., Cincinnati, Ohio.

All of these devices secure to the body wall using two concentric rings that are attached together with vinyl or rubber. One ring is inserted on the undersurface of the abdominal wall and the other ring rests on the outside surface of the body wall. The material holding the two rings together is placed on stretch, maintaining the seal at the body wall and acting as a wound protector. These second-generation devices can be directly inserted into the abdominal cavity without first insufflating, which is a definite time saver.

Advantages of the GelPort (Figure 13.1) device include an excellent seal, flexibility, and comfort offered by the gel. The unique gel-like polymer through which the surgeon inserts his hand is flexible and soft around the wrist. Additionally, this polymer can be temporarily pierced by an instrument or trocar and maintain a seal at the puncture site. Instruments can even be inserted through the gel while the hand is inserted in the device. Other advantages include the fact that removal of the surgeon's hand from

the abdominal cavity does not cause loss of pneumoperitoneum and rarely causes the device to become dislodged. The GelPort device has the largest template or footprint, requiring a large area for application. This is not a problem in most cases, but in small-framed patients the device may be too large to use in a right lower quadrant incision that is commonly used for a right-sided nephrectomy. In these cases the anterior iliac spine may prevent the device from sitting evenly against the body wall, thereby jeopardizing the seal. A smaller version of this device has recently become available to obviate these problems. GelPort is the most expensive hand-access device on the market.

The Lap Disc (Figure 13.2) is the least expensive device on the market and is the easiest to use. There are no pieces

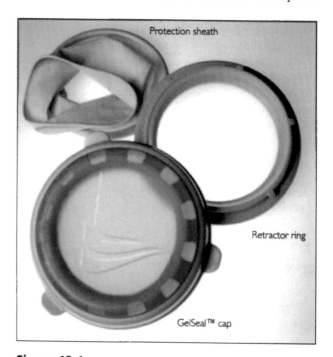

Figure 13.1

The GelPort device is made of a comfortable gel-like polymer which allows insertion of both hand and trocar.

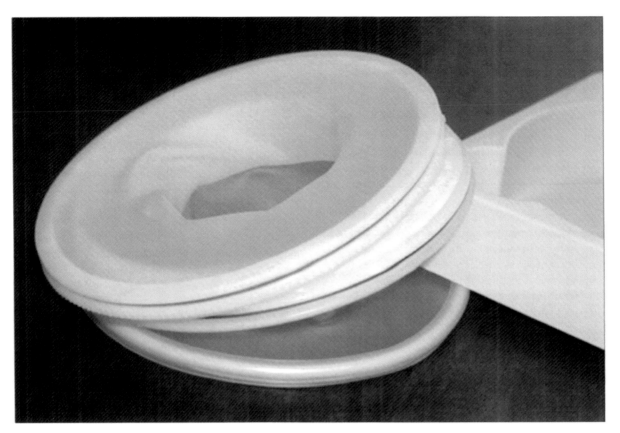

Figure 13.2
The Lap Disc device has an adjustable iris which can tighten around a surgeon's wrist or trocar to develop a seal. This is the least expensive hand-assist device on the market.

that need to be assembled, and insertion of the device is quick and easy. This device has the smallest footprint, fitting almost anywhere on most abdominal walls and rarely interferes with adjacent trocars. An oversized device is available for patients with thicker than normal abdominal walls. The iris that tightens around the surgeon's wrist, to develop the seal, can alternatively be tightened around a trocar or completely closed on itself to maintain the pneumoperitoneum. This iris requires meticulous adjustment around the wrist. If it is too tight, the hand will quickly tire and become painful; if too loose, the device will leak. When removing the hand from the abdomen the iris must be adequately loosened or the Lap Disc will inadvertently be removed. Pneumoperitoneum is lost when the hand is removed but can easily be re-established by quickly closing the iris.

The OmniPort (Figure 13.3) is an inflatable device, which maintains an excellent seal and rarely becomes dislodged once it is inserted. As with the GelPort and Lap Disc, the surgeon can rapidly remove and reinsert his hand, which is a major advantage for resident teaching programs when the teaching surgeon must quickly take over the case to avert or manage a potential complication. The device can be insufflated to maintain pneumoperitoneum without the hand

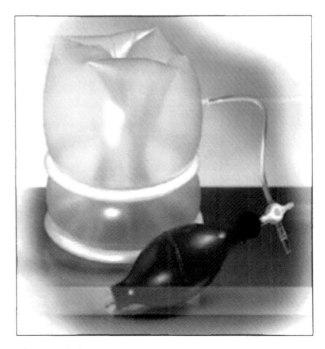

Figure 13.3
The OmniPort device maintains an excellent seal via an inflatable mechanism.

being inserted, but an accessory trocar or instrument cannot be inserted through the device. Unfortunately, the device can be difficult to insert. Additionally, care must be taken to ensure that the bowel or omentum is not caught under the rigid inner ring, which is unforgiving and can easily damage soft tissue.

The inflatable HandPort (Figure 13.4) is probably the most comfortable device, as there are no rigid pieces to rub against the wrist or forearm. Unfortunately, without a rigid inner ring, the device can easily become dislodged. To develop a seal around the arm, the surgeon must wear a sleeve that attaches at the wrist and is covered by a second glove. This sleeve weds the surgeon to the device and makes insertion or removal of the hand and switching surgeons more complicated and time consuming. Additionally, removal of the sleeve from the device does cause immediate loss of pneumoperitoneum. This device has an available insert that can be used to maintain pneumoperitoneum without insertion of the hand and can be used for insertion of an accessory trocar or instrument.

As with all forms of minimally invasive surgery, products will continue to change and improve. It is not practical or cost-effective for any one operating room to have all products available. Surgeons performing hand-assisted laparoscopy should periodically evaluate the hand-access devices available and select the one or two devices they feel are best suited for their needs.

Trocar and hand–port configuration

We have used the following hand incision and trocar configurations successfully in over 500 cases with little modification. Numerous factors must be considered when determining the optimal positioning of trocars and the hand incision. These factors include the specific operation being performed, the patient's anatomy, the surgeon's experience, and the surgeon's hand and forearm size.

The patient is positioned in the semilateral decubitus position and secured to the table with 3 inch cloth tape across the shoulders, hips, and legs (Figure 13.5). At the start of the case, the table is rolled so that the patient is in a near-supine position. Placement of the hand incision is made with the patient in this position, as this allows for easier access to the peritoneal cavity and ensures better cosmetic results, especially in obese patients.

The midline should always be marked, which aids in trocar placement as well as provides a quick and accurate guide if emergent laparotomy is necessary. The use of 12 mm trocars in all port sites enables the camera and endoscopic stapler to be placed through any trocar to allow maximum flexibility. For a right-sided nephrectomy, a 5 mm trocar is used in the right upper quadrant for placement of a liver retractor, as a camera or stapler would never be used at this site.

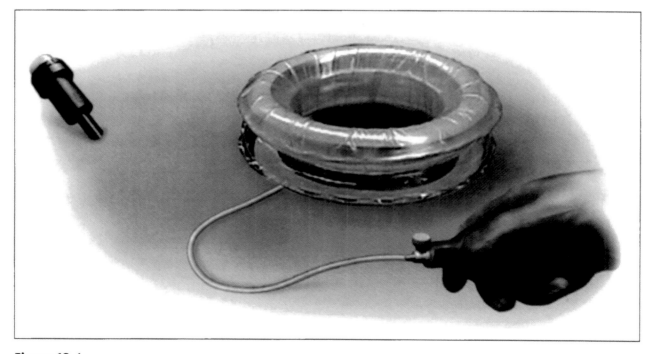

Figure 13.4
The inflatable HandPort device does not have a rigid inner ring, making it very comfortable for the surgeon. However, the HandPort is easily dislodged.

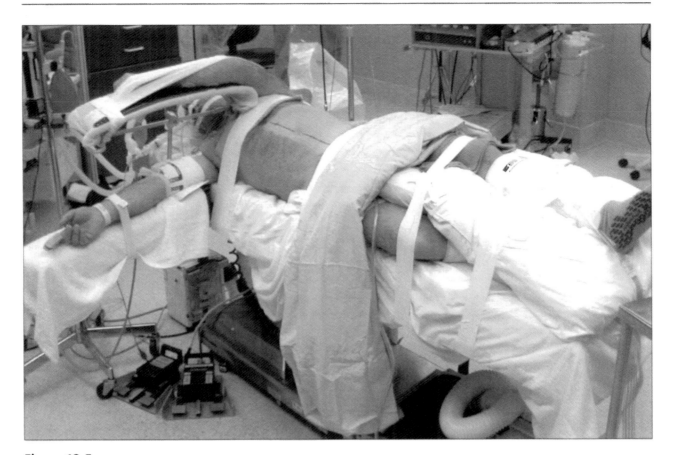

Figure 13.5
Patient positioning for the hand-assist laparoscopic nephrectomy is the semi-lateral decubitus position.

The length of the hand incision in centimeters is usually equal to the surgeon's glove size. Once the incision is made and the peritoneal cavity is entered, test the size and length of the incision for comfort. If the incision is too small, paresthesias and cramping of the surgeon's hand can result, which will make the operation more difficult. Too large of an incision may result in the hand device becoming dislodged and loss of the pneumoperitoneum.

The renal hilum is approximately 8–12 cm superior to the umbilicus, but this distance can vary widely based on the patient's body habitus and vascular anatomy. Examine the patient's computed tomography (CT) scan and calculate this distance by counting the number of tomographic images between the renal hilum and the umbilicus. If the distance is greater than 12 cm, the surgeon has short arms, the patient is obese, or the girth of the abdominal cavity is larger than normal, consider moving the hand incision cephalad, which allows improved access to the renal hilum.

The hand incision should be at such a distance from the operative target as to allow insertion of the entire hand and wrist into the peritoneal cavity. The surgeon's wrist should have free range of motion and the fingertips should comfortably reach the renal hilum (the most important part of the dissection). If the hand incision is placed too close to the kidney, the hand will not be able to be completely inserted into the abdominal cavity, losing maneuverability of the wrist and fingers. The hand will act more as a retractor and less optimally as a dissector.

Attempt to place the hand incision as low as possible on the abdominal cavity, as this will result in decreased postoperative discomfort and respiratory compromise. Additionally, always try to avoid cutting muscle fibers, as this will reduce postoperative morbidity and reduce the risk of incisional hernias. We use a low midline or periumbilical hand incision for a left nephrectomy and a muscle-splitting right lower quadrant incision for a right nephrectomy.

For a right-sided nephrectomy (Figure 13.6), the hand incision is placed in the right lower quadrant lateral to the rectus muscle, just below the level of the umbilicus. The skin is incised in line with the external oblique fascial fibers and the abdominal wall musculature is split. In a small percentage of right-sided cases, the incision is made in line with the internal oblique fibers and shifted more cephalad. This alteration gives the surgeon the option to extend the incision cephalad and medially, creating a low lateral subcostal incision if the case cannot be completed laparoscopically. One must keep in mind that if emergent conversion is required, an incision should be made in a location that will allow most efficient and safe management of the

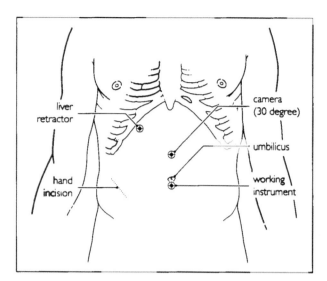

Figure 13.6
Trocar and hand–port placement: right. The hand-assisted device for right-sided nephrectomy is placed in the right lower quadrant lateral to the rectus muscle, just below the level of the umbilicus.

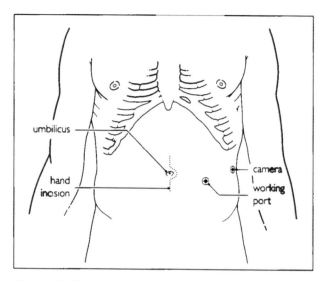

Figure 13.7
Trocar and hand–port placement: left. The hand-assist device for left-sided nephrectomy is placed in the infraumbilical or periumbilical region.

situation at hand. Do not try to manage a complication or difficult case through an extended hand incision if it will not offer optimal exposure.

After insertion of the hand-assist device, the working instrument port is placed just below or above the umbilicus and the camera port is placed in the supra-umbilical midline, approximately 6–8 cm cephalad to the working trocar. The camera and working instruments may be switched at any time to facilitate the dissection. A third port is placed in the right midclavicular line at the costal margin, which allows placement of a liver retractor. Placement of this port more medially will result in the liver retractor leaning against the gallbladder, potentially causing injury.

For a left-sided nephrectomy (Figure 13.7), the hand port is placed midline in the infraumbilical or periumbilical region. The camera port is placed in the anterior axillary line at the level of the umbilicus while the working instrument port is placed in the midclavicular line, just below the level of the umbilicus. For very large upper pole tumors an additional superior midclavicular working port may be used for the most cephalad part of the dissection. Adequate mobilization of the spleen obviates the need for a splenic retraction port.

In morbidly obese patients or patients with very rotund and protuberant abdominal walls, the hand and trocar template is shifted lateral and cephalad. In a left-sided nephrectomy, the hand incision is placed lateral to the rectus muscle belly and the two trocar sites are moved approximately equidistance lateral to their standard locations. In a right-sided nephrectomy, the hand-access incision and trocar sites can be moved lateral any distance, as

the hand-access incision is already lateral to the rectus muscle belly.

In almost all cases we start out by making the hand incision and inserting the hand-access device and trocars prior to establishing a pneumoperitoneum. In cases where there is a high index of suspicion for significant adhesions, the hand incision allows direct visualization of the abdominal cavity and open surgical lysis of adhesions. Taking down extensive intra-abdominal adhesions through the hand incision can save a significant amount of time as compared to using a purely laparoscopic technique.

Another option is to initially establish the pneumoperitoneum using a Hasson trocar or Veress needle and inspect the peritoneal cavity using the laparoscope. This allows the surgeon to identify adhesions and appreciate variations of anatomy that may alter the positioning of the hand-assist device and/or trocars. We stopped using this technique after our first 100 cases as we found that the placement of our hand incision and trocar placement was rarely if ever modified.

Once the pneumoperitoneum is established, it is maintained at a pressure of 12–15 mmHg as per standard laparoscopy.

Stepwise dissection technique
Left radical nephrectomy

The colon is released from the lateral sidewall by incising the white line of Toldt. Dissection is carried out from the splenic flexure to the iliac vessels. The colon is reflected medially using the back of the hand, while the fingertips help dissect the mesocolon off of the anterior aspect of Gerota's fascia. Dissection is continued in the cephalad direction, freeing the splenic flexure and releasing the splenorenal ligaments. The lateral attachments from the body sidewall to the spleen are now released up to the level of the gastric fundus, which allows the entire spleen and splenic flexure to fall medially. Do not release the lateral attachments of the kidney to the body sidewall, as these attachments are used for countertraction, which aids in the medial dissection of the renal hilum. The plane between the tail of the pancreas and the anterior aspect of Gerota's fascia is then developed, which allows the tail of the pancreas to rotate medially with the spleen. The back of the hand is used as an atraumatic retractor on the spleen and the pancreas, while the fingertips aid in dissection. Care is taken to leave the entire anterior aspect of Gerota's fascia intact. The colon and mesocolon are mobilized medially to allow identification of the aorta and renal hilum. Investing tissue overlying the hilar vessels is grasped with the fingertips, retracted anteriorly, and a plane between these tissues and renal vein is developed using the harmonic scalpel or scissors. Once the anterior wall of the renal vein is exposed, meticulous dissection allows identification of both the gonadal vein and left adrenal vein entering the renal vein. These veins are dissected free of their surrounding tissues and doubly clipped both proximally and distally.

In some cases we choose not to clip and divide the gonadal and adrenal vessels at this point in the procedure, as we do not want to have clips potentially interfere with the subsequent firing of the linear stapling device across the renal vein later in the case. In other cases the anatomy may be favorable for dividing the renal vein proximal to the adrenal vein, obviating the need for division of the adrenal and gonadal veins as long as the surgeon plans on removal of the adrenal gland with the kidney.

At this point, the surgeon must not be tempted to continue dissection of the renal vasculature from this anterior approach. The key to the success of the HALN is obtaining the vascular control from a posterior approach, which allows the fingertips to surround the renal hilum, helping with palpation, dissection, and control of the renal artery and vein. In a very rare case the main renal artery will be easily accessible anteriorly and should obviously be ligated and divided at this point in the procedure.

Dissection now continues at the most inferior lateral portion of Gerota's fascia, identifying the body sidewall and psoas muscle. The fingertips and the dissecting instrument of choice, either electrocautery scissors or harmonic scalpel, are used to reflect the perinephric fat in a medial and anterior direction off the psoas muscle. The surgeon works from a lateral to medial direction, coming across the gonadal vein, which is doubly clipped, proximally and

distally with hemoclips and divided. If a radical nephrectomy is performed, the ureter is also identified, clipped and transected. Obviously, during a nephroureterectomy, the ureter is left intact. If a donor nephrectomy is being performed, the periureteral tissue is left adjacent to the ureter as well as leaving the ureter intact, and dissection of the ureter with all of its surrounding tissue is continued into the true pelvis below the iliac vessels.

The surgeon continues reflecting the inferior pole of the kidney, adjacent perinephric fat, and overlying Gerota's fascia anteriorly and medially, releasing the posterior and lateral attachments to the body sidewall and posterior wall. All lateral attachments are now released up to the level of the adrenal gland, as the kidney is reflected anteriorly and medially with the back of the hand. Care must be taken not to enter Gerota's fascia. As the lateral attachments to the inferior aspect of the diaphragm are encountered, the surgeon must be careful not to perforate through the diaphragm. If perforation occurs, rapid loss of pneumoperitoneum will occur, resulting in a tension pneumothorax. Perforations can be closed using hand-assisted laparoscopic suturing techniques; conversion to open nephrectomy may be necessary.

After releasing all lateral and posterior attachments, the kidney can be rolled anteriorly and medially, exposing the posterior aspect of the renal pedicle. The kidney should then be rolled back to its normal position and the tips of the second and third finger are placed just above the exposed anterior aspect of the renal vein. Using the thumb and dissecting instrument, the kidney is now rolled anteriorly and medially and the thumb is placed on the posterior aspect of the renal vessels (Figure 13.8). This maneuver helps identify the renal artery by direct palpation and allows for presentation of the artery to the dissecting instruments. Additionally, if bleeding is encountered, the fingers can compress the pedicle, achieving rapid hemostasis. Using curved electrocautery shears, a Maryland dissector, or a harmonic scalpel to dissect the surrounding lymphatic tissue, the posterior and inferior aspects of the renal artery are exposed. Oftentimes, a lumbar vein is seen coursing across the posterior aspect of the proximal renal artery. This lumbar vein can complicate exposure and dissection of the renal hilum, as it may tether the renal vein or obscure the renal artery. In these situations, the lumbar vein must be clipped and divided. Following this, a right-angle dissector is passed around the renal artery, completely freeing the vessel from all remaining attachments. The artery can be controlled using either three locking clips, two proximally and one distally, or by using an endoscopic linear stapling device.

After the renal artery is divided, the renal vein is freed of all surrounding lymphatic and connective tissues, and controlled using an endoscopic linear stapling device or large hemoclips. When the endoscopic stapler is used, great care must be taken not to engage any previously placed

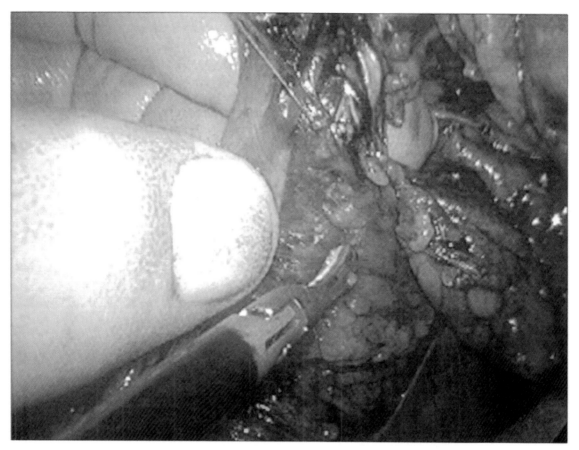

Figure 13.8
The left renal artery is localized by rolling the kidney anteriorly and medially and placing the thumb on the posterior aspect of the renal hilum. With bimanual palpation, the artery can be localized and dissected free of lymphatic tissue.

clips in between the jaws of the stapler. Both visual inspection and palpation with the hand ensures that the stapler has not engaged any extraneous tissue or clips. Engaging clips in the jaws of the stapler will cause the device to misfire, resulting in a disruption of the staple line and significant bleeding.

If the adrenal gland needs to be removed with the left kidney, attention is now directed to the most superior phrenic attachments. With the spleen completely mobilized medially, diaphragmatic attachments are identified and controlled using hemoclips or the harmonic scalpel. There is usually a single artery originating from the diaphragmatic attachment, which must be clipped for adequate control. The remaining vessels can usually be divided using the harmonic scalpel. Care must be taken to identify any accessory phrenic veins that may exist, coursing from the diaphragm along the medial aspect of the adrenal gland toward the renal vein. These structures can be easily mistaken for the adrenal vein when dissecting in the region of the superior aspect of the renal vein. The superolateral attachments from the adrenal gland to the body sidewall are left intact and the medial attachments to the aorta are divided using the harmonic scalpel and clips

when necessary. The remaining superolateral attachments and posterior attachments are now divided using the harmonic scalpel or electrocautery scissors and the specimen is completely freed.

If the adrenal gland is to be left intact, use visual inspection and palpation with the fingertips to locate the groove separating the adrenal gland from the kidney. The attachments between the adrenal gland and the superior aspect of the kidney are divided using the harmonic scalpel. If the adrenal vein has not already been divided, it should be doubly clipped proximally and distally, and sharply transected. Usually, a single large arterial branch originating from the renal artery feeds the most inferior lateral aspect of the adrenal gland. Hemoclips can be used on this vessel for adequate hemostasis.

Once dissection is complete, the kidney is removed through the hand incision. Oncologic principles are no different in the hand-assisted technique than in that of open surgery. The specimen is delivered intact, without the need for morcellation, preserving the pathologic integrity of the specimen. The hand is placed back into the abdomen and pneumoperitoneum is re-established. Adequate hemostasis should be ensured at lower insufflation pressures (5–8 mmHg), confirming vascular control of all arterial and venous structures. Renal hilar vascular stumps are re-examined and any bleeding staple lines or vascular stumps can be controlled with laparoscopic suture ligation.

Right radical nephrectomy

After insertion of the hand device and trocars as previously described, the liver retractor is inserted and the liver is retracted medially. The right lobe of the liver is released from the body sidewall by incising the triangular ligament and, if necessary, the anterior and posterior divisions of the coronary ligaments. There may also be significant attachments between the undersurface of the right lobe of the liver and the anterior/superior aspect of Gerota's fascia that must be released using the harmonic scalpel.

With the liver adequately mobilized medially, the attachments of the hepatic flexure to the overlying Gerota's fascia are released using the fingertips to develop pedicles, which are transected using the harmonic scalpel. The duodenum is now identified. If the vena cava is covered by the duodenum at the level of the renal hilum, a standard Kocher maneuver is performed using sharp dissection, mobilizing the duodenum medially off of the underlying renal hilum and vena cava. Investing tissue over the vena cava and renal vein is released and the anterior wall of the renal vein is skeletonized. The tendency will be to continue dissection on the renal hilum and vasculature at this time, but the surgeon should remember it is imperative to obtain vascular control from the posterior approach.

Posterior exposure of the renal hilum is obtained by releasing all attachments of Gerota's fascia and perinephric fat to the body wall and rotating the kidney anteriorly and medially. We start this part of the dissection by directing our attention to the perinephric fat inferior to the lower pole of the kidney. Using fingertip dissection, the psoas muscle is identified and the fingers are passed lateral to medial, raising the most caudal attachments of the kidney off of the psoas muscle. This large pedicle of tissue may include the right gonadal vein and ureter. The entire pedicle can be divided using an endoscopic linear stapling device. Alternatively, individual pedicles of fat can be divided using the harmonic scalpel, while the gonadal vein and ureter are individually clipped and sharply divided. In some cases the gonadal vein can be gently retracted medially and division of the vein is unnecessary. Attachments of Gerota's fascia and perinephric fat to the lateral and posterior body sidewall are released using the harmonic scalpel or electrocautery shears.

With the hand placed posterior to the kidney, the kidney is elevated. Any remaining inferior medial attachments to the vena cava or lower pole accessory veins are identified

and secured using clips or the harmonic scalpel. The second and third fingers are now curled behind the renal pedicle, allowing identification of the renal artery (Figure 13.9). Using gentle traction with the index finger, the artery can be pulled inferiorly and dissected free of surrounding lymphatic tissue using the harmonic scalpel, Maryland dissector, or right-angle dissector. The artery can be controlled using locking clips or an endoscopic stapling device with a vascular cartridge. The renal vein is dissected free from surrounding lymphatic and investing tissues and transected using the endoscopic stapling device.

If the adrenal gland needs to be removed with the kidney, the liver must be aggressively mobilized medially. The most superior phrenic attachments and vessels feeding the adrenal gland should now be controlled and ligated with clips or the harmonic scalpel. The superolateral attachments should be left intact and dissection should continue along the vena cava, releasing medial attachments. The adrenal vein will now be easily identified and should be ligated using large hemoclips and sharply divided. The remaining posterior and lateral attachments can easily be transected using the harmonic scalpel.

If the adrenal gland does not need to be removed, use visual inspection and palpation with the fingertips to locate the groove separating the adrenal gland from the kidney. The attachments are divided using the harmonic scalpel.

Comparison of open, laparoscopic, and hand-assisted renal surgery

Since the first laparoscopic nephrectomy was reported in 1991, the urologic community has increasingly accepted laparoscopic approaches for many urologic conditions.[9] This acceptance has been fostered by numerous articles demonstrating certain advantages to laparoscopic surgery, particularly decreased postoperative pain and a quicker recovery time to normal activity. In examining whether a new surgical technique is appropriate, one must address the technique's outcomes, morbidities, and costs. Many factors may affect more than one of these criteria: e.g. operative times may affect both morbidity and cost. If outcome, morbidity, and cost results are acceptable, one must then determine whether the new technique is transferable to other surgeons and institutions. Although such comparisons of different procedures are often difficult to interpret, certain trends are apparent when one examines open, laparoscopy, and hand-assisted laparoscopic (HAL) renal surgery.

For a purely ablative procedure, results demonstrate laparoscopic and HAL approaches are as efficacious as

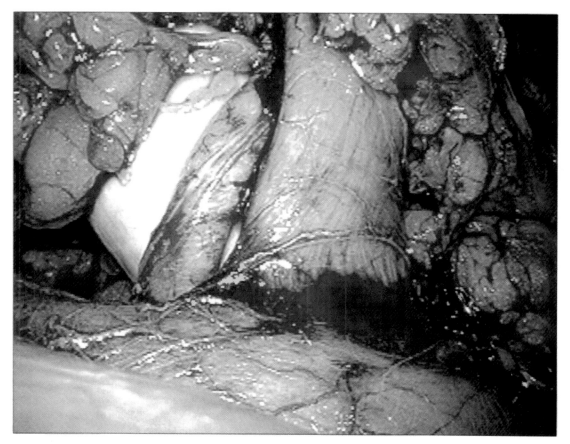

Figure 13.9
Localization of the right renal artery by placing the second and third fingers behind the renal pedicle. Utilizing gentle inferior retraction with the index finger, the artery is freed from its surrounding lymphatic tissue with the harmonic scalpel.

open surgery. With 5 year follow-up, Portis et al demonstrated equal oncologic effectiveness for open and laparoscopic radical nephrectomy.[10] This had also been similarly demonstrated by Ono et al in 2001 for renal masses less than 5 cm.[11] Two-year follow-up data for laparoscopic and HAL nephroureterectomy is also encouraging.[4,12] However, long-term (> 5 years) oncology outcomes are not available for HAL radical nephrectomy.

Laparoscopic partial nephrectomy can be daunting because of the potential for large blood loss and the need for reconstruction, which can be difficult. However, the laparoscopic procedure has been shown to have good pathologic outcomes, and HAL potentially facilitates hemostasis and suturing.[13,14]

Numerous studies have demonstrated equivalent graft function for open, laparoscopic, and HAL donor nephrectomy.[15,16] A randomized trial of HAL vs open donor nephrectomy clearly demonstrated less analgesic use, shorter hospital stay, and quicker return to normal activity in the HAL group.[17] Similarly, shorter hospital stays and quicker returns to normal activity were seen when HAL radical nephrectomy was compared to open radical nephrectomy.[18] Postoperative complications were similar

across all groups in each of these studies. Numerous other studies have similarly shown quicker recoveries for HAL compared to open surgery. The biggest area of controversy is currently whether laparoscopic nephrectomy, particularly with morcellation, offers improved convalescence compared to HAL. Several studies suggest this is not the case.

Despite larger tumors in the HAL group, a nonrandomized study by Nelson and Wolf demonstrated equal recovery and morbidity in the HAL and morcellated laparoscopic groups.[19] A comparison of open, laparoscopic, and HAL donor nephrectomy showed equally shorter recovery times with laparoscopic and HAL nephrectomy.[16] During laparoscopic nephrectomy, no differences are seen in postoperative pain or hospital stay, whether a specimen is morcellated or removed intact.[20] Thus, HAL and laparoscopic renal surgery appear to be equivalent when examining postoperative recovery.

Cost analysis, while important, is a very difficult issue to address. Some studies have demonstrated increased costs associated with laparoscopic procedures due to instrument costs, whereas other studies have shown decreased costs due to decreased hospital stays.[21,22] The issue becomes even more confusing once physician time, patient work hours lost/gained, etc. are entered into the equation. Each element in the process (patient, surgeon, institution, etc.) will have a different cost/benefit ratio that should be considered, although absolute values will always be lacking.

While HAL and laparoscopic renal surgery show similar benefits, HAL is a more easily mastered technique and can be utilized in situations where laparoscopy alone may not be sufficient. Overcoming the lack of three-dimensional viewing is very difficult for the novice laparoscopist; HAL allows the surgeon's hand to be in the operative field and can compensate for the two-dimensional view. Open surgeons are not accustomed to operating with the long instruments and fulcrum points needed for laparoscopy; surgeons are comfortable dissecting and retracting with their open hand. HAL can also be helpful for large renal tumors that might not be as easily removed with straight laparoscopy. We have removed tumors up to 22 cm with HAL and feel nephrectomy under these conditions is more easily performed with HAL than laparoscopy. Together, these factors describe a technique that is more easily learned and can be more widely applied than standard laparoscopy.

References

1. Bannenberg JJ, Meijer DW, Bannenberg JH, Hodde KC. Hand-assisted laparoscopic nephrectomy in the pig: initial report. Minim Invasive Ther Allied Technol 1996; 5:483–7.

2. Nakada SY, Moon TD, Gist M, Mahivi D. Use of the pneumo sleeve as an adjunct in laparoscopic nephrectomy. Urology 1997; 49(4):612–3.

3. Slakey DP, Wood JC, Hender D, et al. Laparoscopic living donor nephrectomy: advantages of the hand-assisted method. Transplantation 1999; 68:581.

4. Stifelman MD, Sosa RE, Andrade A, et al. Hand-assisted laparoscopic nephroureterectomy for the treatment of transitional cell carcinoma of the upper urinary tract. Urology 2000; 56:741.

5. Wolf JS, Seifman BD, Montie JE. Nephron sparing surgery for suspected malignancy: open surgery compared to laparoscopy with selective use of hand assistance. J Urol 2000; 163:1659–64.

6. Wolf JS Jr., Moon TD, Nakada SY. Hand assisted laparoscopic nephrectomy: comparison to standard laparoscopic nephrectomy. J Urol 1998; 160:22.

7. Wolf JS, Jr, Tchetgen MB, Merion RM. Hand-assisted laparoscopic live donor nephrectomy. Urology 1998; 52:885.

8. Clayman RV. Ramon Guiteras Lecture. American Urologic Association Convention, 2000.

9. Clayman R., Kavoussi LR, Soper NJ, et al. Laparoscopic nephrectomy: initial case report. J Urol 1991; 146: 278.

10. Portis AJ, Yan Y, Landman J, et al. Long-term followup after laparoscopic radical nephrectomy. J Urol 2002; 167:1257

11. Ono Y, Kinukawa T, Hattori R, et al. The long-term outcome of laparoscopic radical nephrectomy for small renal cell carcinoma. J Urol 2001; 165:1867.

12. El Fettouh HA, Rassweiler JJ, Schulze M, et al. Laparoscopic radical nephroureterectomy: results of an international multicenter study. Eur Urol 2002; 42:447.

13. Gill IS, Matin SF, Desai MM, et al. Comparative analysis of laparoscopic versus open partial nephrectomy for renal tumors in 200 patients. J Urol 2003; 170:64.

14. Stifelman MD, Sosa RE, Nakada SY, et al. Hand-assisted laparoscopic partial nephrectomy. J Endourol 2001; 15:161.

15. Ratner, LE, Montgomery RA, Kavoussi LR. Laparoscopic live donor nephrectomy. A review of the first 5 years. Urol Clin North Am 2001; 28:709.

16. Ruiz-Deya G, Cheng S, Palmer E, et al. Open donor, laparoscopic donor and hand assisted laparoscopic donor nephrectomy: a comparison of outcomes. J Urol 2001; 166:1270.

17. Wolf JS Jr., Merion RM, Leichtman AB, et al. Randomized controlled trial of hand-assisted laparoscopic versus open surgical live donor nephrectomy. Transplantation, 2001; 72:284.

18. Nakada SY, Fadden P, Jarrard DF, et al. Hand-assisted laparoscopic radical nephrectomy: comparison to open radical nephrectomy. Urology 2001; 58:517.

19. Nelson CP, Wolf JS Jr.. Comparison of hand assisted versus standard laparoscopic radical nephrectomy for suspected renal cell carcinoma. J Urol 2002; 167:1989.

20. Hernandez F, Rha KH, Pinto PA, et al. Laparoscopic nephrectomy: assessment of morcellation versus intact specimen extraction on postoperative status. J Urol 2003; 170:412.

21. Meraney AM, Gill IS. Financial analysis of open versus laparoscopic radical nephrectomy and nephroureterectomy. J Urol 2002; 167:1757.

22. Velidedeoglu E, Williams N, Brayman KL, et al. Comparison of open, laparoscopic, and hand-assisted approaches to live-donor nephrectomy. Transplantation 2002; 74:169.

14

Minimally invasive treatment to treat begign and malignant adrenal disorders

David S Wang, Blake D Hamilton, and Howard N Winfield

Since being first reported by Gagner et al. in 1992,[1] laparoscopic adrenalectomy has become an established procedure. Several comparative studies[2–9] have demonstrated the advantages of the laparoscopic approach to include decreased blood loss, less postoperative pain, shorter hospitalization, faster convalescence, and even cost-effectiveness.[10] As experience with laparoscopic adrenalectomy has been increasing, the indications for this procedure have expanded while the absolute contraindications for its use have diminished. Indeed, laparoscopic adrenalectomy has become a standard of care and the technique of choice for most benign adrenal lesions.

This chapter reviews the preoperative considerations, indications, technique, complications, and results of laparoscopic adrenalectomy.

Diagnosis

Historically, adrenal lesions were diagnosed secondary to clinical manifestations of endocrinopathies. However, widespread use of abdominal ultrasound, computed tomography (CT) scans, and magnetic resonance imaging (MRI) has led to the rather frequent finding of the incidental adrenal mass. Figures 14.1 and 14.2 show typical examples of adrenal lesions diagnosed on CT and MRI, respectively. The differential diagnosis of the incidental adrenal mass is wide and includes the benign nonfunctioning adenoma, hormonally active cortical tumor, myelolipoma, pheochromocytoma, adrenocortical carcinoma, and metastatic lesion.

Tumors diagnosed incidentally on CT scans or MRI are managed according to size and hormone functional status.

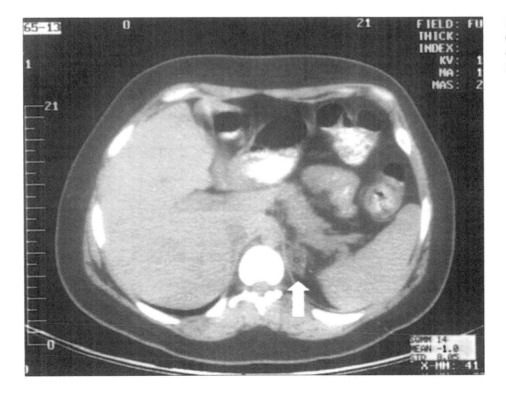

Figure 14.1
CT scan of the abdomen demonstrating left adrenal lesion (arrow).

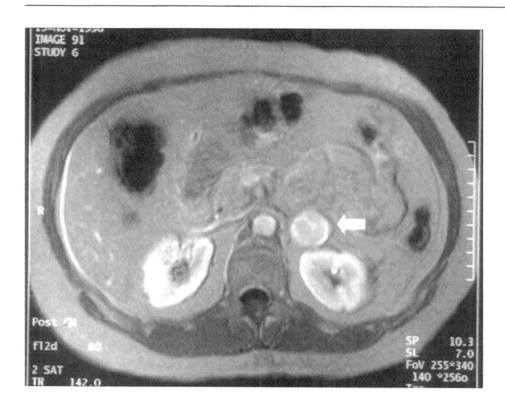

Figure 14.2
MRI of the abdomen demonstrating left adrenal lesion (arrow).

Patients with hormonally active adrenal tumors, such as aldosteronoma, Cushing's syndrome, or pheochromocytoma, should generally undergo surgical removal. Hormonal evaluation of these patients is critical because pre- and postoperative considerations regarding hypertensive control, electrolyte imbalances, and fluid shifts are paramount to ensure good surgical outcomes and minimize complications. A summary of standard laboratory tests in the evaluation of an adrenal lesion is listed in Table 14.1. Most hormonally active tumors should be removed, particularly in the case of pheochromocytoma and cortisol-secreting tumors.[11,12] Occasionally, medical management of aldosteronomas may be satisfactory to circumvent the need for surgical management, particularly in patients who are poor surgical candidates.[13] However side-effects of pharmacotherapy may become intolerable.

Hormonally inactive tumors have traditionally been managed according to size. Tumors less than 3 cm in size are almost always benign adenomas and generally require no further treatment unless clinical signs of hormonal activity develop. Tumors greater than 6 cm in size are worrisome for adrenocortical carcinomas, and thus surgical excision is recommended given the aggressive nature of adrenal cancer.[14] Nonfunctional lesions between 3 and 6 cm in size generally require close follow-up with serial imaging studies every 6 months. These lesions should be removed if tumors demonstrate interval change in appearance or develop endocrine activity.

As mentioned previously, lesions of the adrenal gland greater than 6 cm in size are worrisome for adrenal cancer.

In one meta-analysis, 105 of 114 adrenocortical carcinomas measured 6 cm or greater in diameter.[15] Because a CT scan can underestimate the size of lesions by as much as 1 cm,[16] it is suggested that all lesions on CT scan which

Table 14.1 *Routine laboratory tests useful in the evaluation of adrenal lesions*
Cushing's syndrome
24-hour urine cortisol
Plasma ACTH and plasma cortisol
Low-dose dexamethasone suppression test
High-dose dexamethasone suppression test
Metapyrone stimulation test
Petrosal sinus ACTH measurement
Hyperaldosteronism
Unprovoked hypokalemia
Plasma aldosterone level
Urinary aldosterone level
Aldosterone-to-renin ratio
Postural stimulation test
Adrenal vein sampling of aldosterone
Pheochromocytoma
Plasma catecholamines
Urine catecholamines
Clonidine suppression test
Adrenal vein sampling of catecholamines

ACTH, adrenocorticotropic hormone.

are 5 cm or greater in size be removed. In cases when there is concern for adrenal carcinoma with local extension into adjacent organs such as the kidney, colon, or spleen, open radical adrenalectomy with possible en bloc resection of adjacent organs is the preferred approach.[17,18] More recently, improvements in radiologic imaging techniques such as unenhanced CT with densitometry, delayed enhanced CT with densitometry, chemical-shift MRI, and NP-59 scintigraphy have further assisted in differentiating benign from malignant neoplasms.[19]

Indications for laparoscopic adrenalectomy

The indications for laparoscopic adrenalectomy have expanded as more surgeons have become proficient with the technique and the advantages of this approach have become apparent. Laparoscopic adrenalectomy has in many centers become the surgical procedure of choice for the management of functional tumors less than 6 cm in size. Although the presence of pheochromocytoma was a relative contraindication for laparoscopic adrenalectomy in the past, it is clear that the procedure can be performed safely as long as the same precautions are taken as those for open surgery.[20] The current indications for performing a laparoscopic adrenalectomy are listed in Table 14.2.

There are very few absolute contraindications to laparoscopic adrenalectomy. It is generally felt that a known or suspected primary adrenal carcinoma, particularly with extension into surrounding organs, should be removed by an open technique. Given the aggressive nature of the disease, the open approach allows for en bloc resection and potential removal of surrounding organs.[17] The 5-year survival of completely vs incompletely resected primary adrenocortical carcinoma is 55% vs 5%,[21] respectively. The potential for surgical cure or improved survival should not be compromised for the sake of decreasing patient morbidity. Other contraindications to laparoscopic adrenalectomy include uncorrectable coagulopathy and

cardiopulmonary disease precluding general anesthesia. Patients who will not tolerate an open operation are generally poor candidates for laparoscopic adrenalectomy.

Relative contraindications to laparoscopic adrenalectomy include previous abdominal surgery or significant morbidity. Lesions greater than 8 cm in size, even if not suspected to be primary adrenal carcinomas, should be approached cautiously because of the increased risk of hemorrhage and injury to surrounding viscera. With increasing experience in performing laparoscopic adrenalectomy, relative contraindications become less of a factor. In addition, a variety of approaches to laparoscopic adrenalectomy, including transperitoneal and retroperitoneal, have further decreased some of the relative contraindications.

Occasionally, the urologist will encounter a patient with a suspected solitary metastatic lesion to the adrenal gland. If the lesion is less than 6 cm in size and not obviously adherent to surrounding viscera, a laparoscopic approach is reasonable.[22] The surgeon should be already skilled in laparoscopic adrenalectomy before attempting to remove a solitary metastatic lesion given the more difficult surgical planes that are often present.

Preoperative patient evaluation and preparation

Careful preoperative control and management of hormonally active tumors is critical prior to performing adrenal surgery, whether laparoscopic or open. Inadequate preoperative control of hormonally active lesions can lead to catastrophic intraoperative consequences. Close collaboration with an endocrinologist and anesthesiologist experienced with adrenal disorders is helpful. The urologist should have an understanding of the physiology of adrenal disorders in order to appropriately manage patients in the peri- and postoperative period with regard to fluid management, electrolyte abnormalities, and blood pressure control. Hormonally functional tumors must be adequately

Table 14.2 *Indications for laparoscopic adrenalectomy*

- Adlosterone-secreting adrenal gland, adenoma, or unilateral hyperplasia
- Cushing's syndrome secondary to adrenocortical adenoma
- Nonfunctional adrenal mass ≤ 8 cm with negative metastatic work-up
- Nonfunctional adrenal mass ≤ 8 cm with progressive growth on CT or MRI
- Adrenal pheochromocytoma (benign) ≤ 8 cm
- Solitary adrenal gland metastasis

evaluated and appropriate preoperative interventions initiated in concert with an endocrinologist.

Preoperatively, all patients should receive a mechanical bowel preparation. Clear liquids should be started the day before surgery. A broad-spectrum antibiotic should be administered on call to the operating room.

Aldosteronomas

Primary hyperaldosterononism (Conn's syndrome) is a rare etiology of hypertension (less than 1%). Other clinical manifestations of Conn's syndrome arise from increased total body sodium content and a deficit in total body potassium. Symptoms include lower urinary tract symptoms, muscle weakness, paresthesias, or visual disturbances.[13,23] CT scan or MRI can detect adrenal adenomas as small as 1 cm. Laboratory manifestations include hypokalemia, elevated plasma and urinary aldosterone level, elevated serum aldosterone-to-renin ratio, and suppressed plasma renin activity.[13,23] Once an important part of the evaluation, adrenal vein sampling is now occasionally used to confirm and localize the lesion.

Once the diagnosis is confirmed, medical control of hypertension and correction of hypokalemia should be instituted at least several weeks prior to adrenalectomy. The most effective medication for management of hyperaldosteronism is spironolactone, a competitive antagonist of the aldosterone receptor.[13] Side-effects of spironolactone include hyperkalemia, sexual dysfunction, gynecomastia, gastrointestinal disturbances, and metabolic acidosis.[24] Alternative medications include potassium-sparing diuretics, calcium channel blockers, and converting enzyme inhibitors.[23] Hypertension is improved or cured in more than 90% of patients following adrenalectomy.[25]

Cushing's syndrome

Cushing's syndrome is used to describe the symptom complex that results from excess circulating glucocorticoids, regardless of etiology.[12] Nonadrenal causes of hypercortisolism include pituitary adenomas, ectopic corticotropin production, and exogenous steroid use. The urologist is most often confronted with an adrenal lesion as the etiology of Cushing's syndrome.

Cushing's syndrome manifests with a variety of well-recognized clinical features, including hypertension, truncal obesity, moon facies, easy bruising, and mood disorders. Diagnosis is confirmed by laboratory testing.[12] Hypercortisolism is best diagnosed by 24-hour urinary cortisol measurement. The low-dose dexamethasone suppression test can be used to further diagnose Cushing's syndrome if urinary cortisol measurement is equivocal.

Abdominal CT scan and MRI are used to identify adrenal adenomas or bilateral adrenal hyperplasia.

Adrenal adenomas causing Cushing's syndrome are very amenable to laparoscopic adrenalectomy. Open adrenal surgery is associated with significant perioperative morbidity, which results from the sequelae of chronic hypercortisolism. This presents as compromised wound healing, higher infection rate, diabetes, and increased risk of cardiopulmonary complications.

Pheochromocytoma

Pheochromocytomas can be challenging tumors to treat because of the unique manifestations of chronic and acute catecholamine excess. Once considered a relative contraindication to laparoscopic surgery, laparoscopic adrenalectomy for pheochromocytomas has now been performed successfully and reported in several series.[20,26,27] Successful laparoscopic adrenalectomy for pheochromocytoma involves close collaboration with the surgeon, endocrinologist, and anesthesiologist. Catecholamine excess results in hypertension, tachycardia, and a host of clinical manifestations. Laboratory diagnosis is made by elevated levels of catecholamines in the blood and urine. Radiographic diagnosis is achieved with either CT scan or MRI. MRI imaging classically demonstrates a bright image on a T2-weighted study.

Preoperative medical preparation includes optimal control of blood pressure with alpha blockade or calcium channel antagonists.[11] Beta-blockers may be used to control reflex tachycardia after initiation of the alpha blockade. In addition, aggressive fluid expansion is necessary to increase circulating plasma volume and prevent postoperative hypotension. Close monitoring intraoperatively includes careful attention to blood pressure, central venous pressure, and urinary output. An arterial line and central venous line are routinely used, and occasionally a Swan-Ganz catheter is employed. Severe hypertension can be controlled with sodium nitropusside or phentolamine, and hypotension controlled with fluid resuscitation and norepinephrine.

Surgical technique

Perhaps no other urologic laparoscopic procedure has as many different surgical approaches as does adrenalectomy. Commonly used approaches to the adrenal gland include the transperitoneal approaches, and the posterior and lateral retroperitoneal approaches. Recently, a transthoracic approach has been described for patients who have undergone extensive previous transperitoneal and retroperitoneal surgery.[28] Surgeon preference and experience appear to be the most important factors in determining the approach. Most surgeons are familiar with the anterior transperitoneal approach, but many who have overcome the learning curve of the anterior transperitoneal approach are becoming skilled with the retroperitoneal approach.[29–34] Although each approach has purported advantages and disadvantages, there is no clear-cut evidence that one is superior.[35,36]

Laparoscopic surgical anatomy

A thorough knowledge of the anatomy of the adrenal gland and its relationship to adjacent organs is essential to avoid intraoperative complications. Familiarity with the vascular supply of the adrenal gland is important in minimizing the chances of intraoperative hemorrhage. The adrenal gland, like the kidney, is enveloped by Gerota's fascia; it is, however, located in a distinct fascial compartment that is separate from the kidney. The arterial supply to the adrenal gland arises from the inferior phrenic artery, aorta, and renal artery. A complex arcade of small arteries enters the adrenal gland from the medial and superior border of the gland, and thus the anterior, posterior, and inferolateral surfaces of the adrenal gland are relatively avascular.

The right and left adrenal gland have key anatomic differences in location and vasculature. The main right adrenal vein exits the gland from the superomedial surface and enters the inferior vena cava (IVC) directly. The longer left main adrenal vein exits the inferomedial aspect of the gland and drains into the left renal vein at an oblique angle. The right adrenal gland is more intimately related to the IVC than the left gland is related to the aorta. The capsule surrounding the adrenal gland is very fragile, and direct grasping of the adrenal gland can lead to parenchymal fracture resulting in persistent and troublesome bleeding. The lymphatic drainage of the adrenal gland includes all lateral aortic lymph node tissue between the diaphragm and ipsilateral renal artery. Regional lymphadenectomy is thus very challenging to perform laparoscopically.

Anterior transperitoneal approach for right adrenalectomy

After general anesthesia by agents other than nitrous oxide, the patient is positioned with the right side elevated 45–70° upward and the table slightly flexed at the level of the umbilicus. The patient should be positioned on a beanbag with extensive padding over pressure points. Figure 14.3

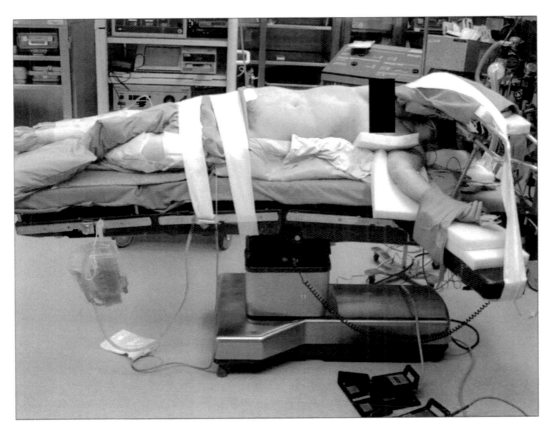

Figure 14.3
Patient positioning for right transperitoneal adrenalectomy.

shows the general modified flank position used for laparo-scopic adrenalectomy. Next, the patient should be secured with tape to allow the table to be tilted side to side to facil-itate exposure. A catheter is placed to drain the bladder, and an orogastric tube to decompress the stomach.

For a right laparoscopic adrenalectomy, four subcostal ports are used and placed two to three fingerbreadths below the costal margin, as depicted in Figure 14.4. Initial entry into the peritoneal cavity is made using the Veress needle just below the costal margin in the midclavicular line. Three additional ports are placed under direct vision; the most medial port is important for upward and medial retraction of the right lobe of the liver. Exposure of the right adrenal gland is dependent upon adequate mobilization of the liver.

Mobilization of the liver is the first step in exposing the right adrenal gland. Unlike laparoscopic nephrectomy, full mobilization of the ascending colon and hepatic flexure is unnecessary. Incision of the posterior peritoneum and extension through the triangular ligaments of the liver allow for upward and medial retraction of the liver (Figure 14.5).

The IVC is eventually identified once there is adequate liver mobilization. Continued and careful dissection along the lateral surface of the IVC will reveal the right adrenal vein (Figure 14.6). The adrenal vein should then be divided between standard clips. Dissection is further continued towards the diaphragm, and the inferior phrenic vessels should next be identified and divided.

The inferior pedicle of the adrenal gland is then released, separating the adrenal gland from the upper pole of the kidney. Gerota's fascia is next incised at the junction of the upper pole of the kidney and the adrenal gland. There is often an arterial branch to the adrenal gland arising from the renal pedicle. Once the kidney is completely mobilized away from the adrenal gland, all that

remains holding the adrenal gland in place is the relatively avascular lateral attachments, which are divided. Use of the harmonic scalpel can facilitate mobilization of the adrenal gland once the main vascular pedicles have been ligated.

Once the adrenal gland is completely separated, it should be placed in a specimen retrieval bag and removed en bloc. Assuming adequate hemostasis, the laparoscopic

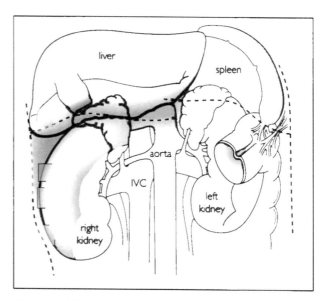

Figure 14.5
T-shaped incision through the posterior peritoneum for left and right adrenalectomy. On the right, incision from second part of the duodenum to triangular ligaments at liver edge and then lateral to hepatic flexure. On the left, incision developed across phrenocolic and splenocolic ligaments and at the inferior border of the spleen. IVC = inferior vena cava.

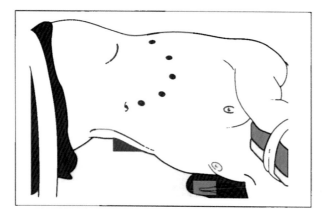

Figure 14.4
Trocar placement for a right transperitoneal adrenalectomy. An umbilical trocar is used for the camera. Other trocars are placed at the anterior axillary line and mid axillary line and are used for resection of the right adrenal gland. A fourth trocar is placed between the midline and anterior axillary line and is used for retraction of the liver.

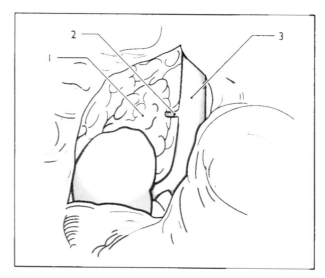

Figure 14.6
Dissection of the right adrenal gland (1). The right adrenal vein (2) is identified with careful dissection along the lateral surface of the inferior vena cava (3).

ports are removed under direct vision and the fascia closed with the Carter–Thomason fascial closure device. A drain is usually not necessary. The orogastric tube is removed at the conclusion of the procedure.

Anterior transperitoneal approach for left adrenalectomy

The patient is positioned with the left side elevated 45–70°, with the table slightly flexed at the level of the umbilicus (Figure 14.7). Three or four trocars are placed in a mirror image as for a right adrenalectomy. The important surrounding structures to identify when performing a transperitoneal left laparoscopic adrenalectomy are the spleen, the tail of the pancreas, the splenic flexure of the colon, and the left kidney. Full mobilization of the splenic flexure of the colon is necessary to provide adequate exposure to the left adrenal gland.

The first step after diagnostic laparoscopy is to incise the posterior peritoneum along the line of Toldt and mobilize the splenic flexure of the colon to allow the colon to fall medially. The splenocolic and lienorenal ligaments are then mobilized to allow the spleen to be safely separated from the field of dissection (see Figure 14.5). This creates an adequate plane between the spleen and the upper pole of the left kidney. If necessary, the tail of the pancreas can be separated away from Gerota's fascia to allow the pancreas to fall away with the spleen to provide more exposure.

Next, Gerota's fascia is incised between the upper pole of the left kidney and the adrenal gland. The left adrenal gland should not be grasped directly, to avoid adrenal

gland fractures, which are associated with troublesome bleeding. Dissection continues through the perirenal fibrofatty tissue. The inferior border of the adrenal gland is defined and the dissection continued medially. Medial dissection will eventually lead to the takeoff of the left adrenal vein emanating directly from the left renal vein. The left adrenal vein is then isolated, clipped, and divided (Figure 14.8). In the case of a pheochromocytoma, early exposure and ligation of the left adrenal vein is ideal to reduce the risk of a hypertensive crisis. We have found it easiest to initially identify the left renal vein and determine the takeoff of the left adrenal vein. Clipping of the adrenal vein at this juncture minimizes catecholamine surges.

The lateral attachments of the left adrenal gland should be saved until the remainder of the gland is mobilized. The superior aspect of the adrenal gland is then mobilized, taking care to divide the phrenic vessels supplying the gland. Once the superior and inferior borders of the gland are dissected adequately, attention is directed to the head of the gland, which is adjacent to the aorta. The left adrenal vein is divided if not previously done. The left adrenal artery arising from the aorta is next divided. The adrenal gland has a highly variable vasculature, especially in larger lesions with increased blood supply. The use of a harmonic scalpel or hook cautery electrode can facilitate adrenal gland mobilization and adequately ligate small blood vessels supplying the gland.

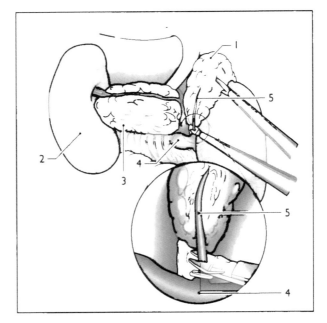

Figure 14.8
Dissection of the left adrenal gland (1). The splenocolic and lienorenal ligaments are mobilized to allow the spleen (2) to be safely separated. If necessary, the tail of the pancreas (3) can be separated from Gerota's fascia. Medial dissection of the inferior border of the adrenal gland will eventually lead to the takeoff of the left adrenal vein (4) from the left renal vein (5).

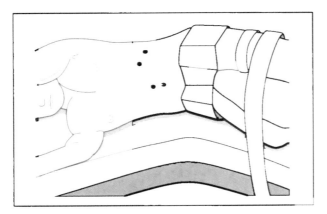

Figure 14.7
Trocar placement for left transperitoneal adrenalectomy. An umbilical trocar is used for the camera. Other trocars are placed at the anterior axillary line and mid axillary line and are used for resection of the left adrenal gland. A fourth trocar is placed between the midline and anterior axillary line and is used for retraction of the spleen.

Lastly, the lateral attachments of the adrenal gland are divided to fully free the gland from all surrounding tissues. The specimen is then placed into a retrieval bag and removed intact. Closure is similar to that for the right adrenalectomy.

Retroperitoneal technique

Patient positioning for the retroperitoneal approach differs from that for the transperitoneal approach. The patient is positioned in the full flank position with the table flexed. The primary port site is a 2 cm incision placed just below the tip of the 12th rib. A Hasson-type port is used here. Two additional ports are routine and a fourth port is optional. The port placement is similar on the right and left sides. Figure 14.9 shows the typical patient positioning and port placement for a laparoscopic retroperitoneal adrenalectomy. The laparoscope is used through the primary port. The second port is placed posterior to the primary site, just below the angle formed by the 12th rib and the vertically-oriented paraspinous muscles. The third

port is placed 3–4 cm medial and slightly superior to the primary site in the anterior axillary line, taking care to avoid the peritoneal reflection. This arrangement allows the camera to sit between the two working ports to optimize orientation. The posterior port must not be too close to the psoas muscle, as the range of motion can be limited. These ports may be 3–10 mm, depending on the surgeon's preference and availability of instruments. We generally use two 5 mm ports, one 10 mm port, and one 12 mm port. This allows for accommodation of dissecting instruments, suction, and a clip applier. The optional fourth port may be used for retraction and is placed in the anterior axillary line, about 5–7 cm inferior to the third port. An alternative is to use the two anterior axillary ports and omit the posterior port site.

Through the primary incision, a muscle-splitting dissection is performed with exposure created by S-retractors. Access into the retroperitoneal space is confirmed by inserting one finger and palpating the inner surface of the 12th rib above and the iliac crest below (Figure 14.10). This finger can also identify the psoas muscle and begin to sweep all anterior structures away. We prefer to create the retroperitoneal working space with a commercial dilating balloon (Origin Medsystems, Menlo Park, California). The trocar-mounted balloon is inflated posteriorly along the abdominal wall and cephalad from the incision, mobilizing Gerota's envelope with its contents away from the back wall. The Hasson port is then secured and the pneumo-retroperitoneum is generated with carbon dioxide under 15 mmHg pressure. Additional ports are placed and secured as needed.

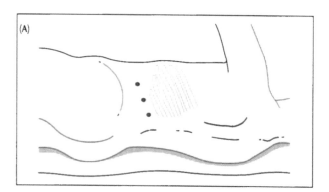

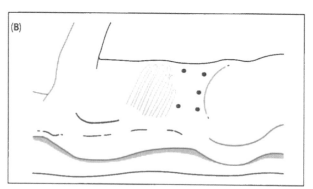

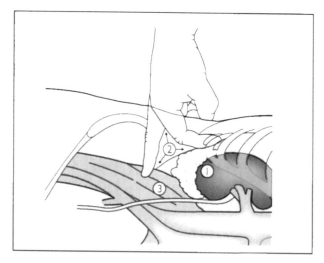

Figure 14.9

The retroperitoneal approach for the left adrenal gland (A) and the right adrenal gland (B). The primary port site is placed just below the tip of the 12th rib for the laparoscope. A posterior port is placed just below the angle formed by the 12th rib and the vertically oriented paraspinous muscles. A third port is placed 3–4 cm medial and slightly superior to the primary site in the anterior axillary line.

Figure 14.10

Retroperitoneal access is obtained by making a 2 inch skin incision between the tip of the 12th rib and the iliac crest. All fascial layers are incised and the retroperitoneal space is digitally entered. The space is then further created by digitally identifying the psoas muscle (3) and the finger begins to sweep the peritoneum (2) medially away from the Gerota's fascia (1).

The key to the retroperitoneal approach is in understanding the orientation, which is distinctly different from the transperitoneal approach. Rather than looking down on the kidney and adrenal from above (very similar to an open transperitoneal view), we approach the kidney from behind with an end-on view of the lower pole. It is helpful if the balloon dissection is positioned up high to gain more rapid access to the adrenal gland. Occasionally it is useful to reposition the balloon up higher and reinflate it. The initial view is nearly always somewhat tattered, but key landmarks can and must be identified. The psoas muscle is easily seen and serves as a guide for longitudinal orientation. Many random veils of tissue near the psoas can be swept aside or divided to clarify the view. Dissecting medially, the great vessels can be identified as they run parallel to the psoas fibers. The renal vessels are found by identifying the pulsations of the posteriorly situated renal artery, although exposure of these vessels is not always necessary. The kidney may be relatively difficult to identify if there is an abundance of perinephric fat. If the patient is thin and the adrenal mass prominent, locating the area of interest may be straightforward. However, a small adrenal mass in the midst of abundant fat can present a challenge. In these cases, intraoperative sonography is helpful.

Left side

Once the initial dissection is complete and the appropriate landmarks identified, the adrenal gland must be located (Figure 14.11). Because there is often scant fatty tissue

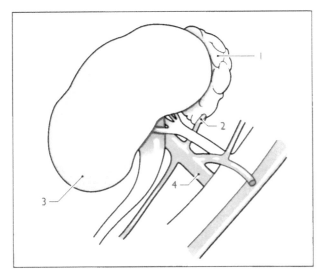

Figure 14.11
The retroperitoneal approach for the left adrenal gland (1). Initial dissection is cephalad along the psoas to the upper pole of the kidney (3). The adrenal vein (2) is often found along the inferomedial border. The adrenal vein can also be found by identifying the left renal vein (4) first.

posterior to the adrenal, the golden hue may be quickly noted. The dissection should be carried cephalad along the psoas to the upper pole of the kidney. We tend to approach the adrenal from a lateral angle and then find the adrenal vein along the inferomedial border, where it can be exposed, clipped, and divided. If locating the adrenal is difficult, or if the mass is a pheochromocytoma, the adrenal vein can be found first by identifying the left renal vessels and locating the junction of the left adrenal vein with the left renal vein. Because the adrenal vein tends to course along the medial aspect of the kidney, the dissection must be kept strictly posterior. This keeps the kidney and adrenal from falling down into the field of view. After division of the adrenal vein, the remainder of the adrenal can be detached, remembering to lift and push, rather than grasp, the adrenal tissue. This reduces the risk of adrenal gland fracture and ensuing hemorrhage.

Once the adrenal is completely mobilized, the laparoscope is placed through one of the secondary ports so that the adrenal may be removed through the largest incision (the primary site). The adrenal is placed in a retrieval bag and removed. The port sites are closed in standard fashion.

Right side

The right retroperitoneal adrenalectomy presents a challenge because of the position of the adrenal and the length of the adrenal vein in relation to the IVC (Figure 14.12). The same principles of retroperitoneal laparoscopy apply. Dissection moves cephalad along the psoas muscle, with careful attention to orientation. The kidney is held anteriorly by its own attachments or by an optional retractor. The adrenal gland must be located by dissection or by ultrasound before the adrenal vein can be approached. Identification and dissection of the IVC above the renal vessels may be helpful, but may also be treacherous. The right adrenal gland rests somewhat more medial to the kidney than the left adrenal gland, and the upper pole of the kidney may interfere with exposure of the adrenal gland. In addition, the right adrenal vein is situated on the far (medial) side of the gland, away from the dissecting instruments. Despite these challenges, once the adrenal is located, it can be mobilized and lifted anteriorly to expose the adrenal vein, which can then be clipped and divided. As with the other approaches, the remainder of the adrenal gland is mobilized with cautery and removed in a retrieval bag. The port sites are then closed.

Transthoracic technique

Recently, the technique of thoracoscopic transdiaphragmatic adrenalectomy has been described.[28] This technique has potential for use when both the transperitoneal and

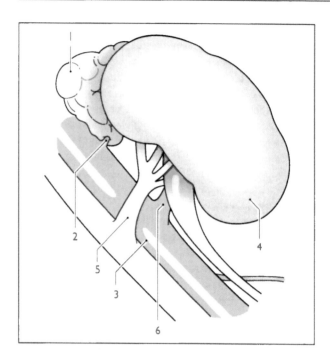

Figure 14.12
The retroperitoneal approach for the right adrenal gland (1).
The adrenal gland must be located by dissection or by
ultrasound before the adrenal vein (2) can be approached.
Identification of the venal cava is helpful (3). The right adrenal
gland rests somewhat more medial to the kidney (4) than the
left adrenal gland. The renal artery (5) and vein (6) are
identified early in the dissection.

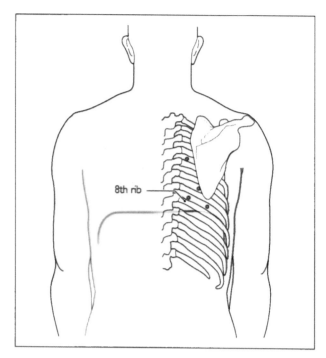

Figure 14.13
Trocar placements for thoracoscopic transdiaphragmatic
adrenalectomy. This technique has potential for use when both
the transperitoneal and retroperitoneal spaces have been
violated by prior surgery. The patient is placed in the prone
position. A four-port transthoracic technique is used.

retroperitoneal spaces have been violated by prior surgery.
Following double-lumen endotracheal intubation, the
patient is placed in the prone position. A four port
transthoracic technique is used (Figure 14.13).

In order to gain exposure to the adrenal gland, the
diaphragm is incised under ultrasonographic guidance
and the retroperitoneum entered. The adrenal gland is
then identified and dissected free. Once the adrenal gland
is removed, the diaphragm is repaired. A chest tube is kept
in place at the conclusion of the procedure.

Postoperative care

The advantages of the laparoscopic approach to the
adrenal gland are immediately apparent in the postoperative period. The orogastric tube is removed immediately
at the end of the case and the Foley catheter removed as
soon as the patient is ambulatory. Postoperative pain is
controlled with parenteral narcotics in the first 24 hours
and ketorolac or oral narcotics thereafter. Supplemental
corticosteroids and appropriate antihypertensive medications are administered as needed, depending on the type of

tumor removed. Postoperative care can be coordinated in
concert with an endocrinologist if necessary. Discharge is
usually within 24–48 hours from surgery and full recovery
requires 10–14 days.

Complications

The most significant intraoperative complication is
hemorrhage. The adrenal gland is highly vascular, which
can result in troublesome bleeding if not adequately
controlled.[37] The use of a harmonic scalpel during dissection of the adrenal gland can limit the amount of hemorrhage. In addition, the adrenal gland itself is very easily
fractured, often resulting in bleeding.

Other intraoperative complications from laparoscopic
adrenalectomy are similar to those for any laparoscopic
procedure, and can include injuries to the colon, small
bowel, liver, gallbladder, spleen, and diaphragm.[37] In
general, major complications occur less often as surgeon
experience increases. Conversion to an open case should be
done if hemorrhage is uncontrollable or intraoperative
injury cannot be repaired through a laparoscopic approach.

Table 14.3 *Selected laparoscopic adrenalectomy series*

Author (year)	No. of cases	Age	Approach	OR time (min)	EBL (ml)	Hospital stay (days)	Conversion rate	Complications
MacGillivray[38] (2002)	60	–	Transperitoneal	183	63	2	0/60	
Valeri[39] (2002)	91	–	Transperitoneal	92–148	–	3.5	2/91	2 postoperative hemorrhage, 1 port-site bleed, 1 UTI, 1 death from myocardial infarction
Kebebew[40] (2002)	176	–	Transperitoneal	168	–	1.7	0/176	5.1%
Lezoche[35] (2002)	216	45.9	149 transperitoneal, 67 retroperitoneal	100	–	–	4/216	1 death, hemoperitoneum, 1 wound infection
Salomon[34] (2001)	115	49.3	115 retroperitoneal	118	77	4	1/118	3.5% intraoperative, 12.1% postoperative
Guazzoni[41] (2001)	161	39.4	Transperitoneal	160	–	2.8	4/161	5.5%
Suzuki[36] (2001)	118	51.7	78 transperitoneal, 40 retroperitoneal	171	96.3	–	6/118	2 paralytic ileus, 4 shoulder tip pain
Soulie[42] (2000)	52	46.9	Retroperitoneal	135	80	5	1/52	5.7% intraoperative, 11.5% postoperative
Mancini[43] (1999)	172	–	Transperitoneal	132	–	5.8	12/172	8.7%, 2 deaths
Schichman[44] (1999)	50	54	Transperitoneal	219	142	3	0/50	10%
Winfield[3] (1998)	21	52.2	Transperitoneal	219	183	2.7	0/21	1 subcutaneous bleed, 2 pneumothorax, 1 pulmonary edema
Yoshimura[4] (1998)	28	42	11 transperitoneal, 17 retroperitoneal	375	370	2.7	0/28	4 blood transfusion, 4 subcutaneous emphysema, 2 postoperative bleeding
Chee[45] (1998)	14	46.2	8 transperitoneal, 6 retroperitoneal	135	Min	3	0/14	1 pneumonia
Gagner[46] (1997)	100	46	Transperitoneal	123	70	3	3/100	12%; 3 DVT, 2 pulmonary embolus
Gasman[33] (1997)	23	49.6	23 retroperitoneal	97	70	3.3	0/23	1 postoperative hematoma
Terachi[47] (1997)	100	–	Transperitoneal	240	77	–	3/100	–
Rutherford[48] (1996)	67	54	Transperitoneal	124	–	5.1	0/67	3 DVT, 2 pulmonary emboli, 1 port-site hernia, 1 postoperative bleed
Average		47.1		153.5	98.6		36/1567 (2.3%)	

DVT, deep vein thrombosis; EBL, estimated blood loss; OR, operating room; UTI, urinary tract infection.

Results

Worldwide experience with laparoscopic adrenal surgery has increased since its introduction in 1992. Several centers have now reported large series in the literature that document the decreased blood loss, shortened hospital stay, and faster return to normal activity. Selected recent series in the literature are summarized in Table 14.3.

Gagner et al reported on 100 consecutive laparoscopic adrenalectomy procedures performed through the transperitoneal approach.[46] The mean operative time was 123 min with an estimated blood loss of 70 ml. In their series, the open conversion rate was 3%, average length of hospital stay was 3 days or less, and morbidity was encountered in 12% of patients. The lesions removed included pheochromocytomas, aldosteronomas, Cushing's lesions, and others.

In the largest published series identified in the literature by Lezoche et al.[35] a total of 216 laparoscopic adrenalectomies were performed through the anterior transperitoneal, lateral transperitoneal, and the posterior retroperitoneal approaches. The study was a combined experience of surgeons in Italy and the Netherlands. The average operating time of all approaches was 100 min with a conversion rate of only 1.9%. Average hospital stay for all approaches was 3–4 days.

Comparison studies have been made between laparoscopic and open adrenalectomy to determine if there are significant benefits in the laparoscopic approach.[2–9] In general, the operative times for laparoscopic surgery are longer than for the open technique, particularly early on in the learning curve. However, the operative times decrease as surgeon experience increases. In addition, the laparoscopic approach offers less blood loss, significantly less postoperative narcotic use, overall shorter hospital stay, and a faster return to normal activity. The cost of a laparoscopic adrenalectomy was shown to be comparable to that of an open adrenalectomy in one study.[10]

Laparoscopic adrenalectomy for malignant tumors

Increased surgeon experience and comfort with laparoscopic adrenalectomies has led to performing laparoscopic adrenalectomies for larger and potentially malignant tumors. Henry et al[50] performed laparoscopic adrenalectomies on 19 patients with potentially malignant tumors, all of which were greater than 6 cm in size. Median operating time was 150 min, and conversion was necessary in 2 patients because of intraoperative evidence of invasive carcinoma. Six of the 19 patients had an adrenocortical carcinoma on pathologic diagnosis. One of these patients presented with a liver metastasis 6 months after surgery

and died. The other 5 patients are alive, with a follow-up ranging from 8 to 83 months. The authors concluded that laparoscopic adrenalectomy can be performed on select patients in experienced hands; however, conversion to open adrenalectomy should be performed if there is evidence of local invasion observed during surgery.

Laparoscopic adrenalectomy has also been safely performed in patients with solitary adrenal metastases. In a recent series by Heniford et al,[22] laparoscopic adrenalectomy was performed in 11 patients, 10 of which had the adrenalectomy performed for metastatic disease. Average operative time was 181 min, and blood loss was minimal at 138 ml. One patient required conversion to an open approach due to local invasion of the tumor into the lateral wall of the vena cava, which was removed with the specimen. Ten of the 11 patients were alive, with a mean follow-up of 8.3 months. This data suggest that the laparoscopic approach to some malignant neoplasms, either originating from or metastasizing to the adrenal gland, is reasonable, but the conversion to an open procedure should be performed if local invasion is present.

Conclusion

Laparoscopic adrenalectomy has become an accepted method for removing benign lesions of the adrenal gland. There is no question that the advantages of the laparoscopic approach include shorter hospitalization and convalescence. In addition, even hormonally active lesions such as pheochromocytomas can be safely approached laparoscopically. Relative contraindications to the laparoscopic approach include very large benign lesions and primary adrenal carcinomas. Both the transperitoneal and retroperitoneal techniques yield satisfactory results.

Laparoscopic adrenalectomy has been shown to be a safe and effective approach to many forms of adrenal pathology. It should be considered the standard of care in the management of benign lesions of the adrenal gland that require surgical removal.

References

1. Gagner M, Lacroix A, Bolte E. Laparoscopic adrenalectomy in Cushing's syndrome and pheochromocytoma. N Engl J Med 1992; 327:1033.

2. Schell SR, Talamini MA, Udelsman R. Laparoscopic adrenalectomy for nonmalignant disease: improved safety, morbidity, and cost-effectiveness. Surg Endosc 1999; 13:30.

3. Winfield HN, Hamilton BD, Bravo EL, Novick AC. Laparoscopic adrenalectomy: the preferred choice? A comparison to open adrenalectomy. J Urol 1998; 160:235.

4. Yoshimura K, Yoshioka T, Miyake O, et al. Comparison of clinical outcomes of laparoscopic and conventional open adrenalectomy. J Endourol 1998; 12:555.

5. Vargas HI, Kavoussi LR, Bartlett DL, et al. Laparoscopic adrenalectomy: a new standard of care. Urology 1997; 49:673.

6. Bolli M, Oertli D, Staub J, Harder F. Laparoscopic adrenalectomy: the new standard? Swiss Med Wkly 2002; 132:12.

7. Hazzan D, Shiloni E, Golijanin D, et al. Laparoscopic vs open adrenalectomy for benign adrenal neoplasm. Surg Endosc 2001; 15:1356.

8. MacGillivray DC, Schichman SJ, Ferrer FA, Malchoff CD. A comparison of open vs laparoscopic adrenalectomy. Surg Endosc 1996; 10:987.

9. Miccoli P, Raffaelli M, Berti P, et al. Adrenal surgery before and after the introduction of laparoscopic adrenalectomy. Br J Surg 2002; 89:779.

10. Ortega J, Sala C, Garcia S, Lledo S. Cost-effectiveness of laparoscopic vs open adrenalectomy: small savings in an expensive process. J Laparoendosc Adv Surg Tech A 2002; 12:1.

11. Walther MM, Keiser HR, Linehan WM. Pheochromocytoma: evaluation, diagnosis, and treatment. World J Urol 1999; 17:35.

12. Goldfarb DA. Contemporary evaluation and management of Cushing's syndrome. World J Urol 1999; 17:22.

13. Blumenfeld JD, Vaughan ED Jr. Diagnosis and treatment of primary aldosteronism. World J Urol 1999; 17:15.

14. Murai M, Baba S, Nakashima J, Tachibana M. Management of incidentally discovered adrenal masses. World J Urol 1999; 17:9.

15. Belldegrun A, Hussain S, Seltzer S, et al. Incidentally discovered mass of the adrenal gland. Surg Gynecol Obstet 1986; 163:203.

16. Cerfolio RJ, Vaughan ED Jr, Brennan TG Jr, Hirvela ER. Accuracy of computed tomography in predicting adrenal tumor size. Surg Gynecol Obstet 1993; 176:307.

17. Schulick RD, Brenna MF. Adrenocortical carcinoma. World J Urol 1999; 17:26.

18. Vaughan ED Jr. Surgical options for open adrenalectomy. World J Urol 1999; 17:40.

19. Teeger S, Papanicolaou N, Vaughan ED Jr. Current concepts in imaging of adrenal masses. World J Urol 1999; 17:3.

20. Edwin B, Kazaryan AM, Mala T, et al. Laparoscopic and open surgery for pheochromocytoma. BMC Surg 2001; 1:2.

21. Schulick RD, Brennan MF. Long-term surival after complete resection and repeat resection in patients with adrenocortical carcinoma. Ann Surg Oncol 1999; 6:719.

22. Heniford BT, Arca MJ, Walsh RM, Gill IS. Laparoscopic adrenalectomy for cancer. Sem Surg Oncol 1999; 16:293.

23. Ferriss JB, Beevers DG, Brown JJ, et al. Clinical, biochemical and pathological features of low-renin ('primary') hyper-aldosteronism. Am Heart J 1978; 95:375.

24. deGasparo M, Whitebread SE, Preiswerk G, et al. Antialdosterones: incidence and prevention of sexual side effects. J Steroid Biochem 1989; 32(1B):223.

25. Blumenfeld JD, Sealey JE, Schlussel Y, et al. Diagnosis and treatment of primary aldosteronism. Ann Intern Med 1994; 121:877.

26. Salomon L, Rabii R, Soulie M, et al. Experience with retroperitoneal laparoscopic adrenalectomy for pheochromocytoma. J Urol 2001;165:1871.

27. Gotoh M, Ono Y, Hattori R, et al. Laparoscopic adrenalectomy for pheochromocytoma: morbidity compared with adrenalectomy for tumors of other pathology. J Endourol 2002; 16:245.

28. Gill IS, Meraney AM, Thomas JC, et al. Thoracoscopic transdiaphragmatic adrenalectomy: the initial experience. J Urology 2001; 165:1875.

29. Bonjer HJ, Sorm V, Berends FJ, et al. Endoscopic retroperitoneal adrenalectomy: lessons learned from 111 consecutive cases. Ann Surg 2000; 232:796.

30. Suzuki K. Laparoscopic adrenalectomy: retroperitoneal approach. Urol Clin North Am 2001; 28:85.

31. Soulie M, Mouly P, Caron P, et al. Retroperitoneal laparoscopic adrenalectomy: clinical experience in 52 procedures. Urology 2000; 56:921.

32. Baba S, Ito K, Yanaihara H, et al. Retroperitoneoscopic adrenalectomy by a lumbodorsal approach: clinical experience with solo surgery. World J Urol 1999; 17:54.

33. Gasman D, Droupy S, Koutani A, et al. Laparoscopic adrenalectomy: the retroperitoneal approach. J Urol 1998; 159:1816.

34. Salomon L, Soulie M, Mouly P, et al. Experience with retroperitoneal laparoscopic adrenalectomy in 115 procedures. J Urol 2001; 166:38.

35. Lezoche E, Guerrieri M, Feliciotti F, et al. Anterior, lateral, and posterior retroperitoneal approaches in endoscopic adrenalectomy. Surg Endosc 2002; 16:96.

36. Suzuki K, Kageyama S, Hirano Y, et al. Comparison of 3 surgical approaches to laparoscopic adrenalectomy: a nonrandomized, background matched analysis. J Urol 2001; 166:437.

37. Henry JF, Defechereux T, Raffaelli M, et al. Complications of laparoscpoic adrenalectomy: results of 169 consecutive procedures. World J Surg 2000; 24:1342.

38. MacGillivray DC, Whalen GF, Malchoff CD, et al. Laparoscopic resection of large adrenal tumors. Ann Surg Oncol 2002; 9:480.

39. Valeri A, Borrelli A, Presenti L, et al. The influence of new technologies on laparoscopic adrenalectomy. Surg Endosc 2002; 16:1274.

40. Kebebew E, Siperstein AE, Duh QY. Laparoscopic adrenalectomy: the optimal surgical approach. J Laparoendosc Adv Surg Tech A 2001; 11:409.

41. Guazzoni G, Cestari A, Montorsi F, et al. Eight-year experience with transperitoneal laparoscopic adrenal surgery. J Urol 2001; 166:820.

42. Soulie M, Mouly P, Caron P, et al. Retroperitoneal laparoscopic adrenalectomy: clinical experience in 52 procedures. Urology 2000; 56:921.

43. Mancini F, Mutter D, Peix JL, et al. Experience with adrenalectomy in 1997. Apropros of 247 cases: a multicenter prospective study of the French-speaking Association of Endocrine Surgery. Chirurgie 1999; 124:368.

44. Shichman SJ, Herndon CD, Sosa RE, et al. Lateral transperitoneal laparoscopic adrenalectomy. World J Urol 1999; 17:48.

45. Chee C, Ravinthiran T, Cheng C. Laparoscopic adrenalectomy: experience with transabdominal and retroperitoneal approaches. Urology 1998; 51:29.

46. Gagner M, Pomp A, Heniford BT, et al. Laparoscopic adrenalectomy: lessons learned from 100 consecutive procedures. Ann Surg 1997; 226:238.

47. Terachi T, Matsuda T, Terai A, et al. Transperitoneal laparoscopic adrenalectomy: experience in 100 patients. J Endourol 1997; 11:361.

48. Rutherford JC, Stowasser M, Tunny TJ, et al. Laparoscopic adrenalectomy. World J Surg 1996; 20:758.

49. Marescaux J, Mutter D, Wheeler MH. Laparoscopic right and left adrenalectomies. Surg Endosc 1996; 10:912.

50. Henry JF, Sebag F, Iacobone M, Mirallie E. Results of laparoscopic adrenalectomy for large and potentially malignant tumors. World J Surg 2002; 26:1043.

15

Laparoscopic retroperitoneal lymph node sampling for testicular cancer

Gunter Janetschek and Mohamed El Ghoneimy

Laparoscopic surgical techniques were first introduced to the field of urology a decade ago. Initial applications for benign diseases showed decreased postoperative pain, quicker convalescence, and improved cosmetic results as compared to open surgery. These successful results have provided the impetus for its introduction to the field of urologic oncology. In this chapter, we present the role of laparoscopic lymphadenectomy as a minimally invasive tool in the management of testicular tumors.

Pathology of testicular neoplasm

Testicular cancer, although relatively rare, is the most common malignancy in men in the 15- to 35-year-old age group and evokes widespread interest for several reasons. The dramatic improvement in survival resulting from the combination of effective diagnostic techniques, improved tumor markers, effective multidrug chemotherapeutic regimens, and modifications of surgical technique has led to a decrease in patient mortality from more than 50% before 1970 to less than 5% in 1997.[1]

Histologic classification of germ cell tumors

Histologic classifications, grading systems, and staging evaluations have traditionally provided a major clinical basis for therapeutic decisions. There have been at least six major attempts since 1940 to classify germinal tumors. The World Health Organization (WHO) standardized pathologic criteria for diagnosis of testis cancer, which has gone a long way toward eliminating confusion associated with various histologic staging systems.[2] Germ cell tumors

(GCTs) are composed of five basic cell types: seminoma, embryonal cell carcinoma, yolk sac tumor, teratoma, and choriocarcinoma. More than half of GCTs contain more than one cell type and are therefore known as mixed GCTs. Heterogeneity among germ cell neoplasms is an expected consequence of their pluripotential origin. Biochemical marker 'probes' can provide a means of delineating tumor heterogeneity, which may be useful in treatment selection.

Classification of germ cell neoplasms according to morphologic appearance is invaluable in treatment selection. The broad distinction between seminomas and nonseminomas has been particularly important in determining management strategies for retroperitoneal lymph node metastasis.

In general, survival of patients with GCT is related to the stage at presentation and therefore to the amount of tumor burden as well as to the effectiveness of subsequent treatment. Patients who present with advanced disease (stage III) generally have a much poorer prognosis than do those with disease confined to the testis or those with regional nodal involvement only. Delay in diagnosis of 1–2 months or more is not uncommon in these patients and seems to be related directly to patient factors such as ignorance, denial, and fear as well as physician factors such as misdiagnosis.[3]

Patterns of spread of germ cell tumors

The principles that underlie (the) modern surgical treatment of GCT of the testis are based on the fact that testis cancer spreads in a predictable and stepwise fashion, with the notable exception of choriocarcinoma. This will be explained later through the work of Weissbach and Boedefeld, who described templates that include practically all the primary landing sites of lymph node metastases and which were modified later by Hoeltl and colleagues.

Clinical staging

A convenient division for staging systems is between patients with seminomas and those with nonseminomatous tumors. Patients with pure seminoma are usually staged by clinical means, whereas staging in patients with nonseminomatous germ cell tumors (NSGCTs) sometimes employs surgical techniques such as retroperitoneal lymph node dissection (RPLND) as well. The extent of staging is determined in part by decisions for therapy; for example, if surveillance protocols are to be considered, every effort should be made to exclude patients with any evidence of retroperitoneal disease. If retroperitoneal lymphadenectomy is likely to be elected as the primary treatment for low-stage, nonseminomatous tumors, efforts should be directed toward delineation of regional and nodal vs distant metastases.

Staging systems

A variety of clinical staging systems have been advocated since the 1960s (Tables 15.1 and 15.2).

Table 15.1	*Royal Marsden Hospital staging for testicular cancer*	
Stage		**Definition**
I		No evidence of metastases
	M	Rising serum markets with no other evidence of metastases
II		Abdominal node metastases
	A	< 2 cm diameter
	B	2–5 cm diameter
	C	> 5 cm diameter
III		Supradiaphragmatic nodal metastases
	M	Mediastinal
	N	Supraclavicular, cervical, or axillary
	O	No abdominal disease
IV		Extralymphatic metastases
	L1	< 3 lung metastases
	L2	> 3 lung metastases all < 2 cm in diameter
	L3	> 3 lung metastases, one or more > 2 cm in diameter
	H+	Liver metastases
	Br+	Brain metastases
	Bo+	Bone metastases

Source: reproduced with permission from Hendry WF. Testicular cancer. In: Kirby RS, Kirby MG, Farah RN, eds. Men's health. Oxford: Isis Medical Media, 1999: 27.

In 1997, an internationally agreed-on consensus classification applicable to both seminoma and nonseminoma was published. The American Joint Committee on Cancer (AJCC) staging for GCTs is unique because, for the first time, a serum tumor marker category (S) is used to supplement the prognostic stages defined by anatomy alone. This tumor, nodes, and metastasis staging (TNMS) system should replace all prior staging systems and should, it is hoped, standardize patient reporting.[4,5]

The AJCC TNMS system subdivides stage I disease into stages Ia and Ib, depending on the T (tumor) stage, as well as into stage S (serum tumor markers), according to serum tumor marker levels; stage II is subdivided into stages IIa, IIb, and IIc, depending on volume of retroperitoneal lymph node involvement; and stage III is subdivided into stages IIIa, IIIb, and IIIc, according to the degree of metastatic involvement and serum tumor marker levels.

Removal of the testicular tumor is via an inguinal approach, the so-called *radical orchiectomy*, and remains the definitive procedure for pathologic diagnosis as well as for local treatment of testicular neoplasms. Transscrotal biopsy is to be avoided.

Imaging studies

Chest X-ray study

Posteroanterior and lateral chest X-ray studies should be the initial radiographic procedures performed.

Computed tomography

Chest computed tomography (CT) scans are now routinely used, as they further increase the sensitivity for detection of pulmonary metastases. Abdominal CT scans have been advertised as being the most effective means to identify retroperitoneal lymph node involvement. CT scanning, however, is not sufficiently accurate to distinguish fibrosis, teratoma, or malignancy by size criteria alone.[6] It also yields a good percentage of false-positive and at the same time false-negative results.

Positron emission tomography

The use of positron emission tomography (PET) in the evaluation of retroperitoneal lymph nodes and radiographic abnormalities after chemotherapy in patients with testis cancer has been reported. No apparent advantage over CT scans has been demonstrated, mainly because neither PET nor CT has the ability to detect microscopic nodal disease.[7,8]

Table 15.2 *AJCC TNMS staging system for testis cancer.*[4,5]

Primary tumor (T)

PT_x	unknown
PT_0	no evidence of cancer
PT_1	confined to testis
PT_2	invades beyond tunica
PT_3	invades paratesticular structures (rete testis) and/or epididymis
PT_{4a}	invades cord structure
P_4	invades scrotal structures

Regional lymph nodes (N)
Clinical:

N_x	cannot be assessed
N_0	no regional lymph node involvement
N_1	lymph node tissue < 2 cm diameter
N_2	lymph node tissue 2–5 cm diameter
N_3	lymph node tissue > 5 cm diameter
Pathologic	same as above with pathologic
PN_0–PN_4	confirmation

Distant metastases (M)

M_0	no evidence of distant metastases
M_1	nonregional nodal or pulmonary metastases
M_2	nonpulmonary visceral masses

Serum tumor markers (S)

	LDH	hCG (m/u/ml)	AFP (ng/ml)
S_0	≤ normal	≤ normal	≤ normal
S_1	< 1.5 × normal	< 5000	< 1000
S_2	1.5–10 × normal	5000–50,000	1000–10,000
S_3	> 10 × normal	> 50,000	> 10,000

AFP = alpha fetoprotein; hCG = human chorionic gonadotropin; LDH = lactic acid dehydrogenase

Tumor markers

Germinal testis tumors are among a select group of neoplasms identified as producing so-called marker proteins that are relatively specific and readily measurable in minute quantities using highly sensitive radio-immunoassay technology (Table 15.3). The study of biochemical marker substances, particularly alpha fetoprotein (AFP) and human chorionic gonadotropin (hCG), is clinically useful in the diagnosis, staging, and monitoring of treatment response in patients with germ cell neoplasms, and may be useful as a prognostic index. GCT markers belong to two main classes:

1. oncofetal substances associated with embryonic development (AFP and hCG) and

2. certain cellular enzymes, such as lactic acid dehydrogenase (LDH) and placental alkaline phosphatase (PLAP).

Tumor marker levels have to be evaluated before orchiectomy, especially when one is considering a surveillance protocol. Persistent serum tumor marker elevations after radical inguinal orchiectomy must be interpreted with caution to avoid unnecessary adjuvant treatment. Elevation of serum levels of AFP in patients with GCTs can be produced by liver dysfunction, and serum elevations of hCG can occur in hypogonadotropic patients. However, in general, persistently elevated tumor markers after orchiectomy reflect systemic metastases rather than tumor confined to retroperitoneal nodes, and for this reason chemotherapy is recommended for this subset of patients.

The rate of tumor marker decline relative to expected marker half-life after treatment has been proposed as a prognostic index. Patients whose values decline according to negative half-lives after treatment are more likely to be disease free than those whose marker decline is slower or whose markers never return to normal levels[4,9] (see Table 15.3).

Treatment options

Non-seminomatous germ cell tumors

Clinical stage I

Three treatment modalities are advocated by various urologists for the management of clinical stage I non-seminomatous testicular cancer: surveillance, risk-adapted chemotherapy, and retroperitoneal lymph node dissection.

Twenty-five to thirty percent of patients with clinical stage I have occult lymph node metastases, which cannot be diagnosed by the most sensitive imaging techniques available.[10,11] This group of patients will be at higher risk if surveillance strategy is followed, as they will be diagnosed later after the tumor has substantially increased in size, thereby requiring a higher dose of chemotherapy for treatment. Furthermore, as patient compliance is usually not perfect, some tumor-bearing patients might be lost during follow-up. Surveillance without prior lymph node dissection has a relapse rate of 19–40%[12–14] vs 5–10% for pathologic stage I testicular cancer after RPLND.[15–18] Moreover, the most serious drawback of surveillance is not only the high relapse rate but also the associated death rate of

approximately 10% among those patients who do relapse.[11] The primary advantage of surveillance was the avoidance of RPLND and its attendant morbidity as, before the introduction of modified unilateral dissection and nerve-sparing techniques, the majority of the patients suffered ejaculatory disturbances with resultant loss of fertility.[19]

Recently, risk-adapted chemotherapy has been introduced as a measure to overcome the above-mentioned problems.[20] However, there is no general consensus about risk factors and their clinical relevance, except for vascular invasion and embryonal carcinoma.[21] We have performed a retrospective analysis on 88 consecutive patients undergoing RPLND. Because the definition of risk factors varies greatly, the patients were evaluated using a highly specific risk factor (70% or more embryonal carcinoma together with vascular invasion) as an example of the many possibilities of calculating the risk. Even though the risk factor used was specific (present in 25% of the patients), 52% of patients who would have been considered candidates for chemotherapy did not have retroperitoneal tumors. On the other hand, 50% of patients with retroperitoneal tumors would have been considered low risk and left without treatment. Another staging study has also shown that 20% of patients with suspicious findings on CT actually have pathologic stage I disease.[22] These individuals might have unnecessarily been subjected to the side-effects of adjuvant chemotherapy: the acute ones (nausea, mucositis and nadir sepsis) as well as the long-term more morbid ones (pulmonary fibrosis and impaired spermatogenesis).[23,24]

RPLND is the only reliable method that permits the verification of small positive lymph nodes and the exclusion of false-negative ones. However, the morbidity of open RPLND is too high for a diagnostic procedure: the short-term morbidity of major intra-abdominal surgery

Table 15.3 *Testicular tumor markers*[5]

Tumor marker	Half-life ($t_{1/2}$)	Clinical source of production
Alpha fetoprotein	5–7 days	Pure embryonal carcinoma Terato carcinoma Yolk sac tumor Combined tumors
Beta-human chorionic gonadotropin	24–36 hours	Syncytiotrophoblastic cells Pure seminoma Castration
Lactic acid dehydrogenase (isoenzymes I–IV)	N/A	Common cellular enzyme found elevated when high tumor burden present (especially advanced pure seminoma)
Placental alkaline phosphatase	N/A	Fetal isoenzyme elevated in advanced testicular cancer

and the long-term ones, which are much less tolerated because of loss of antegrade ejaculation and a lifelong scar that impairs the quality of life of a usually young patient.

Since knowledge of the definite lymph node status is a prerequisite for adequate stage-adapted treatment, RPLND is retained as a diagnostic and in a way therapeutic tool, its morbidity being substantially reduced by the use of laparoscopy.

Our recent data, as well as the data from other centers, will show that laparoscopy shares the same efficacy as open RPLND. Relapse rates after open RPLND alone are as high as 8–29% for stage IIa tumors[25,26] and 34–55% for stage IIb tumors.[26,27] This rate falls to as low as 0–1% if two cycles of adjuvant chemotherapy are given.[27,28] Laparoscopic RPLND, thereby, reduces the high morbidity of the combination of open RPLND and adjuvant chemotherapy in node-positive patients.

Clinical stage II

Neither retroperitoneal lymphadenectomy[25–27,29] nor chemotherapy[30,31] alone can be expected to be curative in all patients in this stage. A combination of both is expected to achieve the most effective results. Most urologists prefer the strategy of primary chemotherapy followed by RPLND for residual masses. In this case, RPLND is performed in a diagnostic intent, i.e. to exclude the residual mass containing active tumor, but sometimes can be curative, i.e. if a mature teratoma is found and removed. Again, the advantage of laparoscopy here rises by reducing the (double) morbidity of chemotherapy and open surgery. In an attempt to further reduce the morbidity of this combined treatment, we have reduced the dose of chemotherapy to two cycles for stage IIb, which is obviously the minimum dose required for complete tumor control.[32] However, this approach is experimental at present, which makes the evaluation of the effect of chemotherapy by laparoscopic RPLND mandatory in each patient. RPLND can be performed as a first step in a therapeutic intent. In this case, it has to be done bilaterally to remove not only the primary landing site but also all possible sites of tumor spread. By laparoscopy, bilateral RPLND is only feasible as a staged procedure, which decreases efficiency and increases the morbidity. Other studies have found laparoscopic RPLND for residual masses to be not recommendable, owing to the intense desmoplasia in the vicinity of the great vessels after chemotherapy,[33] but our results have shown it to be technically feasible not only in stage IIb but also in stage IIc. However, in the latter stage, the risk of contralateral tumor spread is high and, as laparoscopy allows for unilateral dissection only, we have now restricted it to stage IIb.[32,34]

Seminoma

Since the morbidity of carboplatinum monotherapy is low and its efficacy is very high, we feel there is no place for laparoscopy in the management of stage I seminoma.[35] The only exception we consider is the removal of residual masses after chemotherapy.

Technique
Preoperative measures

Bowel preparation, including a clear liquid diet and oral laxatives, is performed day 1 preoperatively. All patients receive low-dose antibiotic coverage. Typing and cross-matching are performed for two units of blood. Preoperative preparation now also includes a low-fat diet for 1 week that is continued 2 weeks postoperatively so as to prevent chylous ascites, which was observed in some patients after postchemotherapy laparoscopic RPLND. We have not seen this complication since.

Template

Weissbach and Boedefeld have described templates that include practically all the primary landing sites of lymph node metastases.[36] If all the metastatic tissue is resected within these templates, there is only minimal risk of metastases to be overlooked. The templates for the left and right sides differ substantially; only the templates for right-sided tumors include the interaortocaval tissues (Figures 15.1 and 15.2).

However, there is still some controversy as to whether to remove the tissues behind the lumbar vessels, the vena cava, and the aorta. There is currently no study available investigating whether this area is among the primary landing sites of lymph node metastases. We have developed a laparoscopic split and roll technique that enables transection of all lumbar vessels and enables us to perform the same radical dissection as with open surgery. Meanwhile, we have investigated the primary landing sites as regards their ventrodorsal location. All solitary metastases, and at least, in one patient, multiple metastases, were detected ventral to the lumbar vessels. Therefore, it can be concluded that the primary landing sites are invariably located ventrally, whereas dorsal metastases result from further tumor spread.[37] Consequently, we no longer routinely transect the lumbar vessels to remove the tissues behind them, as it is not required in diagnostic RPLND for clinical stage I tumors. This makes the laparoscopic procedure considerably easier, faster, and safer.

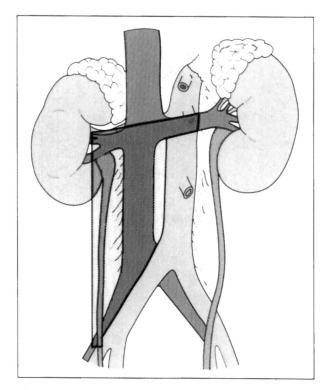

Figure 15.1
Template for right-sided dissection.

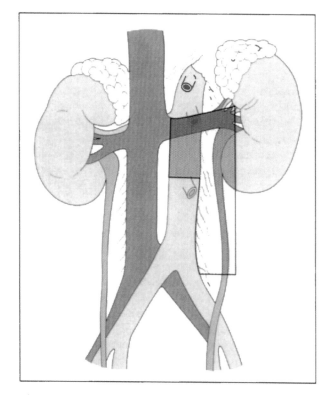

Figure 15.2
Template for left-sided dissection.

The same procedure is performed in clinical stage II disease following chemotherapy. All tissue in which tumor was detected before chemotherapy is removed and the ipsilateral template is dissected in the same fashion as in clinical stage I disease.

Equipment

The following tools have proved useful additions to the standard laparoscopic equipment. We exclusively use a 3-chip video camera and a 30° laparoscope. The laparoscope is held and maneuvered by a robotic arm (Computer motion, Inc., Santa Barbara, California). This robot is used to replace one assisting surgeon and has the advantage of providing stable video images even in lengthy procedures. Insufflation with a high flow rate has proved helpful because it prevents the pneumoperitoneum from collapsing during suction.

A small surgical sponge held with an atraumatic grasper is used for retraction, dissection, and hemostasis (Figure 15.3). A right-angled dissector (Aesculap; Karl Storz, Tuttlingen, Germany) is applied for dissection of the vessels. We prefer the use of reusable clips because their small branches allow for more precise placement of the clips.

Operative technique

Clinical stage I: right side

The patient is placed on the operating table with the right side elevated 45° upwards so that the patient can be brought into a supine or lateral decubitus position by rotating the table. In addition the table is flexed at the umbilicus. If necessary, the Trendelenburg or anti-Trendelenburg position is used. The patient is secured to the table.

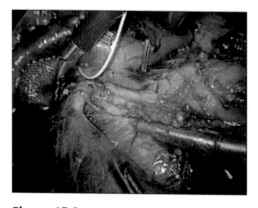

Figure 15.3
Blunt dissection and retraction with sponge.

A Veress needle is used for the initial stab incision to create the pneumoperitoneum, whereas the Hasson cannula is preserved for patients who have previously undergone abdominal surgery. Only 10 mm trocars are used. The first trocar for the laparoscope is placed at the site of the umbilicus. Two secondary trocars for the surgeon are placed at the lateral edge of the rectus muscle, approximately 8 cm above and below the umbilicus. One more trocar is positioned in the anterior axillary line to facilitate retraction.

Wide access to the retroperitoneum is a prerequisite for laparoscopic RPLND. Excellent access can be gained by wide dissection of the right colon and the duodenum in the plane of Toldt. As a first step, the peritoneum is incised along the line of Toldt from the cecum to the right colic flexure. This incision is then carried cephalad parallel to the transverse colon and lateral to the duodenum along the vena cava all the way up to the hepatoduodenal ligament. Caudally, the incision is carried along the spermatic vessels down to the internal inguinal ring. Next, the colon, the duodenum, and the head of the pancreas are reflected medially until the anterior surface of the vena cava, the aorta, and the origin of the left renal vein are exposed.

At this point, the entire template described by Weissbach and Boedefeld for right-sided tumors is accessible. This template includes the interaortocaval lymph nodes, the preaortic tissue (between the left renal vein and the inferior mesenteric artery), and all the tissue ventral and lateral to the vena cava and the right iliac vessels (between the renal vessels and the crossing of the ureter with the iliac vessels). The lateral limit of the template is the ureter. As mentioned previously, the tissues behind the lumbar vessels and the vena cava are no longer removed. The spermatic vein is then dissected along its entire course, starting from the internal inguinal ring.

Special care must be taken while dissecting its insertion into the vena cava, because at this point the vein is easily ruptured. Cranially, the spermatic artery takes a separate course; it is clipped and transected at its crossing with the vena cava, whereas its origin from the aorta is approached later (Figure 15.4).

Next, the lymphatic tissue overlying the vena cava is split open cranially to caudally and its anterior and lateral surfaces are dissected free. Both renal veins are freed from surrounding lymphatic tissue. It is important to dissect the lower border of the left renal vein at this point of the procedure. When dissecting the interaortocaval package from caudal in a cephalad direction, the left renal vein can be easily injured if it is not clearly visible. The lymphatic tissue overlying the common iliac artery is incised up to the bifurcation and further to the origin of the inferior mesenteric artery. In this area, the lymphatic tissue is very dense and care must be taken not to injure the mesenteric artery. Cephalad to the artery, the lymphatic tissue is split along the left border of the aorta so that the ventral surface

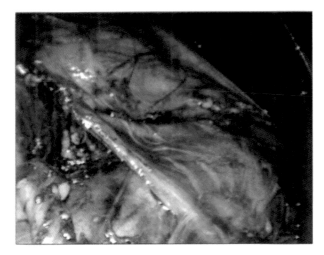

Figure 15.4
Right RPLND: spermatic artery and vein; the artery crosses the vena cava.

of the aorta is completely freed. The spermatic artery is now clipped and transected at its origin from the aorta. When dissecting the cranial portions of the template, the liver has to be retracted with a fan retractor. Now, the right renal artery can be identified as it courses above the interaortocaval space, and the cranial border of the dissection is well delineated. The dissection is carried down to the lumbar vessels and the interaortocaval package is removed step by step.

The ureter, which defines the lateral border of the dissection, is usually identified during excision of the spermatic vessels. It is separated from the nodal package down to its crossing with the iliac artery (Figure 15.5). This point delineates the distal border of the dissection, and the lymph node package is clipped and transected.

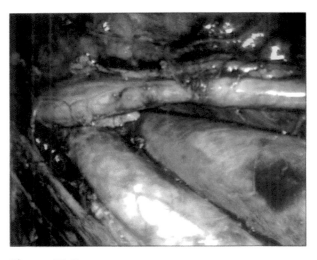

Figure 15.5
Right RPLND: lower limit of dissection; ureter crossing common iliac artery and vein.

From here, the lymph nodes are dissected free in a cephalad direction. The lumbar veins are exposed, but they are transected in exceptional cases only to facilitate removal of the lymph nodes (Figure 15.6). Cranially, the ureter enters Gerota's fascia, which can also be differentiated clearly from the lymphatic tissue. In addition to the right renal vein, the right renal artery is exposed lateral to the vena cava, which delineates the cranial border of the dissection (Figures 15.7 and 15.8).

Now, the nodal package is completely free and can be removed inside a specimen retrieval bag. A drain is not required. Finally, the colon and the duodenum are returned to their anatomic positions and secured with one suture, which is tied extracorporeally.

Left side

The patient is in a right decubitus position. The trocars are placed as for right-sided tumors but in a mirror image array. Usually three or four 10 mm trocars will suffice, because the bowel has to be retracted in rare cases only.

The peritoneum is incised along the line of Toldt from the left colonic flexure to the pelvic brim and distally along the spermatic vein to the internal inguinal ring. It is essential also to incise the splenocolic ligament.

The dissection of the colon must be continued until the anterior surface of the aorta is exposed completely in the plane of Toldt. Normally, the colon falls away from the operative site because of gravity, and a retractor is required only in a few exceptional cases (Figure 15.9).

Then, the spermatic vein is dissected free along its entire course from the internal inguinal ring to its opening into the renal vein and removed (Figure 15.10). The ureter, which defines the lateral border of the template, is identified and separated from the lymphatic tissue. Care must be taken to preserve the connective tissue that provides the blood supply of the ureter. Now, the renal vein can be freed completely. Next, the lymphatic tissue overlying the common iliac artery is split open. The dissection is started

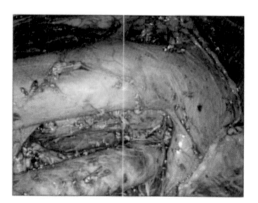

Figure 15.6
Right RPLND: interaortocaval space.

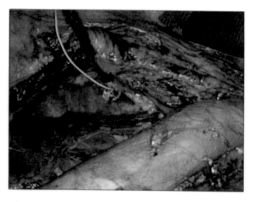

Figure 15.8
Right RPLND: operative field lateral to vena cava after completion of dissection.

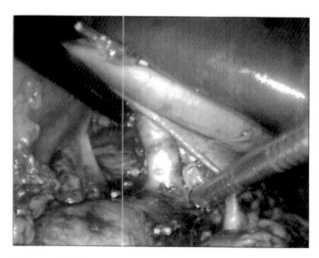

Figure 15.7
Right RPLND: renal artery and vein.

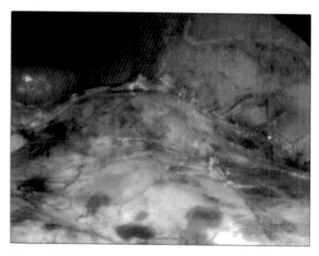

Figure 15.9
Left RPLND: plane of Toldt after colon reflection.

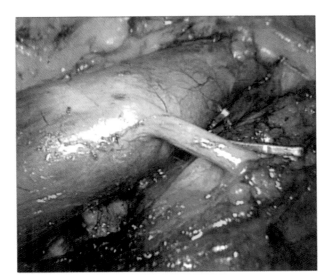

Figure 15.10
Left RPLND: left renal vein with the opening of spermatic vein.

at the crossing of the artery with the ureter, which delineates the distal border of the template. From there, the dissection is continued cephalad. The inferior mesenteric artery is circumvented on the left and preserved. Directly above the mesenteric artery, the dissection is continued along the medial border of the aorta up to the level of the renal vein, which has been identified before.

The spermatic artery is secured with clips at its origin from the aorta and transected. The lateral surface of the aorta is dissected down to the origin of the lumbar arteries. Next, the lumbar vein, which passes caudal to the left renal artery, is approached as it enters the renal vein and transected between clips. This provides access to the renal artery, which lies directly underneath (Figure 15.11). As a last step, the lumbar vessels are separated from the lymphatic tissue to the point at which they disappear in the layer between the spine and the psoas muscle.

Directly lateral to that point, the sympathetic chain is encountered. The postganglionic fibers, although readily identified in most cases, are not preserved. Now, the nodal package is completely free and can be retrieved (Figure 15.12). Finally, the colon is returned to its normal anatomic position and secured in place with one extracorporeally tied suture.

Laparoscopic retroperitoneal lymph node dissection for stage II after chemotherapy

Unilateral RPLND is performed within the same template as is used for clinical stage I disease. Bilateral RPLND is not attempted; in all of our 58 patients, the residual tumor was located within the unilateral template. Displacement of the bowel was feasible in all cases, although chemotherapy rendered identification of the tissue layers more difficult. Mature teratoma is usually well delineated, whereas tumor-free residuals after embryonal carcinoma may be tightly adherent to the surrounding structures (Figure 15.13). This is particularly true for the vena cava. Small venous branches draining the tumor have to be meticulously dissected before they are clipped and transected.

Technique of dissection and hemostasis

The most useful tools for achieving bloodless dissection and adequate hemostasis are bipolar coagulation forceps and the harmonic scalpel (Ethicon, Endo-surgery, Cincinnati, Ohio). Ever since the authors have been using these tools, dissection has become easier, safer, and faster. A small clamp for bipolar coagulation (Johnson and Johnson, New Brunswick, New Jersey) allows for meticulous dissection

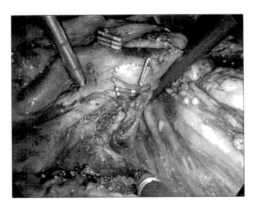

Figure 15.11
Left RPLND: left renal artery and vein (cranial limit of dissection).

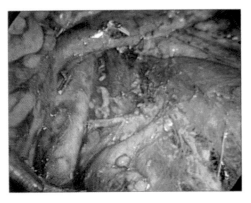

Figure 15.12
Left RPLND: operative field after completion of dissection.

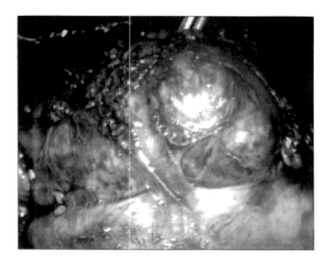

Figure 15.13
Right RPLND: residual mass after chemotherapy overlying the vena cava.

of delicate structures, whereas broader bipolar forceps provide highly efficient hemostasis. In our hands, these tools have proved very efficient.

In open surgery, acute bleeding can be stopped instantaneously with the index finger of the surgeon. In laparoscopy, a small surgical sponge that is held with an atraumatic grasper can be used to substitute for the surgeon's finger. Once the bleeding has been stopped with this technique, the surgeon needs not act in a hurry but has plenty of time to undertake the necessary steps. Furthermore, our animal studies and clinical experience have shown that most venous bleedings, including those resulting from small leaks in the vena cava, can be stopped with the help of the fibrin glue (Tisseel; Baxter-Immuno, Deerfield, Illinois). A special laparoscopic applicator is available (from the manufacturer) with two separate channels for the two components of fibrin glue. The edges of larger defects are approximated with a grasper or clips and then sealed with fibrin glue. In addition, a strip of oxidized regenerated cellulose or other hemostatic agents can be used to enhance the tightness of the repair.

Using these hemostatic techniques, only 3 out of 122 laparoscopic RPLNDs had to be converted to open surgery. No late bleeding was observed.

Results

Between August 1992 and October 2002, 159 consecutive patients underwent laparoscopic RPLND. No patients were excluded because of body habitus or previous operations (Tables 15.4 and 15.5).

Stage I

RPLND was performed for 101 patients with clinical stage I testicular tumor. Mean age was 29.9 years old (16–51). In 64 patients, the tumor was located on the right side and in 37 on the left side. Patient selection was not based on assessment of risk factors or histologic findings.

Surgical efficacy

Laparoscopy is a technically challenging procedure, that requires a steep learning curve. However, once this obstacle is overcome, its results are comparable to and sometimes even better than open surgery. This can be demonstrated by our operative time, which fell from an average of 276 min to 217 min on exclusion of the first 30 patients. This time is now shorter than the mean operative time reported for open RPLND[40,41] and comparable to operative

Table 15.4 *Demographic and perioperative data for laparoscopic RPLND*		
	Clinical stage I	Stage II after chemotherapy
Patients No.	101	58
Mean age (years)	29.9	29.1
Tumor side	Right: 64 Left: 37	Right: 32 Left: 26
Operative time	Overall: 276 min (140–360) After 1st 30 cases: 217 min (140–300)	IIb: 216 min (135–300) IIc: 281 min (145–360)
Blood loss	144 ml (10–470)	165 ml (20–350)
Conversion rate	3/101 (3%)	No conversion
Hospital stay	3.6 days (2–8)	3.8 days (3–10 days)

Table 15.5 *Outcome data for laparoscopic RPLND*

	Clinical stage I	Stage II after chemotherapy
Mean follow-up	47 months (4–97)	38 months (3–73)
Patients No.	96/101	58/58
No. of relapses	2	None
Antegrade ejaculation	98/98 (100%)	56/58 (96.5%)

time in other series.[38,39] Mean blood loss was 144 ml (range 10–470), not including 2600 ml in a converted patient with horseshoe kidney. We had three conversions: one due to injury of a small aortic branch, another due to injury of a renal vein in a horseshoe kidney, and the third due to injury of a left renal vein ventral to the aorta (conversion rate 3%). Four other minor intraoperative complications were encountered, including vena caval, renal, and lumbar vein injury. All were controlled laparoscopically with either clips or fibrin glue; a left renal vein injury was controlled via laparoscopic suturing. Few minor complications occurred postoperatively, including three asymptomatic lymphoceles, a transient irritation of the genitofemoral nerve, and a spontaneously resolving retroperitoneal hematoma. Other groups have reported ureteral stenosis following ureteric stenting, which was abandoned later on, as well as the need for temporary ureteric drainage in some cases.[38] Mean postoperative hospitalization was 3.6 (2–8 days).

Oncologic efficacy

Histologic findings were positive in 25 of the 101 patients (25%). Some groups have reported the number of resected lymph nodes but this doesn't appear practical, since to our knowledge there are no data to indicate how many lymph nodes a specimen must contain to prove the completeness of the dissection in a given template.

Follow-up data are available on 96 of our 101 patients; 5 patients were lost during follow-up. Of 96 pathologic stage I patients on a mean follow-up of 47 months, 2 relapses were reported (see Table 15.5). One retroperitoneal recurrence occurred on the contralateral side outside the surgical field. Further investigations revealed that the tumor in the primary landing site had been removed at surgery but was missed on histologic examination. This patient was cured with two cycles of chemotherapy and contralateral laparoscopic RPLND. Another patient developed lung recurrence during follow-up. No further relapses occurred, which clearly demonstrates the oncologic efficacy of the procedure. Rassweiler et al.[38] and

Gerber et al.[39] also reported pulmonary relapses in 4 cases, but no retroperitoneal relapses.

The rate of retroperitoneal relapse after open RPLND was reported to be 6.8% in 88 clinical stage I patients; 37 of the 88 patients had pathologic stage I lesions.[40] By comparison, the relapse rate in our series is extraordinarily low, a fact that cannot be explained. Nevertheless, it is tempting to speculate that at least some of the recurrences in the literature may be due to false-negative findings on histologic examination.

The mean follow-up in 25 clinical stage I pathologic stage II patients who received two cycles of adjuvant chemotherapy (all except 1 patient with mature teratoma) is currently 47 months. Over this time period, no relapse has been seen.

Stage II after chemotherapy

Between February 1995 and October 2002, 58 patients with clinical stage II underwent RPLND (42 stage IIb and 16 stage IIc). The mean age was 29.1 years old (15–56). The procedure was performed on the right side in 32 patients and on the left in 26. The mean operative time was 234 min (135–360) and the mean blood loss was 165 ml (20–350). No conversion occurred and the spectrum of complications was almost the same as in stage I patients with a higher incidence of chylous ascites in stage II. Postoperative hospital stay averaged 3.8 days (3–10 days).

Histologic analysis of the specimens revealed necrosis in 36 patients, mature teratoma in 20 patients, active tumor in 1 patient and seminoma in 1 patient (Table 15.6). To date, this was our only seminoma case for which RPLND was performed. The patient had a residual tumor 6 cm in size following three cycles of chemotherapy (20% of the original tumor size). A PET scan showed no reduction in size between the second and third course and no signs of vital tumor. RPLND was performed on the left side; the procedure was quite difficult owing to a large tumor mass and numerous venous interconnections. Histology revealed small foci of a vital tumor. On a mean

Table 15.6 *Postoperative pathology for residual mass (laparoscopic resection)*	
Stage II after chemotherapy: postoperative pathology	No. of patients
Total number	58 patients
Necrosis	36 cases (62%)
Mature teratoma	20 cases (34.5%)
Active tumor	1 case (1.7%)
Seminoma	1 case (1.7%)

follow-up of 38 months (3–73), no relapse was detected in any of these 58 patients.

Antegrade ejaculation

Loss of antegrade ejaculation (see Table 15.5) is the major morbidity encountered after RPLND. This drawback can be overcome either by performing a template dissection, as described by Weissbach and Boedefeld[36] or by nerve sparing RPLND.[14] The template dissection, although downscaling the operative field, maintains acceptable sensitivity and, more importantly doesn't increase relapse rate. We have followed this strategy in our work, and in 98 of our stage I patients, antegrade ejaculation rate was 100% (3 patients were lost during follow-up). In stage II patients, antegrade ejaculation was preserved in 56 out of 58 patients.

With the introduction of nerve-sparing RPLND, Donohue was able to improve the ejaculation rate from 70 to almost 100%. Donohue did not only introduce nerve-sparing dissection but also simultaneously limited the dissection to the unilateral template.[15,19] It has been known since 1964 that destruction of the sympathetic chain on one side doesn't result in aspermia as long as the contralateral side is intact.[42] Therefore, nerve-sparing, in addition to a unilateral dissection, is not necessary and cannot improve the already good results. Recently, Peschel et al published the results of laparoscopic nerve sparing RPLND in 5 patients, showing an operative time of 3.2 hours average, a blood loss of 66 ml, and a hospital stay of 3.7 days (results comparable to the standard procedure). This required meticulous dissection and identification of the sympathetic chain and the postganglionic fibers in the retrocaval, the interaortocaval, and the para-aortic regions. Although, as we mentioned earlier, antegrade ejaculation is routinely preserved when a nerve-sparing dissection is limited to a unilateral template, the development of a unilateral laparoscopic nerve-sparing technique is a step towards bilateral laparoscopic dissection.[43]

Quality of life

A major issue to be considered when comparing various treatment modalities is the patient's quality of life thereafter. Thus, a quality of life study has been performed in coordination with a psychiatric group at our center. A questionnaire was distributed to 119 patients and completed by personal interviews with 118 (the open group consisted of 53 patients and the laparoscopic group 59). The questionnaire included questions about the patient's satisfaction with the information about the disease, and his experience of treatment and its side-effects. Patients were asked about the time it took them

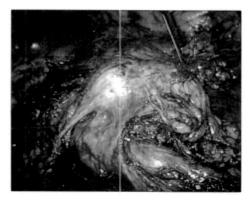

Figure 15.14
Seminoma: residual mass after chemotherapy, overlying the aorta.

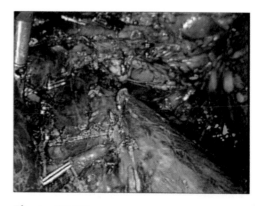

Figure 15.15
Seminoma: operative field after excision of residual mass (lateral edge of aorta, lumbar artery, and psoas muscle).

until they were able to perform moderate physical exercise, return to normal activities, and were free of symptoms. Other questions – regarding sexual activity, whether the patient felt lovable, experienced any problems in his partnership, psyche, or social life, and whether he was anxious about losing his job or had emotional problems associated with the loss of testicle or the RPLND procedure – were also addressed. Surprisingly, the patients better tolerated not only laparoscopic RPLND but also open RPLND rather than chemotherapy. Open RPLND was found to impair the quality of life more than laparoscopic RPLND. There is not a single item where open RPLND was superior to laparoscopy. The patients who participated in the study preferred RPLND to all other treatment modalities.[44]

Cost-effectiveness

Although costs are not a primary issue, they have to be taken in consideration. In our series, the surgical procedure itself was found to be less expensive if done by the open rather than by the laparoscopic approach, but adding the hospital stay to the surgical costs brings the latter down in the case of laparoscopy so that the total hospital costs in both groups are almost equal. Another factor that has not been taken into account in most studies is the time to convalescence, especially considering that most of our patients are young productive individuals. If this factor were to be added, laparoscopy would definitely be the clear winner.[32]

Extraperitoneal approach

Two centers have described an extraperitoneal approach for laparoscopic RPLND. One group strongly supports the procedure, arguing that it is more safe to the bowel and other viscera, and suggesting that it provides better access to the retrovascular areas, thereby facilitating nerve-sparing dissection.[45] However, based on our experience, the risk of bowel injury is minor during transperitoneal RPLND, as it is totally out of the operative field. On the other hand, access to the retrovascular area is not really required, as it is not included in the template dissection, since lymph node metastases were found to be exclusively ventral to the lumbar vessels. In addition, we feel that the transperitoneal route gives a better access to the inter-aortocaval area, for the right-side RPLND. Although this first group did not report any incidence of lymphocele, it is expected to occur once a larger group of patients is evaluated.[32] In short, we are not convinced that retroperitoneoscopy offers any major advantage over the transperitoneal approach.

Summary

In our hands, laparoscopic RPLND has demonstrated its surgical and oncologic efficacy. The morbidity and the complication rate are low. Adherence to the templates described above allows for preservation of antegrade ejaculation in virtually all patients. It is a difficult procedure indeed, but once the long and steep learning curve has been overcome, operative times are equal to or even shorter than those of open surgery. Thereafter, the costs will be in the range of open surgery. The recurrence rate of laparoscopic RPLND is at least as low and survival is equal to that of open surgery and chemotherapy. Patient satisfaction, however, is clearly higher with laparoscopic RPLND, which the authors demonstrated in a recent extensive quality of life study.

References

1. Bosl GJ, Motzer RJ. Testicular germ-cell cancer. N Engl J Med 1997; 337:242–53.

2. Mostofi FK, Sesterhenn IA, Sobin LH. Histological typing of testicular tumors. In: World Health Organization: international histological typing of tumors, 2nd edn. Berlin: Springer-Verlag, 1998.

3. Bosl GJ, Vogelzang NJ, Goldman A, et al. Impact of delay in diagnosis on clinical stage of testicular cancer. Lancet 1981; 2: 970–3.

4. Steele GS, Kantoff PW, Richie JP. Staging and imaging of testis cancer. In: Vogelzang NJ, Scardino PT, Shipley WU, Coffey DS eds. Genitourinary oncology. Philadelphia: Lippincott, Williams and Williams, 2000: 939–49.

5. Ritchie JP, Steele GS. Neoplasms of the testis. In: Walsh PC, Retik AB, Vaughan ED Jr, Wein AJ, eds. Campbell's urology, 8th edn, Vol. 4, Philadelphia, WB Saunders, 2002: 2876–919.

6. Stomper PC, Jochelson MS, Garnick MB, Richie JP. Residual abdominal masses following chemotherapy for nonseminomatous testicular cancer: correlation of CT and histology. AJR Am J Roentgenol 1985; 145(4):743–6.

7. Cremerius U, Wildberger JE, Borchers H, et al. Does positron emission tomography using 18-fluoro-2-deoxyglucose improve clinical staging of testicular cancer? Results of a study in 50 patients. Urology 1999; 54: 900–4.

8. Ganjoo KN, Chan RJ, Sharma M, Einhorn LH. Positron emission tomography scans in the evaluation of postchemotherapy residual masses in patients with seminoma. J Clin Oncol 1999; 17: 3457–60.

9. Lange, Raghavan. Clinical application of tumor markers in testicular cancer. In: Donohue JP, ed. Testis tumor. Baltimore: Williams & Wilkins, 1983:111–30.

10. Freedman LS Parkinson MC Jones WG, et al. Histopathology in the prediction of relapse of patients with stage I testicular teratoma treated by orchidectomy alone. Lancet 1987; 2 (8554):294–8.

11. Nicolai N, Pizzocaro G. A surveillance study of clinical stage I nonseminomatous germ cell tumors of the testis: 1-year follow up. J Urol 1995; 154 (4):1045–9.

12. Jewett MAS, Herman JG, Stugeron JFP, et al. Expectant treatment for clinical stage A nonseminomatous germ cell testicular tumors. World J Urol 1984; 2:57.

13. Sogani PC, Perrotti M, Herr HW, et al. Clinical stage I testis cancer: long-term outcome of patients on surveillance. J Urol 1998; 159(3):855–8.

14. Thompson PI, Nixon J, Harvey VJ. Disease relapse in patients with stage I nonseminomatous germ cell tumors of the testis on active surveillance. J Clin Oncol 1988; 6:1597–603.

15. Donohue JP, Foster RS, Rowland RG. Nerve-sparing retroperitoneal lymphadenectomy with preservation of ejaculation. J Urol 1990; 144:287–91.

16. Fossa SD, Ous S, Stenwig AE, et al. Distribution of retroperitoneal lymph node metastases in patients with nonseminomatous testicular cancer. Eur Urol 1990; 17:107–12.

17. Richie JP. Clinical stage I testicular cancer: the role of modified retroperitoneal lymphadenectomy. J Urol 1990; 144(5):1160–3.

18. Weissbach L, Boedefeld EA, Hostmann-Dubral B. Surgical treatment of stage I nonseminomatous germ cell testis tumor. Eur Urol 1990; 17(2):97–106.

19. Donohue JP, Thornhill JA, Foster RS, et al. Retroperitoneal lymphadenectomy for clinical stage A testis cancer (1965 to 1989): modification of technique and impact on ejaculation. J Urol 1993; 149:237–43.

20. Böhlen D, Borner M, Sonntag RW, et al. Long-term results following adjuvant chemotherapy in patients with clinical stage I testicular non-seminomatous malignant germ cell tumors with high risk factors. J Urol 1999; 161:1148–52.

21. Heidenreich A, Sesterhenn IA, Mostofi FK, et al. Prognostic risk factors that identify patients with clinical stage I nonseminomatous germ cell tumors at low risk and high risk for metastasis. Cancer 1998; 83:1002–111.

22. Bussar-Matz R, Weissbach L. Retroperitoneal lymph node staging of testicular tumors. TNM Study Group. Br J Urol 1993; 72:234–40.

23. Albert H, Heidenreich A, Engelmann U. Primary adjuvant carboplatin monotherapy in clinical stage I seminoma. Eur Urol 1999; 35(Suppl 2):35.

24. Albers P, Siener R, Hartmann M, et al. Prospective randomized multicenter trial in clinical stage I NSGCT – preliminary results. Eur Urol 1999; 35 (Suppl 2):121.

25. Richie JP, Kantoff PW. Is adjuvant chemotherapy necessary for patients with stage B1 testicular cancer? J Clin Oncol 1991; 9:1393–6.

26. Donohue JP, Thornhill JA, Foster RS, et al. The role of retroperitoneal lymphadenectomy in clinical stage B testis cancer: the Indiana University experience (1965 to 1989). J Urol 1995; 153:85–9.

27. Williams SD, Stablein DM, Einhorn LH, et al. Immediate adjuvant chemotherapy versus observation with treatment at relapse in pathological stage II testicular cancer. N Engl J Med 1987; 317:1433–8.

28. Javadpour N. Predictors of recurrence in stage II nonseminomatous testicular cancer after lymphadenectomy: implications for adjuvant chemotherapy. J Urol 1985; 134(3):629.

29. Pizzocaro G, Nicolai N, Salvioni R. Evolution and controversies in the management of low-stage nonseminomatous germ-cell tumors of the testis. World J Urol 1994; 12: 113–19.

30. Nelson JB, Chen RN, Bishoff JT, et al. Laparoscopic retroperitoneal lymph node dissection for clinical stage I nonseminomatous germ cell testicular tumors. Urology 1999; 54: 1064–7.

31. Socinski MA, Gernick MB, Stomper PC, et al. Stage II nonseminomatous germ cell tumors of the testis: an analysis of treatment options in patients with low volume retroperitoneal disease. J Urol 1988; 140:1437–41.

32. Janetschek G. Laparoscopic retroperitoneal lymph node dissection. Urol Clin North Am 2001; 28:107–14.

33. Rassweiler JJ, Seemann O, Henkel TO, et al. Laparoscopic retroperitoneal lymph node dissection for nonseminomatous germ cell tumors: indications and limitations. J Urol 1996; 156:1108–13.

34. Janetschek G, Hobisch A, Hittmair A, et al. Laparoscopic retroperitoneal lymphadenectomy after chemotherapy for stage IIB nonseminomatous testicular carcinoma. J Urol 1999; 151:477–81.

35. Steiner H, Holtl L, Wirtenberger W, et al. Long-term experience with carboplatin monotherapy for clinical stage I seminoma: a retrospective single-center study. Urology 2002; 60(2):324–8.

36. Weissbach L, Boedefeld EA. Testicular Tumor Study Group: localization of solitary and multiple metastases in stage II nonseminomatous testis tumor as basis for a modified staging lymph node dissection in stage I. J Urol 1987; 138: 77–82.

37. Holtl L, Peschel R, Knapp R, et al. Primary lymphatic metastatic spread in testicular cancers occurs ventral to the lumbar vessels. Urology 2002; 59:114–18.

38. Rasweiler JJ, Frede T, Lenz E, et al. Long-term experience with laparoscopic retroperitoneal lymph node dissection in the management of low-stage testis cancer. Eur Urol 2000; 37:251–60.

39. Gerber GS, Bissada NK, Hulbert JK, et al. Laparoscopic retroperitoneal lymphadenectomy: multi-institutional analysis. J Urol 1994; 152:1188–91.

40. Cespedes RD, Peretsman SJ. Retroperitoneal reccurrences after retroperitoneal lymph node dissection for low-stage nonseminomatous germ cell tumors. Urology 1999; 54:548–52.

41. Janetschek G, Hobisch A, Höltl L, et al. Retroperitoneal lymphadenectomy for clinical stage I nonseminomatous testicular tumor: laparoscopy versus open surgery and impact of learning curve. J Urol 1996; 156:89–93.

42. Whitelaw GP, Smithwick RH. Some secondary effects of sympathectomy with particular reference to disturbance of sexual function. New E J Med 1951; 245:212.

43. Peschel R, Gettman MT, Neururer R, et al. Laparoscopic retroperitoneal lymph node dissection: description of the nerve sparing technique. Urology 2002; 60:339–43.

44. Hobisch A, Tönnemann J, Janetschek G. Morbidity and quality of life after open versus laparoscopic retroperitoneal lymphadenectomy for testicular tumour – the patient's view. In: Jones WG, Appleyard 1, Harnden P, Joffe JK, eds. Germ cell tumours VI. London: John Libbey, 1998: 277.

45. LeBlanc E, Caty A, Dargent D, et al. Extraperitoneal laparoscopic para-aortic lymph node dissection for early stage nonseminomatous germ cell tumors of the testis with introduction of a nerve sparing technique: description and results. J Urol 2001; 165:89–92.

16

Minimally invasive treatments for bladder cancer – from transurethral resection to laparoscopic radical cystectomy

John W Davis, Ingolf Arthur Tuerk, Serdar Deger and Stefan A Loening

Introduction

Overview of bladder cancer presentation

De-novo bladder cancer most commonly presents with gross or microscopic hematuria. As cystoscopy is a mandatory part of any complete work-up for hematuria, this is the most common test that confirms the diagnosis. Bladder cancers may also create filling defects that are visible on an intravenous pyelogram (IVP), ultrasound, and/or computed tomography (CT) scan. However, sensitivity is poor when tumors are less than 2 cm, and therefore incidental detection of bladder cancer is unusual.

Currently there is no commonly accepted screening test for bladder cancer, other than urinalysis to detect microscopic hematuria. Cytology has been used to detect preclinical cancer in high-risk populations, i.e. those subjects involved in chemical industrial exposure. Again, cystoscopy provides visual confirmation and the avenue for securing tissue for histopathology. Interval cystoscopy is also indicated for individuals with a history of bladder cancer or a history of upper tract transitional cell carcinoma. Another high-risk group includes those with a chronic suprapubic catheter where a transitional or squamous transitional or pure squamous cancer occurs with increased frequency. They should undergo yearly cystoscopy and cytology studies. For individuals with a history of bladder cancer undergoing routine cystoscopy, urinary cytology is an adjunct surveillance study that is standard. Cytology is sensitive for carcinoma-in-situ and high-grade transitional cell carcinoma, but notoriously insensitive for detecting low-grade tumors. Several urinary marker tests such as BTA and NMP-22 have been investigated that are more sensitive in detecting low-grade tumors, but none have such accuracy that cystoscopy can

be safely omitted in the face of normal urine marker tests. Thus, the use of newer urine markers has yet to become standard, and the standard of care remains cystoscopy to detect papillary tumors of all grades, and cytology to assist with the diagnosis of carcinoma-in-situ and high-grade invasive recurrence, and to alert for possible upper tract tumor occurrence.

Physical examination

A complete history and physical examination is an important part of any evaluation of bladder cancer. As transurethral resection (TUR) is the mainstay of initial diagnosis and treatment, patients must be judged safe to undergo a general anesthetic. Patients with bladder cancer often have a significant smoking history, and must therefore be screened for other smoking-related conditions such as coronary artery disease, peripheral vascular disease, lung cancer, emphysema, and chronic obstructive pulmonary disease. A complete genitourinary examination surveys for the presence of other conditions such as prostate cancer, urethral masses, and in females any adnexal masses.

The most important part of the physical examination specific to bladder cancer is the pelvic examination under anesthesia before and at the conclusion of the TUR. The physician should perform bimanual examination with one hand on the abdomen and an examining finger in the rectum (males) or vagina. With the patient maximally relaxed by the anesthesiologist, the bladder walls are compressed between the examining hand and finger and systematically palpated laterally and medially. Again, patient muscular relaxation is critical to being able to adequately feel for bladder masses. Optimally, the examination should be repeated with the opposite hand on the abdomen/finger in the rectum or vagina. Any induration or two-dimensional mass that persists after the tumor resection may represent unresected tumor more deeply invasive in a primary case, or possibly scar in a patient after a recent transurethral resection of bladder tumor (TURBT). A three-dimensional mass is highly indicative of a locally advanced muscle invasive tumor.

Diagnostic work-up and staging

Given that bladder cancer is commonly related to smoking and occurs in older individuals, diagnostic work-up will turn towards appropriate preparation for transurethral resection. Complete blood counts, electrolytes, chest X-ray, and electrocardiogram (ECG) are obtained and possible medical/cardiac clearance in appropriate patients. While spinal anesthesia is an option, many prefer a general anesthetic so that the patient can be maximally relaxed with muscular paralytic agents for bimanual examination, and avoid an obturator reflex during lateral resection. When histopathology reveals high-risk superficial disease or muscle invasive disease, further staging for metastatic disease is done with a CT of the abdomen and pelvis, and serum liver function tests. A chest CT is obtained for any suspicious chest X-ray finding, and nuclear bone scans are obtained if alkaline phosphatase is elevated or if the patient complains of bone pains (excluding chronic conditions).

Transurethral technique

While TURBT is a routine procedure for urologists, many surgical goals require careful attention to detail and technique. Pre-existing urinary infections are treated before surgery and uninfected patients are given prophylactic antibiotics. In general, TURBT is a low-risk procedure with few major complications or mortalities. Patients are advised of the risks of bleeding and bladder perforation. The aim of resection is complete removal of visible cancer and harvest of tissue for accurate staging, while controlling bleeding and avoiding perforation. While not technically 'complications,' several untoward outcomes occur after TURBT. First and foremost, bladder tumors recur, regardless of initial grade and stage. A field defect and tumor cell reimplantation are certainly among the causes, while other causes are missed or inadequately resected tumors. Pathologic examination of the specimens may also identify problems with the technique of resection that prevents ideal characterization and management. The two most common problems are excessive cautery artifact in the specimen and a lack of muscularis propria in the specimen. When either of these situations occurs in the setting of a high-grade lesion, the urologist cannot reliably stage

the patient as superficial vs muscle invasive, and re-resection becomes mandatory. At the other extreme, excessively deep resection may lead to bladder perforation, which may, in theory, allow tumor cells to implant in the pelvis, and which necessitates additional catheter time to heal the injury. Furthermore, perforation along the posterior wall of the bladder may penetrate the intraperitoneal abdominal cavity and require open or laparoscopic repair.

With these issues in mind, the technique of TURBT starts with equipment. A full range of resectoscopes and dilators are needed to negotiate the urethra safely with minimal trauma, thereby avoiding postoperative stricture formation. The use of continuous flow is popular with some urologists and may aid in visualization with bleeding, prevents the need for repetitive interruption to drain the bladder, and keeps the bladder wall in a relatively 'stable' position of distention throughout resection. Complete inspection of the bladder is best achieved with use of a 12° or 30° lens and a 70° lens. Inspection at different filling levels and with manual suprapubic pressure helps visualize the more acute angles of view along the anterior walls and bladder neck. Photographs and/or bladder maps help document the number, location, and size of tumors for future reference.

The technique of resection varies with the size and location of the tumor. Small, papillary lesions may often be removed by a cold-cup biopsy grasper alone. Larger tumors require a standard resectoscope loop using cutting current to preserve tissue for pathology. When more aggressive pathology is suspected, the tumor specimen should be fractionated into superficial and deep layers. The deeper layers should include resected muscularis propria under the tumor, and possibly cold-cup biopsies of the area to exclude invasive disease. With higher-risk tumors, random bladder biopsies and prostate urethral biopsies are obtained to identify surrounding carcinoma-in-situ and/or prostatic urethral involvement.

Post-procedure, a large catheter is placed, and the duration varies depending on the difficulty and depth of resection performed. Evidence is now available that a single post-TURBT instillation of a chemotherapeutic agent such as mitomycin C or Adriamycin (doxorubicin) will help reduce recurrences with minimal morbidity. Routine use is incorporated in the European Association of Urology Guidelines on Bladder Cancer (download from their website www.uroweb.org), and can now be recommended unless perforation occurred – even when further therapy with BCG (bacille Calmette-Guérin) is anticipated.[1,2]

Transurethral outcome

Outcomes after transurethral resection for superficial pTa or pT1 tumors are measured in terms of tumor recurrence and tumor progression. Both outcomes are predicted by tumor stage, grade, presence of carcinoma-in-situ, initial tumor size, and multiplicity.[3] Allard et al[4] evaluated adverse predictors of recurrence, including tumor multiplicity, diameter > 3 cm, stage T1, and grade 2–3. They reported a strong relationship between the number of adverse predictors and subsequent recurrence/progression. For patients without adverse predictors, recurrence-free survival was 86% at 1 and 69% at 2 years; no patients progressed. For 3–4 adverse predictors, recurrence-free survival was 30% at 1 and 19% at 2 years; 7% of patients progressed.[4] Parmer et al[5] demonstrated the adverse prognostic significance of tumor recurrence at the initial 3-month surveillance cystoscopy. As stated, a single intravesical dose of chemotherapy after resection as well as an induction course can reduce recurrences but not alter progressions.[1,6]

If histopathology from TURBT shows high-risk features for recurrence/progression, i.e. grade 3, stage T1, ± presence of carcinoma-in-situ, intravesical therapy with BCG becomes standard. Long-term data are emerging that support durable disease-free survival in most patients, yet approximately 20–30% of patients will progress to muscle invasive disease, and approximately 15% will develop upper tract recurrences.[7,8] Lifelong surveillance is critical, and early cystectomy for patients progressing or recurring with high-risk disease. Maintenance BCG has been shown to reduce recurrences and lengthen worsening-free survival in patients with carcinoma-in-situ and select patients with high-risk Ta/T1 disease,[9] and should be considered in patients who can tolerate the treatment. Newer treatment strategies are also available for patients not tolerating or failing BCG, which combines lower doses of BCG with interferon (IFN). O'Donnell reported efficacy in 40 patients previously deemed BCG refractory, and this finding held true in patients failing one or two 6-dose inductions of BCG.[10] At the very least, BCG/IFN allows for the reduction in dose of BCG for patients with significant symptoms on full dose, and the combination immune response may be superior.

In sum, TURBT is the starting point for all treatments for bladder cancer, and for superficial disease is the mainstay of bladder-sparing treatment. However, as stated, patients with high-risk disease can progress despite therapy, while others have a durable response. Thus, patients can be undertreated if they undergo repeated TURBTs and intravesical therapy, but later progress to invasive disease and are at significant risk for dying of metastatic disease. On the other hand, immediate cystectomy is overtreatment in the majority of T1G3 tumors. The benefits of bladder preservation must be balanced with long-term cancer control. The pendulum may be swinging in favor of earlier cystectomy in cases of BCG failures. Herr and Sogani reported on 307 patients with high-risk transitional cell carcinoma who underwent

cystectomy during follow-up after initial BCG and found improved long-term survival when cystectomy was performed early (< 2 years) vs late.[11] Solsona et al[12] found that the 3-month response to intravesical therapy predicted for progression–T1G3 recurrences at 3 months after induction BCG had a 66% 1-year and 96% 2-year progression rate. Molecular markers are urgently needed to predict which patients will respond to TURBT plus BCG, and which patients are better served with early cystectomy. Examples of such research include the report from Bernardini et al, who evaluated combining T1 microstaging and p53 expression.[13]

Bladder-sparing strategies for muscle invasive disease: transurethral resection of bladder tumor, trimodal therapy, partial cystectomy

Cystectomy is the gold standard for muscle invasive disease, and as reviewed, is indicated for high-risk superficial disease failing intravesical therapy. For patients presenting with limited muscle invasive disease, TUR alone can be effective. Herr has reported a series of patients treated by TUR alone if re-resection showed pT0 or pT1 residual disease. For pT0, 10-year survival was similar to immediate cystectomy.[14] Solsona et al[15] have reported similar success with select patients with invasive transitional cell carcinoma treated by aggressive TUR alone.

Trimodal therapy has been evaluated as a bladder-sparing treatment for muscle invasive disease: deep TUR, cisplatin-based chemotherapy, and external beam radiation. In their most recent update, Shipley et al[16] reported cancer-specific survival by pathologic stage that was comparable to radical cystectomy at 5 and 10 years: pT2, 74%/66%; pT3–T4a, 53%/52%. The findings of an initial complete resection, absence of hydronephrosis, and no evidence of cancer on restaging resection after 4000 rad selects patients most likely to respond to the chemoradiation regimen. Of note, one-third of patients eventually required a cystectomy, but none for bladder morbidity alone. Thus, trimodal therapy is a valid bladder-preserving option in patients refusing or inappropriate for cystectomy. The extent to which all three treatments are needed is unclear, however, as neoadjuvant cisplatin chemotherapy and TUR is known to produce a P0 response at cystectomy[17] and aggressive TUR alone can be successful.[14]

A more invasive, but bladder-sparing treatment strategy is partial cystectomy. As reviewed by Feneley and Schoenberg,[18] partial cystectomy is feasible but has strict selection criteria that limit its use. The ideal candidate has a solitary lesion located in the dome or anterior wall, well away from the bladder neck and/or trigone. Contraindications include multifocal disease, prostatic involvement, and carcinoma-in-situ. Pelvic lymph node dissection may be performed, and outcomes by stage may match radical cystectomy. However, local recurrence rates of 30–80% have been reported.[18] Other applications of this technique are for tumors arising in diverticula (TUR alone are often inadequate), and adenocarcinoma of the urachus.[18]

Laparoscopic radical cystectomy

Radical cystectomy with urinary diversion remains the gold standard treatment for muscle invasive bladder carcinoma. Constant advances in anesthesiology and surgical technique, and a more sophisticated postoperative care, have decreased the risk of such major surgery. However, radical cystectomy remains an aggressive procedure, with significant morbidity and mortality. The complication rate in the early postoperative period after radical cystectomy and urinary diversion is still 25–35%.[19] This remaining morbidity of open cystectomy has stimulated interest in treatment alternatives with less morbidity without compromising the oncologic outcome.

Advances in laparoscopic surgery have resulted in a notable decrease in patient morbidity, with speedier recovery and shorter hospital stay. Since the first report of a laparoscopic nephrectomy by Clayman and coworkers in 1991,[20] the role of laparoscopy in urology has been expanding. Laparoscopic radical nephrectomy has been established in the last 5 years, with reports of equivalent oncologic results, and the traditional benefits of less postoperative pain, improved cosmesis, shorter hospital stay, and faster return to full activity.[21,22] Recently, laparoscopic radical prostatectomy seems to be as efficacious as the open procedure. Early oncologic data look similar to open series, but only short-term observation is available. However, new benefits are evident with the laparoscopic approach: improved visualization of the operative field with more surgical precision, and significantly lower blood loss.[23–25]

The next logical step is the utilization of the laparoscopic approach for the surgical treatment of muscle invasive bladder cancer. Application of laparoscopy in the field of cystectomy started in 1992 when Parra et al[26] reported a laparoscopic simple cystectomy in a 27-year-old female with symptomatic pyocystitis of a retained bladder after previous urinary diversion. The operating time was 130 min, the blood loss was 115 ml, and the hospital stay was 5 days. In 1993, De Badajoz et al were the first to use the laparoscopic approach to cystectomy for invasive cancer in a 64-year-old female.[27] Operating room time was 8 hours, blood loss was minimal, and the postoperative course was

free of complications. Puppo et al[28] performed laparoscopically assisted transvaginal radical cystectomy in 5 female patients with bladder cancer. Operating times were between 6 and 9 hours. Four of the 5 patients were discharged from hospital free of complications on days 7–11. The largest series of laparoscopic radical cystectomy was published by an Egyptian group. Denewer et al[29] reported on 10 patients with invasive bladder cancer, who underwent laparoscopically assisted cystectomy and urinary diversion. They demonstrated that the laparoscopic access involves less morbidity and earlier recovery as well as shorter hospital stay.

The Department of Urology at Charité Hospital in Berlin began its experience with laparoscopic radical cystectomy and urinary diversion in March 2000 to treat patients with muscle invasive bladder cancer.

Technique of laparoscopic radical cystectomy

Preoperative preparation includes a bowel preparation with a clear liquid diet starting preoperative day 2; a 3 liters mechanical bowel on pre-operative day 1; and a cephalosporin and metronidazole on call to the operating room. The patient is placed supine with steep Trendelenburg position, and a six-port transperitoneal laparoscopic access is established (Figure 16.1). As in the open procedure, the right-handed surgeon stands to the patient's left. Camera monitors are positioned at the patient's feet. In our experience, dissection is best accomplished via laparoscopic scissors attached to

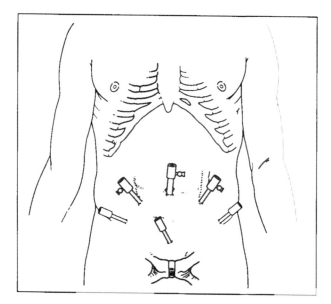

Figure 16.1
Number and placement of trocars.

monopolar cautery in one hand of the surgeon, and graspers attached to bipolar cautery in the other. The first assistant utilizes suction in one hand and graspers for retraction in the other. We commonly utilize the Aesop robotic arm and voice recognition to give control of the camera to the surgeon. However, if the first assistant is being instructed, it is best to have a second assistant operate the camera.

Bilateral pelvic lymph node dissections are performed, removing tissue from the obturator fossa, and external iliac vein and artery from the obturator fossa up to the bifurcation of the aorta. The ureters are mobilized from the iliac vessel crossover to their entry into the bladder. Next, the peritoneum over the pouch of Douglas is incised and the vasa deferentia (in male) identified. Each vas is dissected towards the seminal vesicles, which are completely mobilized. The vasa deferentia and seminal vesicles are lifted anterior-superiorly, so that Denonvilliers' fascia can be incised, and the plane between the prostate and the rectum can be developed. In females, the pouch of Douglas is incised, and the posterior wall of the vagina is mobilized from the rectum. Also both ovaries are mobilized after transection of the ovarian vessels.

The dissection now turns anterior, where the peritoneum over the umbilical ligaments is incised, and the ligaments transected. The space of Retzius is developed as in the open procedure, with the urinary bladder dissected off the anterior abdominal wall, and the endopelvic fascia exposed. The endopelvic fascia is incised bilaterally, and the puboprostatic or pubourethral (women) ligaments divided. The dorsal vein complex is sutured with an 0-Vicryl purse-string, but not divided at this point.

The posterior and anterior pedicles of the bladder and the pedicles of the prostate or uterus are divided by serial applications of the Endo-GIA stapler (Figure 16.2). The dorsal vein complex is now divided just proximal to the suture. The urethra is divided close to the pelvic floor, the catheter is removed, and the bladder neck is closed with a suture to avoid spillage of urine into the peritoneal cavity with the risk of tumor seeding. In men, the remaining attachments are divided to completely free the specimen (bladder, prostate, and seminal vesicles), which is secured in an endobag for later removal during the urinary diversion. In women, the bladder with the anterior wall of the vagina are removed to complete the dissection, and the specimen is entrapped in an endobag for immediate removal through the vaginal opening. The vagina is then closed by a running 0-Vicryl suture.

Urinary diversion

Once laparoscopic radical prostatectomy has been mastered, the only additional simple steps radical cystec-

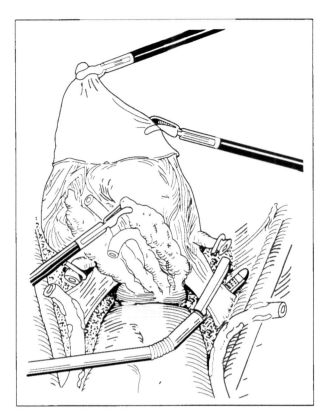

Figure 16.2
Transection of the bladder pedicles with an Endo-GIA stapler.

tomy involves are taking down the lateral pedicles with the Endo-GIA stapler. The challenge is the urinary diversion.

The ileal loop urinary diversion has been the standard type of urinary diversion since it was described by Bricker in 1950.[30] The first laparoscopic ileal loop urinary conduit was reported by Kozminski and Partamian.[31] Their procedure did not include a cystectomy. A total of five port sites were used, one of which served as the stoma site. Laparoscopically, both ureters were mobilized and transected. The bowel anastomosis was performed extracorporeally by gently elevating a small loop of ileum through a port site. The initial operation took 6 hours and 20 min. De Badajoz et al[27] and Puppo et al[28] provided their patients with an ileal conduit after a laparoscopic cystectomy, as described before.

To date, most authors perform a laparotomy after laparoscopic cystectomy to remove the specimen and construct the urinary diversion (ileal conduit). However, Gill et al[32] have recently reported on an ileal conduit urinary diversion by laparoscopy alone, performed in two men: the surgical times of the complete procedure (laparoscopic cystectomy and ileal conduit) were 11.5 and 10 hours and blood losses were 1200 and 1000 ml. However, most patients motivated and healthy enough to undergo a 10-hour laparoscopic procedure will also be the type of patients desiring the long-term quality of life aspects of a continent urinary diversion as well as the short-term recovery benefits of a laparoscopic approach. Most patients willing to accept the longer operative time required for a laparoscopic approach will also desire a continent urinary diversion because of the better quality of life and cosmesis.

The first experimental laparoscopic ureterosigmoidostomy for urinary diversion using pigs was reported by Trinchieri et al.[33] Anderson et al[34] published their experience constructing a laparoscopically assisted sigma rectum pouch as a continent urinary diversion in an animal model (pig). The laparoscopically mobilized sigma was extracorporeally positioned via a laparotomy. The pouch was formed by side-to-side anastomosis of the opened bowel segment with a stapler, and the ureterocolonic anastomoses were done extracorporeally. Postoperative function of the pouch was good. However, in 44% of the cases the formation of stones was diagnosed in the area of titan clips and in 33% stenosis of the ureterocolic anastomosis occurred. Denewer et al[29] used the same technique in 1999 for continent urinary diversion after laparoscopic cystectomy in his 10 patients. An 8 cm long incision in the lower abdomen was required to construct the sigma rectum pouch extracorporeally using a stapling technique, and the ureters were implanted in an antireflux fashion. No postoperative follow-up information was provided regarding stone formation.

The most noticeable benefit of the sigma rectum pouch diversion is the easy construction and the nearly 100% day- and night-time continence of properly selected patients. The sigma rectum pouch is a modification of the ureterosigmoidostomy and was first described by Fisch et al[35] as an alternative continent urinary diversion. Several authors reported excellent functional results of this continent urine reservoir after open radical cystectomy.[36-38]

To our knowledge, we performed the first continent urinary diversion completely laparoscopically in April 2000 at Charité Hospital, Berlin, using the Mainz pouch II technique.[39] Another issue of the laparoscopic procedure is how to remove the cystectomy specimen. Until now, laparoscopists have made a minilaparotomy for specimen removal. The opening of the sigmoid and rectum or the vagina also allows removal of the specimen without enlarging any of the abdominal port sites.

Technique – laparoscopic Mainz II pouch (rectum sigma pouch)

Prior to surgery, patients undergo outpatient sigmoidoscopy to exclude diverticulosis or other abnormalities. Further selection criteria include a competent anal sphincter, assessed by the ability to hold a 200–300 ml water enema for 2 hours, and adequate renal function (serum creatinine < 1.5 mg/Dl).

An antimesenteric enterotomy is made with an electric hook at the recto-sigmoid junction and extended 10 cm proximally and 10 cm distally (Figure 16.3). In men, this allows for transanal removal of the specimen (Figure 16.4). The posterior walls of the rectum and sigmoid are then anastomosed side-to-side with a running 3-0 Maxon suture to form the posterior wall of the pouch (Figure 16.5). Nonrefluxing ureteral anastamoses are formed by preparing a 3 cm submucosal bed in the posterior plate of the pouch, and then drawing the mobilized ureters through the pouch plate and securing them with 3–4 sutures in this previously formed bed. After insertion of 8F monopigtail ureteral catheters (via the opened rectum), the submucosal tunnels are completed by suturing the mucosa over the ureters (Figure 16.6). The ureteral stents are brought out of the anus and the pouch is drained with a transanal 26F Nélaton catheter. The anterior wall of the pouch is closed with a running 3–0 Maxon suture (Figure 16.7). The pelvis is drained with a single Jackson–Pratt (JP) drain through one of the lateral 5 mm trocar incisions. Hemostasis is checked, all trocars are removed under vision, and the trocar sites closed with running sutures.

Results

From April 2000 until October 2002, 13 patients (7 male, 6 female) diagnosed with clinical T2N0M0 transitional cell carcinoma of the bladder were selectively offered

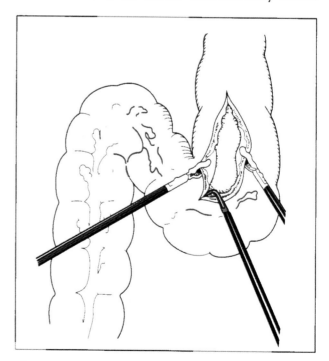

Figure 16.3
Opening of the sigmoid intestine (antimesenterically) with electric hook.

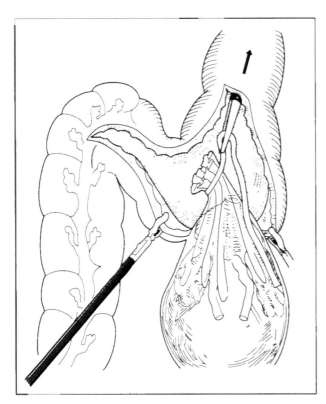

Figure 16.4
Removal of the specimen in the endobag via the opened
rectum.

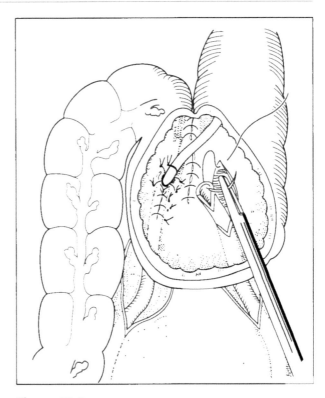

Figure 16.6
Suturing of the mucosa of the sigmoid over the already
implanted ureter to create the submucosal tunnel
(nonrefluxing anastomosis).

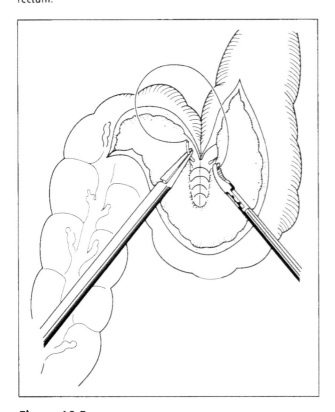

Figure 16.5
Side-to-side anastomosis of rectum and sigmoid to form the
posterior wall of the pouch.

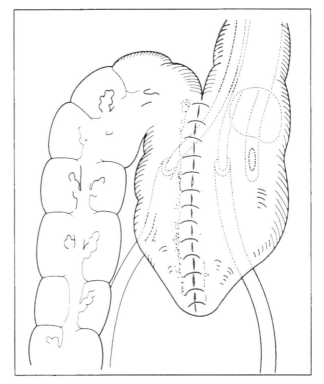

Figure 16.7
The anterior wall of the pouch is closed with running suture
(Maxon 3 × 0). Both ureters were stented with 8F ureteral
catheters and the pouch was drained with a 26F Nélaton catheter.

laparoscopic radical cystectomy with continent urinary diversion – the Mainz II sigma rectum pouch. Prior to initiating this laparoscopic approach, 36 open cystectomies with Mainz II pouch diversions had been performed at Charité Hospital in Berlin. The mean age was 64.7 years old (range 58–69). The Mainz II diversion was selected for males with tumors infiltrating the prostatic urethra (orthotopic neobladder therefore contraindicated) or because they preferred this procedure to open surgery. In females the Mainz II pouch had already been our continent urinary diversion of choice before we started with the laparoscopic approach.

All 13 procedures were completed laparoscopically without intraoperative complications. Conversion to open surgery was required in no case. The median operating time was 6.3 hours (range 5.5–7.9). The median estimated blood loss was 220 ml (range 150–300 ml, 0 transfusions), and approximately 2500 ml of combined crystalloid/colloid intravenous fluids were required per the discretion of the anesthesiologist. In general, liquids were tolerated on postoperative day (POD) 2, the JP drain was removed POD 4, the ureteral stents were removed POD 8, and the pouch drain was removed POD 9. On POD 10, IVPs were performed, demonstrating normal upper tracts and no leakage from the pouch. Patients were discharged POD 10–12 (median 11), significantly earlier than patients after comparable open surgery in the German context. All patients are fully continent (day/night) of urine and stool. The only complication was a pouch leak at 3 weeks followup, repaired by open suturing. Histopathologic examination of the specimens revealed transitional cell carcinoma: pT1 G3 + carcinoma-in-situ ($n = 1$); pT2b G2–3 ($n = 4$); pT3a G3 ($n = 5$); and pT3b G3 ($n = 3$). The resection margins were free of tumor in all specimens. Positive lymph nodes were detected in 1 patient, who was treated with adjuvant chemotherapy. Follow-up ranges are 1–27 months and has shown no local or systemic recurrence so far. In all patients, the upper urinary tract is still well preserved without any evidence of hydronephrosis. The renal function is normal and a mild hypercloremic acidosis, compensated with oral sodium bicarbonate, occurred in 11/13 cases.

In our experience, the laparoscopic sigma rectum pouch has significant technical advantages as a 'first-step' continent urinary diversion. The sigmoid and rectum have posterior attachments that keep them fixed and facilitate laparoscopic suturing. Also, suture lines are significantly shorter than for an ileal neobladder. The rectum has a capacity of approximately 400 ml, and therefore only a 20 cm opening is needed along the sigmoid and rectal surface to form a detubularized, low-pressure pouch. Although endostapler devices could speed up the bowel closure, we only use absorbable sutures to minimize the chance of future stone formation.

It is important to emphasize that the sigma rectum pouch is not a traditional ureterosigmoidostomy, nor

should it be associated with the significant complications and secondary cancers in connection with that abandoned procedure. Gumus et al have demonstrated, by filling cystometry, that the sigma rectum pouch holds 400 ml of urine without reflux into the descending colon or ureters.[40] In reports of the classic ureterosigmoidoscopy, urine and stool were stored together in the rectum, and it was thought that urine frequently refluxed up the colon caused by frequent contractions that led to frequent fecaluria. Chronic irritation of the ureteral anastamoses with fecal material was thought to predispose future cancer growths.[41]

The sigma rectum pouch provides the fixation of the left descending colon to the rectal ampulla in order to keep the colon in line with the rectum. The result is that the majority of our patients reported separately passing urine and feces at convenient intervals and with good anal control. Since urine and stool are not constantly mixed because ureteral anastomoses are away from the path of stool, it has been proposed that the risk of carcinogenesis should be significantly lower.[42] Nevertheless, long-term follow-up to determine the incidence of colonic carcinogenesis and ureteral strictures is limited.

Despite the advantages of continence and ease of construction with the sigma rectum pouch, the ileal neobladder remains the favored continent urinary diversion. In cases where it is not appropriate or desired to divert to the urethra, the sigma rectum pouch is a viable alternative and feasible to construct laparoscopically. Further functional follow-up and quality of life studies will be needed to determine its equivalence or superiority. In the meantime, Kaouk et al[43] have recently reported success with laparoscopic construction of an ileal neobladder in a pig model, and we anticipate working towards this clinical goal in the near future. Regardless of the form of laparoscopic diversion, the relatively low intravenous fluid requirements during these procedures (2500 ml combined crystalloid/colloid) suggests the intriguing possibility of less fluid shifts and electrolyte loss, and overall cardiovascular stress to the patient is reduced, which is another potential benefit that needs further study.

Summary

The last decade has seen promising advances in laparoscopic urologic surgery. What once was thought technically impossible is now becoming a reality. While early laparoscopy was mostly used for ablation of diseased tissue, it has changed and has now become a tool for reconstruction as well. While reconstructive laparoscopy still remains challenging, advances in clip and suture technology have been of great benefit. These advances have enabled radical cystectomy and construction of a continent urinary diversion to be performed by the laparoscopic approach alone, while established oncologic and reconstructive principles are maintained. But laparoscopic cystectomy and urinary diversion are still in their infancy. A number of problems will need to be addressed before such complicated procedures become commonplace. The future will surely see further improvements in instruments for reconstruction plus the application of novel energy sources to achieve more rapid, yet accurate approximation of tissue.

References

1. Bouffioux Ch, Kurth KH, Bono A, et al. Intravesical adjuvant chemotherapy for superficial transitional cell bladder carcinoma: results of 2 European Organization for Research and Treatment of Cancer randomized trials with Mitomycin C and Doxorubicin comparing early versus delayed instillations and short-term versus long-term treatment. J Urol 1995; 153:934–41.

2. Oosterlinck W, Kurth KH, Schroder F, et al. A prospective European Organization for Research and Treatment of Cancer Genitourinary Group randomized trial comparing transurethral resection followed by a single intravesical instillation of epirubicin or water in single stage Ta, T1 papillary carcinoma of the bladder. J Urol 1993; 149:749–52.

3. Heney NM, Ahmed S, Flanagan MJ, et al. Superficial bladder cancer: progression and recurrence. J Urol 1983; 130:1083–6.

4. Allard P, Bernard P, Fradet Y, Tetu B. The early clinical course of primary Ta and T1 bladder cancer: a proposed prognostic index. Br J Urol 1998; 81:692–8.

5. Parmar MKB, Freedman LS, Hargreave TB, Tolley DA. Prognostic factors for recurrence and followup policies in the treatment of superficial bladder cancer: report from the British Medical Research Council Subgroup on Superficial Bladder Cancer (Urological Cancer Working Party). J Urol 1989; 142:284–8.

6. Tolley DA, Parmar MK, Grigor KM, et al. The effect of intravesical mitomycin on recurrence of newly diagnosed superficial bladder cancer: a further report with 7 years of follow-up. J Urol 1996; 155:1233.

7. Davis JW, Sheth SI, Doviak MJ, Schellhammer PF. Superficial bladder carcinoma treated with bacillus Calmette-Guerin: progression-free and disease specific survival with minimum 10-year follow-up. J Urol 2002; 167:494–501.

8. Cookson MS, Herr HW, Zhang ZF, et al. The treated natural history of high risk superficial bladder cancer: 15 year outcome. J Urol 1997; 158:62.

9. Lamm DL, Blumenstein BA, Crissman JD, et al. Maintenance bacillus Calmette-Guerin immunotherapy for recurrent TA, T1 and carcinoma in situ transitional cell carcinoma of the bladder: a randomized Southwest Oncology Group Study. J Urol 2000; 163:1124–9.

10. O'Donnell M, Krohn J, DeWolf WC. Salvage intravesical therapy with interferon-alpha 2b plus low dose bacillus Calmette-Guerin is effective in patients with superficial bladder cancer in whom bacillus Calmette-Guerin alone previously failed. J Urol 2001; 166:1300–5.

11. Herr H, Sogani PC. Does early cystectomy improve the survival of patients with high risk superficial bladder tumors? J Urol 2001; 166:1296–9.

12. Solsona E, Iborra I, Dumont R, et al. The 3-month clinical response to intravesical therapy as a predictive factor for progression in patients with high-risk superficial bladder cancer. J Urol 2000; 164:685–9.

13. Bernardini B, Billerey C, Martin M, et al. The predictive value of muscularis mucosae invasion and p53 overexpression on progression of stage T1 bladder carcinoma. J Urol 2001; 165:42–6.

14. Herr HW. Transurethral resection of muscle-invasive bladder cancer: 10-year outcome. J Clin Oncol 2001; 19:89–93.

15. Solsona E, Iborra I, Ricos JV, et al. Feasibility of transurethral resection for muscle infiltrating carcinoma of the bladder: long-term followup of a prospective study. J Urol 1998; 159:95–8,

16. Shipley WU, Kaufman DS, Zehr E, et al. Selective preservation by combined modality protocol treatment: long-term outcomes of 190 patients with invasive bladder cancer. Urology 2002; 60:62–7.

17. Millikan R, Dinney C, Swanson D, et al. Integrated therapy for locally advanced bladder cancer: final report of a randomized trial of cystectomy plus adjuvant M-VAC versus cystectomy with both preoperative and postoperative M-VAC. J Clin Oncol 2001; 19:4005–13.

18. Feneley MR, Schoenberg M. Bladder-sparing strategies for transitional cell carcinoma. Urology 2000; 56:549–60.

19. Malavaud B, Vaessen C, Mouzin M, et al. Complications for radical cystectomy. Eur Urol 2001; 39:79–84.

20. Clayman RV, Kavoussi LR, Soper NJ, et al. Laparoscopic nephrectomy: initial case report. J Urol 1991; 146:278–82.

21. Kavoussi LR, Kerbl K, Capelonto CC, et al. Laparoscopic nephrectomy for renal neoplasms. Urology 1993; 42:603–9.

22. Gill IS. Laparoscopic radical nephrectomy for cancer. Urol Clin North Am 2000; 27:707–19.

23. Turk I, Deger S, Winklemann B, et al. Laparoscopic radical prostatectomy – technical aspects and experience with 125 cases. Eur Urol 2001; 40:46–53.

24. Guillonneau B, Vallancien G. Laparoscopic radical prostatectomy: the Montsouris experience. J Urol 2000; 163:418–22.

25. Jacob F, Salomon L, Hoznek A, et al. Laparoscopic radical prostatectomy: preliminary results. Eur Urol 2000; 37:615–20.

26. Parra RO, Andrus CH, Jones JP, et al. Laparoscopic cystectomy: initial report on a new treatment for retained bladder. J Urol 1992; 148:1140–4.

27. De Badajoz ES, Perales JLG, Rosado AR, et al. Laparoscopic cystectomy and ileal conduit: case report. J Endourol 1995; 8:59–62.

28. Puppo P, Perachino M, Ricciotti G, et al. Laparoscopically assisted transvaginal radical cystectomy. Eur Urol 1995; 27:425–8.

29. Denewer A, Kotb S, Hussein O, et al. Laparoscopic assisted cystectomy and lymphadenectomy for bladder cancer: initial experience. World J Surg 1999; 23:608–11.

30. Bricker EM. Bladder substitution after pelvic evisceration. Surg Clin North Am 1950; 30:1511.

31. Kozminski M, Partamian KO. Case report of laparoscopic ileal loop conduit. J Endourol 1992; 6:147–50.

32. Gill IS, Fergany AMR, Klein EA, et al. Laparoscopic radical cystectomy with ileal conduit performed completely intracorporally: the initial 2 cases. Urology 2000; 56:26–9.

33. Trinchieri A, Zannetti G, Montanari E, et al. Experimental and clinical urinary diversion. Ann Urol 1995; 29:113–16.

34. Anderson KR, Fadden PT, Kerbl K, et al. Laparoscopic assisted continent urinary diversion in the pig. J Urol 1995; 154:1934–8.

35. Fisch M, Wammack R, Steinbach F, et al. Sigma-rectum pouch (Mainz pouch II). Urol Clin North Am 1993; 20:561–9.

36. Fisch M, Wammack R, Hohenfellner R. The sigma rectum pouch (Mainz pouch II). World J Urol 1996; 14:68–72.

37. Gerharz EW, Kohl UN, Weingartner K, et al. Experience with the Mainz modification of ureterosigmoidostomy. Br J Surg 1998; 85:1512–16.

38. Gilja I, Kovacic M, Radej M, et al. The sigmoidorectal pouch (Mainz Pouch). Eur Urol 1996; 29:210–15.

39. Tuerk I, Deger S, Winkelmann B, et al. Laparoscopic radical cystectomy with continent urinary diversion (rectal sigmoid pouch) performed completely intracorporeally: the initial 5 cases. J Urol 2001; 165:1863–6.

40. Gumus E, Miroglu C, Saporta L, et al. Rectodynamic and radiological assessment in modified Mainz Pouch II cases. Eur Urol 2000; 38:316–22.

41. Berg NO, Fredlund P, Mansson W, et al. Surveillance colonoscopy and biopsy in patients with ureterosigmoidostomy. Endoscopy 1987; 19:60–3.

42. Atta MA. Detubularized isolated ureterosigmoidostomy: description of a new technique and preliminary results. J Urol 1996; 156:915–19.

43. Kaouk JH, Gill IS, Desai MM, et al. Laparoscopic orthotopic ileal neobladder. J Endourol 2001; 15:131–42.

17

Minimally invasive uses of intestinal segments for urinary diversion

Sidney C Abreu and Inderbir S Gill

History of urinary diversion:

Bowel segments have been used throughout the years for various reconstructive urologic applications. The stomach, jejunum, ileum, and colon have been successfully employed for bladder augmentation and bladder replacement. The initial clinical attempts to drain urine into the rectosigmoid were performed in the 19th century.[1] As the indications for cystectomy increased, so did the necessity to develop an optimal technique of urinary diversion. Remarkable surgical innovation has recently made possible the development and widespread use of orthotopic neobladder techniques.[1] Approaching the beginning of this new millennium, urologists have begun to explore minimally invasive techniques to urinary diversion.[2,3] Laparoscopy has been applied in an attempt to reduce the morbidity resulting from bladder removal and substitution. To date, various techniques of urinary diversion have been performed laparoscopically, either completely intracorporeally or by laparoscopic-assisted techniques.[4,5]

In this chapter, we describe the morphologic and physiologic aspects related to urinary diversion in general. Following this, the worldwide available clinical experience with laparoscopic use of various bowel segments is reviewed. Finally, experimental minimally invasive approaches related to urinary diversion are also presented briefly.

Applied anatomy of the stomach, and small and large bowel, as used for urinary diversion

Stomach

The stomach is a well-vascularized organ that receives most of its blood supply from the celiac axis. Maintaining the gastroepiploic vessels that supply the greater curvature of the stomach as a pedicle, a vascularized stomach patch consisting of the entire antrum pylori or a wedge of the fundus can be mobilized to the pelvis. Furthermore, the stomach has a thick seromuscular layer that can be separated from the mucosa, thus facilitating a submucosa ureteral reimplantation when required.

Colon

The colon requires mobilization from its fixed position to achieve the mobility necessary for the reconstructive procedures. The larger diameter of the colon when compared to the ileum may be an advantage. Preservation of an intact ileocecal valve may help to avoid diarrhea and excessive bacterial colonization of the ileum.

Ileum

The ileum is a preferred segment of bowel that has been employed in various types of urologic reconstructive procedures. It is mobile, has a constant blood supply, its shape is ideal for conduit formation, and it has enough redundancy to allow various lengths of segments to be used without compromising the host. Occasionally, the mesentery may be short, which makes its mobilization into the deep pelvis difficult.

Physiologic considerations

Selection of the appropriate intestinal segment must consider the physiologic properties unique to the stomach, jejunum, ileum, and colon. In each case, the ideal bowel segment must fit the patient's condition, the renal function status, and type of diversion required.

Metabolic implications

Ileum and colon

Reabsorption of urinary ammonia and ammonium chloride by the ileal and colonic segments produces hyperchloremic metabolic acidosis. Although such acidosis occurs in most patients, it is generally of minor degree.[6,7] Severity of hyperchloremic metabolic acidosis depends on the period of contact between the urine and the intestinal mucosa, as well as the length of bowel segment used. Severe metabolic acidosis is manifested by patient weakness, fatigue, polydipsia, and anorexia. Chronic metabolic acidosis causes mobilization of calcium carbonate from bone. The carbonate combines with hydrogen while the calcium is excreted in urine, whereas can result in osteomalacia.[8]

Stomach

When the stomach is employed, the gastric mucosa acts as a barrier to chloride and acid reabsorption. However, due to the secretory nature of the gastric mucosa, hypochloremic hypokalemic metabolic alkalosis may occur. Also, in cases of gastrocystoplasty, hematuria–dysuria syndrome may occur.[9] However, in most patients these symptoms are intermittent and mild, and do not require treatment.

Jejunum

The jejunum is usually not employed for reconstruction of the urinary system because it potentially can cause severe electrolyte disorders such as hyponatremia, hypochloremia, hyperkalemia, azotemia, and acidosis. Rarely, when the jejunum is the only segment available, a portion of the jejunum as distal as possible should be used to minimize problems with electrolyte imbalance.[10]

Mechanics of tubular and detubularized bowel

Volume–pressure considerations

Configuration of the selected segment of bowel directly impacts upon the reservoir volume–pressure characteristics. Laplace's law states (for a sphere) that the tension of its wall is proportional to the product of the radius and pressure. Thus, theoretically, for a given wall tension, the greater the radius, the smaller the generated pressure. Therefore, detubularization of the bowel segment along its antimesenteric border and creation of a spherical reservoir should be the goal, aiming to preserve the upper urinary tract and to prevent incontinence.

Motor activity

The impact of detubularization upon motor activity of the bowel is unclear. Theoretically speaking, splitting the bowel along its antimesenteric border should discoordinate its motor activity, thus decreasing the intraluminal pressure. Experimental and clinical data suggest that the motor activity is markedly interrupted following the detubularization, resulting in fewer or ineffective contractions of the reservoir walls. However, over a period of 3 months, peristaltic waves reappear, returning to their normal coordinated status.[12]

Renal functional considerations

Although urinary diversion in and of itself may compromise renal function, a certain robust baseline renal reserve is necessary to efficiently eliminate the excess of urinary solutes reabsorbed by the employed intestinal segment in order to prevent potentially serious metabolic side-effects.[12] The level of renal function required to safely perform a urinary diversion depends on the amount of bowel used for the diversion as well as the length of time that the urine stays in contact with intestinal mucosa. Thus, a higher baseline renal reserve is necessary for continent reservoirs than for short conduits. However, as a general rule, patients with serum creatinine below 2.0 mg/dl tolerate intestinal interposition in the urinary tract well.[12]

Patient selection for laparoscopic urinary diversion

Proper patient selection is crucial to achieve good surgical outcomes. The criteria for selection of the type of urinary diversion have been outlined above. Furthermore, the criteria for selection of a laparoscopic approach in general should be followed. Contraindications include patients with acute intraperitoneal infection process and uncorrected coagulopathy. Although previous abdominal surgery is not an absolute contraindication, significant peritoneal adhesions should be factored into the decision-making process, which should be made on a case-by-case basis. Obesity is not, in itself, a contraindication to the laparoscopic approach; however, difficulty may be encountered during instrument manipulation, bowel mobilization, and while constructing an ileal conduit through the thicker abdominal wall.

Preoperative patient assessment and preparation

The preoperative assessment for patients undergoing laparoscopic urinary diversion is similar to that for the open surgery. In brief, patients undergo a complete physical examination, routine blood tests (complete blood count, renal panel, alkaline phosphatase, liver function tests, and calcium), and radiographic testing to rule out metastatic disease. On the day prior to surgery, the bowel is prepared mechanically using 4 liters of GoLYTLEY, and chemically with neomycin and metronidazole. Broad-spectrum intravenous antibiotics and subcutaneous low-molecular-weight heparin (2500 units) are given prior to surgery.

Port placement

Laparoscopic cystectomy, discussed elsewhere in this book, precedes the urinary diversion. The same five-port transperitoneal configuration is employed for both procedures, with one additional port in the left iliac fossa for the laparoscopic bowel work (Figure 17.1). A primary 10 mm port is placed at the umbilicus for the 0° laparoscope. Four secondary ports are placed under visualization: a 12 mm port to the left of the umbilicus, lateral to the rectus muscle, and two 10 mm ports in the left and right lower quadrants, approximately 2 fingerbreadths to the ipsilateral anterior superior iliac spines. In the case of an ileal conduit, another 12 mm port is placed at the preselected stoma site in the right rectus muscle; otherwise, this 12 mm port is placed at the lateral border of the rectus

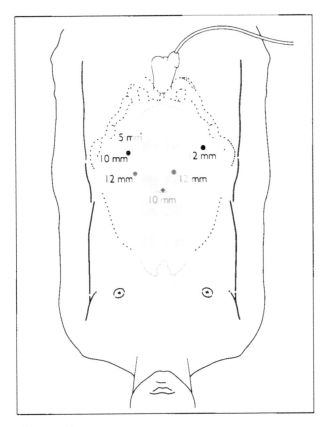

Figure 17.1
Transperitoneal six-port approach.

muscle, approximately 2 fingerbreadths caudal to the umbilicus. Finally, a 5 mm port is placed in the midline infraumbilical location, approximately 2 fingerbreadths cephalad to the symphysis pubis.

It is important to note that during the initial bowel manipulation (ileal segment isolation, ileal–ileal anastomosis) the laparoscope is inserted through the left lateral port while the surgeon works through the midline infraumbilical and the pararectal ports. If an ileal conduit is selected, this same triangular port configuration is used for the ureterointestinal anastomosis. However, if a continent reservoir is to be performed, the laparoscope is moved back to the umbilical port upon completion of bowel detubularization.

Laparoscopic ileal conduit
Ileal conduit creation

After the cystectomy and pelvic lymphadenectomy are completed, attention is focused on the urinary diversion. When an ileal conduit is selected for urinary diversion, a 15–20 cm segment of ileum is identified 20 cm away from the ileocecal junction. All bowel manipulations are performed completely intracorporeally.[13, 14] In this manner, division of the selected segment of bowel and mesentery is performed using the EndoGIA stapler. Staple heights of 3.5 mm are used for bowel and 2 mm or 2.5 mm (vascular load) for the mesentery. Two firings are used to complete the distal mesenteric division and one firing is used to complete the proximal division (Figure 17.2). As in open surgery, care is taken not to compromise the main mesenteric vessels feeding the conduit. Ileoileal continuity is re-established by creating a generous side-to-side anastomosis with two sequential firings of the Endo-GIA stapler. The open ileal ends are closed with two transverse firings of the Endo-GIA stapler. The mesenteric window is closed with 3-0 silk sutures. The distal end of the conduit is exteriorized through the preselected stoma site at the rectus muscle and an end-ileal stoma is fashioned using conventional techniques.

Ureteroileal anastomosis

Technical difficulty in performing laparoscopic freehand suturing was the main reason why the initial reports of laparoscopic ileal conduit urinary diversion employed conventional open techniques to perform the ureteroileal anastomosis. In these early 1990s reports, ureteral reimplantation was performed extracorporeally through either a minilaparotomy incision or by delivering the ends of the conduit and both ureters outside the abdomen through an enlarged port-site incision.[2,3] In our view, such an extracorporeal anastomosis through a limited incision, as described, may create problems as regards tissue orientation and positional distortion.[13] Moreover, it may be difficult or even impossible to extract the ileum and the ureters to the skin level in obese patients. One decade later, with advances in intracorporeal free-hand suturing, Gill et al reported the initial two cases of laparoscopic ileal conduit where the ureterointestinal anastomosis was performed completely intracorporeally.[4] In this technique, a 90 cm, 7F single-J stent is grasped with a laparoscopic right-angle clamp and inserted into the conduit lumen. It is then used to tent the conduit wall at the desired site of ureteroileal anastomosis. Using an electrical J hook, a small ileotomy is created and the stent is delivered into the abdominal cavity. The ureteral rim is freshened and spatulated. A 4-0 Vicryl (RB-1 needle) stitch is placed outside-in at the apex of the ureteral spatulation and is anchored to the desired site of the ileotomy. A running suture is then performed to approximate 80% of the posterior (far) wall and the J stent is fed into the ureter up to the renal pelvis. The remainder of the posterior wall anastomosis is completed. The anterior (near) wall is sutured in a running fashion with a second 4-0 suture to complete the anastomosis. The contralateral ureteral anastomosis is performed in a similar manner (Figure 17.3).

Laparoscopic orthotopic neobladder

Following cystectomy and lymphadenectomy, a 65 cm ileal segment is selected and isolated in a similar manner as described above for the ileal conduit.[4,15] Bowel segment length is precisely measured by inserting a malleable footruler into the abdomen through a 12 mm port. The proximal 10–15 cm of the excluded ileal segment is reserved for the isoperistaltic Studer limb of the neobladder. The remaining length of the ileal segment is detubularized along its antimesenteric border using endoshears with electrocautery or the harmonic scalpel. The posterior wall of the neobladder is created by continuous intracorporeal suturing of adjacent edges of the U-shaped ileal segment using 2-0 Vicryl suture on a CT-1 needle.[4,15] The segment is then brought into the pelvis, avoiding any undue tension or torsion of the mesentery. The previously confirmed most-dependent portion of the ileal segment is selected for urethroileal (neobladder) anastomosis. A running circumferential suture is performed using 2-0 Vicryl on a UR-6 needle. Prior to completing the anastomosis, a 22F silicone Foley catheter is inserted per urethra. In female patients, two 90 cm single-J stents are inserted via the external urethral meatus alongside the Foley catheter and delivered into the neobladder. In the male,

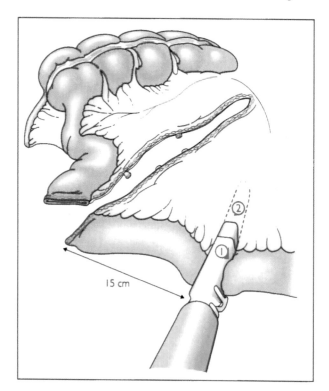

Figure 17.2
Division of the isolated bowel segment and mesentery is performed with serial firings of the Endo-GIA stapler.

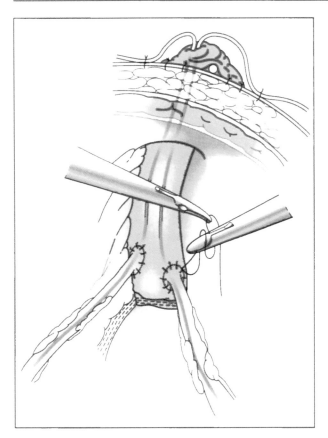

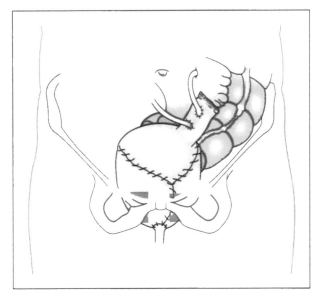

Figure 17.4
Orthotopic neobladder urinary diversion. After isolation of the ileal segment and detubularization of the distal portion, the posterior plate is created and urethroileal anastomosis is completed using a running suture. The anterior wall of the neobladder is folded to achieve a spherical configuration of the neobladder.

Figure 17.3
Ileal conduit urinary diversion. The distal end of the ileal loop is exteriorized through the preselected stoma site and is secured to the skin using the standard technique. Stented bilateral ureteroileal anastomoses are completed.

these two stents are inserted through the right lateral port into the neobladder. The anterior wall of the neobladder is folded forward and the free edges are sutured to achieve a spherical configuration. Prior to completion of the neobladder suturing, a 5 cm incision is performed in the anterior wall of the Studer limb and the stents are delivered through it. Two small ileotomies are created at the side of the Studer limb, and one ureter is pulled inside the Studer limb through each ileotomy. The ureters are then freshened and spatulated. A full-thickness anchoring stitch affixes the edge of the ureter to the apex of the ileotomy. The single-J stent is delivered up to the renal pelvis and two additional stitches are placed between the ureter and the ileum wall. Finally, the anterior wall of the Studer limb is closed with a running suture (Figure 17.4). All suturing and knot tying is performed intracorporeally using a freehand laparoscopic technique.[4,15] The neobladder is irrigated through the Foley catheter and any obvious sites of leakage are specifically repaired with figure-of-eight stitches. A suprapubic catheter is inserted into the neobladder through the midline port-site incision.

Laparoscopic rectal sigmoid (Mainz II) pouch

Türk and colleagues were the first to report a laparoscopic rectal sigmoid pouch.[16] This rectal sphincter-based continent type of urinary diversion was successfully performed in 5 patients completely intracorporeally. Upon completion of cystectomy, the rectosigmoid colon was incised open along its antimesenteric border with a hook electrocautery. This incision was then extended for 10 cm, respectively, proximally and distally from the rectosigmoid junction. The adjacent posterior walls of the rectum and sigmoid were anastomosed side to side with absorbable running suture, forming the posterior wall of the pouch. Subsequently, the mobilized ureters were brought into the pouch and sutured to the pouch plate in a pre-prepared 3 cm submucosal bed. Single-J 8F stents were inserted through the anus into the pouch and then passed up to the renal pelvis. A submucosal tunnel was formed by suturing the mucosa over the ureters. Finally, the anterior wall of the pouch was closed with a running suture of 3-0 Vicryl. The pouch was drained transanally with a Nelaton catheter. In the female patient the specimen was extracted intact through the vagina, while in the male patient the specimen was placed in an endoscopic bag and extracted transanally.

Laparoscopic-assisted reconstruction of pouch/enterocystoplasty

Alternatively, during laparoscopic procedures, bowel manipulation as well as construction of complex enteric pouches or enterocystoplasty can be performed extracorporeally (Figure 17.5). Generally, a 2–5 cm incision is performed to exteriorize the preselected bowel segment. Several advantages can accrue:

- bowel mesentery can be precisely incised after ensuring good vascularity using transillumination
- side-to-side bowel anastomosis can be performed rapidly

- contamination of the abdominal cavity can be prevented during detubularization of the loop
- overall this approach allows considerable savings in operative times.[17]

Recently, we reported a laparoscopic-assisted continent Indiana pouch urinary diversion in a patient with muscle invasive bladder cancer.[4] Due to urethral involvement, orthotopic diversion was contraindicated in this case. The pouch and continent catheterizable ileal limb were created extracorporeally by standard open techniques after the selected ileocecal segment was extruded through a 2–3 cm extension of the right pararectal port incision. Subsequently, the bowel was reinserted into the abdomen, and the bilateral uretero-ileal anastomoses were created intracorporeally by freehand laparoscopic techniques.

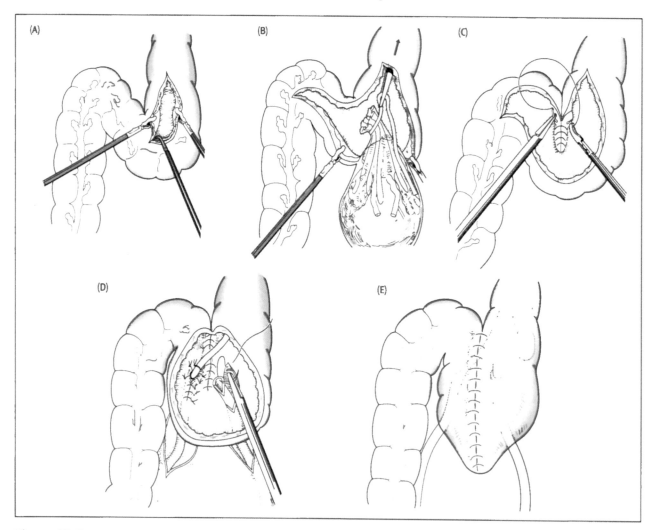

Figure 17.5

Construction of a rectosigmoid pouch: (A) the rectosigmoid is incised at the antimesentery border; (B) the cystectomy specimen is extracted through the rectum; (C) the posterior wall is anastomosed side to side; (D) the ureters are implanted via a submucosal posterior tunnel; (E) the ureters are stented with ureteral catheters and the pouch is drained with a 26F Nelaton catheter. The anterior wall of the pouch is closed.

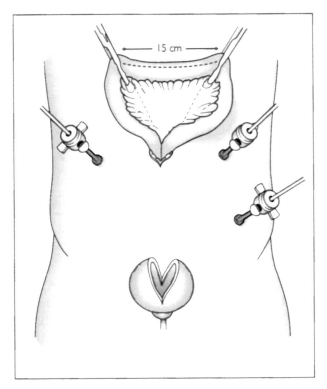

Figure 17.6
During laparoscopic procedures, bowel work can be performed through an extended port-site incision.

Laparoscopic gastroileal neobladder

Although demanding more complex gastrointestinal resection, the combination of bowel and stomach to create a pouch may have metabolic advantages compared to the use of intestinal segments alone. The tendency to metabolic acidosis when ileum or colon is used in urinary reconstruction can be counterbalanced by the combined use of stomach, due to its tendency towards metabolic alkalosis. Thus, metabolic neutrality may be achieved in highly selected cases. These composite reservoirs may be employed judiciously in the setting of metabolic acidosis, short bowel syndrome, and renal failure. To date, no clinical reports of laparoscopic use of stomach for urinary diversion have been reported. Experimentally, Carvalhal et al described the construction of a gastroileal composite reservoir in a porcine model.[18] Briefly, the surgical steps were:

1. gastric mobilization and right gastroepiploic pedicle dissection
2. wedge resection of the greater curvature (8–12 cm × 4 cm) with Endo-GIA stapler (Figure 17.7)
3. isolation of a 20 cm ileal segment
4. stapled restoration of ileoileal continuity
5. cystectomy and ureteral dissection
6. construction of the composite gastrointestinal plate (gastric patch and U-shaped ileum) with freehand laparoscopic suturing

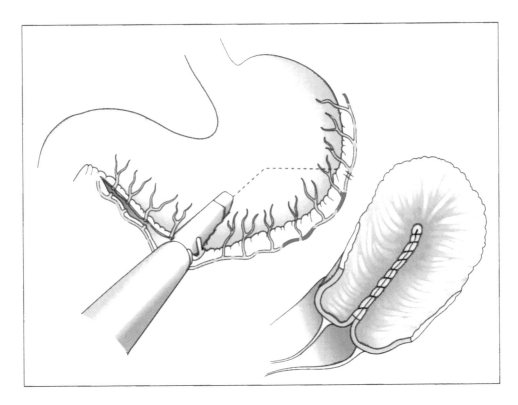

Figure 17.7
Laparoscopic wedge resection of the greater curvature of the stomach is performed to create a composite pouch with an ileal segment.

7. urethroileal anastomosis
8. bilateral reimplantation into the gastric patch
9. closure of the composite plate in a spherical manner.

Intracorporeal laparoscopic freehand suturing was employed exclusively. The complexity of the procedure explains the long mean operative time of 7.1 hours in this experimental model.

Laparoscopic ureterocystoplasty using balloon-expanded normal ureter

Despite all the technical advances with minimally invasive use of intestine for urinary diversion, the problems inherent to the contact of urine with bowel mucosa have not been overcome and continue to be a source of morbidity. Perhaps the ureter, with its transitional epithelium, may be the ideal tissue for bladder augmentation or replacement. However, the use of ureteral tissue for this purpose is limited to the rare patient with a megaureter subtending a nonfunctional kidney. The concept of ureteral tissue expansion was initially proposed by Hensle and colleagues.[19] Recently, we have completed an experimental study wherein a balloon device was used to expand the normal ureter.[20] This balloon (Microvasive, Natick, Massachusetts) is mounted in a dual-channel catheter: one for balloon inflation and the other for proximal nephrostomy drainage. Using a porcine model, a percutaneous renal tract was dilated, followed by the passage of the expansion balloon device. The balloon was then manipulated antegradely into the juxtavesical ureter (Figure 17.8). The ureteral balloon was gradually inflated over a 2–3 week period by instillation of dilute contrast solution. The inflation was performed without anesthesia, while the animal was eating. The mean daily inflation volume was 1.8, 5.5, 9.5, and 16.1 ml/day respectively in the first, second, third and final week. Total balloon volumes averaged 12.9, 60.3 and 171.8 ml respectively, at 1, 2, and 3 weeks. After completion of ureteral balloon expansion, laparoscopic ureterocystoplasty was performed. Over a follow-up ranging from 15 days to 3 months, a mean augmented bladder capacity of 574 ± 221.3 ml was achieved. In the future, such expanded ureteral tissue may be successfully used to augment or replace the bladder using minimally invasive techniques.

References

1. Stenzl A, Ninkovic M. Urinary diversion in the new millennium. World J Urol 2000; 18:303–4.

2. Badajoz ES, Perales G, Rosado R, et al. Laparoscopic cystectomy and ileal conduit: case report. J Endourol 2000; 9:59–62.

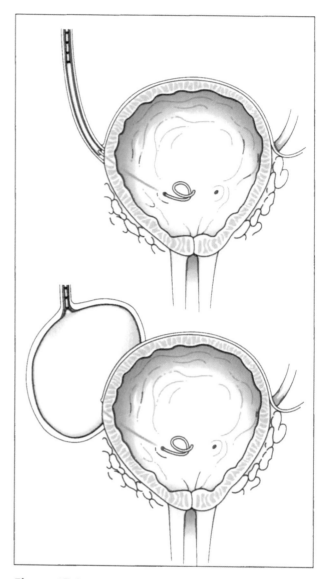

Figure 17.8
A balloon catheter is inserted antegradely into the juxtavesical ureter to gradually expand the normal ureter.

3. Kozminski M, Partamian KO. Case report of laparoscopic ileal loop conduit. J Endourol 1992; 6:147–50.

4. Gill IS, Kaouk JH, Meraney AM, et al. Laparoscopic radical cystectomy and continent orthotopic ileal neobladder performed completely intracorporeally: the initial experience. J Urol 2002; 168:13–18.

5. Gaboardi F, Simonato A, Galli S, et al. Minimally invasive laparoscopic neobladder. J Urol 2002; 168:1080–3.

6. Castro JE, Ram MD. Electrolyte imbalance following ileal urinary diversion. Br J Urol 1970; 42:29–32.

7. Whitmore WF, Gittes RF. Reconstruction of the urinary tract by cecal and ileocecal cystoplasty: review of a 15 year experience. J Urol 1983; 129:494–8.

8. Harrison AR. Clinical and metabolic observations on osteomalacia following ureterosigmoidostomy. Br J Urol 1958; 30: 455–61.

9. Nguyen DH, Bain MA, Salmonson KL. The syndrome of dysuria and hematuria in pediatric urinary reconstruction with stomach. J Urol 1993; 150: 707–9.

10. Klein EA, Montie JE, Montague DK. Jejunal conduit urinary diversion. J Urol 1986; 135:244–6.

11. Concepcion RS, Koch MO, McDougal WS, Richards WO. Detubularized intestinal segments in urinary tract reconstruction: Why do they work? Abstr Am Urol Assoc, 1988; 592.

12. McDougal WS.Use of intestinal segments and urinary diversion. In Campbell's urology, 7th edn. Philadelphia: WB Saunders, 1998.

13. Gill IS, Fergany A, Klein EA, et al. Laparoscopic radical cystoprostatectomy with ileal conduit performed completely intracorporeally: the initial 2 cases. Urology 2000; 56:26–30.

14. Fergany A, Gill IS, Kaouk J, et al. Laparoscopic intracorporeally constructed ileal conduit after porcine cystoprostatectomy. J Urol 2001; 166:285–8.

15. Kaouk J, Gill IS, Desai M, et al. Laparoscopic orthotopic ileal neobladder. J Endourol 2001; 15:131–42.

16. Türk I, Deger S, Winkelmann B, et al. Laparoscopic radical cystectomy with continent urinary diversion (rectal sigmoid pouch) performed completely intracorporeally: the initial 5 cases. J Urol 2001; 165:1863–6.

17. Gill IS, Rackley R, Meraney A, et al. Laparoscopic Enterocystoplasty. Urology 2000; 55:178–81.

18. Carvalhal EF, Kaouk JH, Desai MM, et al. Laparoscopic gastroileal bladder augmentation: technical feasibility in a porcine model. J Endourol, 2000; 14 (Suppl) 1: A124.

19. Stifelman MD, Ikeguchi EF, Hensle TW. Ureteral tissue expansion for bladder augmentation: a long-term prospective controlled trial in a porcine model. J Urol 1998;160: 1826–9.

20. Desai M, Gill IS, Goel M, et al. Laparoscopic ureterocystoplasty using balloon-expanded normal ureter: chronic porcine study. J. Endourol (in press).

18

Minimally invasive techniques to diagnosis and stage carcinoma of the prostate

Mark L Gonzalgo, Li-Ming Su, and Alan W Partin

Prostate cancer is the most commonly diagnosed malignancy and the second leading cause of cancer death in the male population over the age of 40 in the United States. Approximately 198,000 American men were diagnosed with prostate cancer, and almost 32,000 men died from the disease in the year 2001.[1] Adenocarcinoma of the prostate most frequently arises in the periphery of the gland, thus making it more easily detected by digital rectal examination (DRE). The predisposition for prostate cancer to originate from the peripheral zone increases the likelihood that patients with early stages of the disease will remain asymptomatic. The presence of obstructive or irritative voiding symptoms rarely suggests locally advanced or metastatic disease resulting from growth of the cancer into the urethra or bladder neck and is often the result of benign prostatic hyperplasia (BPH). Other less common findings that may be elicited from the history of a patient with more advanced disease include hematospermia (rare), decreased ejaculate volume, impotence, bone pain, anemia, and lower extremity edema.[2]

Diagnosis

In the past, diagnosis of prostate cancer was primarily accomplished by obtaining a thorough history of the patient and from physical examination findings. Over the last two decades, there has been increased utilization of serum prostate-specific antigen (PSA) to aid in diagnosis in addition to its use for monitoring progression following definitive therapy. The so-called 'PSA era' and changes in prostate cancer incidence and mortality have been associated with widespread acceptance of PSA testing by clinicians.[3,4] Perhaps the most compelling evidence that suggests a benefit from early detection of prostate cancer using PSA is the observation of a decline in prostate cancer mortality rates to below those which existed prior to its

diagnostic use. In 1997, prostate cancer mortality rates in the United States for men 60–79 years of age were the lowest in almost 50 years, and for white men less than 85 years of age prostate cancer mortality rates decreased to levels below those observed in 1986 (the year PSA testing was approved).[4] The reduction in overall mortality may be attributed to an increased number of high-grade cancers being detected before metastasis. A concomitant decrease in the incidence of distant-stage disease at an annual rate of almost 18% over the past decade also supports the argument that PSA testing has resulted in lower prostate cancer mortality.[3,5] Further evidence supporting the beneficial impact of early disease detection with PSA was provided in a unique natural study that compared prostate cancer mortality in Tyrol, Austria, where PSA testing was introduced at no charge, with the rest of Austria, where it was not introduced.[6] The trends in prostate cancer mortality rates since 1993 were significantly lower in Tyrol compared to the rest of Austria. The combination of DRE and serum PSA represents the most useful initial diagnostic tool for the assessment of prostate cancer at the present time.[7–9]

Digital rectal examination

DRE is considered to be an essential component of the urologic evaluation and has been the primary method for assessment of the prostate. An abnormal DRE, regardless of PSA level, warrants further work-up, especially in men with risk factors for prostate cancer (i.e. older age, family history, race, elevated PSA, symptoms). The positive predictive value of DRE has been shown to be dependent upon age, race, and PSA level.[10,11] Prostate biopsy is recommended for all patients who have an abnormal DRE, regardless of serum PSA, since up to 25% of men with prostate cancer will have PSA levels < 4.0 ng/ml.[2] The reproducibility of DRE is limited even among experienced clinicians, and a significant number of cancers may still be missed.[12] This variability may result in detection of cancer at a more advanced stage. In fact, there is often a significant amount of clinical understaging by DRE compared with pathologic stages of radical prostatectomy specimens.[13–15] Over 50% of patients in screened and unscreened populations were found to have more pathologically advanced disease when their prostate cancer was detected by DRE.[16,17] The sensitivity and specificity for detection of organ-confined prostate cancer by DRE alone have been estimated to be approximately 52% and 81%, respectively.[18]

Prostate-specific antigen

PSA is a 33 kDa serine protease that facilitates liquefaction of the seminal coagulum shortly following ejaculation.[19,20] The majority of PSA found in serum is complexed either to alpha$_1$-antichymotrypsin (ACT) or alpha$_2$-macroglobulin (MG).[21–23] The most detectable form of PSA in serum (65–90%) is bound to ACT. Approximately 10–35% of detectable PSA found in the circulation exists either as unbound or free.[22,23] Free PSA lacks proteolytic activity and circulates as an inactive molecule. Protease complexes are typically metabolized in the liver. The large size of complexed PSA may prevent filtration at the level of the glomerulus.[24]

Secretion of PSA normally occurs via the prostatic ductal epithelium in mg/ml concentrations and it is found in low serum concentrations (ng/ml). Changes in prostate tissue architecture during tumorigenesis may result in secretion of PSA into blind-ending ducts, thereby causing an increase in leakage into the circulation and raising serum concentrations. Diffusion of PSA into the prostatic tissue and an increase in serum PSA levels may also occur in benign conditions (e.g. BPH, prostatitis) or after manipulation (e.g. prostate massage, biopsy).[25–28] The presence of prostatic disease (benign or malignant) remains the most important factor influencing serum PSA levels. Therefore, elevation of PSA is not necessarily specific for cancer.[2]

Administration of a 5-alpha reductase inhibitor such as finasteride (Proscar) for the treatment of BPH has been shown to decrease PSA levels by as much as 50% after 12 months.[29] It is recommended that a baseline PSA level be obtained prior to initiation of finasteride in men who undergo treatment for BPH. Interpretation of PSA levels should always take into consideration the presence of benign prostatic disease, prostatitis, and manipulation. Failure of PSA to decrease by 50% or a rise in PSA while taking finasteride should raise suspicion of the existence of occult prostate cancer.[2]

Clinical utility of prostate-specific antigen

Comparison of the various methods for prostate cancer detection has demonstrated that PSA elevation has the highest positive predictive value for the presence of malignancy.[2] A higher percentage of patients will have cancer found at biopsy in the presence of a markedly elevated serum PSA (> 10.0 ng/ml) compared to an abnormal DRE or transrectal ultrasound (TRUS).[7,30] The use of PSA has been shown to increase the predictive value of DRE for cancer detection.[10,31,32] Therefore, combined use of DRE and PSA for assessment of prostate cancer risk remains the most effective method for early detection of malignancy.[2] Recent results have shown little difference in the overall characteristics of prostate cancer cases detected by utilizing a PSA cutoff of 3.0 ng/ml compared to cases detected with a regimen based on PSA, DRE, and TRUS.[33] This indicates a possible role for PSA measurement alone as a baseline screening test for prostate cancer.

Various PSA threshold levels have been proposed above which further evaluation (i.e. biopsy) is warranted to rule out cancer. This area remains highly controversial, but the most commonly used threshold value is a PSA of 4.0 ng/ml.[34,35] Age- and race-specific PSA ranges have been previously established (Table 18.1).[36,37] Threshold PSA levels for detection of approximately 95% of prostate cancers among men aged 40–50 years are lower than 4.0 ng/ml. For Caucasian and African-American men 50–69 years of age, threshold PSA levels are very close to 4.0 ng/ml. It has been suggested that a PSA threshold of 4.0 ng/ml should be utilized, regardless of age or race.[38] African-American men may have higher PSA levels overall compared to Caucasian males, and race-specific threshold levels have been established at higher levels for this population. Utilization of a PSA threshold of 4.0 ng/ml, regardless of age or race, may lead to earlier disease diagnosis and increase the chance for curative intervention, particularly for African-Americans, since this population often has more aggressive disease at the time of presentation.[38] While the utility of PSA screening remains controversial, an unvalidated strategy of PSA testing (with a threshold of 4.0 ng/ml) at ages 40, 45, and then biennially after 50 has been recommended. This strategy has been shown to be more cost-effective compared with annual testing after age 50.[2,39]

Prostate-specific antigen density and velocity, and free prostate-specific antigen

Over 80% of men with an elevated PSA will have a level between 4.0 and 10.0 ng/ml due to the high prevalence of BPH in the population.[7] Adjustment of PSA level by determination of prostate size via ultrasound has been proposed

Table 18.1 *PSA thresholds based on age and race*

Age (years)	'Normal' PSA ranges (ng/ml)			
	Based on 95% specificity[a]		Based on 95% sensitivity[b]	
	White males[c]	Black males[d]	White males[d]	Black males[d]
40	0–2.5	0–2.4	0–2.5	0–2.0
50	0–3.5	0–6.5	0–3.5	0–4.0
60	0–4.5	0–11.3	0–3.5	0–4.5
70	0–6.5	0–12.5	0–3.5	0–5.5

[a]Upper limit of normal prostate-specific antigen (PSA) determined from 95th percentile of PSA among men without prostate cancer.
[b]Upper limit of normal PSA required to maintain 95% sensitivity for cancer detection.
[c]From Oesterling et al 1993.[36]
[d]From Morgan et al 1996.[37]
Source: reprinted with permission from Carter and Partin.[2]

as a means of identifying patients with elevated PSA levels resulting from BPH vs prostate cancer.[40,41] The quotient of PSA and ultrasound measured prostate volume is termed PSA density (PSAD). A PSAD of ≥ 0.15 has been proposed as a threshold for recommending prostate biopsy in patients with PSA levels between 4.0 and 10.0 ng/ml and no evidence of prostate cancer on DRE or TRUS.[42,43] However, the utility of PSAD for detection of prostate cancer is limited, since up to 50% of cancers found in men following the above guidelines would have been missed.[7] Furthermore, PSAD has not been shown to increase the ability to predict cancer in men with a normal DRE and PSA level between 4.0 and 10.0 ng/ml compared to using PSA alone.[44]

A change in the level of serum PSA over a period of time is known as PSA velocity.[45] It has been shown that a rate of change in PSA ≥ 0.75 ng/ml per year is a specific marker for the presence of prostate cancer.[45] PSA velocity is highly valuable in detecting prostate cancer and distinguishing it from BPH early in the course of the disease. Several studies have demonstrated that men with prostate cancer have a more rapid rise in PSA compared to men without prostate cancer up to 10 years before diagnosis.[46–48] The minimum length of time over which PSA velocity can be determined is 18 months, and three repeated PSA measurements have been shown to optimize the accuracy of PSA velocity for detection of cancer.[46,47,49,50] Parameters such as PSAD, PSA velocity, or age- and race-specific PSA ranges have been partially successful in enhancing the specificity of PSA.[51]

The majority of PSA in circulation is bound to either ACT or MG; however, in men with prostate cancer there is a higher proportion of serum PSA complexed to ACT compared to men without malignancy.[52–55] This results in a lower percentage of free PSA found in the serum of men with prostate cancer. Initial studies suggested that a

threshold level of free/total PSA of 0.18 has been shown to significantly improve the ability to distinguish between patients with and without cancer compared to the use of total PSA alone.[53] It has also been suggested that PSA should be approximately 10% (no higher than 15%) of the total prostate weight (PSAD of 0.1–0.15) in benign disease.[38] The threshold value for free PSA that is optimal for both sensitivity and specificity of prostate cancer detection is dependent upon prostate size, since overlap in the percentage of free PSA is greatest in men with and without cancer who have enlarged prostates.[56,57] A free PSA threshold value of 25% has been shown to detect up to 95% of prostate cancer in both Caucasian and African-American men.[58] This finding indicates that race may not be a significant factor when using free PSA for detection of cancer. The utility of percent free PSA for distinguishing those men with and without prostate cancer is highest when total PSA levels are between 4.0 and 10.0 ng/ml.[59] Recent results also support a similar role of percent free PSA for detecting prostate cancer at lower PSA levels between 2.6 and 4.0 ng/ml.[60]

Other serum markers: complexed PSA, pPSA, BPSA, hK-2, and PAP

Measurement of PSA bound to other proteins such as ACT (complexed PSA) has also been used to identify men with prostate cancer.[61] Assays that measure complexed PSA have recently been approved by the Food and Drug Administration (FDA) for prostate cancer detection.[62–65] However, there are controversies about the replacement of percent free PSA by complexed PSA.[66] An alternative molecular form of free PSA known as BPSA has been isolated from the nodular BPH tissue in the transition zone of the prostate.[67] Purified BPSA contains two distinct cleavages at lysine 145 and lysine 182, and it is increased in the prostatic transition zone. The utility of this test for prostate cancer screening and detection is at present limited, however, because BPSA may in fact serve as a better marker for the severity of BPH than cancer. A proportion of uncomplexed PSA is found in circulation as the inactive zymogen precursor pro PSA (pPSA).[68] Elevated levels of pPSA are more highly correlated with prostate cancer than with BPH.[69] Serum pPSA may represent a more cancer-specific form of PSA; however, further studies are warranted to determine if pPSA is clinically useful for distinguishing prostate cancer from BPH.[69,70]

Human glandular kallikrein (hK2) is a serine protease that has approximately 78% amino acid sequence homology to PSA.[71] The activity of PSA may in part be regulated by hK2, since hK2 has been shown to cleave the precursor form of PSA.[72,73] The hK2 protein is found almost exclusively in the prostate and is up-regulated in poorly differentiated prostate cancer cells compared to normal tissues.[74–76] Although the ratio of hK2 to free PSA may increase the sensitivity of PSA to identify men with prostate cancer, the use of hK2 as a serum marker remains limited.[77–79]

Prostatic acid phosphatase (PAP) was the most widely used serum marker for prostate cancer prior to the availability of PSA.[80] Enzymatic phosphatase activity is not restricted to the prostate, and the use of PAP for monitoring prostate cancer has been largely supplanted by PSA, since PAP levels are often detectable even after complete removal of prostate tissue.[2] Preoperative PAP levels have been shown to be predictive of patient outcome after radical prostatectomy; however, the lower sensitivity and specificity of PAP in detection of prostate cancer compared to PSA has led to its significantly decreased use in clinical practice.[81] Serum PAP levels may provide important confirmatory information in patients in whom advanced disease is suspected.[82]

Histologic grading of prostate cancer

The Gleason histologic score is the most commonly used grading system for prostate cancer.[83,84] The Gleason system is based on microscopic analysis of tissue architecture (Figure 18.1).[85] A Gleason pattern of 1–5 is assigned as a primary grade (most common pattern) and a secondary grade (second most common pattern). A Gleason sum of 2–10 is then obtained by addition of the primary grade to the secondary grade. The presence of a primary or secondary Gleason grade ≥ 4 or Gleason sum ≥ 7 has been

associated with poorer prognosis.[86–89] Table 18.2 shows the distribution of Gleason grades found on prostate biopsy according to final pathologic stage in 2096 men who underwent surgery for clinically localized prostate cancer (Johns Hopkins series of 1982–1999).[2] Higher biopsy grade is associated with worse pathologic stage; however, on an individual basis, grade information alone does not accurately predict pathologic stage.

Prostate cancer staging systems

Whitmore developed the initial clinical staging system for prostate cancer in 1956 which was subsequently modified by Jewett. The tumor, node, metastases (TNM) staging system adopted by the American Joint Committee for Cancer (AJCC) is currently the most widely used staging system.[90,91] The TNM system has undergone numerous revisions over the past several years, with the most recent update occurring in 2002 (Table 18.3). The most significant change in the 2002 TNM clinical staging system was stratification of palpable (T2) lesions into three different groups as follows: T2a, palpable tumor confined to less than one-half of one lobe; T2b, palpable tumor involving more than half of one lobe but not both lobes; and T2c, tumor involving both lobes (Figure 18.2). This modification was readopted, because the recurrence-free survival following treatment was significantly different using this system compared to the 1997 guidelines that combined clinical stages T2a and T2b.[92,93] The Gleason scoring system has also been emphasized as the grading system of choice and use of the terms well differentiated, moderately differentiated, and poorly differentiated is no longer recommended.[94]

Assessment of the extent of disease based on DRE, serum tumor markers, tumor grade, and imaging studies is termed clinical staging. Pathologic staging is more accurate in predicting disease involvement, since it is based upon histologic examination of the prostate specimen and lymph nodes after surgical removal. Prostate tumor grade, status of surgical margins, presence of extracapsular disease, seminal vesicle invasion, and pelvic lymph node involvement are the most important pathologic findings that are predictive of prognosis after radical prostatectomy.[2] Poor outcomes and recurrence with metastatic disease are associated with seminal vesicle invasion or lymph node metastases.[13,88,95,96] Perineural invasion (PNI) found in radical prostatectomy specimens has limited prognostic utility; however, an increased risk of non-organ confined disease at prostatectomy is associated with the presence of PNI in pretreatment biopsy cores.[97] The finding of PNI on biopsy is also associated with increased PSA level, poor tumor differentiation, and higher pathologic stage.[98]

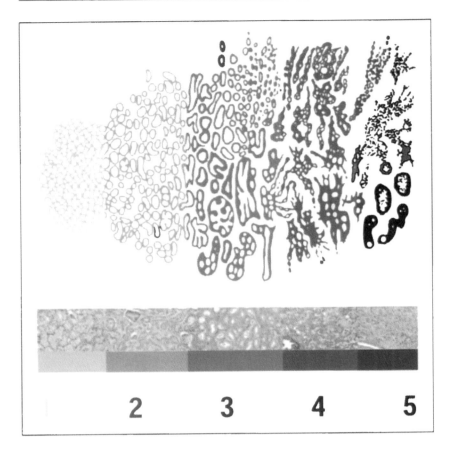

Figure 18.1
The Gleason scoring system: prostatic adenocarcinoma histologic grades.[84] Integrated design, R Sean Fulton. (Courtesy of Pittsburgh Supercomputing Center.)

Table 18.2 *Comparison of biopsy Gleason grade and pathologic stages in 2096 men who underwent radical prostatectomy (Johns Hopkins series 1982–1999)*

Grade	Organ confined No. (%)	Capsular penetration No. (%)	Seminal vesical status No. (%)	Lymph node status No. (%)
2–4	54 (68)	26 (30)	2 (2)	0 (0)
5	162 (54)	133 (44)	3 (1)	4 (1)
6	756 (59)	434 (34)	42 (3)	45 (4)
7	105 (29)	181 (51)	28 (8)	43 (12)
8–10	31 (29)	36 (33)	11 (10)	30 (28)

Source: reprinted with permission, from Carter and Partin.[2]

Diagnostic imaging modalities

Transrectal ultrasound

TRUS has become the most commonly used imaging modality for the prostate; however, the utility of TRUS as a screening method for localization of early prostate cancer remains limited.[99] Most hypoechoic lesions are not malignant and 50% of nonpalpable tumors larger than 1 cm in greatest dimension are not visualized by ultra-

sound.[30,100,101] Although hypoechoic areas on TRUS are more than twice as likely to contain cancer compared to isoechoic areas, up to 50% of cancers can potentially be missed if only hypoechoic areas are biopsied.[2,30,32] TRUS-guided biopsy of the prostate (Figure 18.3) can be utilized to obtain histologic confirmation of cancer once an individual has been identified as being at risk for the disease.[102] Systematic needle biopsy with TRUS is recommended to ensure accurate sampling of prostatic tissue in men who have an increased likelihood of harboring cancer.[2] Routine

Table 18.3 *Prostate cancer staging systems*

TNM 2002	Description	Whitmore-Jewett	Description
TX	Primary tumor cannot be assessed	None[*]	None
T0	No evidence of primary tumor	None	None
T1	Nonpalpable tumor not evident by imaging	A	Same as TNM
T1a	Tumor found in tissue removed at TUR; 5% or less is cancerous and histological grade ≤ 7	A1	Same as TNM
T1b	Tumor found in tissue removed at TUR; > 5% is cancerous or histologic grade > 7	A2	Same as TNM
T1c	Tumor identified by needle biopsy (e.g. because of elevated PSA)	None	None
T2	Palpable tumor confined to the prostate[a]	B	Same as TNM
T2a	Tumor involves less than one-half of one lobe	B1N	Tumor involves one-half lobe – surrounded by normal tissue on all sides
T2b	Tumor involves more than one-half of a lobe but not both lobes	B1	Same as TNM
T2c	Tumor involves both lobes	B2	Same as TNM
T3	Tumor extends through the prostate capsule[b]	C1	Tumor < 6 cm in diameter
T3a	Extracapsular extension (unilateral or bilateral)	C1	Same as TNM
T3b	Tumor invades seminal vesicle(s)	C1	Same as TNM
T4	Tumor is fixed or invades adjacent structures (not seminal vesicles): bladder neck, external sphincter, rectum, levator muscles, and/or pelvic wall.	C2	Same as TNM
None	None	D0	Elevated prostatic acid phosphatase
NX	Regional lymph nodes cannot be assessed	None	None
N0	No lymph node metastases	None	None
N1	Metastases in regional lymph node(s)	D1	Same as TNM
MX	Distant metastases cannot be assessed	None	None
M0	No evidence of distant metastases	None	None
M1	Distant metastases	D2	Same as TNM
M1a	Involvement of nonregional lymph nodes	D2	Same as TNM
M1b	Involvement of bones	D2	Same as TNM
M1c	Involvement of other distant sites with or without bone disease	D2	Same as TNM
None	None	D3	Hormonal refractory disease

[a] Tumor found in one or both lobes by needle biopsy, but not palpable or reliably visible by imaging is classified as T1c.
[b] Invasion into the prostatic apex or into (but not beyond) the prostatic capsule is classified not as T3 but as T2. TNM, tumor – node – metastases staging system; TUR, transurethral resection; PSA, prostate-specific antigen.
Source: adapted with permission from Carter and Partin.[2]

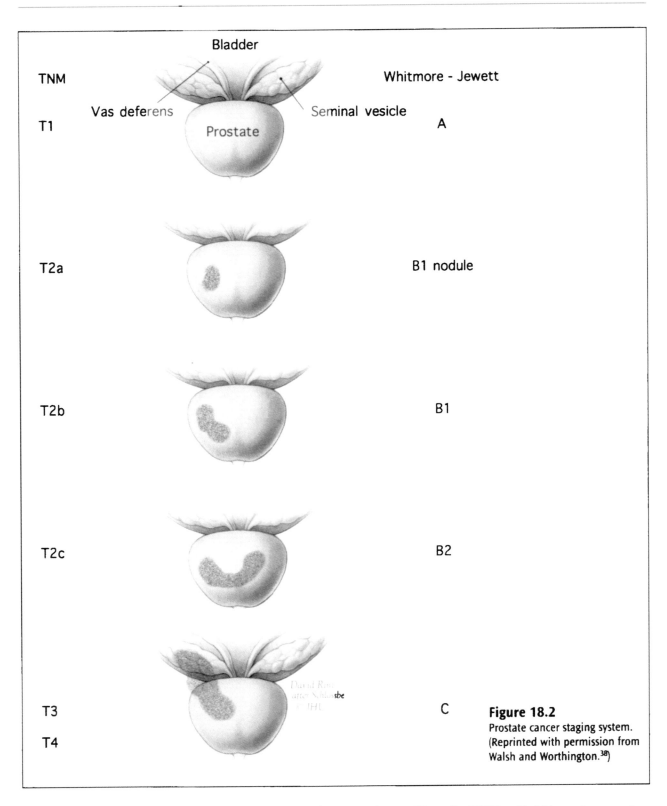

Figure 18.2
Prostate cancer staging system.
(Reprinted with permission from
Walsh and Worthington.[38])

sampling of sextant and posterolateral aspects of the gland with 12 cores sampled per patient is suggested. The combination of both sextant and posterolateral needle biopsies maximizes the detection of cancer, since up to 25% of prostate cancers may be missed if only routine sextant needle biopsy is performed.[103] Some patients, however, may not be candidates for TRUS-guided biopsy (e.g. previous history of bowel/rectal surgery or inflammatory disease process). An alternative, yet not commonly utilized, method for obtaining prostatic tissue for pathologic diagnosis of cancer is via the transperineal approach under ultrasound or magnetic resonance imaging (MRI) guidance.[104,105]

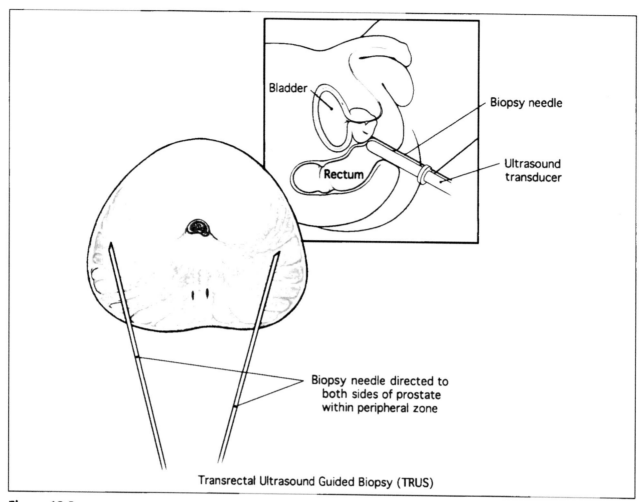

Figure 18.3
Transrectal ultrasound (TRUS)-guided biopsy of the prostate. (Reprinted with permission from Walsh and Worthington.[38])

Radionuclide bone scan

The utility of radionuclide bone scan in patients with localized disease is rather limited. Bone scintigraphy is not recommended for preoperative prostate cancer staging in patients with PSA values < 10 unless symptomatic bone pain is present.[106] On the other hand, radionuclide bone scan has been shown to be the most sensitive method for detecting bone metastases.[107,108] Bone scans may provide more useful information for patients with advanced disease (PSA > 10, Gleason score > 7, clinical stage T3 or higher). An appropriate treatment algorithm including hormonal therapy can be initiated if bone metastases are detected. Positive findings on bone scan are not always specific for prostate cancer, since any inflammatory or wound healing processes (e.g. recent fracture, osteomyelitis) may be interpreted as a false-positive result. Radionuclide bone imaging has also been shown to be helpful in detecting urinary tract obstruction (including upper tracts) and assessing bilateral renal function.[109]

Computed tomography, magnetic resonance imaging, magnetic resonance spectroscopic imaging, and ProstaScint™

Abdominal and pelvic computed tomography (CT) scanning provides little useful diagnostic or staging information, especially in patients with PSA < 20 ng/ml.[110–112] Use of pelvic CT would not benefit the majority of patients whose prostate cancers were detected by DRE and PSA testing, and may be of some limited value only in patients with advanced disease.[2] Diagnosis of lymph node metastases by CT scan is based primarily on size with any node > 1 cm in diameter (short axis) considered abnormal. The sensitivity of positive lymph node detection based on size criteria (> 1 cm) is approximately 25–78% and specificity is approximately 90%.[113,114]

Endorectal coil MRI has limited value in staging localized disease at the present time. Pelvic phase-arrayed coil MRI has been shown to predict positive surgical margins with up to 75% accuracy in some studies.[115,116] The sensitivity and specificity of pelvic coil MRI for prediction of capsular penetration and seminal vesicle invasion has been reported to be approximately 50% and 92%, respectively. MRI for prostate cancer staging may be more useful in the detection of lymph node metastases in men who are at high risk. MRI may provide additional information in patients with PSA levels between 10 and 20 ng/ml, Gleason score ≤ 7, and $\geq 50\%$ positive biopsies on sextant sampling.[106]

Quantitative magnetic resonance spectroscopic imaging (MRSI) is a recent advance in MR technology that permits evaluation of cellular metabolism and anatomy of the prostate. MRSI can be utilized to define tumor volume through functional or metabolic imaging differences compared to normal prostate tissue. Detection of extraprostatic disease can be significantly improved by combining MRI findings with estimates of metabolic abnormalities provided by MRSI.[117] MRSI has been shown to be significantly better than TRUS and MRI in differentiating among prostate cancer, BPH, and necrosis in patients suspected of having recurrent disease after cryosurgery.[118] The addition of MRSI to MRI has also been reported to increase the overall accuracy of prostate cancer tumor volume measurement; however, MRSI is not routinely used for pretreatment prostate cancer staging at the present time.

Capromab pendetide scanning (ProstaScint™) utilizes an Indium[111]-radiolabeled antibody (capromab pendetide or CYT-356) directed against prostate-specific membrane antigen (PSMA) for detection of cancer. This test may be most useful when other diagnostic studies have failed to identify metastatic disease in high-risk patients or in patients with evidence of biochemical recurrence after radical prostatectomy. ProstaScint has been approved by the FDA for evaluation of newly diagnosed patients at high risk for metastases. Patients who are appropriate candidates for ProstaScint typically have a Gleason score ≥ 7 and PSA > 20 ng/ml; Gleason score of 8–10 regardless of PSA value; or Gleason score ≥ 6 and clinical stage T3 disease.[106]

Prediction of pathologic stage

The accuracy of prostate cancer staging is significantly enhanced by considering the following parameters: extent of local disease (T stage), serum PSA level, and Gleason grade obtained from biopsy.[18,119–122] An increasing number of men over the past decade have presented with nonpalpable (stage T1c) disease, PSA levels < 10 ng/ml, and well to moderately differentiated tumors (Gleason score 4–6).

This downward stage migration which may be attributed to the utility of PSA and better screening strategies has resulted in approximately 60% of newly diagnosed cases presenting with localized or regional disease.[1] Staging nomograms (Table 18.4) have been constructed and further validated based on clinical stage, serum PSA level, and Gleason grade from the biopsy specimen.[123] The nomograms are also referred to as the Partin tables and values represent the percent probability of having the indicated final pathologic stage based on logistic regression analyses for all three variables combined.

The Partin tables were designed in order to provide patients with information that could be used for treatment decision making based on prediction of pathologic stage before definitive therapy. The likelihood of having organ-confined disease, capsular penetration, cancer in the seminal vesicles, and cancer in the lymph nodes is predicted with 95% accuracy. The 2001 Partin tables reflect the improvement in cancer control that has occurred with earlier diagnosis of disease and stage migration.[122] Important factors that must be considered in disease management include age, race, and the presence of low-volume (stage T1c) disease.[38] Older men tend to have larger-volume tumors and more aggressive disease (Gleason score ≥ 7).[124] Ethnic background is important, since African-American men are more likely to develop prostate cancer and are also more likely to die from the disease than other ethnic groups.[38] Approximately 25% of men diagnosed with nonpalpable (T1c) disease will have low-volume disease (< 0.2 cm^3).[125] Consideration of factors such as specific findings on needle biopsy, PSA density, and percentage of free PSA may be useful in determining whether stage T1c cancer is significant (Table 18.5).[38]

Clinical staging procedures

Clinical staging procedures such as laparoscopic or mini-laparotomy (mini-lap) pelvic lymphadenectomy should be reserved for situations in which it is unclear whether a patient has localized disease. Appropriate candidates for such staging procedures would have clinically localized prostate cancer and have high risk for extraprostatic lymph node involvement. These staging procedures should not be performed on men with clear evidence of advanced disease (i.e. positive bone scan). The probability of disease recurrence after radical prostatectomy in a patient with Gleason score 8 disease and positive lymph nodes is approximately 85% within 5 years.[38] Histologic examination of lymph nodes may be less important in men with Gleason score ≤ 7 cancers, because positive lymph nodes in this group are unlikely and associated with a $< 15\%$ probability of metastatic disease at 5 years.[38] Therefore, staging pelvic lymphadenectomy is recommended for men with

Table 18.4 *Prostate cancer staging nomograms (2001 Partin tables)*

PSA range (ng/ml)	Pathologic stage	Gleason score				
		2–4	5–6	3 + 4 = 7	4 + 3 = 7	8–10
Clinical stage T1c (nonpalpable, PSA elevated)						
0–2.5	Organ confined	95 (89–99)	90 (88–93)	79 (74–85)	71 (62–79)	66 (54–76)
	Extraprostatic extension	5 (1–11)	9 (7–12)	17 (13–23)	25 (18–34)	28 (20–38)
	Seminal vesicle (+)	–	0 (0–1)	2 (1–5)	2 (1–5)	4 (1–10)
	Lymph node (+)	–	–	1 (0–2)	1 (0–4)	1 (0–4)
2.6–4.0	Organ confined	92 (82–98)	84 (81–86)	68 (62–74)	58 (48–67)	52 (41–63)
	Extraprostatic extension	8 (2–18)	15 (13–18)	27 (22–33)	37 (29–46)	40 (31–50)
	Seminal vesicle (+)	–	1 (0–1)	4 (2–7)	4 (1–7)	6 (3–12)
	Lymph node (+)	–	–	1 (0–2)	1 (0–3)	1 (0–4)
4.1–6.0	Organ confined	90 (78–98)	80 (78–83)	63 (58–68)	52 (43–60)	46 (36–56)
	Extraprostatic extension	10 (2–22)	19 (16–21)	32 (26–36)	42 (35–50)	45 (36–54)
	Seminal vesicle (+)	–	1 (0–1)	3 (2–5)	3 (1–6)	5 (3–9)
	Lymph node (+)	–	0 (0–1)	2 (1–3)	3 (1–5)	3 (1–6)
6.1–10.0	Organ confined	87 (73–97)	75 (72–77)	54 (49–50)	43 (35–51)	37 (28–46)
	Extraprostatic extension	13 (3–27)	23 (21–25)	36 (32–40)	47 (40–54)	48 (39–57)
	Seminal vesicle (+)	–	2 (2–3)	8 (6–11)	8 (4–12)	13 (8–19)
	Lymph node (+)	–	0 (0–1)	2 (1–3)	2 (1–4)	3 (1–5)
> 10.0	Organ confined	80 (61–95)	62 (58–64)	37 (32–53)	27 (21–34)	22 (16–30)
	Extraprostatic extension	20 (5–39)	33 (30–36)	43 (38–48)	51 (44–59)	50 (42–59)
	Seminal vesicle (+)	–	4 (3–5)	12 (9–17)	11 (6–17)	17 (10–25)
	Lymph node (+)	–	2 (1–3)	8 (5–11)	10 (5–17)	11 (5–18)
Clinical stage T2a (palpable <½ of one lobe)						
0–2.5	Organ confined	91 (79–98)	81 (77–85)	64 (56–71)	53 (43–63)	47 (35–59)
	Extraprostatic extension	9 (2–21)	17 (13–21)	29 (23–36)	40 (30–49)	42 (32–53)
	Seminal vesicle (+)	–	1 (0–2)	5 (1–9)	4 (1–9)	7 (2–16)
	Lymph node (+)	–	0 (0–1)	2 (0–5)	3 (0–8)	3 (0–9)
2.6–4.0	Organ confined	85 (69–96)	71 (66–75)	50 (43–57)	39 (30–48)	33 (24–44)
	Extraprostatic extension	15 (4–31)	27 (23–31)	41 (35–58)	52 (43–61)	53 (44–63)
	Seminal vesicle (+)	–	2 (1–3)	7 (3–12)	6 (2–12)	10 (4–18)
	Lymph node (+)	–	0 (0–1)	2 (0–4)	2 (0–6)	3 (0–8)

Table 18.4 *Continued*

PSA range (ng/ml)	Pathologic stage	Gleason score				
		2–4	5–6	3 + 4 = 7	4 + 3 = 7	8–10
Clinical stage T2a (palpable <½ of one lobe) *continued*						
4.1–6.0	Organ confined	81 (63–95)	66 (62–70)	44 (39–50)	33 (25–41)	28 (20–37)
	Extraprostatic extension	19 (5–37)	32 (28–36)	46 (40–52)	56 (48–64)	58 (49–66)
	Seminal vesicle (+)	–	1 (1–2)	5 (3–8)	5 (2–8)	8 (4–13)
	Lymph node (+)	–	1 (0–2)	4 (2–7)	6 (3–11)	6 (2–12)
6.1–10.0	Organ confined	76 (56–94)	58 (54–61)	35 (30–40)	25 (19–32)	21 (15–28)
	Extraprostatic extension	24 (6–44)	37 (34–41)	49 (43–54)	58 (51–66)	57 (48–65)
	Seminal vesicle (+)	–	4 (3–5)	13 (9–18)	11 (6–17)	17 (11–26)
	Lymph node (+)	–	1 (0–2)	3 (2–6)	5 (2–8)	5 (2–10)
> 10.0	Organ confined	65 (43–89)	42 (38–46)	20 (17–24)	14 (10–18)	11 (7–15)
	Extraprostatic extension	35 (11–57)	47 (43–52)	49 (43–55)	55 (46–64)	52 (41–62)
	Seminal vesicle (+)	–	6 (4–8)	16 (11–22)	13 (7–20)	19 (12–29)
	Lymph node (+)	–	4 (3–7)	14 (9–21)	18 (10–27)	17 (9–29)
Clinical stage T2b (palpable >½ of one lobe, not on both lobes)						
0–2.5	Organ confined	88 (73–97)	75 (69–81)	54 (46–63)	43 (33–54)	37 (26–49)
	Extraprostatic extension	12 (3–27)	22 (17–28)	35 (28–43)	45 (35–56)	46 (35–58)
	Seminal vesicle (+)	–	2 (0–3)	6 (2–12)	5 (1–11)	9 (2–20)
	Lymph node (+)	–	1 (0–2)	4 (0–10)	6 (0–14)	6 (0–16)
2.6–4.0	Organ confined	80 (61–95)	63 (57–69)	41 (33–48)	30 (22–39)	25 (17–34)
	Extraprostatic extension	20 (5–39)	34 (28–40)	47 (40–55)	57 (47–67)	57 (46–68)
	Seminal vesicle (+)	–	2 (1–4)	9 (4–15)	7 (3–14)	12 (5–22)
	Lymph node (+)	–	1 (0–2)	3 (0–8)	4 (0–12)	5 (0–14)
4.1–6.0	Organ confined	75 (55–93)	57 (52–63)	35 (29–40)	25 (18–32)	21 (14–29)
	Extraprostatic extension	25 (7–45)	39 (33–44)	51 (44–57)	60 (50–68)	59 (49–69)
	Seminal vesicle (+)	–	2 (1–3)	7 (4–11)	5 (3–9)	9 (4–16)
	Lymph node (+)	–	2 (1–3)	7 (4–13)	10 (5–18)	10 (4–20)
6.1–10.0	Organ confined	69 (47–91)	49 (43–54)	26 (22–31)	19 (14–25)	15 (10–21)
	Extraprostatic extension	31 (9–53)	44 (39–49)	52 (46–58)	60 (52–68)	57 (48–67)
	Seminal vesicle (+)	–	5 (3–8)	16 (10–22)	13 (7–20)	19 (11–29)
	Lymph node (+)	–	2 (1–3)	6 (4–10)	8 (5–14)	8 (4–16)
> 10.0	Organ confined	57 (35–86)	33 (28–38)	14 (11–17)	9 (6–13)	7 (4–10)
	Extraprostatic extension	43 (14–65)	52 (46–56)	47 (40–53)	50 (40–60)	46 (36–59)
	Seminal vesicle (+)	–	8 (5–11)	17 (12–24)	13 (8–21)	19 (12–29)
	Lymph node (+)	–	8 (5–12)	22 (15–30)	27 (16–39)	27 (14–40)

Table 18.4 *Continued*

PSA range (ng/ml)	Pathologic stage	Gleason score				
		2–4	5–6	3 + 4 = 7	4 + 3 = 7	8–10
Clinical stage T2c (palpable on both lobes)						
0–2.5	Organ confined	86 (17–97)	73 (63–81)	51 (38–63)	39 (26–54)	34 (21–48)
	Extraprostatic extension	14 (3–29)	24 (17–33)	36 (26–48)	45 (32–59)	47 (33–61)
	Seminal vesicle (+)	–	1 (0–4)	5 (1–13)	5 (1–12)	8 (2–19)
	Lymph node (+)	–	1 (0–4)	6 (0–18)	9 (0–26)	10 (0–27)
2.6–4.0	Organ confined	78 (58–94)	61 (50–70)	38 (27–50)	27 (18–40)	23 (14–34)
	Extraprostatic extension	22 (6–42)	36 (27–45)	48 (37–59)	57 (44–70)	57 (44–70)
	Seminal vesicle (+)	–	2 (1–5)	8 (2–17)	6 (2–16)	10 (3–22)
	Lymph node (+)	–	1 (0–4)	5 (0–15)	7 (0–21)	8 (0–22)
4.1–6.0	Organ confined	73 (52–93)	55 (44–64)	31 (23–41)	21 (41–31)	18 (11–28)
	Extraprostatic extension	27 (7–48)	49 (32–50)	50 (40–60)	57 (43–68)	57 (43–70)
	Seminal vesicle (+)	–	2 (1–4)	6 (2–11)	4 (1–10)	7 (2–15)
	Lymph node (+)	–	3 (1–7)	12 (5–23)	16 (6–32)	16 (6–33)
6.1–10.0	Organ confined	67 (45–91)	46 (36–56)	24 (17–32)	16 (10–24)	13 (8–20)
	Extraprostatic extension	33 (9–55)	46 (37–55)	52 (42–61)	58 (46–69)	56 (43–69)
	Seminal vesicle (+)	–	5 (2–9)	13 (6–23)	11 (4–21)	16 (6–29)
	Lymph node (+)	–	3 (1–6)	10 (5–18)	13 (6–25)	13 (5–26)
> 10.0	Organ confined	54 (32–85)	30 (21–38)	11 (7–17)	7 (4–12)	6 (3–10)
	Extraprostatic extension	46 (15–68)	51 (42–60)	42 (30–55)	43 (29–50)	41 (27–57)
	Seminal vesicle (+)	–	6 (2–12)	13 (6–24)	10 (3–20)	15 (5–28)
	Lymph node (+)	–	13 (6–22)	33 (18–49)	38 (20–58)	38 (20–59)

PSA = prostate-specific antigen.
Source: reprinted with permission of Elsevier Science from Partin et al.[122]

Table 18.5 *Determination of significant vs insignificant stage T1c (nonpalpable) disease.*[38]

Significant T1c cancer	Insignificant T1c cancer
Cancer identified in 3 needle cores, or	Cancer identified in only 1 or 2 needle cores, and
Cancer present in greater than half of any one core, or	Cancer present in less than half of each core, and
Gleason score ≥ 7, or	Gleason score ≤ 6, and
PSA density > 0.1–0.15, or	PSA density < 0.1–0.15, and
Free PSA < 15%	Free PSA > 15 %

These factors apply only if cancer is nonpalpable and if biopsies have included at least six cores.

PSA ≥ 15 ng/ml, Gleason score ≥ 8 disease, or TNM stage T2b or greater who are candidates for surgery, and who are potentially curable.

Operative technique for limited laparoscopic pelvic lymphadenectomy

The use of laparoscopic pelvic lymphadenectomy for prostate cancer staging was first introduced in 1991.[126] Transperitoneal laparoscopic pelvic lymphadenectomy may be accomplished using either the diamond or fan configurations for trochar placement (Figure 18.4). The diamond configuration is formed by placement of trochars as follows: two 10 mm ports at the umbilicus and 4–6 cm superior to the pubic symphysis in the midline; two 5 mm ports located near McBurney's point in the midclavicular line bilaterally. The fan configuration may be utilized for obese patients or men with a dense urachus.[127] The fan configuration comprises 5 trochars placed in the following locations: a 10 mm umbilical trochar for the laparoscope; two trochars at the level of the umbilicus and lateral to the inferior epigastric vessels in line with the anterior superior iliac crest (a 10 mm trochar on the left side and a 5 mm trochar on the right side); and two 5 mm trochars placed laterally and midway between the umbilicus and pubic symphysis.

After insufflation of the abdomen and division of the vas deferens, the external iliac vein is identified to define the lateral extent of the dissection. Pulsations of the external iliac artery can serve as a helpful landmark in identifying the location of the external iliac vein (Figure 18.5). The fatty tissue inferior to the arterial pulsation is elevated and gently dissected in order to expose the

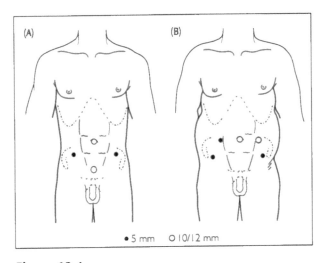

• 5 mm   ○ 10/12 mm

Figure 18.4
Placement of trochars for laparoscopic pelvic lymphadenectomy. (A) Diamond configuration: two 10 mm trochars at umbilicus and 4–6 cm above the pubic symphysis in the midline; two 5 mm trochars near McBurney's point in the midclavicular line bilaterally. (B) Fan configuration: 10 mm umbilical trochar; 10 mm on left and 5 mm trochar on right at the level of the umbilicus, lateral to the inferior epigastric vessels in line with the anterior superior iliac crest; two 5 mm trochars are also placed laterally and midway between the umbilicus and pubic symphysis.

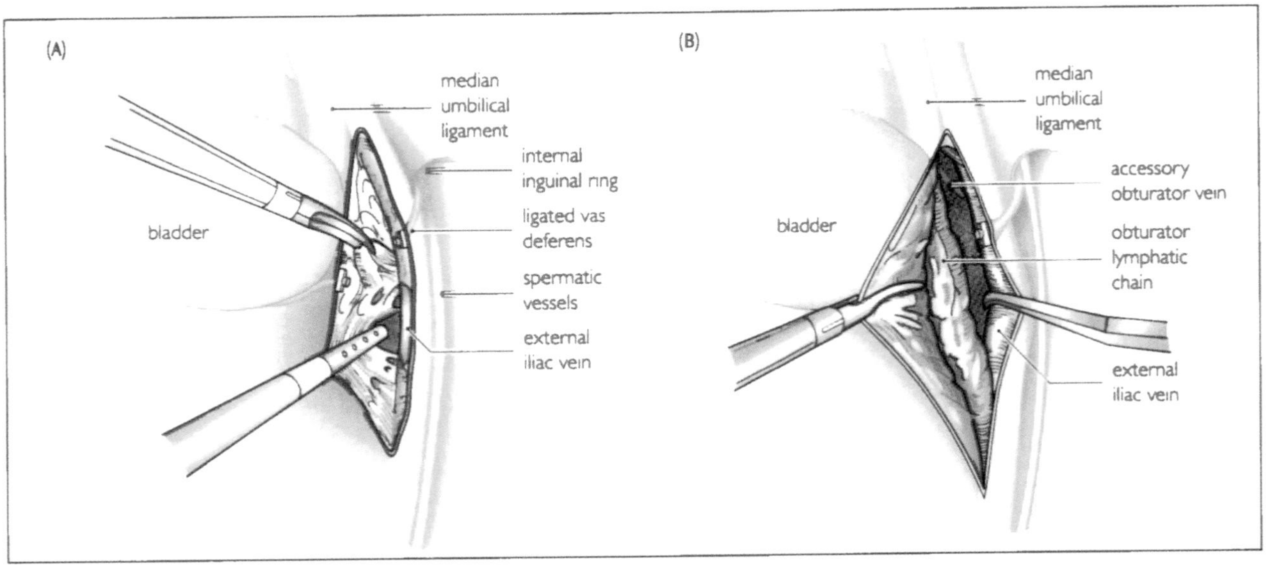

Figure 18.5
Laparoscopic pelvic lymphadenectomy. (A) The pulsation of the external iliac artery is used to identify the external iliac vein. Blunt dissection with the irrigator-aspirator is used to facilitate mobilization of the lymph node packet from the anterior surface of the vein. (B) The lymphatic tissue is mobilized free from the bifurcation of the common iliac vein to the pubis and medially until the obturator internus muscle is visualized.

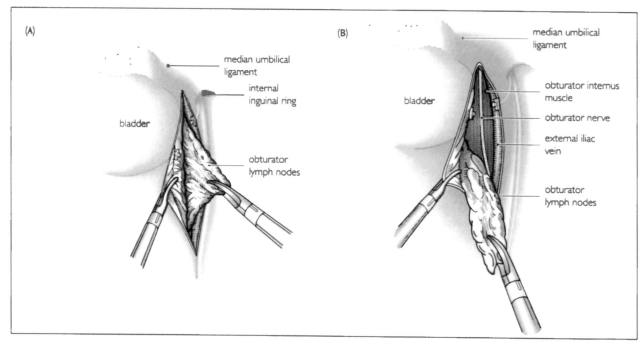

Figure 18.6
Laparoscopic pelvic lymphadenectomy (continued). (A) The inferior portion of the lymph node packet is isolated and divided near the circumflex iliac artery in order to avoid injury to the obturator nerve. (B) The lymph node packet is gently freed from the obturator nerve and pelvic sidewall using blunt dissection. The remaining pedicle is clipped in addition to any open lymphatic channels and small blood vessels prior to removal of the lymph node packet.

external iliac vein. The lymphatic tissue is then mobilized free from the bifurcation of the common iliac vein to the pubis and medially until the obturator internus muscle is visualized. The dissection proceeds along the lateral pelvic sidewall to the inferior portion of the iliac vein. Once this portion of the dissection is completed, the inferior aspect of the lymph node packet is divided near the circumflex iliac artery and femoral canal to avoid injury to the obturator nerve (Figure 18.6). Removal of the lymph node packet is facilitated by blunt dissection and retraction in a cephalad direction. Sharp dissection should be avoided to minimize iatrogenic nerve and vascular injury. Hemoclips can be applied to any small lymphatic structures or vessels coursing between the pelvic sidewall and the lymph node packet. Following removal of the lymph node packet, hemostasis should be assessed under low insufflation pressures (i.e. 5–10 mmHg).

Operative technique for minilaparotomy pelvic lymphadenectomy

The mini-lap approach was first introduced in 1992 as an alternative to laparoscopic pelvic lymphadenectomy.[128]

This technique has proven to be versatile in lymph node sampling in patients at risk for harboring metastatic disease. In the mini-lap approach, a 6 cm lower midline abdominal incision is made approximately 2 cm above the pubic symphysis (Figure 18.7). The anterior rectus fascia and transversalis fascia are sharply incised in the midline between the rectus muscles to enter the space of Retzius. The peritoneum is then mobilized off the external iliac vessels up to the bifurcation of the common iliac arteries. Removal of the lymph node packet is initiated by incision of the lymphatic tissue overlying the medial aspect of the external iliac vein (Figure 18.8). A metal clip is placed proximal to the node of Cloquet, followed by an incision proximal to the clip in order to remove the distal node packet. Care should be taken to avoid injury to the accessory obturator vein which may present and coursing from the obturator foramen to the external iliac vein. The lymph node packet is removed en bloc from the pelvic sidewall with preservation of the obturator nerve and vessels.

The mini-lap procedure has been reported to be more cost-effective and have less morbidity than the laparoscopic approach. In a community practice setting, operative time was shorter and complication rates were lower for patients undergoing mini-lap vs laparoscopic pelvic lymph node dissection.[129] A comparison of the modified open approach to laparoscopic and mini-lap procedures demonstrated equal staging efficacy with no difference in

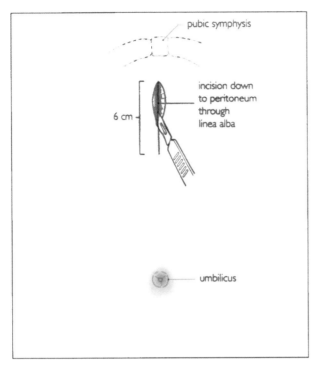

Figure 18.7
Minilaparotomy (mini-lap) pelvic lymphadenectomy. A 6 cm lower midline abdominal incision is made approximately 2 cm above the pubic symphysis. The anterior rectus fascia and transversalis fascia are sharply incised in the midline between the rectus muscles to enter the space of Retzius.

terms of the number of harvested lymph nodes.[130] The laparoscopic approach required significantly more operative time compared to the modified open and mini-lap techniques. Postoperative hospital recovery was similar for patients undergoing the mini-lap and laparoscopic pelvic lymph node dissection. The mini-lap approach has therefore been favored at institutions that are inexperienced with laparoscopic techniques.

Future directions: molecular markers for prostate cancer detection

Most cancer detection assays are based on antibody interactions with marker proteins that are up-regulated in patients with prostate cancer. Advances in diagnostic techniques have resulted in the ability to detect circulating tumor cells in the blood of patients with prostate cancer. This may ultimately lead to diagnosis at earlier stages of disease when the primary lesion is potentially more curable. Molecular techniques such as polymerase chain reaction (PCR) and reverse transcriptase PCR (RT-PCR) are highly sensitive methods that have been utilized for detection of cancer cells. Over the past few years, numerous clinical studies have used PCR technology to detect genetic alterations, including mutations, deletions,

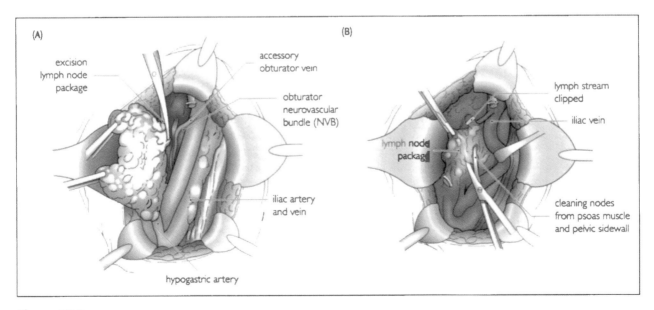

Figure 18.8
Mini-lap pelvic lymphadenectomy. (A) Removal of the lymph node packet is initiated by incision of the lymphatic tissue overlying the medial aspect of the external iliac vein. A clip is placed next to the external iliac vein and Cooper's ligament followed by incision of the lymph node packet boundary proximal to the clip. The distal lymph node packet is then mobilized. (B) The lymph node packet is removed en bloc from the obturator fossa.

translocations, and amplifications. RT-PCR is a sensitive method for detecting the presence of tumor-specific mRNA in cells isolated from peripheral blood. Several studies have characterized the presence of PSA-mRNA-bearing cells in the circulation of prostate cancer patients without evidence of metastatic disease.[131] A higher frequency of PSA-mRNA-expressing cells in the peripheral blood is correlated with extent of disease and has been shown to be an independent predictor of disease-free survival after radical prostatectomy.[132] The RT-PCR assay for PSA has been reported to be a better predictor of pathologic stage in men undergoing radical prostatectomy compared to PSA and Gleason score.[133]

PSMA is a 100 kDa type II transmembrane glycoprotein expressed in normal prostatic epithelium, BPH, prostatic intraepithelial neoplasia, and carcinoma.[134,135] Detectable PSMA levels have also been identified in duodenal mucosa and proximal renal tubules. The primary method for detection of PSMA expression has been with a monoclonal antibody (7E11) that binds a six amino acid intracellular epitope of PSMA near the amino terminus.[136] Immunohistochemical staining of PSMA has been observed in vascular endothelium associated with tumors, which suggests a potential relationship between PSMA expression and angiogenesis.[137] Expression of PSMA may be dependent upon the degree of tumor differentiation, since lower levels have been observed in advanced prostate cancers.[136] The use of RT-PCR has been applied for detection of PSMA-expressing cells in blood with a reported sensitivity of 62–67%.[138] The potential clinical significance of detecting hematogenous micrometastatic disease remains promising; however, current RT-PCR strategies are not sensitive or accurate enough and in some cases may overpredict the extent of disease in early-stage cancer.

Prostate stem cell antigen (PSCA) is a homologue of the Thy-1/Ly-6 family of glycosylphosphatidylinositol (GPI)-anchored cell surface antigens and is expressed in the basal cells of normal prostate and in > 80% of prostate cancers.[139] PSCA mRNA is up-regulated in both androgen dependent and independent prostate cancer xenografts. Increased PSCA expression measured by immunohisto-chemical analysis was observed in approximately 94% of primary prostate tumors and 100% of bone metastases.[140] PSCA expression was found to be increased with higher Gleason score, higher tumor stage, and progression to androgen independence. Although there have been no reports of PSCA detection in the circulation of patients with prostate cancer, further characterization of PSCA is needed to evaluate the prognostic utility of PSCA in prostate cancer.

The process of angiogenesis describes the dependence of solid tumors on development of new blood vessels required for growth, invasion, and metastasis.[141] Angiogenesis can be quantitated immunohistochemically by determination of microvessel density (MVD) and may be of prognostic significance. The overall utility of angiogenesis as a prognostic tool for prostate cancer, however, remains controversial. Normal prostate tissue and prostate adenomas typically have low MVD, whereas the MVD in prostate cancer has been shown to increase significantly with tumor stage and grade.[142] MVD has also been shown to be an independent predictor of progression after radical prostatectomy in patients with Gleason score 5–7 disease.[143] In other studies, MVD was not associated with Gleason sum, tumor stage, surgical margin status, or seminal vesicle invasion.[144,145] Further investigation to assess the prognostic utility of angiogenesis markers is warranted, and may facilitate the development of antiangiogenic treatment strategies that target tumor vasculature.

DNA methylation is an epigenetic phenomenon that may also be used as a marker for prostate cancer. Methylation of gene promoter regions has been associated with transcriptional silencing. This process can affect many genes during tumorigenesis, including those involved in control of cellular growth.[146] Abnormal methylation of regulatory sequences at the glutathione S-transferase pi (GSTP1) gene locus is found in the majority (> 90%) of prostate carcinomas but not in normal prostate tissue.[147,148] This methylation change has also been detected in urine and ejaculate specimens from patients with prostate cancer.[149,150] Aberrant methylation occurring in multiple genes has been shown to be correlated with poor clinical outcomes and may serve as a potentially useful tool for disease prognostication.[151] The clinical utility of methylation markers for prostate cancer detection or surveillance remains promising, but has not been validated at the present time.

Routine use of serum PSA and improvements leading to early detection have had a profound impact on the diagnosis and management of patients with prostate cancer. Current methods for preoperative assessment of disease prognosis are based on classic parameters such as clinical tumor stage, Gleason grade, and serum PSA level. Scientific advances over the past decade have led to the characterization of new molecular markers that may eventually prove to be more useful than PSA. An ideal marker is one with high sensitivity and specificity that could not only detect the presence or recurrence of prostate cancer but could also differentiate between an indolent tumor and an aggressive tumor with metastatic potential. Development of more sensitive and accurate measures of outcome is needed to improve upon existing treatments, and can only be achieved through a better understanding of the molecular basis of prostate cancer pathogenesis.

References

1. Greenlee RT, Hill-Harmon MB, Murray T, Thun M. Cancer statistics, 2001. CA Cancer J Clin 2001; 51:15–36.

2. Carter HB, Partin AW. Diagnosis and staging of prostate cancer. In: Walsh PC, Retik AB, Vaughan ED, Wein AJ, eds Campell's urology. Vol. 4. Philadelphia: WB Saunders, 2002:3055–79.

3. Hankey BF, Feuer EJ, Clegg LX, et al. Cancer surveillance series: interpreting trends in prostate cancer – part I: evidence of the effects of screening in recent prostate cancer incidence, mortality, and survival rates. J Natl Cancer Inst 1999; 91:1017–24.

4. Tarone RE, Chu KC, Brawley OW. Implications of stage-specific survival rates in assessing recent declines in prostate cancer mortality rates. Epidemiology 2000; 11:167–70.

5. Gann PH. Interpreting recent trends in prostate cancer incidence and mortality. Epidemiology 1997; 8:117–20.

6. Bartsch G, Horninger W, Klocker H, et al. Prostate cancer mortality after introduction of prostate-specific antigen mass screening in the Federal State of Tyrol, Austria. Urology 2001; 58:417–24.

7. Catalona WJ, Richie JP, Ahmann FR, et al. Comparison of digital rectal examination and serum prostate specific antigen in the early detection of prostate cancer: results of a multicenter clinical trial of 6,630 men. J Urol 1994; 151:1283–90.

8. Littrup PJ, Kane RA, Mettlin CJ, et al. Cost-effective prostate cancer detection. Reduction of low-yield biopsies. Investigators of the American Cancer Society National Prostate Cancer Detection Project. Cancer 1994; 74:3146–58.

9. Bangma CH, Kranse R, Blijenberg BG, Schroder FH. The value of screening tests in the detection of prostate cancer. Part I: results of a retrospective evaluation of 1726 men. Urology 1995; 46:773–8.

10. Schroder FH, van der Maas P, Beemsterboer P, et al. Evaluation of the digital rectal examination as a screening test for prostate cancer. Rotterdam section of the European Randomized Study of Screening for Prostate Cancer. J Natl Cancer Inst 1998; 90:1817–23.

11. Carvalhal GF, Smith DS, Mager DE, et al. Digital rectal examination for detecting prostate cancer at prostate specific antigen levels of 4 ng./ml. or less. J Urol 1999; 161:835–9.

12. Smith DS, Catalona WJ. Interexaminer variability of digital rectal examination in detecting prostate cancer. Urology 1995; 45:70–4.

13. Walsh PC, Jewett HJ. Radical surgery for prostatic cancer. Cancer 1980; 45:1906–11.

14. Friedman GD, Hiatt RA, Quesenberry CP Jr, Selby JV. Case-control study of screening for prostatic cancer by digital rectal examinations. Lancet 1991; 337:1526–9.

15. Chodak GW, Keller P, Schoenberg HW. Assessment of screening for prostate cancer using the digital rectal examination. J Urol 1989; 141:1136–8.

16. Thompson IM, Rounder JB, Teague JL, et al. Impact of routine screening for adenocarcinoma of the prostate on stage distribution. J Urol 1987; 137:424–6.

17. Epstein JI, Walsh PC, Carmichael M, Brendler CB. Pathologic and clinical findings to predict tumor extent of nonpalpable (stage T1c) prostate cancer. JAMA 1994; 271:368–74.

18. Partin AW, Yoo J, Carter HB, et al. The use of prostate specific antigen, clinical stage and Gleason score to predict pathological stage in men with localized prostate cancer. J Urol 1993; 150:110–14.

19. Lilja H. A kallikrein-like serine protease in prostatic fluid cleaves the predominant seminal vesicle protein. J Clin Invest 1985; 76:1899–903.

20. McGee RS, Herr JC. Human seminal vesicle-specific antigen is a substrate for prostate-specific antigen (or P-30). Biol Reprod 1988; 39:499–510.

21. Christensson A, Laurell CB, Lilja H. Enzymatic activity of prostate-specific antigen and its reactions with extracellular serine proteinase inhibitors. Eur J Biochem 1990; 194:755–63.

22. Stenman UH, Leinonen J, Alfthan H, et al. A complex between prostate-specific antigen and alpha 1-antichymotrypsin is the major form of prostate-specific antigen in serum of patients with prostatic cancer: assay of the complex improves clinical sensitivity for cancer. Cancer Res 1991; 51:222–6.

23. Lilja H, Christensson A, Dahlen U, et al. Prostate-specific antigen in serum occurs predominantly in complex with alpha 1-antichymotrypsin. Clin Chem 1991; 37:1618–25.

24. Pizzo SV, Mast AE, Feldman SR, Salvesen G. In vivo catabolism of alpha 1-antichymotrypsin is mediated by the Serpin receptor which binds alpha 1-proteinase inhibitor, antithrombin III and heparin cofactor II. Biochim Biophys Acta 1988; 967:158–62.

25. Stamey TA, Yang N, Hay AR, et al. Prostate-specific antigen as a serum marker for adenocarcinoma of the prostate. N Engl J Med 1987; 317:909–16.

26. Yuan JJ, Coplen DE, Petros JA, et al. Effects of rectal examination, prostatic massage, ultrasonography and needle biopsy on serum prostate specific antigen levels. J Urol 1992; 147:810–14.

27. Crawford ED, Schutz MJ, Clejan S, et al. The effect of digital rectal examination on prostate-specific antigen levels. JAMA 1992; 267:2227–8.

28. Chybowski FM, Bergstralh EJ, Oesterling JE. The effect of digital rectal examination on the serum prostate specific antigen concentration: results of a randomized study. J Urol 1992; 148:83–6.

29. Guess HA, Heyse JF, Gormley GJ, et al. Effect of finasteride on serum PSA concentration in men with benign prostatic hyperplasia. Results from the North American phase III clinical trial. Urol Clin North Am 1993; 20:627–36.

30. Ellis WJ, Chetner MP, Preston SD, Brawer MK. Diagnosis of prostatic carcinoma: the yield of serum prostate specific antigen, digital rectal examination and transrectal ultrasonography. J Urol 1994; 152:1520–5.

31. Cooner WH, Mosley BR, Rutherford CL Jr, et al. Prostate cancer detection in a clinical urological practice by ultrasonography, digital rectal examination and prostate specific antigen. J Urol 1990; 143:1146–52.

32. Hammerer P, Huland H. Systematic sextant biopsies in 651 patients referred for prostate evaluation. J Urol 1994; 151:99–102.

33. Schroder FH, Roobol-Bouts M, Vis AN, et al. Prostate-specific antigen-based early detection of prostate cancer – validation of screening without rectal examination. Urology 2001; 57:83–90.

34. Carter HB. A PSA threshold of 4.0 ng/mL for early detection of prostate cancer: the only rational approach for men 50 years old and older. Urology 2000; 55:796–9.

35. Catalona WJ, Partin AW, Slawin KM, et al. Percentage of free PSA in black versus white men for detection and staging of prostate cancer: a prospective multicenter clinical trial. Urology 2000; 55:372–6.

36. Oesterling JE, Jacobsen SJ, Chute CG, et al. Serum prostate-specific antigen in a community-based population of healthy men. Establishment of age-specific reference ranges. JAMA 1993; 270:860–4.

37. Morgan TO, Jacobsen SJ, McCarthy WF, et al. Age-specific reference ranges for prostate-specific antigen in black men. N Engl J Med 1996; 335:304–10.

38. Walsh PC, Worthington JF. Dr. Patrick Walsh's guide to surviving prostate cancer. New York: Warner Books, 2001:462.

39. Ross KS, Carter HB, Pearson JD, Guess HA. Comparative efficiency of prostate-specific antigen screening strategies for prostate cancer detection. JAMA 2000; 284:1399–405.

40. Benson MC, Whang IS, Olsson CA, et al. The use of prostate specific antigen density to enhance the predictive value of intermediate levels of serum prostate specific antigen. J Urol 1992; 147:817–21.

41. Benson MC, Whang IS, Pantuck A, et al. Prostate specific antigen density: a means of distinguishing benign prostatic hypertrophy and prostate cancer. J Urol 1992; 147:815–16.

42. Seaman E, Whang M, Olsson CA, et al. PSA density (PSAD). Role in patient evaluation and management. Urol Clin North Am 1993; 20:653–63.

43. Bazinet M, Meshref AW, Trudel C, et al. Prospective evaluation of prostate-specific antigen density and systematic biopsies for early detection of prostatic carcinoma. Urology 1994; 43:44–51.

44. Brawer MK, Aramburu EA, Chen GL, et al. The inability of prostate specific antigen index to enhance the predictive value of prostate specific antigen in the diagnosis of prostatic carcinoma. J Urol 1993; 150:369–73.

45. Carter HB, Morrell CH, Pearson JD, et al. Estimation of prostatic growth using serial prostate-specific antigen measurements in men with and without prostate disease. Cancer Res 1992; 52:3323–8.

46. Smith DS, Catalona WJ. Rate of change in serum prostate specific antigen levels as a method for prostate cancer detection. J Urol 1994; 152:1163–7.

47. Kadmon D, Weinberg AD, Williams RH, et al. Pitfalls in interpreting prostate specific antigen velocity. J Urol 1996; 155:1655–7.

48. Lujan M, Paez A, Sanchez E, et al. Prostate specific antigen variation in patients without clinically evident prostate cancer. J Urol 1999; 162:1311–13.

49. Carter HB, Pearson JD, Metter EJ, et al. Longitudinal evaluation of prostate-specific antigen levels in men with and without prostate disease. JAMA 1992; 267:2215–20.

50. Carter HB, Pearson JD, Waclawiw Z, et al. Prostate-specific antigen variability in men without prostate cancer: effect of sampling interval on prostate-specific antigen velocity. Urology 1995; 45:591–6.

51. Nixon RG, Brawer MK. Enhancing the specificity of prostate-specific antigen (PSA): an overview of PSA density, velocity and age-specific reference ranges. Br J Urol 1997; 79(Suppl 1):61–7.

52. Leinonen J, Lovgren T, Vornanen T, Stenman UH. Double-label time-resolved immunofluorometric assay of prostate-specific antigen and of its complex with alpha 1-antichymotrypsin. Clin Chem 1993; 39:2098–103.

53. Christensson A, Bjork T, Nilsson O, et al. Serum prostate specific antigen complexed to alpha 1-antichymotrypsin as an indicator of prostate cancer. J Urol 1993; 150:100–5.

54. Lilja H. Significance of different molecular forms of serum PSA. The free, noncomplexed form of PSA versus that complexed to alpha 1-antichymotrypsin. Urol Clin North Am 1993; 20:681–6.

55. Stenman UH, Hakama M, Knekt P, et al. Serum concentrations of prostate specific antigen and its complex with alpha 1-antichymotrypsin before diagnosis of prostate cancer. Lancet 1994; 344:1594–8.

56. Catalona WJ, Smith DS, Wolfert RL, et al. Evaluation of percentage of free serum prostate-specific antigen to improve specificity of prostate cancer screening. JAMA 1995; 274:1214–20.

57. Stephan C, Lein M, Jung K, et al. The influence of prostate volume on the ratio of free to total prostate specific antigen in serum of patients with prostate carcinoma and benign prostate hyperplasia. Cancer 1997; 79:104–9.

58. Catalona WJ, Ramos CG, Carvalhal GF, Yan Y. Lowering PSA cutoffs to enhance detection of curable prostate cancer. Urology 2000; 55:791–5.

59. Catalona WJ, Partin AW, Slawin KM, et al. Use of the percentage of free prostate-specific antigen to enhance differentiation of prostate cancer from benign prostatic disease: a prospective multicenter clinical trial. JAMA 1998; 279:1542–7.

60. Roehl KA, Antenor JA, Catalona WJ. Robustness of free prostate specific antigen measurements to reduce unnecessary biopsies in the 2.6 to 4.0 ng./mL. range. J Urol 2002; 168:922–5.

61. Allard WJ, Zhou Z, Yeung KK. Novel immunoassay for the measurement of complexed prostate-specific antigen in serum. Clin Chem 1998; 44:1216–23.

62. Stamey TA, Yemoto CE. Examination of the 3 molecular forms of serum prostate specific antigen for distinguishing negative from positive biopsy: relationship to transition zone volume. J Urol 2000; 163:119–26.

63. Okegawa T, Kinjo M, Watanabe K, et al. The significance of the free-to-complexed prostate-specific antigen (PSA) ratio in prostate cancer detection in patients with a PSA level of 4.1-10.0 ng/mL. BJU Int 2000; 85:708–14.

64. Filella X, Alcover J, Molina R, et al. Measurement of complexed PSA in the differential diagnosis between prostate cancer and benign prostate hyperplasia. Prostate 2000; 42:181–5.

65. Jung K, Elgeti U, Lein M, et al. Ratio of free or complexed prostate-specific antigen (PSA) to total PSA: which ratio improves differentiation between benign prostatic hyperplasia and prostate cancer? Clin Chem 2000; 46:55–62.

66. Stephan C, Jung K, Diamandis EP, et al. Prostate-specific antigen, its molecular forms, and other kallikrein markers for detection of prostate cancer. Urology 2002; 59:2–8.

67. Mikolajczyk SD, Millar LS, Wang TJ, et al. 'BPSA,' a specific molecular form of free prostate-specific antigen, is found predominantly in the transition zone of patients with nodular benign prostatic hyperplasia. Urology 2000; 55:41–5.

68. Mikolajczyk SD, Grauer LS, Millar LS, et al. A precursor form of PSA (pPSA) is a component of the free PSA in prostate cancer serum. Urology 1997; 50:710–14.

69. Mikolajczyk SD, Millar LS, Wang TJ, et al. A precursor form of prostate-specific antigen is more highly elevated in prostate cancer compared with benign transition zone prostate tissue. Cancer Res 2000; 60:756–9.

70. Peter J, Unverzagt C, Krogh TN. Identification of precursor forms of free prostate-specific antigen in serum of prostate cancer patients by immunosorption and mass spectrometry. Cancer Res 2001; 61:957–62.

71. Schedlich LJ, Bennetts BH, Morris BJ. Primary structure of a human glandular kallikrein gene. DNA 1987; 6:429–37.

72. Lovgren J, Rajakoski K, Karp M, et al. Activation of the zymogen form of prostate-specific antigen by human glandular kallikrein 2. Biochem Biophys Res Commun 1997; 238:549–55.

73. Takayama TK, Fujikawa K, Davie EW. Characterization of the precursor of prostate-specific antigen. Activation by trypsin and by human glandular kallikrein. J Biol Chem 1997; 272:21582–8.

74. Morris BJ. hGK-1: a kallikrein gene expressed in human prostate. Clin Exp Pharmacol Physiol 1989; 16:345–51.

75. Darson MF, Pacelli A, Roche P, et al. Human glandular kallikrein 2 (hK2) expression in prostatic intraepithelial neoplasia and adenocarcinoma: a novel prostate cancer marker. Urology 1997; 49:857–62.

76. Tremblay RR, Deperthes D, Tetu B, Dube JY. Immunohistochemical study suggesting a complementary role of kallikreins hK2 and hK3 (prostate-specific antigen) in the functional analysis of human prostate tumors. Am J Pathol 1997; 150:455–9.

77. Kwiatkowski MK, Recker F, Piironen T, et al. In prostatism patients the ratio of human glandular kallikrein to free PSA improves the discrimination between prostate cancer and benign hyperplasia within the diagnostic 'gray zone' of total PSA 4 to 10 ng/mL. Urology 1998; 52:360–5.

78. Partin AW, Catalona WJ, Finlay JA, et al. Use of human glandular kallikrein 2 for the detection of prostate cancer: preliminary analysis. Urology 1999; 54:839–45.

79. Becker C, Piironen T, Pettersson K, et al. Clinical value of human glandular kallikrein 2 and free and total prostate-specific antigen in serum from a population of men with prostate-specific antigen levels 3.0 ng/mL or greater. Urology 2000; 55:694–9.

80. Lowe FC, Trauzzi SJ. Prostatic acid phosphatase in 1993. Its limited clinical utility. Urol Clin North Am 1993; 20:589–95.

81. Han M, Piantadosi S, Zahurak ML, et al. Serum acid phosphatase level and biochemical recurrence following radical prostatectomy for men with clinically localized prostate cancer. Urology 2001; 57:707–11.

82. Burnett AL, Chan DW, Brendler CB, Walsh PC. The value of serum enzymatic acid phosphatase in the staging of localized prostate cancer. J Urol 1992; 148:1832–4.

83. Gleason DF. Classification of prostatic carcinomas. Cancer Chemother Rep 1966; 50:125–8.

84. Gleason DF. The Veterans Administration Cooperative Urological Research Group: histological grading and clinical staging of prostate carcinoma. In: Tannenbaum M, ed. Urologic pathology: the prostate. Philadelphia: Lea & Febiger, 1977:171–97.

85. Gleason DF. Histologic grading of prostate cancer: a perspective. Hum Pathol 1992; 23:273–9.

86. Stein A, deKernion JB, Smith RB, Dorey F, Patel H. Prostate specific antigen levels after radical prostatectomy in patients with organ confined and locally extensive prostate cancer. J Urol 1992; 147:942–6.

87. Epstein JI, Pizov G, Walsh PC. Correlation of pathologic findings with progression after radical retropubic prostatectomy. Cancer 1993; 71:3582–93.

88. Partin AW, Pound CR, Clemens JQ, et al. Serum PSA after anatomic radical prostatectomy. The Johns Hopkins experience after 10 years. Urol Clin North Am 1993; 20:713–25.

89. Stamey TA, McNeal JE, Yemoto CM, et al. Biological determinants of cancer progression in men with prostate cancer. JAMA 1999; 281:1395–400.

90. Wallace DM, Chisholm GD, Hendry WF. T.N.M. classification for urological tumours (U.I.C.C.) – 1974. Br J Urol 1975; 47:1–12.

91. Schroder FH, Hermanek P, Denis L, et al. The TNM classification of prostate cancer. Prostate Suppl 1992; 4:129–38.

92. Iyer RV, Hanlon AL, Pinover WH, Hanks GE. Outcome evaluation of the 1997 American Joint Committee on Cancer staging system for prostate carcinoma treated by radiation therapy. Cancer 1999; 85:1816–21.

93. Han M, Walsh PC, Partin AW, Rodriguez R. Ability of the 1992 and 1997 American Joint Committee on Cancer staging systems for prostate cancer to predict progression-free survival after radical prostatectomy for stage T2 disease. J Urol 2000; 164:89–92.

94. Greene FL, Page DL, Fleming ID, et al. AJCC cancer staging manual. New York: Springer, 2002:480.

95. Catalona WJ, Smith DS. 5-year tumor recurrence rates after anatomical radical retropubic prostatectomy for prostate cancer. J Urol 1994; 152:1837–42.

96. Pound CR, Partin AW, Epstein JI, Walsh PC. Prostate-specific antigen after anatomic radical retropubic prostatectomy. Patterns of recurrence and cancer control. Urol Clin North Am 1997; 24:395–406.

97. Egan AJ, Bostwick DG. Prediction of extraprostatic extension of prostate cancer based on needle biopsy findings: perineural invasion lacks significance on multivariate analysis. Am J Surg Pathol 1997; 21:1496–500.

98. de la Taille A, Katz A, Bagiella E, et al. Perineural invasion on prostate needle biopsy: an independent predictor of final pathologic stage. Urology 1999; 54:1039–43.

99. Littrup PJ, Bailey SE. Prostate cancer: the role of transrectal ultrasound and its impact on cancer detection and management. Radiol Clin North Am 2000; 38:87–113.

100. Flanigan RC, Catalona WJ, Richie JP, et al. Accuracy of digital rectal examination and transrectal ultrasonography in localizing prostate cancer. J Urol 1994; 152:1506–9.

101. Carter HB, Hamper UM, Sheth S, et al. Evaluation of transrectal ultrasound in the early detection of prostate cancer. J Urol 1989; 142:1008–10.

102. Hodge KK, McNeal JE, Terris MK, Stamey TA. Random systematic versus directed ultrasound guided transrectal core biopsies of the prostate. J Urol 1989; 142:71–4.

103. Epstein JI, Walsh PC, Carter HB. Importance of posterolateral needle biopsies in the detection of prostate cancer. Urology 2001; 57:1112–16.

104. Vis AN, Boerma MO, Ciatto S, et al. Detection of prostate cancer: a comparative study of the diagnostic efficacy of sextant transrectal versus sextant transperineal biopsy. Urology 2000; 56:617–21.

105. D'Amico AV, Cormack RA, Tempany CM. MRI-guided diagnosis and treatment of prostate cancer. N Engl J Med 2001; 344:776–7.

106. Moul JW, Kane CJ, Malkowicz SB. The role of imaging studies and molecular markers for selecting candidates for radical prostatectomy. Urol Clin North Am 2001; 28:459–72.

107. Gerber G, Chodak GW. Assessment of value of routine bone scans in patients with newly diagnosed prostate cancer. Urology 1991; 37:418–22.

108. Terris MK, Klonecke AS, McDougall IR, Stamey TA. Utilization of bone scans in conjunction with prostate-specific antigen levels in the surveillance for recurrence of adenocarcinoma after radical prostatectomy. J Nucl Med 1991; 32:1713–17.

109. Narayan P, Lillian D, Hellstrom W, et al. The benefits of combining early radionuclide renal scintigraphy with routine bone scans in patients with prostate cancer. J Urol 1988; 140:1448–51.

110. Rifkin MD, Zerhouni EA, Gatsonis CA, et al. Comparison of magnetic resonance imaging and ultrasonography in staging early prostate cancer. Results of a multi-institutional cooperative trial. N Engl J Med 1990; 323:621–6.

111. Tempany CM, Zhou X, Zerhouni EA, et al. Staging of prostate cancer: results of Radiology Diagnostic Oncology Group project comparison of three MR imaging techniques. Radiology 1994; 192:47–54.

112. Wolf JS Jr, Cher M, Dall'era M, et al. The use and accuracy of cross-sectional imaging and fine needle aspiration cytology for detection of pelvic lymph node metastases before radical prostatectomy. J Urol 1995; 153:993–9.

113. Oyen RH, Van Poppel HP, Ameye FE, et al. Lymph node staging of localized prostatic carcinoma with CT and CT-guided fine-needle aspiration biopsy: prospective study of 285 patients. Radiology 1994; 190:315–22.

114. Rorvik J, Halvorsen OJ, Albrektsen G, Haukaas S. Lymphangiography combined with biopsy and computer tomography to detect lymph node metastases in localized prostate cancer. Scand J Urol Nephrol 1998; 32:116–19.

115. Soulie M, Aziza R, Escourrou G, et al. Assessment of the risk of positive surgical margins with pelvic phased-array magnetic resonance imaging in patients with clinically localized prostate cancer: a prospective study. Urology 2001; 58:228–32.

116. Yu KK, Hricak H, Alagappan R, et al. Detection of extracapsular extension of prostate carcinoma with endorectal and phased-array coil MR imaging: multivariate feature analysis. Radiology 1997; 202:697–702.

117. Yu KK, Scheidler J, Hricak H, et al. Prostate cancer: prediction of extracapsular extension with endorectal MR imaging and three-dimensional proton MR spectroscopic imaging. Radiology 1999; 213:481–8.

118. Palumbo F, Bettocchi C, Selvaggi FP, et al. Sildenafil: efficacy and safety in daily clinical experience. Eur Urol 2001; 40:176–80.

119. Humphrey PA, Walther PJ, Currin SM, Vollmer RT. Histologic grade, DNA ploidy, and intraglandular tumor extent as indicators of tumor progression of clinical stage B prostatic carcinoma. A direct comparison. Am J Surg Pathol 1991; 15:1165–70.

120. Kleer E, Larson-Keller JJ, Zincke H, Oesterling JE. Ability of preoperative serum prostate-specific antigen value to predict pathologic stage and DNA ploidy. Influence of clinical stage and tumor grade. Urology 1993; 41:207–16.

121. Partin AW, Kattan MW, Subong EN, et al. Combination of prostate-specific antigen, clinical stage, and Gleason score to predict pathological stage of localized prostate cancer. A multi-institutional update. JAMA 1997; 277:1445–51.

122. Partin AW, Mangold LA, Lamm DM, et al. Contemporary update of prostate cancer staging nomograms (Partin Tables) for the new millennium. Urology 2001; 58:843–8.

123. Blute ML, Bergstralh EJ, Partin AW, et al. Validation of Partin tables for predicting pathological stage of clinically localized prostate cancer. J Urol 2000; 164:1591–5.

124. Carter HB, Epstein JI, Partin AW. Influence of age and prostate-specific antigen on the chance of curable prostate cancer among men with nonpalpable disease. Urology 1999; 53:126–30.

125. Epstein JI, Chan DW, Sokoll LJ, et al. Nonpalpable stage T1c prostate cancer: prediction of insignificant disease using free/total prostate specific antigen levels and needle biopsy findings. J Urol 1998; 160:2407–11.

126. Schuessler WW, Vancaillie TG, Reich H, Griffith DP. Transperitoneal endosurgical lymphadenectomy in patients with localized prostate cancer. J Urol 1991; 145:988–91.

127. West DA, Moore RG. Laparoscopic pelvic lymphadenectomy. In: Bishoff J, Kavoussi LR, eds. Atlas of laparoscopic retroperitoneal surgery. Vol. 1. Philadelphia: WB Saunders, 2000:225–236.

128. Steiner MS, Marshall FF. Mini-laparotomy staging pelvic lymphadenectomy (minilap). Alternative to standard and laparoscopic pelvic lymphadenectomy. Urology 1993; 41:201–6.

129. Lezin MS, Cherrie R, Cattolica EV. Comparison of laparoscopic and minilaparotomy pelvic lymphadenectomy for prostate cancer staging in a community practice. Urology 1997; 49:60–3.

130. Herrell SD, Trachtenberg J, Theodorescu D. Staging pelvic lymphadenectomy for localized carcinoma of the prostate: a comparison of 3 surgical techniques. J Urol 1997; 157:1337–9.

131. Moreno JG, Croce CM, Fischer R, et al. Detection of hematogenous micrometastasis in patients with prostate cancer. Cancer Res 1992; 52:6110–12.

132. de la Taille A, Olsson CA, Buttyan R, et al. Blood-based reverse transcriptase polymerase chain reaction assays for prostatic specific antigen: long term follow-up confirms the potential utility of this assay in identifying patients more likely to have biochemical recurrence (rising PSA) following radical prostatectomy. Int J Cancer 1999; 84:360–4.

133. Katz AE, Olsson CA, Raffo AJ, et al. Molecular staging of prostate cancer with the use of an enhanced reverse transcriptase-PCR assay. Urology 1994; 43:765–75.

134. Israeli RS, Powell CT, Corr JG, et al. Expression of the prostate-specific membrane antigen. Cancer Res 1994; 54:1807–11.

135. Silver DA, Pellicer I, Fair WR, et al. Prostate-specific membrane antigen expression in normal and malignant human tissues. Clin Cancer Res 1997; 3:81–5.

136. Troyer JK, Beckett ML, Wright GL Jr. Detection and characterization of the prostate-specific membrane antigen (PSMA) in tissue extracts and body fluids. Int J Cancer 1995; 62:552–8.

137. Liu H, Moy P, Kim S, et al. Monoclonal antibodies to the extracellular domain of prostate-specific membrane antigen also react with tumor vascular endothelium. Cancer Res 1997; 57:3629–34.

138. Israeli RS, Miller WH Jr, Su SL, et al. Sensitive nested reverse transcription polymerase chain reaction detection of circulating prostatic tumor cells: comparison of prostate-specific membrane antigen and prostate-specific antigen-based assays. Cancer Res 1994; 54:6306–10.

139. Reiter RE, Gu Z, Watabe T, et al. Prostate stem cell antigen: a cell surface marker overexpressed in prostate cancer. Proc Natl Acad Sci USA 1998; 95:1735–40.

140. Gu Z, Thomas G, Yamashiro J, et al. Prostate stem cell antigen (PSCA) expression increases with high gleason score, advanced stage and bone metastasis in prostate cancer. Oncogene 2000; 19:1288–96.

141. Folkman J. Seminars in Medicine of the Beth Israel Hospital, Boston. Clinical applications of research on angiogenesis. N Engl J Med 1995; 333:1757–63.

142. Strohmeyer D, Rossing C, Strauss F, et al. Tumor angiogenesis is associated with progression after radical prostatectomy in pT2/pT3 prostate cancer. Prostate 2000; 42:26–33.

143. Silberman MA, Partin AW, Veltri RW, Epstein JI. Tumor angiogenesis correlates with progression after radical prostatectomy but not with pathologic stage in Gleason sum 5 to 7 adenocarcinoma of the prostate. Cancer 1997; 79:772–9.

144. Gettman MT, Bergstralh EJ, Blute M, et al. Prediction of patient outcome in pathologic stage T2 adenocarcinoma of the prostate: lack of significance for microvessel density analysis. Urology 1998; 51:79–85.

145. Rubin MA, Buyyounouski M, Bagiella E, et al. Microvessel density in prostate cancer: lack of correlation with tumor grade, pathologic stage, and clinical outcome. Urology 1999; 53:542–7.

146. Jones PA, Baylin SB. The fundamental role of epigenetic events in cancer. Nat Rev Genet 2002; 3:415–28.

147. Lee WH, Morton RA, Epstein JI, et al. Cytidine methylation of regulatory sequences near the pi-class glutathione S-transferase gene accompanies human prostatic carcinogenesis. Proc Natl Acad Sci USA 1994; 91:11733–7.

148. Lee WH, Isaacs WB, Bova GS, Nelson WG. CG island methylation changes near the GSTP1 gene in prostatic carcinoma cells detected using the polymerase chain reaction: a new prostate cancer biomarker. Cancer Epidemiol Biomarkers Prev 1997; 6:443–50.

149. Cairns P, Esteller M, Herman JG, et al. Molecular detection of prostate cancer in urine by GSTP1 hypermethylation. Clin Cancer Res 2001; 7:2727–30.

150. Goessl C, Muller M, Straub B, Miller K. DNA alterations in body fluids as molecular tumor markers for urological malignancies. Eur Urol 2002; 41:668–76.

151. Maruyama R, Toyooka S, Toyooka KO, et al. Aberrant promoter methylation profile of prostate cancers and its relationship to clinicopathological features. Clin Cancer Res 2002; 8:514–19.

19

Perineal prostatectomy for treatment of localized prostate cancer

J Brantley Thrasher and HJ Porter II

Introduction

In the age of laparoscopy and other minimally invasive procedures, a discussion of the treatment of localized prostate cancer would be incomplete without the inclusion of radical perineal prostatectomy (RPP). The perineal prostatectomy is the oldest means of prostate resection and at one time was the standard of care for surgical treatment of localized prostate cancer. However, the procedure became less popular during the 1970s after studies published by Walsh and Donker demonstrated the advantages of a nerve-sparing technique using a retropubic approach.[1] The radical retropubic prostatectomy (RRP) became the urologist's preferred approach and the latest generation of surgeons was trained in this technique.

There has been a renewed interest in the perineal approach in recent years for a number of reasons. First, the research of Weldon and Tavel in the late 1980s applied Walsh's anatomic discoveries to the perineal approach, and opened the era of nerve-sparing RPP.[2] Secondly, concerns about the pelvic lymph nodes have been minimized as risk-assessment tables such as the Partin nomogram have clearly outlined which patients are at low risk for lymph node metastasis.[3] Couple this with the well-documented stage migration of prostate cancer and you have a large number of patients presenting with organ-confined disease and little chance of nodal involvement.

Since RPP has been practiced for decades, long-term data regarding the procedure are readily available.[4,5] Margin positivity, biochemical failure rates, and disease-specific mortality compare quite favorably with those reported in RRP series. Overall, early and late complications are equivalent between the two procedures, with the exception of an increased risk of rectal injury with RPP and a higher blood loss with RRP. Postoperative continence and potency rates are likewise quite similar.[6,7]

Perhaps the most compelling reason for the resurgence of the RPP is the introduction of laparoscopic prostatectomy. As the search for a minimally invasive, low-morbidity technique is evolving in the laparoscopic arena, other urologists are returning to RPP, a well-known, proven operation for the control of prostate cancer associated with very low estimated blood loss (EBL), shorter hospital stay, and quicker return to daily activities.

Historical perspective

The perineal approach to the prostate dates back to the first century AD, when Celsus described a curvilinear incision anterior to the anus for removal of bladder stones.[8] In the modern era, credit is given to Bilroth for performing the first planned perineal prostatectomy in 1867.[9] In 1882, Leisrink modified the original technique of a median perineal incision by adding a curve over the region of the prostate. In addition, he described reconstruction of the urethra and the bladder neck.[10] All of these earlier advances culminated in the work of Hugh Hampton Young. Using a curvilinear approach, Young enucleated adenomatous tissue through the perineum to relieve bladder outlet obstruction. After finding evidence of carcinoma in several of these specimens, he undertook the task of perfecting a prostatectomy through the perineum with the intent of curing the disease. He performed autopsy studies and, with the assistance of Dr Halsted, performed the first radical perineal prostatectomy in 1904.[11] Young's technique is the foundation of the modern procedure and has undergone few modifications since its original description.

Vest described a modification of the closure of the wound, whereby the sutures passed through the vesicle neck and urethra and were subsequently tacked to the apex of the perineal wound to provide additional support for the anastomosis.[12] In a similar vein, Jewett described placement of a figure-of-eight suture along the posterior aspect of the vesicourethral anastomosis.[13] This suture began at the bladder neck, incorporated the urethra, and also gathered the urogenital diaphragm with the intent of providing extra support to the posterior aspect of the anastomosis.

Another significant contribution was introduced by Elmer Belt in 1939.[14] Belt described a new approach to perineal prostatectomy between the longitudinal fibers of the rectum and the circular fibers of the external anal sphincter. By approaching the surgery in this fashion, the prostate was exposed in a relatively bloodless field. However, he further modified Young's procedure in two key areas and was openly criticized by Young for these changes. First, he recommended leaving behind the apex of the prostate to achieve better urinary control. Secondly, he recommended opening the anterior layer of Denonvilliers' fascia during the dissection to expose the ampulla and seminal vesicles. Young considered these changes in violation of the principles of cancer surgery and recommended against their use in RPP.[15]

Perhaps the most relevant modification came after the sentinel work of Walsh and Donker with regard to RRP and the preservation of the cavernosal nerves and, thus, potency.[1] Modifying the principles described, Weldon and Tavel were able to successfully translate the nerve-sparing technique used in RRP to the perineal approach.[2] The modification entailed making a vertical incision in Denonvilliers' fascia as opposed to the classic transverse incision. This allowed reflection of the layer laterally over the apex of the gland and thus preservation of the neurovascular bundles.

Patient selection

With renewed interest in the technique of perineal prostatectomy, the urologist must have a clear understanding of which patients are best suited for this technique. Prostatectomy is curative only if all of the cancer is removed; therefore, it should be reserved for those patients with organ-confined disease, a life expectancy longer than the natural history of the cancer (typically 10 years with prostate cancer), and no significant surgical risk factors. This includes patients with clinical stages T1b, T1c, or T2 tumors. A disqualifying age of approximately 75 years is reasonable given that a 75-year-old male has a survival of roughly 10.5 years.[16] Surgery should be delayed for 2 weeks following prostate biopsy and longer if the procedure was associated with any significant bleeding or infection.

Anatomy

Pelvic fascia

Surgeons preparing to undertake an RPP must have a clear understanding of the pelvic fascia, whether they intend to use the nerve-sparing technique or a wide dissection. The pelvic fascia is a single continuous layer

that envelops all pelvic organs above the levator ani. Denonvilliers' fascia extends inferiorly from the peritoneal cul-de-sac, often to the level of the prostatic apex, while laterally it extends to envelop the neurovascular bundles. Typically, it is densely adherent to the posterior capsule of the prostate and becomes somewhat more tenuous overlying the seminal vesicles. It is separated from the rectum by the ventral rectal fascia, or the posterior lamella of Denonvilliers'.

Neurovascular bundles

Knowledge of the course of the cavernous nerves is paramount when undertaking a nerve-sparing dissection. The nerves course caudally and ventrally as part of the neurovascular bundles. They lie within the lateral pelvic fascia and over the dorsolateral aspect of the prostate and membranous urethra (Figure 19.1). Most often these bundles are surrounded by a fatty layer that serves to make them readily identifiable visually. The nerves penetrate the urogenital diaphragm to reach their respective corpora.

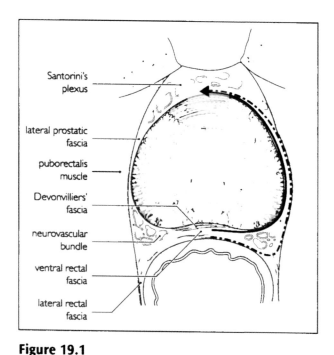

Figure 19.1

Transverse section through the perineum at the level of the verumontanum. The ventral rectal fascia is the key to the modern nerve-sparing dissection. The solid line represents the plane for a nerve-sparing approach on Denonvilliers' fascia and underneath the ventral rectal fascia. The dashed line lies outside all fascial planes and is followed for a wide, extended dissection.

Advantages and disadvantages of the two techniques

Comparative data suggest that RPP and RRP offer equivalent cancer control rates for localized carcinoma of the prostate. Short- and long-term complication rates of the procedures are likewise very similar, with the exception of higher blood loss associated with RRP and an increased incidence of rectal injuries for RPP.[7] Further details are discussed at length later in the chapter.

RPP provides the distinct advantage of accessing the prostate at its most superficial location through a small perineal incision. Because of this, patients experience low morbidity, minimal postoperative pain, and thus have a short hospital stay. Published reports by Ruiz-Deya et al and Parra have documented discharge within 24 hours in 91% and 82% of patients, respectively.[17,18] The second major advantage is direct visualization and easy access to the apex and membranous urethra. This allows not only for improvement in dissection but also for direct visualization of the vesicourethral anastomosis. A third advantage is that the perineal resection is carried out underneath the dorsal venous complex and thus results in significantly less blood loss. Anecdotally, the authors believe that salvage prostatectomy after radiation is often easier via the perineal approach, as it allows for a direct access to the prostate and sharp dissection of the rectum away from the overlying prostate gland.

Disadvantages likewise exist. Of concern historically was the inability to access the lymph nodes through the same incision. Recent studies, however, outline specific guidelines using prostate-specific antigen (PSA), clinical stage, and grade to determine which patients do not routinely need lymph node dissection. Pelvic lymph node dissection can safely be omitted in patients with PSA $\leq$ 10 ng/mL, Gleason sum $\leq$ 6, and clinical stage T2b or less.[19] Another disadvantage is the exaggerated lithotomy position. While generally well tolerated, patients with conditions such as hip ankylosis, morbid obesity, and lower extremity amputations may not be candidates for this technique. A simple office test involves having the patient lie supine on the examination table and bringing his knees to his chest. If the patient is able to tolerate this test, he will probably be able to tolerate the position for RPP. However, after positioning in the operating room, ventilatory pressures > 40 cmH$_2$O, or difficulties oxygenating the patient will infrequently result in the inability to perform RPP.

A third disadvantage of RPP is the difficulty performing the procedure on patients with very large prostate glands and a narrow pelvis. Because of the small incision, glands > 120 g can be difficult to resect, particularly if associated with a narrow pelvis; however, glands > 180 g have been removed via this approach.[20] A good rule of thumb is that if the base of the gland is not palpable on rectal examination, or if the gland fills the pelvis from side to side, it may foreshadow a difficult resection. Perhaps the most significant disadvantage of RPP is that the current generation of urologists lack familiarity with the perineal technique.

Preoperative preparation

Although the incidence of rectal injury is quite low in skilled hands, RPP does require extensive dissection near the rectal wall. Therefore, we routinely perform a mechanical bowel preparation and provide antibiotic prophylaxis for all patients. A well-tolerated cleansing that avoids enemas includes a clear liquid diet the day before surgery, 45 ml oral buffered sodium biphosphate, and 1 g of erythromycin and neomycin as described by Nichols et al.[21] Preoperatively, a single intravenous dose of cefazolin 1 g is given. Since we transfuse < 1% of our RPPs, type and cross, or even, type and screen are usually not performed. In addition, we do not routinely recommend autologous blood donation to our patients because of its cost and because it is seldom needed.

Anesthesia

This procedure has been performed using a variety of anesthetics, ranging from a spinal or epidural to general endotracheal anesthesia. We routinely have all of our patients undergo a general anesthetic, as we have found that spinal anesthesia is often incomplete and, perhaps more importantly, the patients are prone to move during the surgery.

Patient positioning

For ideal operative conditions to be met, the patient must be placed in an exaggerated lithotomy position with the buttocks brought down slightly beyond the end of the table. Lower-extremity elastic compression stockings (TED hose) are placed, although, because of positioning, the venous drainage of the lower extremities is already maximal. The legs are then secured in Yellofins stirrups (OR Direct, Acton, Massachusetts) and elevated into the lithotomy position. Once the legs have been elevated, the foot of the bed is lowered completely. The perineum is then elevated to a position essentially parallel to the floor by placing rolled blankets underneath the sacrum. When properly positioned, the scrotum should fall forward onto the abdomen and the surgeon should have excellent access to the anal verge (Figure 19.2). All pressure points are well padded. The arms should be abducted as little as possible to prevent injury to the brachial plexus. Once the patient is properly positioned, broad tape is attached to the stirrups and placed over the buttocks to maintain this position. In

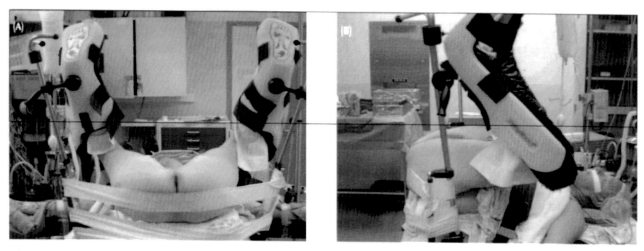

Figure 19.2
(A and B) Patient positioned in the exaggerated lithotomy position with Yellofins stirrups. Note that after proper positioning, the perineum is parallel to the floor.

addition, we routinely place a loose belt across the abdomen to prevent patient migration during the operation. The hair of the posterior scrotum and perineum is shaved and an antiseptic surgical scrub is performed.

Special instruments

- Young retractor.
- Lowsley retractor.
- Thorek scissors.

Special instruments (Figure 19.3) greatly facilitate this procedure but are not required. The most useful of these are the prostatic retractors designed by Young and Lowsley. Both of these retractors allow for manipulation of the gland during various portions of the operation. In addition, Thorek scissors aid in dissection of the bladder neck and the vascular pedicles during dissection under the pubic bone. Another instrument we find particularly useful, but not mandatory, is a multifunction self-retaining retractor, such as the Thompson perineal retractor.

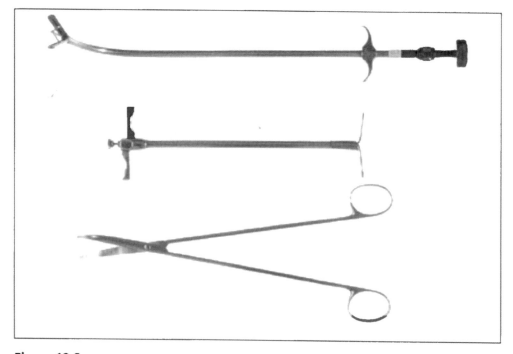

Figure 19.3
From top to bottom: Lowsley retractor, Young retractor, and Thorek scissors. Although not essential for RPP, each greatly facilitates the procedure.

Operative procedure

Incision

Prior to incision, the Lowsley prostatic retractor is placed in the bladder and the wings opened. An inverted U or horseshoe-shaped incision is made just inside the ischial tuberosities (Figure 19.4). The apex of the incision is typically located 2–3 cm anterior to the anal verge; usually, a color change in the skin denotes the proper location. The vertical arms of the incision lie medial to the ischial tuberosities and are extended posteriorly to a point lateral to the sphincter at the 3 and 9 o'clock positions. The incision can be carried further posteriorly without side-effects if large flaps are needed. The incision is then carried down 1–2 cm into the subcutaneous fat.

The ischiorectal fossa is developed next. Small stab incisions are made through the ischiorectal fascia bilaterally at the superior aspect of each vertical arm of the incision. Once a defect has been created, these spaces are developed bluntly with the index fingers directed inferiorly and perpendicular to the floor (Figure 19.5). The spaces are opened with electrocautery. Once the pockets have been adequately developed, the index fingers are brought together toward the midline. A space is then created under the central tendon connecting the ischiorectal fossae. This space overlies the anterior rectal wall and is superior to the anal sphincter. The central tendon is then divided with cautery (Figure 19.6). At this point, the rectum is draped out of the field by applying four Alice clamps to the developed flap and attaching them to a ¾ inch surgical drape.

Rectal mobilization

After division of the central tendon, the rectal sphincter will be seen as an arch overlying the rectum. Dissection is then carried out between the longitudinal rectal fibers on the ventral aspect of the rectal wall and the external anal sphincter. We prefer a modified Belt approach, as described by Hudson and Lilien, whereby bilateral spaces are created through the mid-portion of the sphincter with the remaining central tendon between the two (Figure 19.7).[22] This allows the external anal sphincter to be lifted up and away from the underlying rectum. A Young prostatic bifid retractor is then placed beneath the sphincter and the external anal sphincter is elevated superiorly (Figure 19.8). Using the nondominant hand, two of the previously placed Alice clamps are grasped in the palm while the index finger is placed into the rectum. This allows for downward traction on the rectum. The remaining central tendon is sharply incised with Metzenbaum scissors (Figure 19.9).

The longitudinal fibers of the rectum are then followed to the rectourethralis muscle, which attaches the rectum to the posterior urogenital diaphragm. The depth of dissection is greatly facilitated by the finger in the rectum to constantly monitor the level of resection relative to the anterior rectal wall. The rectum can be mobilized on either side of the rectourethralis with blunt dissection to the level of the prostatic apex. The rectourethralis itself is variably developed, ranging from a few rudimentary fibers to a substantial fibromuscular structure several centimeters long. Once thoroughly isolated, the muscle should be divided sharply, as blunt dissection will invariably result in rectal injury.

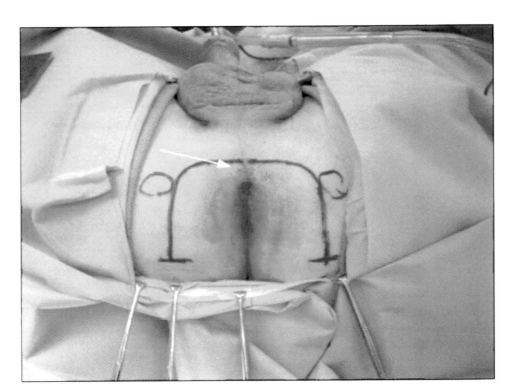

Figure 19.4
Line of incision marked on the perineum. The apex of the incision lies ~ 2 cm anterior to the sphincter and the lateral wings lie within the ischial tuberosities. A slight change in skin color denotes the area and is marked by the arrow.

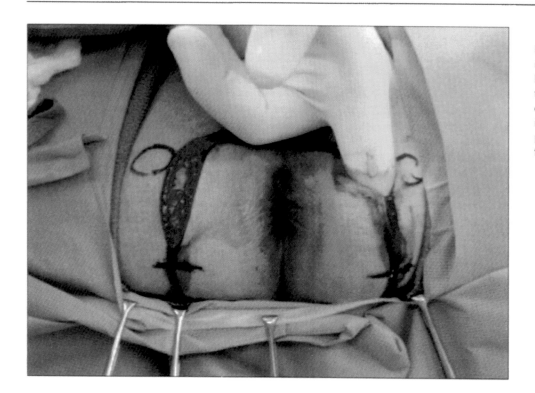

Figure 19.5
Development of the ischiorectal fossa using blunt dissection. Note the direction of dissection should be inferior and perpendicular to the floor.

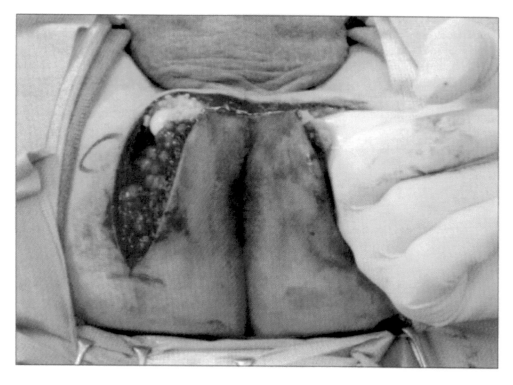

Figure 19.6
The central tendon has been isolated and is elevated away from the underlying rectum prior to its division with electrocautery

After division of the rectourethralis, the Thompson perineal retractor is placed (Figure 19.10).

At this point the ventral rectal fascia should be visible, and is identified by its white, shiny appearance. The space between it and the rectal wall should be developed and can usually be done with gentle, blunt finger dissection. It is important to note that the plane of dissection changes

at this point to the vertical from the horizontal. The space must be developed to the base of the prostate, which is identified by palpation of the wings of the retractor. The rectal wall is then gently retracted with a padded retractor to provide optimum exposure. At this point the decision must be made whether to proceed with the nerve-sparing technique or with wide dissection. The posterior lamella is

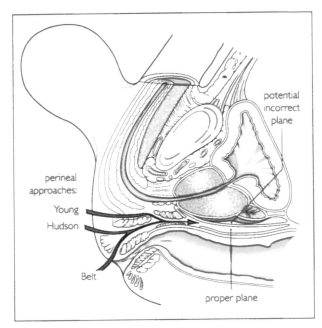

Figure 19.7
The three described perineal approaches to the prostate. The Young approach is the most direct, but risks injury to the urinary spincter. The Hudson and Belt approaches allow for early visualization of the longitudinal fibers of the rectum. The anterior wall of the rectum can then be followed directly to the prostate.

the key, and how it is handled from this point forward will define each separate technique. If a nerve-sparing technique is to be used, the fascia should be incised vertically, and the neurovascular bundles mobilized. If extended dissection is intended, the neurovascular bundles can be ligated at their superior edge and the fascia incised transversely to free the rectum (Figure 19.11).

Extended dissection

The intent of the extended dissection lies not only in the removal of the neurovascular bundles but also in the widest possible resection of the posterolateral fascia. It may be performed either unilaterally or bilaterally. If a unilateral technique is employed, a vertical incision should be made in the ventral fascia just off midline on the side and medial to the neurovascular bundle to be spared. Entry into Denonvilliers' fascia should be avoided. If a bilateral extended dissection is performed, the ventral fascia should be maintained. The fascia is opened transversely at the level of the membranous urethra and the base of the prostate if possible. The neurovascular bundle is then ligated at both ends, and the dissection continued laterally to the base of the bladder.

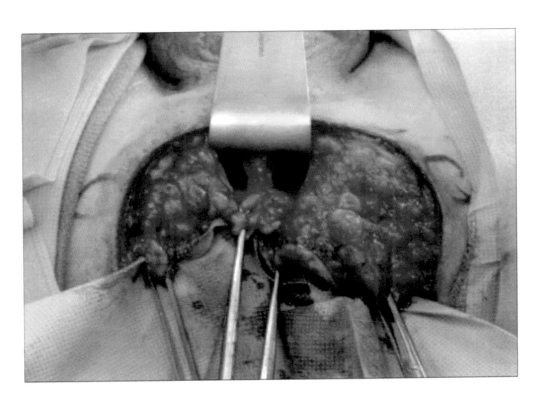

Figure 19.8
The external anal sphincter has been entered on both sides of the remaining central tendon and is elevated away from the field with a Young bifid retractor.

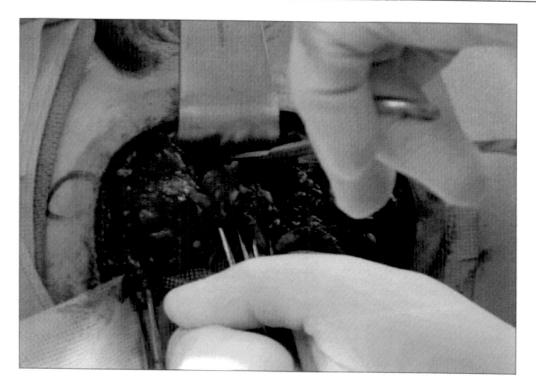

Figure 19.9
The central tendon is sharply divided with Metzenbaum scissors. Note a finger of the non-dominant hand in the rectum, which is used to direct the underlying rectum away from possible injury.

Nerve-sparing technique

The key to a nerve-sparing technique lies in the understanding that this dissection is carried out in a plane completely different from the one dissected in the extended approach. Preservation of the neurovascular bundles demands a dissection plane that is inside the ventral rectal fascia of Denonvilliers' fascia. Once the

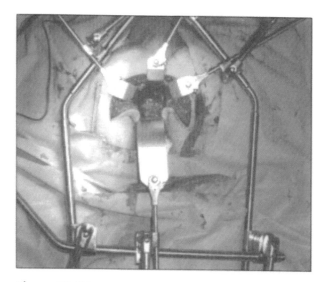

Figure 19.10
The Thompson perineal retractor has been placed. We use a grooved retractor superiorly, two 1 inch double-angled retractors laterally, and a 1½ inch malleable retractor inferiorly. This provides optimum exposure.

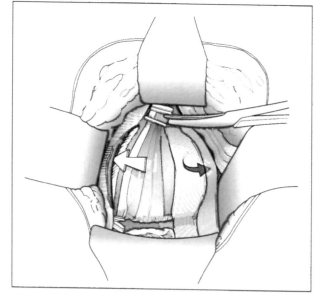

Figure 19.11
An extended dissection has been performed on the right. The ventral rectal fascia and neurovascular bundle have been clipped and divided at the base of the prostate. The lateral rectal fascia has been incised, exposing the proper plane for a wide dissection (white arrow). The left neurovascular bundle and ventral rectal fascia have been mobilized off of Denonvilliers' fascia, exposing the proper plane for a nerve-sparing technique (black arrow).

rectum is mobilized, the neurovascular bundles can be visualized running within the lateral aspect of the ventral rectal fascia. If a bilateral dissection is to be carried out, a vertical incision should be made in the midline. If one intends a unilateral dissection, the incision should be made 1 cm lateral to the midline on the side to be saved. The medial edge of the divided fascia is then carefully elevated and separated from the underlying prostatic capsule (Figure 19.12). Perforating vessels usually found entering the prostate from the neurovascular bundles at the superior and inferior neural pedicles are ligated with clips. The neurovascular bundles must be mobilized at least 1 cm over the membranous urethra and sufficiently proximal to the base to ensure enough laxity as to avoid traction injury during removal of the gland. The dissection is then continued laterally and ventrally on the prostatic capsule beneath the dorsal venous complex.

Apical dissection

Blunt and sharp dissection is continued until the junction of the membranous urethra and apex of the prostate are visualized (Figure 19.13). The urethra is then surrounded by a right-angle clamp and hemitransected with a scalpel. At this point we preplace the posterior anastomotic sutures at the 4, 6, and 8 o'clock positions with 2-0 Monocryl. Next, the Lowsley retractor is removed and the remainder of the urethra is sharply transected. The Young prostatic retractor is then placed through the prostatic urethra directly into the bladder and the blades are extended.

Puboprostatic ligament division

The Young retractor is used as the prostate is rotated ventrally to expose the anterior prostatic capsule and the puboprostatic ligaments that lie in the midline beneath the dorsal venous complex (Figure 19.14). It is advisable to divide the ligaments sharply since they are avascular, and this helps to avoid a potential tear in the prostate capsule

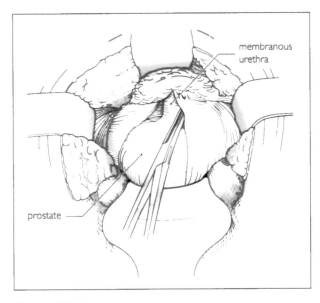

Figure 19.13
Meticulous dissection reveals the junction of the membranous urethra and the prostatic apex. Here the nerves have been spared on the left side and a wide dissection performed on the right. The right-angle clamp should be kept in close approximation to the urethra to avoid injury to the overlying neurovascular bundle.

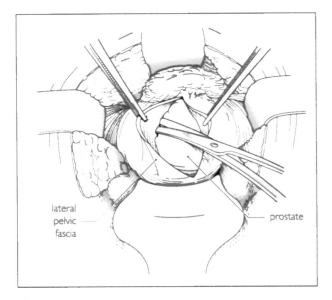

Figure 19.12
Here the periprostatic fascia (ventral rectal fascia) is split in the midline and a plane developed between it and the capsule of the prostate. The neurovascular bundles course within this fascia.

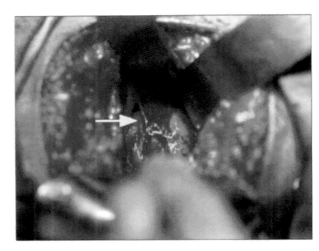

Figure 19.14
The Young retractor is used to rotate the prostate ventrally, which exposes the puboprostatic ligaments (arrow). They are avascular and thus can be sharply divided.

from traction and a positive anterior margin. Dissection is carried back until one can readily visualize the circular fibers of the bladder neck (Figure 19.15). Troublesome bleeding from the dorsal venous complex can be handled by grasping the offending vessels with vascular forceps and cauterizing. Generally, however, oozing is handled by placing an open gauze sponge against the plexus and compressing it with a retractor until the prostate is removed. Bleeding is minimal and controlled with pressure and has usually ceased after removal of the prostate.

Bladder neck division

Typically, the muscles of the bladder neck are easily visualized and can be transected with the Thorek scissors. Routine wide excision is not advisable, as cancerous invasion of the bladder neck is rare (3%) and invariably associated with positive margins at another site.[23] The correct plane of transection is identified by palpating the contour of the gland and visualizing the circular fibers of the bladder neck. The anterior bladder neck is transected by cutting down onto the Young retractor until urine begins to flow out of the incision. The Young retractor is removed and subsequent traction applied with the assistance of a ⅜ inch Penrose drain, which is passed through

the division between the base of the prostate and the bladder neck and brought out through the apex of the prostate using a right-angle clamp (Figure 19.16). The posterior bladder neck is then divided using Thorek scissors. Next, attention is turned to the vascular pedicles, which serve as the primary attachments that restrict mobilization of the gland (Figure 19.17). The pedicles are carefully isolated with a right-angle clamp and ligated with surgical clips using a right-angle clip applier. Care is taken to avoid the overlying neurovascular bundles if a nerve-sparing technique was performed.

Seminal vesicle dissection

With the majority of attachments released, the prostate is now anchored only by the seminal vesicles and ampulla of the vas deferens. An Allis clamp is placed through the prostatic urethra and clamped to provide better posterior exposure. The prostate is then elevated anteriorly so the seminal vesicles may be approached posteriorly. The respective ampulla and seminal vesicle are isolated, ligated with surgical clips, and transected (Figure 19.18). Once this step is complete, the prostate is handed off the surgical field and the anastomotic repair begun.

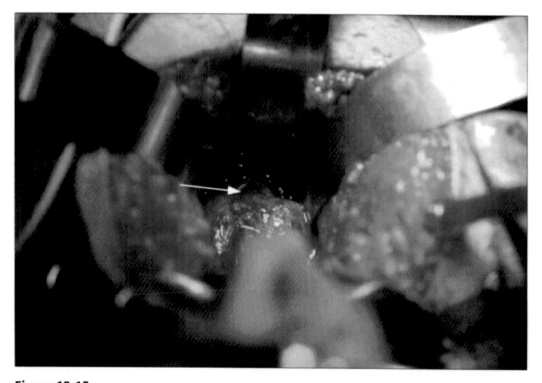

Figure 19.15
The circular fibers of the bladder neck (arrow) are readily seen after division of the puboprostatic ligaments. Thorek scissors are then used to cut down onto the Young retractor and open the bladder.

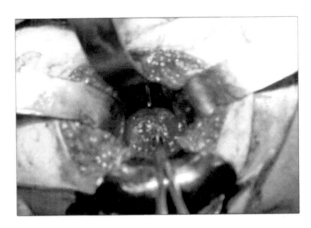

Figure 19.16
Here the anterior urethra has been divided and a right-angle clamp has been placed through the prostatic urethra to grasp a ⅜ inch Penrose drain. The drain will be passed through and used for retraction.

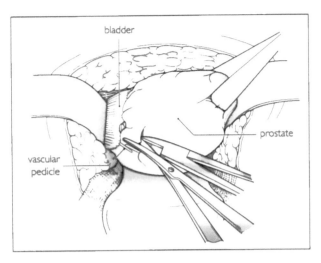

Figure 19.17
The vascular pedicle has been isolated with a right-angle clamp and clipped.

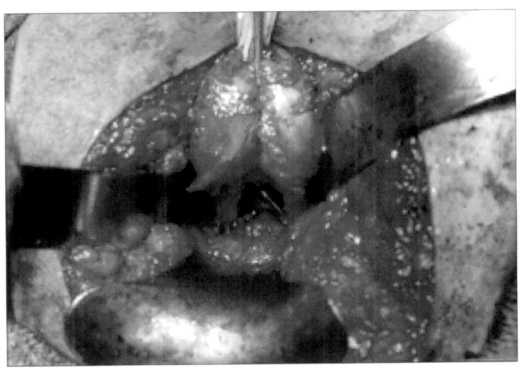

Figure 19.18
The prostate is reflected anteriorly with an Alice clamp to aid in posterior dissection of the seminal vesicles and ampulla of the vas deferens. Here, the ampullae have been ligated, leaving only the seminal vesicles intact.

Vesicourethral anastomosis

The bladder neck is carefully inspected and trimmed as needed. A 20F Silastic catheter is placed in the urethral stump, and 2-0 Monocryl sutures are placed from the urethral stump at the 10 and 2 o'clock positions into the anterior bladder neck at the 10 and 2 o'clock positions and they are snapped to the drape for later use (Figure 19.19).

The catheter is then advanced into the bladder. Redundant posterior bladder neck is closed vertically in a racquet handle technique with interrupted 2-0 chromic sutures. Because of excellent exposure and direct visualization, it is unnecessary to evert the mucosal edges prior to anastomosis. At this point the preplaced posterior sutures are placed through the bladder neck. The anastomosis is then completed by tying all sutures down in a sequential

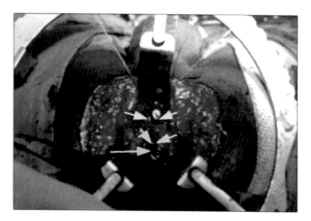

Figure 19.19
The 20F Silastic catheter is seen exiting through the membranous urethra. The bladder neck is identified by the solid arrow. At this point we place our anterior anastomotic sutures through the membranous urethra (white arrows) and directly into the bladder neck (yellow arrows). The catheter is then advanced into the bladder and the bladder neck reconstructed.

fashion, beginning anteriorly and ending with the posterior sutures.

Closure

Because unrecognized rectal injuries are associated with significant morbidity, we routinely place a finger in the rectum prior to closure to ensure there are no proctotomies. If encountered they should be repaired using a standard two-layer closure with 3-0 Vicryl for the mucosa and 3-0 silk Lembert sutures for the seromuscular layer. A ⅜ inch Penrose drain is placed anterior to the rectal surface and brought out through one of the corners of the incision. The perineal wound is closed in three layers. The perineal body is reconstituted, connecting the deep and superficial portions of the muscle with 2-0 chromic suture. The subcutaneous perineal fascia is closed with interrupted 2-0 chromic suture and the skin edges approximated with 2-0 chromic horizontal mattress suture (Figure 19.20). The sutures should be kept on the outside of the wound. We leave tails of approximately 1 inch to prevent complaints from the patients about the sutures bothering them. Others have described closing the skin using a subcuticular suture, but we find that the horizontal mattress is better as it provides more support at the apex of the wound where a breakdown is likely to occur.

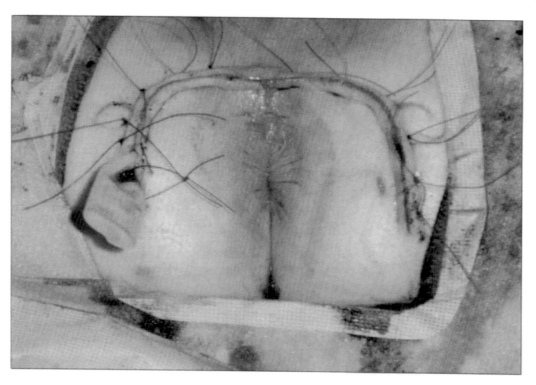

Figure 19.20
Final closure of the wound with interrupted 2-0 chromic sutures in a horizontal mattress. Note the Penrose drain exiting from the lateral aspect of the wound.

Postoperative care

We have developed a postoperative pathway for RPPs at our institution (Table 19.1). Clear liquids are given to the patient immediately postoperatively, and the diet is advanced to regular the following morning. Patients are out of bed the evening of surgery and ambulate on postoperative day 1. The Penrose drain is usually removed on the first postoperative day. Ketorolac is routinely given for analgesia and, more times than not, patients do not require narcotics, although they are available as part of our routine postoperative orders. Young, healthy patients are usually discharged within 24 hours, and 95% will be out of hospital by day 2. Nothing is given per rectum. Patients are discharged home with prophylactic antibiotics while the catheter is in place, and the catheter is typically removed 10–14 days after surgery.

Complications

Proctotomy

Rectal injuries are generally not problematic if they are noted at the time of surgery, are repaired intraoperatively, and the patient has undergone a bowel prep.[24] We repair the injury with a two-layer closure of 3-0 Vicryl for the first layer, followed by 3-0 silk Lembert stitches for the second layer. The wound is then copiously irrigated with 1 liter of antibiotic irrigation. We perform a two-finger anal dilation to reduce sphincter tone. Large rectal tears, prior radiation, or unpreped bowel are best managed with diverting colostomy. This is generally performed laparoscopically with the assistance of a general surgeon. If a rectal injury has occurred, broad-spectrum antibiotics covering both aerobic and anaerobic bacteria are given for 48 hours. We use the combination of ceftriaxone (rocephin) and metronidazole (flagyl) at our institution. A low-residue liquid diet is encouraged for 5 days. Unrecognized injuries will usually present within the first

Table 19.1 *Radical perineal prostatectomy postoperative clinical pathway*

	Pre-admission	Day of surgery	Post-op day 1	Post-op day 2
Treatment and lab	CBC, Chem 7, UA EKG CXR	bilat SCDs at all times IS q1° RA SaO$_2$ ≥92% Foley to DD Penrose – leave in 'NPR' sign above bed change perineal dressing pm promise pants on at all times	H&H this AM	d/c Penrose after 1st BM Sitz bath after 1st BM
Diet	clear liquids to start with bowel prep	sips of clears	advance to regular	regular
Activity		OOB to chair for 30 min this night	OOB must walk 4 times a day	OOB and walking D/C home
Meds	Fleet's Phosphosoda Nichol's Prep	IVF as maintenance Toradol 30 mg IV × 48° Levsin 0.125 mg PRN Colace 100 mg BID Ancef 1 gram IV × 3 doses Percocet 1–2 q4° PRN	HLIV start PO Abx at dinner	D/C IV PO pain meds only cont Levsin PRN cont Colace D/C home with PO meds
Patient education	Review clinical pathway		leg bag & catheter care perineal care	review D/C instructions
Discharge planning		begin D/C planning and assessing home needs	continue assessing home needs	Discharge home

CBC, Complete blood count; UA, urinalysis; EKG, electrocardiogram; CXR, chest x-ray; SCD, sequential compression device; IS, incentive spirometry; RA, room air; DD, dependent drainage; NPR, nothing per rectum; OOB, out of bed; IVF, intravenous fluids; D/C, discharge H&H, hemoglobin and hematocrit; HLIV, heparin lock IV.

few days and are manifest as fecal drainage from the perineal wound. These are best treated by reopening the incision and repairing the rectum. If the injuries present later, it may be advisable to proceed with a diverting colostomy.

Catheter displacement

If the Foley catheter should fall out in the first 4–5 days, it can usually be replaced by careful passage of a catheter with a coude tip. Any resistance or catheter displacement in the first few days is best handled by cystoscopic replacement of the catheter. After the first week, if the catheter falls out we leave it out and have rarely had any complications.

Vesicourethral-perineal urine leak

This is usually the result of disruption of the racquet handle closure of the posterior bladder neck secondary to bladder spasm. These invariably resolve with prolonged catheter drainage and should be monitored with intermittent cystograms to insure complete healing prior to catheter removal, especially in the case of a salvage prostatectomy. If an anastomotic perineal fistula occurs, replacing the catheter for an additional week has corrected the problem in all cases.

Fecal soilage

This particular complication was not reported until recently. In 1998, Bishoff et al reported this complication in a study of 1200 patients.[25] Each had been mailed a 26-question quality of life instrument to assess fecal and urinary incontinence after prostatectomy. The instrument used was not a validated tool for clinically localized prostate cancer patients. Of the 1200 patients surveyed, 907 returned the surveys; of these, 784 came from patients who had undergone RRP and 123 came from patients who had undergone RPP. In their investigation, Bishoff et al discovered a higher incidence of fecal incontinence (daily, weekly, monthly, or less than monthly) after RPP than after RRP (3, 9, 3, and 16% compared with 2, 5, 3, and 8% ($p = 0.002$)). In addition RPP patients were more likely to wear pads ($p = 0.013$), experienced more accidents ($p = 0.001$), had larger volumes of stool leakage ($p = 0.002$), and had more loosely formed stools ($p = 0.001$).

These data are contrary to the experience at our institution. We recently mailed the UCLA-RAND Prostate Cancer Index, a validated questionnaire, to 184 patients (107 RRP and 77 RPP). This was not a randomized comparison, and the patients were not matched. The survey was completed by 76/107 RRP patients (71%) and 58/77 RPP patients (75.3%). Of interest is the information relayed from the patients regarding bowel function. When asked if they never or rarely experienced rectal urgency, 31.5% of RRP patients and 20.6% of RPP patients answered positively. Furthermore, 85.5% of RRP and 82.8% of RPP patients reported no bowel-related quality of life effect due to the procedure. To provide a wider perspective, two surgeons with extensive experience in performing RPP were contacted. Dr David Paulson at Duke University has performed over 2000 RPPs and has not seen fecal soilage or incontinence except in those patients previously irradiated prior to salvage perineal prostatectomy. Dr Robert Gibbons from Virginia Mason states that only 1–2% of patients experience fecal soilage, and he has not seen fecal incontinence in any of his patients.[7]

The actual prevalence of this problem remains debatable. Nevertheless, we do routinely counsel patients regarding this potential complication prior to RPP, with the qualifier that it has been reported but that we have not experienced the problem in our practice. Further investigation is certainly warranted, since it was originally reported to occur in both RPP and RRP patients. We are, accordingly, reviewing a large longitudinal database to assess the incidence, prevalence, and severity of fecal incontinence after radical prostatectomy.

Lower extremity neuropraxia

This is a unique morbidity associated with the perineal approach and is due to positioning. The etiology is presumed to be undue pressure on the sural nerve due to pressure points just lateral to the head of the fibula. Price et al reported that 43 of 111 patients undergoing RPP experienced some degree of lower extremity neuropraxia, although it was of short duration and in all cases resolved.[26] Typically, patients complain of 2–3 days of sensory loss in the leg or foot and may have associated paresthesias. Until 2 years ago we experienced similar problems at our institution. At that time we began using Yellofins Stirrups and have not had a problem subsequently. These stirrups provide superior padding and eliminate any pressure points at the knee in contrast to the conventional Allen or candy-cane stirrups.

Comparison of RPP to RRP

Few studies can be found that directly compare the results of RRP to RPP. One of the first reports comparing the two techniques was from Boxer et al in the late 1970s.[27] The study involved 329 patients, with 265 undergoing a perineal approach and 64 cases undergoing a procedure performed retropubically. The study was flawed by inconsistencies with pelvic lymphadenectomy and perioperative estrogen therapy, but overall, when the morbidity associated with the two techniques was directly compared, the only difference noted was that the RRP group had an EBL 700 ml greater than the RPP group.

A study by Frazier et al provided the first contemporary analysis directly comparing the two techniques.[28] The population consisted of 122 patients undergoing RPP vs 51 with RRP. The particular technique chosen depended upon surgeon preference. An extensive number of variables were reviewed, including operative time, transfusions, length of hospital stay, length of catheter drainage, both short- and long-term complications, and evidence of disease extension. Of note, no difference were found between the two groups with regard to positive margins, urethral or bladder neck involvement, and short- vs long-term complications. The only statistically significant differences noted were an increased EBL and a greater number of transfusions associated with RRP. Critics of this study are quick to point out that patients were not matched based upon preoperative data and that, while all RPPs were performed by a single surgeon, the RRPs were divided amongst three.

Haab et al published results of a similar, but smaller study soon thereafter.[29] This study evaluated 71 patients with clinically localized prostate cancer: 35 patients underwent RPP vs 36 undergoing RRP. Each group had similar age, preoperative PSA, and clinical stage. Measured variables included operative time, blood transfusions, length of hospital stay, complication rates, incontinence, sexual function, and pathologic extent of disease. Ultimately, the only statistical differences noted were a higher transfusion rate with the retropubic approach (100% with RRP vs 54% with RPP) and the number of anastomotic strictures (2 in the RRP and 0 in the RPP). Organ-confined rates, incontinence, and PSA failures were similar in the two groups. The authors concluded that the two techniques were identical in their ability to control organ-confined disease.

The largest comparison trial to date was reported by the Uniformed Services Urology Research Group.[30] This study pooled data from five military installations and identified 1698 men who had undergone radical prostatectomies between 1988 and 1997. Of these 1382 underwent RRP and 316 were treated by RPP. In order to provide a more meaningful comparison, patients were retrospectively stratified according to race, clinical stage, Gleason sum, and preoperative PSA. A total of 190 patients were identified in each group who met matching criteria. Data points examined included age, race, PSA, Gleason sum, clinical stage, pathologic stage, EBL and transfusion rate, organ-confined rate, margin positivity, PSA failures, and short- and long-term complications.

No significant differences were noted in matched patient characteristics such as race, mean preoperative PSA, or clinical stage between the patient populations. Overall, the authors found no statistical differences in either PSA failures, margin-positive, or organ-confined rates in this matched group analysis. The only significant differences found were higher EBL in the RRP group ($p < 0.001$) and a higher rectal injury rate in the RPP group ($p = 0.03$). No differences were noted in regard to incontinence, impotence, bladder neck contractures, or other postoperative complications.

Conclusion

In this modern era of minimally invasive urology, radical perineal prostatectomy holds great promise. It is a time-tested surgical technique with well-proven cancer control rates and both short- and long-term complication rates comparable to those with the retropubic approach. As with laparoscopic procedures, patients are generally in the hospital for a very short stay and are quick to return to their daily activities. It provides an attractive alternative to the laparoscopic approach.

References

1. Walsh PC, Donker PJ. Impotence following radical prostatectomy: insight into etiology and prevention. J Urol 1982; 128:492.

2. Weldon VE, Tavel FR. Potency-sparing radical perineal prostatectomy: anatomy, surgical technique, and initial results. J Urol 1988; 140:559–62.

3. Partin AW, Kattan MW, Subong EN et al. Combination of prostate-specific antigen, clinical stage, and Gleason score to predict pathologic stage of localized prostate cancer: A multi-institutional update. JAMA 1997; 277:1445–51.

4. Gibbons RP, Correa RJ, Brannen GE, Mason JT. Total prostatectomy for localized prostate cancer. J Urol 1984; 131:73–6.

5. Paulson DF. Impact of radical prostatectomy in the management of clinically localized disease. J Urol 1994; 152:1826–30.

6. Walsh PC, Partin AW, Epstein JI. Cancer control and quality of life following anatomical radical retropubic prostatectomy: results at 10 years. J Urol 1994; 152:1831–6.

7. Thrasher JB, Robinson JJ, Lance R. Comparison of radical perineal prostatectomy to radical retropubic prostatectomy for localized prostate cancer. Lesson 2. American Urological Association Update Series. Baltimore: American Urological Association, Vol. 20, 2001; 10–15.

8. Celsus. De medicina (translated) Paris: Chemin des Etangs, 1846.

9. Belt E, Ebert CE, Surber AC Jr. A new anatomic approach in perineal prostatectomy. J Urol 1939; 41:482–97.

10. Leisrink H. Tumor prostatae: totale exstirpation der prostata. Arch Klin Chir 1883; 28:578.

11. Young HH. The early diagnosis and radical cure of carcinoma of the prostate. Bull Johns Hopkins Hosp 1905; 16:315.

12. Vest SA. Radical perineal prostatectomy, modification of closure. Surg Gynec Obstet 1940; 40:935–7.

13. Paulson DF. The surgical technique of radical perineal prostatectomy. Lesson 38. American Urological Association Update Series. Baltimore. American Urological Association, Vol. 5, 1986:1–7.

14. Belt E, Ebert CE, Surber AC Jr. A new anatomic approach in perineal prostatectomy. J Urol 1939; 482–97.

15. Young HH. The cure of cancer of the prostate by radical perineal prostatectomy (prostatoseminal vesiculectomy): history, literature, and statistics of Young's operation. J Urol 1945; 53:188–256.

16. Lew EA, Garfinkel L. Mortality at ages 75 and older in the cancer prevention study. CA Cancer J Clin 1990; 40:210–24.

17. Ruiz-Deya G, Davis R, Srivastav SK, et al. Outpatient radical prostatectomy: impact of standard perineal approach on patient outcome. J Urol 2001; 166:1270–3.

18. Parra RO. Analysis of an experience with 500 radical perineal prostatectomies in localized prostate cancer. J Urol 2000; 163(suppl)284–5, abstract 1265.

19. Bluestein DL, Bostwick DG, Bergstrahl EJ, et al. Eliminating the need for bilateral pelvic lymphadenectomy in select patients with prostate cancer. J Urol 1994; 151:1315.

20. Weldon VE. Radical perineal prostatectomy. In: Crawford ED, Das S, eds. Current genitourinary cancer surgery, 2nd edn. Baltimore: Williams and Wilkins, 1997:258–7.

21. Nichols RL, Condon RE, Gorback SL, Nyhus LM. Efficacy of preoperative antimicrobial preparation of the bowel. Ann Surg 1972; 176:227–32.

22. Hudson PB, Lilien OM. Perineal surgery for benign conditions of the prostate. In: Droller MJ, ed. Surgical management of urologic disease. St. Louis: Mosby-Year Book, 1992:713–19.

23. Weldon VE, Tavel FR, Neuwirth H, Cohen R. Patterns of positive specimen margins and detectable prostate-specific antigen after radical perineal prostatectomy. J Urol 1995; 153:1565–9.

24. Lassen PM, Kearse WS Jr. Rectal injuries during radical perineal prostatectomy. Urology 1995; 45:266–79.

25. Bishoff JT, Motley G, Optenberg SA, et al. Incidence of fecal and urinary incontinence following radical perineal and retropubic prostatectomy in a national population. J Urol 1998; 160:454–8.

26. Price DT, Vieweg J, Roland F, et al. Transient lower extremity neuropraxia associated with radical perineal prostatectomy: a complication of the exaggerated lithotomy position. J Urol 1998; 160(4):1376–8.

27. Boxer RJ, Kaufman JJ, Goodwin WE. Radical prostatectomy for carcinoma of the prostate: 1971–1976. A review of 329 patients. J Urol 1977; 117:208–13.

28. Frazier HA, Robertson JE, Paulson DF. Radical prostatectomy: the pros and cons of the perineal versus retropubic approach. J Urol 1992; 147:888–90.

29. Haab F, Boccon-Gibod L, Delmas V, et al. Perineal versus retropubic radical prostatectomy for T1, T2 prostate cancer. Br J Urol 1994; 74:626–9.

30. Lance RS, Freidrichs PA, Kane C, et al. A comparison of radical retropubic with perineal prostatectomy for localized prostate cancer within the Uniformed Services Urology Research Group. BJU Int 2001; 87:61–5.

20

Laparoscopic prostatectomy for the treatment of localized prostate cancer

Bertrand Guillonneau and Tullio Sulser

Introduction

The first laparoscopic radical prostatectomy was performed by Schuessler et al in 1992.[1] It took 6 more years for this technique to become standardized, and reproducible, owing to the strong commitment of several French teams. This approach is now used worldwide by many urologic teams, and thousands of patients have been operated on laparoscopically for treatment of localized prostate cancer. This chapter summarizes the outcomes data on the application of laparoscopic prostatectomy for localized prostate cancer.

Operative technique

Specific contraindications

There is no strict anatomic specific contraindication for laparoscopic radical prostatectomy. There are certain case scenarios that will potentially make this operation more diffcult.

From the anatomic point of view, a high body mass index (BMI > 30) definitively makes this procedure more difficult. The distance to the operative field is greater than the length of standard laparoscopic instruments available, and often necessitates increasing the number of access ports.

A large prostate (> 60 g) makes lateral prostatic dissection more difficult secondary to poor vision, particularly when the pelvis is deep and narrow. Moreover, large glands often have a prominent prostatic median lobe that makes bladder neck dissection difficult.

A previous history of prostate surgery (transurethral incision of the prostate, transurethral resection of the prostate or even open prostatectomy) is not a contraindication for the laparoscopic approach but it does make the surgery more difficult. Finally, previous history of intra-abdominal surgery can potentially preclude the transperitoneal route, making the extraperitoneal route the preferred method.

Preoperative care

Antibiotic prophylaxis, by a single intravenous dose of third-generation cephalosporin is initially prescribed 2 hours before the operation.

Prevention of thrombosis remains an essential element of perioperative care. Compression stockings are mandatory during the surgery and hospital stay. Bowel preparation with or without oral antibiotic is optional and dependent on surgeon preference.

Installation

Positioning of the patient is an essential step of the procedure. The surgeon should supervise all the steps of position to prevent positioning injuries.

The patient is placed in the dorsal supine position and secured to the operative table via a thoracic wrap of elastic adhesive tape. The arms are abducted along the body in a way to avoid risk of brachial plexus injury, while the legs are positioned in a modified frog-leg position with foam support. Generous padding of the lower extremities is recommended to prevent muscular ischemic injury to the calves. The buttocks are positioned at the end of the operative table to allow for intraoperative rectal and urethral access.

Standard skin preparation is carried out from the costal margins to the perianal region. The patient is draped medially, with each leg draped individually. An 18F Foley catheter is inserted on the sterile field and the bladder is drained.

The monitor is placed between the patient's legs, as close as possible to the surgeon's eye level. A right-handed surgeon stands on the patient's left with his assistant on the opposite side. The scrub nurse stands on the surgeon's left with the instrument table.

After inferior umbilical incision, a Verres needle is introduced intraperitoneally. Insufflation is started after confirmation that the needle is within the abdominal cavity.

A 10 mm trocar is then inserted into the umbilicus for passage of the 0° laparoscopic lens. The patient is repositioned in the Trendelenburg position, so as to improve the access to the pelvic region, with spontaneous gravity mobilization of the intestine and sigmoid colon. The operating table is lowered to an ergonomic position for the surgeon.

Four other 5 mm trocars are inserted: one into the left lower quadrant, one in the midline half-way between the umbilicus and the pubis, one at the level of the umbilicus in the mid-clavicular line, and one in the right lower quadrant at McBurney's point. The surgeon uses the two upper ports close to the camera port in order to have a triangular approach to the operative field. The assistant has at his disposal the lateral right and the suprapubic ports (Figure 20.1).

The operative technical steps

Transperitoneal pelvic lymph node dissection is performed according to the usual[2] or the extended lymph node dissection.[3] As to our experience, the number of removed nodes was 19 (range 6–42), the mean operative time for the extended lymph node dissection was 55 (37–73) min, and no complications occurred (Figure 20.2). A descriptive narrative of pelvic lymph node dissection is given in Chapter 40.

Six standardized steps can be individualized during laparoscopic radical prostatectomy.[4]

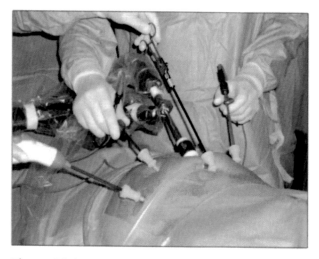

Figure 20.1
Four 5 mm trocars are used for instrumentation. The individual surgeon works with two trocars on each side of the scope in order to optimize the triangulation of his instruments. The scope is held by a voice-controlled robotic arm, allowing the assistant to assist with both hands.

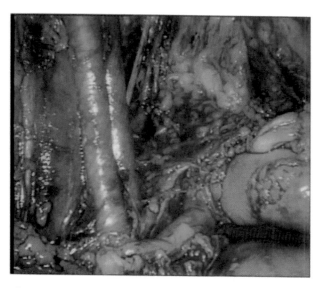

Figure 20.2
After the extended lymph node dissection is performed, the left external iliac artery, hypogastric artery, obturator nerve, and the ureter are clearly visible.

First step: posterior approach to the seminal vesicles

Incising the pouch of Douglas. The sigmoid colon may be held gently by the assistant, retracting the rectum cranially. The surgeon will then notice the appearance of two peritoneal arches in the pouch of Douglas. The superior one represents the approximate location of the ureters and the trigone. The inferior arch, just above the peritoneal reflection, is created by the merger of the vasa deferentia in the midline.

The posterior peritoneum is incised transversally along the inferior peritoneal arch (Figure 20.3). The dissection follows the inferior peritoneal flap and enters into an avascular plane that should be developed. This exposes Denonvilliers' fascia, which is easily recognizable by vertical fibers.

Freeing the seminal vesicles. Once Denonvilliers' fascia is identified, the outlines of the seminal vesicles and vasa deferentia are clearly visible. Denonvilliers' fascia is transversally incised, allowing for clear identification of the vasa deferentia, which are coagulated with bipolar forceps and then transected. One must be aware of the presence of the deferential artery of the vas that runs along the vas and that must be carefully coagulated. Transection of the vasa deferentia provides for direct access to the seminal vesicles. They should be dissected along their surface to isolate the two vascular pedicles, one at the tip and the second at the base. These arteries are meticulously coagulated by bipolar forceps to prevent thermal injury of the neurovascular bundle (Figure 20.4). The vesicles are then completely mobilized to their respective bases.

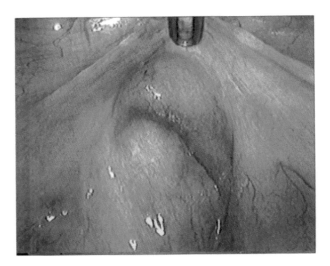

Figure 20.3
The assistant holds up the bladder to facilitate opening of the pouch of Douglas. The seminal vesicles are revealed, generally 2 cm above Douglas' pouch, recognizing an arch.

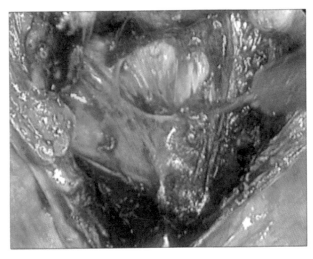

Figure 20.5
Holding up the seminal complex reveals Denonvilliers' fascia, which is transected transversally, demonstrating the prerectal fat and the posterior aspect of the prostate.

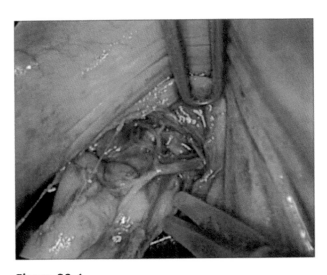

Figure 20.4
The seminal vesicles are located immediately behind the peritoneum. This direct access leads to a close dissection of the seminal vesicles complex. The entire surrounding vascular network is clearly visible, allowing for precise dissection with minimal damage to the nervous plexus when a nerve-sparing technique is considered.

Opening Denonvilliers' fascia. Incision of Denonvilliers' fascia allows an easier and safer dissection later in the operation, by separating the rectum away from the prostatic pedicles. To facilitate the exposure, the assistant can, by pulling the vasa deferentia upward, place Denonvilliers' fascia on tension. It will appear to have longitudinal striations under the magnification of the laparoscope. Denonvilliers' fascia is then incised medially and horizontally on the line of reflection between the prostatic base

and the posterior surface of the seminal vesicles. As soon as a shallow incision is made, prerectal fat is revealed (Figure 20.5).

No attempt is made to dissect the prostatic apex from this posterior approach. Further dissection is not necessary and can be dangerous, since the rectum appears usually vertical. In case of difficulties differentiating the rectum, the use of a Hegar bougie inserted into the rectum is helpful, to improve tactile perception of the anterior rectal wall.

Second step: anterior approach to the prostate

Entering Retzius' space. The bladder is filled with approximately 120 ml of saline to help identify the contours of the bladder. The anterior parietal peritoneum is incised from one umbilical ligament to the other just above the distended bladder. If a lymph node dissection has been performed, it is easier to follow the pubic bone that is already exposed to enter Retzius' space, and then to transect the umbilical ligaments as high as necessary; otherwise, the medial umbilical ligaments are preserved. By staying close to the medial aspect of the medial umbilical ligaments and heading medially, the pubic arches are encountered. This dissection allows for clear identification of the urachus that is divided last, thus minimizing the risk of injuring the bladder. It is essential to free the bladder well from its anterior and lateral attachments in order to create a large working space and to permit a tension-free vesicourethral anastomosis at the end of the operation. After the bladder is freed anteriorly and laterally, it is emptied with a syringe. Since the patient is in Trendelenburg position, spontaneous emptying is never complete.

Exposing the endopelvic fascia. The fat over the fascia covering the prostate must be gently swept away in order to clearly expose the intrapelvic fascia and the puboprostatic ligaments (Figure 20.6). The superficial dorsal vein is identified and coagulated with bipolar forceps. The endopelvic fascia is visualized lateral to the prostate, and incised at its

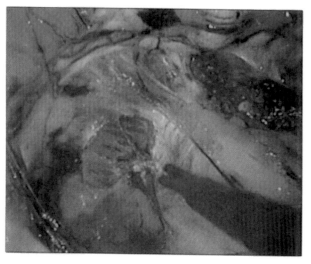

Figure 20.6
After developing the space of Retzius, the endopelvic fascia is opened (here on the left side) and the fibers of the levator ani are pushed away to free the lateral aspect of the prostate.

line of reflection with the pelvic floor muscles (Figure 20.7). An adherent zone between the muscle and the prostate is often found. These attachments correspond to vascular penetration. The veins, once identified, are coagulated and transected, allowing complete opening of the area lateral to the apex. Occasionally, an artery runs cephalad to the veins, which is preserved, since it runs toward the sphincter complex. Incision of the puboprostatic ligaments is done under visual control, taking care to avoid the veins of Santorini's plexus. The endopelvic fascia incision can be extended toward the fascia that covers the veins laterally. This lateral incision will facilitate further dissection and exposure of the dorsal venous complex.

Ligating the dorsal venous complex. Santorini's plexus is ligated with a 2-0 absorbable suture, passed with a # 26 needle underneath the venous plexus from one side to the other of the distal side of Santorini's plexus (Figure 20.8). For a right-handed surgeon, the needle is passed from the right side of the plexus to the left side with backhand, the needle being situated such that the curve of the needle follows the curve of the symphysis.

Depending on the size of the plexus, a second separate suture or a figure-of-eight stitch may be placed to make the ligation more hemostatic. At this point of the operation, transection of the complex is unnecessary and will be done later.

A back-bleeding stitch, ligating the preprostatic venous drainage, is placed, since it is helpful during the subsequent bladder neck dissection and section of the venous complex.

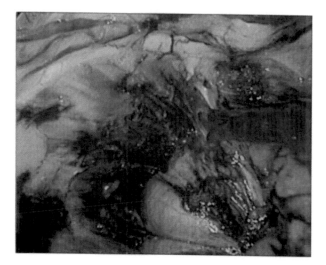

Figure 20.7
Towards the apex, the fibers of the external sphincter are freed from the prostate, preserving them as much as possible. This operative maneuver reveals the lateral and inferior aspects of the deep venous prostatic complex.

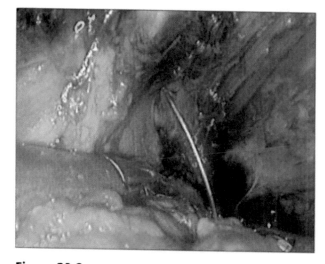

Figure 20.8
The venous complex is ligated with a 2-0 SH stitch under close vision (here from the right to the left side).

Third step: bladder neck dissection

This step is considered the most difficult since the anatomic landmarks are not well defined. To identify the bladder neck area, the anterior prevesical fat must be retracted superiorly, causing a faint outline of the prostatovesical plane. The cranial retraction of the preprostatic fat is possible because the superficial dorsal vein had been previously transected. The prostatic vesical junction is generally located where the fat becomes adherent. The fascial covering at this point is transversally incised at this landmark, which needs coagulation of several veins running in this layer.

It is then generally easier to find an avascular plane between bladder and prostate that is developed by sharp and blunt dissection. The prostatic urethra is identified by a change in the orientation of the muscular fibers, which become longitudinal rather than circular. The urethra is dissected laterally on each side. The bladder is checked again to be empty and the catheter balloon is deflated.

The urethra is incised transversally and the tip of the catheter is pulled up by a grasper via the suprapubic port, to expose the posterior urethral wall that is incised at the level of the bladder neck (Figure 20.9). Since the bladder neck is thus preserved, the ureteral orifices are far away from the bladder incision and are not specially identified. While the assistant pulls up the prostate via the catheter, the surgeon exposes the posterior face of the bladder neck, grasping the posterior bladder incision.

As one proceeds to incise the posterior junction between the prostate and the bladder, it is important to direct the dissection straight posterior, following the posterior bladder wall. This way one enters the 'anterior layer' of Denonvilliers' fascia. This fascia is recognized by the vertical muscular fibers between the prostate base and the bladder neck. The fascia is incised in order to gain access to the previously dissected retrovesical space. The vasa deferentia and the seminal vesicles are then simply brought into the operating field by the assistant. This maneuver exposes both sides of the prostatic pedicles, since they have been already completely dissected medially and laterally (Figure 20.10).

Fourth step: lateral dissection of the prostate

Preserving the neurovascular bundles: the intrafascial technique.
The assistant grasps the vas and the seminal vesicle through the space of dissection between the prostate and the posterior bladder neck, and pulls them upward.

The inferior and medial landmarks are identified by the posterior layer of Denonvilliers' fascia that had been already dissected during the first step of the procedure. The superior and medial landmarks require making an incision in the periprostatic fascia, on the prostate, from the base toward the apex (Figure 20.11).

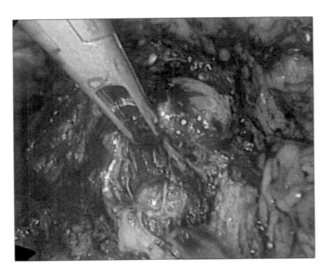

Figure 20.9
After opening the bladder neck, the superficial layer of Denonvilliers' fascia should be opened to create access to the already freed seminal vesicles. A grasper holds up the posterior aspect of the prostate while the scissors retract down the posterior wall of the bladder neck, revealing Denonvilliers' fascia, already open here.

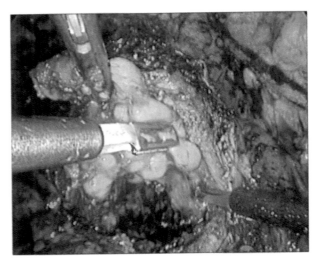

Figure 20.10
The direct access to the seminal vesicles exposes the pedicle of the prostate (here the right side) where the seminal vesicle is grasped and held up. The lateral part of Denonvilliers' fascia is visible and should be incised to identify safely the medial aspect of the neurovascular bundle (here on the right side).

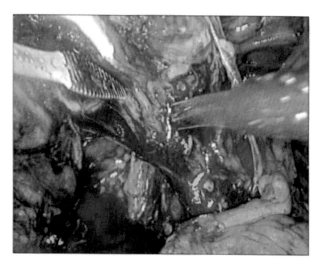

Figure 20.11
The perforating vessels should be identified accurately before any transection. Here, a pedicle artery is coagulated with slender bipolar forceps on the prostate side, far removed from the neurovascular pedicle to avoid thermal injury.

Finally, the medial landmark requires the transection of the prostatic pedicle. This is made easier by the previous dissections that exposed the pedicle high on the prostate, theoretically at a safe distance from the nervous and vascular components of the bundles. Due to the magnification, the pedicle vessels are well visualized and must be systematically controlled (Figure 20.12). Because of the traction on the seminal vesicles, the vessels appear to rise vertically, which facilitates their exposure but is a distortion of their natural orientation. One must remember that the neurovascular bundles are attached. It could be helpful

for the surgeon to reorientate himself periodically during the dissection of the pedicles to keep the location of the posterolateral neurovascular bundle in view.

Once the pedicle is transected, the two fascial incisions (the superior, periprostatic, and the inferior, Denonvilliers' fascia) can be joined. It is then possible to develop, with careful and blunt dissection, an avascular intrafascial plane of the periprostatic (lateral prostatic) fascia pushing the neurovascular bundle lateral and posterior (Figure 20.13). Thus, the incision/dissection of the periprostatic (lateral prostatic) fascia displaces the neurovascular bundle away from the lateral prostatic pedicle. This intrafascial dissection is extended toward the apex. Depending on the size of the gland, dissection is more difficult at the distal third of the gland as it approaches the bladder neck. It is preferable to continue the apical dissection of the bundle after transecting Santorini's plexus and the urethra, which gives mobility to the gland and facilitates the exposure of the distal third of the prostate. At the apex, the neurovascular bundles are divergent from the prostate, but must be followed until their entrance into the pelvic floor, below and lateral to the urethra, to avoid the risk of injury. Due to the magnification, the pulses of the arterial component of the bundle are often visible, which could be a good anatomic guide to the functional integrity of the bundle. Hemorrhage around the bundles is always minor and, for the sake of neurovascular integrity, should not be controlled.

Non nerve-sparing procedure.   If nerve sparing is not considered, the procedure is easier. The prostate pedicles are transected far from the prostate and the posterolateral attachments of the prostate are not dissected but simply controlled (by bipolar coagulation or clips) and transected.

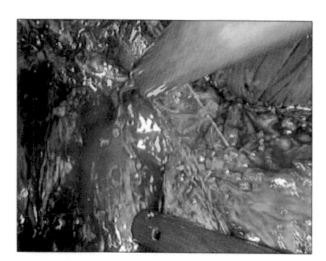

Figure 20.12
The neurovascular bundle (here on the left side) is freed all along the prostate. Particular attention is paid to the apex where the bundle could be very close and adherent to the apical edge of the prostate.

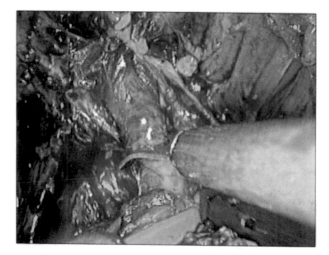

Figure 20.13
Once the bundles are freed and away from the urethra, the latter is transected.

It is important to remember that, if this step looks easier, the risk to enter into the rectum is higher because the dissection is performed close to it, in the perirectal fat.

Fifth step: apical dissection of the prostate

At this time, only three structures are attached to the prostate: Santorini's complex, the urethra, and the rectourethralis muscle.

Sectioning the dorsal venous complex. Because the superficial dorsal vein has been ligated and the pedicles have been controlled, there is little bleeding when the dorsal complex is incised. The incision is tangential to the prostate to avoid capsular incision at this place. Gradually, the dorsal vein complex is retracted anteriorly to reach an avascular plane of dissection, situated between the venous complex and the urethra. This plane must be developed to perfectly expose the anterior and lateral urethral wall.

Incising the urethra. Laterally, the urethra must be dissected free from surrounding fibrotic structures. A Béniqué catheter (metal sound with an 'S' shape) is introduced to tactilely identify the urethra. The urethral wall is then incised with scissors or a retractable cold knife. The urethral bougie is pushed through the anterior urethrotomy and into the pelvis to expose the lateral and posterior urethral walls (Figure 20.14). The posterior wall of the urethra is similarly incised with scissors.

Transection of Denonvilliers' fascia. After complete transection of the urethra, the distal attachment of Denonvilliers' fascia is on stretch and represents the final attachments of the prostate. In order to avoid injury to the neurovascular bundles, it is necessary to cut these fibers from lateral to medial. This division of the distal part of Denonvilliers' fascia close to the prostate completely frees the specimen, which is placed into a laparoscopic bag (Figure 20.15), under the control of a 5 mm scope through a lateral port.

The specimen is then extracted through an enlargement of the 10 mm umbilical incision, depending on the size of the specimen. The gland is macroscopically checked, and sent to the pathologist for frozen section if necessary. The umbilical incision is carefully closed around a 10 mm trocar and the abdomen is reinsufflated.

Sixth step: urethrovesical anastomosis

Eversion of the bladder mucosa and reconstruction of a wide bladder neck, traditionally performed during open radical retropubic, are not necessary during laparoscopic prostatectomy. However, occasionally, reconstruction of a very large bladder neck is necessary to make the anastomotic approximation smaller and more continent, and a posterior tennis racquet rather than an anterior racket is performed. This maneuver moves the ureteral orifices away from the suture line.

Throughout this portion of the procedure, the surgeon works with two needle-holders. The anastomosis is made with interrupted stitches of 3-0 absorbable suture with a

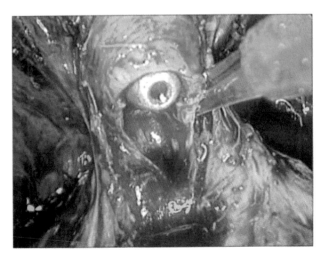

Figure 20.14
Particular attention is required for the transection of the posterior wall of the urethra, to avoid any opening into the posterior aspect of the prostate that could lead to positive margins or incomplete resection of the prostate.

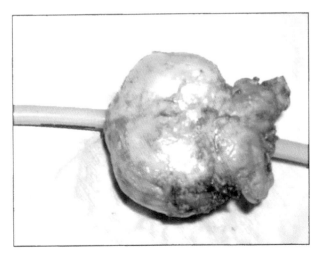

Figure 20.15
After completion of the prostatectomy, the specimen is extracted in a laparoscopic bag through an enlargement of the umbilical incision. The operative specimen is inspected to rule out positive margins.

18 mm half-circle needle. All ties are made intracorporeally. The metal sound (Béniqué catheter with a depressed tip) helps to guide the needle into the urethra and to place the sutures, at precise locations around the urethra (Figure 20.16).

The three first sutures are placed posterior at 5, 6, and 7 o'clock, going inside-out on the urethra and outside-in on the bladder neck. The 5 o'clock stitch goes inside-out on the urethra (right hand, forehand) and outside-in on the bladder (right hand, forehand); the 5 and 6 o'clock stitches go inside-out on the urethra (right hand, forehand) and outside-in on the bladder (left hand, forehand). These stitches are tied intraluminal.

Four other sutures are symmetrically placed at 4 and 8, then 2 and 10 o'clock, and tied outside the lumen. As a rule, for a right-handed surgeon, the right-sided stitches go outside-in on the bladder (right hand, forehand) and inside-out on the urethra (left hand, backhand); the left-sided stitches are symmetrical, going outside-in on the bladder (left hand, forehand) and inside-out on the urethra (right hand, backhand).

Three final anterior stitches are placed at 11, 12, and 1 o'clock, symmetrically to the posterior stitches. The 11 and the 12 o'clock stitches go outside-in on the urethra (right hand, forehand) and inside-out on the bladder (right hand, forehand), while the 1 o'clock stitch goes outside-in on the urethra (right hand, forehand) and inside-out on the bladder (left hand, forehand). Once the stitches are tied, the Foley catheter is inserted. The bladder is filled with 180 ml of saline to check the water tightness of the anastomosis and to confirm the correct position of the catheter. Finally, the balloon is inflated with 10 ml.

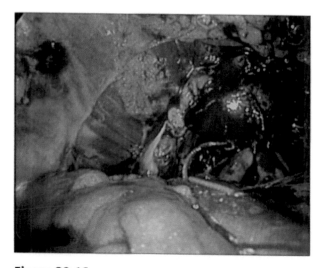

Figure 20.16
Performance of the anastomosis is facilitated with the use of a 'Béniqué bougie'. This device directs the anastomotic needle to encompass the full thickness of the urethra.

Completing the operation

The abdominal pressure is lowered to 5 mmHg, to check for venous bleeding. The peritoneal incisions are left open and two suction drains are placed, one anteriorly in Retzius' space and one posteriorly through the incision of the pouch of Douglas, on contact with the rectum. The 5 mm trocars are removed under visual control and are checked to exclude vascular injury, particularly of the epigastric vessels. Finally, the incisions are conventionally closed and dressed.

Operative variants

Technical points

Extraperitoneal approach. The extraperitoneal approach has been described[5,6] and is currently used by several teams. The theoretical advantages are the absence of risk of injury of intra-abdominal organs, less peritoneal irritation, and a quicker development of Retzius' space. On the other hand, the operative room is narrower, reducing the ergonomic conditions of the procedure. During this procedure, posterior mobilization of the bladder is not as great as with the transperitoneal approach, making the anastomosis much more difficult, with tension that necessitates some technical tricks (anterior and/or posterior racquet stitches to reconstruct the bladder neck). But, above all, it appears that a key point of the nerve-sparing operation lies in the initial approach to the seminal vesicle, since the seminal vesicles complex is more easily accessible via the transperitoneal approach, thus potentially preserving the neurovascular bundles better than the extraperitoneal approach.

Operative strategy. Different strategies have been developed, mainly with a direct approach to Retzius' space without preliminary dissection of the seminal vesicles complex.[7] The theoretical objection is the same as for the extraperitoneal approach, if a nerve-sparing procedure is planned. The retrograde technique of retropubic prostatectomy,[8] mimicking Walsh's technique, has been described, but doesn't seem to have the advantage of the benefit of an axis of dissection identical to the vision. However, this technique has proven to have excellent results for preserving the neurovascular bundles via the traditional open approach. If the laparoscopic counterpart can replicate the open approach, this may become the preferred approach.

The anastomosis: The urethrovesical anastomosis can be correctly performed with a running suture, and several teams prefer to use a continuous suture rather than an interrupted one.[9] An advantage of the interrupted sutures is that they are theoretically less ischemic, they can always be done in all situations, the help of the assistant is not necessary, and the manipulation of short stitches is easier when one starts. On the other hand, a running suture needs less knots, and could be a simpler way for the less-experienced surgeon.

The trocars

Placement of trocars.   The trocars can be placed in any array, according to the habits of the surgeon. In particular, they can be arranged 'like a fan' round the umbilicus, with two trocars in the left iliac fossa and two trocars in the right iliac fossa. In the absence of an arm holding the camera, this set-up is certainly more surgical assistant-friendly, since the assistant is not bothered by the surgeon's movements. It allows the surgeon to operate seated, with the two trocars in front of him, but is theoretically less ergonomic since the triangular operating range of the instruments is reduced. The dissection on the opposite side of the prostate can be impractical, and the sutures necessitate modifying the instrument set-up anyway into a triangular configuration.

The size and number of the trocars.   Except for the umbilical port, an additional 10 mm port is not always necessary. In addition to the 10 mm trocar for the scope, four other ports are sufficient.

Instrumentation

The use of various different instruments is technically possible. In particular, endoscopic staplers can be used for transection and hemostatic control of the prostatic pedicles when a non-nerve-sparing procedure is planned.[7] Apart from the cost, the major critical point is that the rectum can be pulled into the line of section.

The use of harmonic scissors is advocated to theoretically decrease the extent of the heat diffusion at the level of the capsular arteries and thus protect the neurovascular bundles from thermal injury. With the same goal, the use of clips to control pedicular vessels has been advocated.

Outcome data are not presently available to confirm this theoretical advantage over bipolar coagulation.

The use of the 'robotics'

Voice-controlled robotic arm.   The use of a voice-controlled robotic arm enables the surgeon to control the laparoscopic lens. This device allows the surgical assistant to fully assist the primary surgeon and also ensures excellent stability of the image.

Remote-controlled laparoscopic surgery.   The feasibility of a remote robotic device to perform laparoscopic radical prostatectomies has been demonstrated and confirmed by several teams.[10–12] Although this technology may enable an experienced surgeon to perform this complex procedure from a remote site, the increased cost and legality of this form of telesurgery has not been worked out.

Postoperative care

Analgesics

The usual analgesic protocol for the first 24 hours consists of anti-inflammatory drugs. Often no intravenous analgesia is requested by the patient from the second postoperative day. Major analgesics are rarely necessary; in those cases postoperative complications must be suspected and ruled out.

Nutrition

Oral intake is usually resumed 12 hours after the operation and intravenous perfusion is generally stopped between the 12th and 24th hour after operation.

Antithrombosis care

Antithrombosis precautions are of major importance given the increased risk of a pelvic cancer operation and a laparoscopic approach, which diminishes the venous return to the heart. Preoperative and postoperative prevention is based on thrombosis prophylaxis started before the operation (low molecular weight heparin) and continued for 2 weeks after the operation in the form of compression stockings while in hospital and early mobilization of the patient on the first day after operation. This essential preventive element is favored by the absence of postoperative pain, allowing for early mobility.

Bladder catheter removal

As a rule, if the bladder neck has been preserved and if the anastomosis was watertight during the operation, the bladder catheter can be removed as early as the 3rd day after operation. If the quality of the anastomosis is uncertain, the bladder drainage should be prolonged. In such a situation, a cystogram is necessary to assess the anastomotic integrity. The Foley catheter must not be removed if urine is present in the pelvic drain.

Technical feasibility

Surgical conversion

Surgical conversion to a conventional open retropubic approach can be indicated in case of intraoperative complications and/or technical difficulties.

The intraoperative complications are generally due to hemorrhage of Santorini's venous plexus. In this event, vascular control should be attempted by compressing the plexus with a clamp and placing a new ligature. From our experience, the use of bipolar coagulation or the application of a clip is a transient and unsatisfactory solution. If hemostasis seems impossible and if the decision to convert is taken, it is always possible to compress the plexus with a laparoscopic clamp or by the insertion of a sponge through the 10 mm trocar to compress the bleeder, while the laparotomy is performed.

Dissection planes that are difficult to identify may result in technical problems. This can be potentially due to an extracapsular tumor (pT3 or pT4) adhering to the posterior surface of the prostate, which may make the posterior dissection plane difficult. Dissection planes are difficult to define in patients treated with prior endocrine therapy. The prostate is of reduced size, with ill-defined surgical borders. Another cause of operative difficulties may be a history of prostatic surgery: transurethral resection of the prostate (TURP) or open prostatectomy. Obviously, the preservation of the bladder neck in these cases is impossible.

The patient needs to be informed beforehand that there is always a risk of open surgical conversion. Although the conversion rate decreases with experience and now tends towards zero, there will always be difficult cases for which laparoscopic surgery cannot be completed. One must keep in mind that the surgical benefit is for the patient and the primary goal is patient safety.

Finally, it is important to stress the technical difficulty of a correct and watertight urethrovesical anastomosis. When the urethrovesical anastomosis cannot be achieved correctly, a minilaparotomy must be done to perform the anastomosis in the conventional way, and take advantage of the incision to extract the operative specimen.

Operative time

Laparoscopic prostatectomy is an ambitious operation that makes high demands on the technical skills and anatomic knowledge of the surgeon. At the end of the operation the anastomosis is a very important surgical step, always difficult, that determines the quality of the postoperative results. Obviously, with experience, the surgical time decreases. At present, the mean operative time reported by several different teams is around 200 min, which is more or less comparable to the operative time required for the retropubic procedure.[4,8,13,14]

Specific complications

Despite the technical difficulties and long learning curve, in our experience the morbidity of laparoscopic radical prostatectomy is low.

Hemorrhage

The dorsal venous complex

Vascular injury mainly results from the inability to surgically control Santorini's venous plexus. A laparoscopic procedure cannot be continued in case of bleeding as hemorrhage interferes considerably with vision. One needs to revert to conventional surgery if adequate hemostasis cannot be obtained. This complication occurred early in our experience when a secure ligation of the dorsal venous complex was not correctly placed. Presently, control of the venous complex presents no technical problem and is always perfectly performed, according to the technique we have described above.

The epigastric injury

Another potential vascular injury is to the epigastric artery, which occurs during insertion of the ports. On completion of the procedure, it is essential to carefully examine the point of entry of each secondary sheath into the abdomen. Unrecognized bleeding related to an epigastric injury can lead to an extensive hematoma, requiring transfusion and sometimes even surgical repair.

Transfusion

Altogether the transfusion rate in many different series is low, and averages less than 5% of the patients.[14,15] This low transfusion rate is clearly related to the reduction of the estimated blood loss to an average of less than 500 ml in these series. There are several explanations for this reduction. The pressure of the pneumoperitoneum (12 mmHg or less) certainly contributes to occlusion of small veins, but the other element concerns the technique itself. Since a laparoscopic procedure cannot be continued in case of insufficient vision, one of the objectives is to ensure excellent vision of the operative site, which requires systematic coagulation of all small vessels that are generally neglected in an open procedure. Finally, the quality of vision is improved by magnification of the operative field and the various camera angles optimizes the visualization of vascular structures.

Bowel complications

Rectal injury

Rectal injury may occur during two different steps of the procedure: firstly, when Denonvilliers' fascia is incised too far posterior at the base of the seminal vesicles; secondly, during the lateral dissection of the prostate at the apex, where Denonvilliers' fascia is in close proximity to the rectum and space for dissection becomes limited. In this situation, the use of an intrarectal bougie may facilitate optical and tactile detection of the plane of Denonvilliers' fascia as well as the limits of the rectal wall. In our experience, all cases of rectal injury occurred at the end of the procedure during transection of the distal attachments of Denonvilliers' fascia, when the dissection of the posterior aspect of the prostate was not completed. Once the injury is recognized, it can be accurately repaired with two layers of suture line. This can be meticulously achieved laparoscopically, and colostomy is not required. The operative site should be disinfected, and antibiotic therapy prescribed. Oral intake is delayed (after the 3rd day) and the bladder catheter should be removed on the 8th postoperative day. A cystogram should be obtained to confirm a watertight anastomosis.[16]

Peritonitis

This is related to unrecognized bowel injury. Although this trauma is rare, it requires immediate diagnosis and treatment.[17]

Urologic complications

Bladder injury

Bladder injury occurs during the approach to the space of Retzius. Because the bladder extends towards the umbilicus, the urachus must be transected as high as possible. A bladder injury is easily identified (appearance of vascular mucosa; gas in urinary bladder). It is repaired by extramucosal sutures of the bladder. The bladder catheter is left in place for 5 days.

Ureteral injury

Ureteral injury can occur during the freeing of the seminal vesicles through the pouch of Douglas, when the peritoneal incision is made too high, and the ureter is mistaken for the vas deferens. This complication is rare. The best way to avoid this complication is to follow the vas to the ampulla and the seminal vesicle, which identifies clearly the structure as the vas deferens. An injured ureter should be accurately sutured via the laparoscope over a ureteral stent, and the healing process checked postoperatively with an intravenous pyelogram (IVP).

The ureter can also be damaged during the closure of the urethral anastomosis. This danger is greater after previous prostate surgery (TURP or open prostatectomy) or a large median prostatic lobe. To prevent this complication, indigo carmine should be utilized to identify the ureteral orifice. Laparoscopic reintervention may be necessary to correct this problem.

Urinary fistula

Urine in the pelvic drains documents anastomosic leakage. A few milliliters of urine by suction drainage frequently subsides within 24 hours and has no sequelae. Large amounts of urinary drainage, however, may cause clinical signs of a urinoma in the peritoneal cavity (rising serum creatinine, metabolic acidosis, decreased urine output). During these situations, the bladder catheter is left in place until urine drainage from the pelvic drains is zero. The Foley catheter can be removed after a radiologic control documents an intact anastomosis.

Performing a new anastomosis due to a persisting fistula is sometimes necessary, particularly when a ureteral orifice is inadvertently included in the anastomosis. This secondary anastomosis can be successfully performed laparoscopically without difficulties.

Anastomotic stricture

With the present follow-up, only 1 of the patients developed a stricture of the anastomosis that required an additional endoscopic procedure. This stricture resolved after endoscopic incision. Anastomotic stricture after laparoscopic radical prostatectomy is rare in our hands.

Pelvic lymph node dissection

Obturator nerve injury

One patient developed a mild obturator nerve paralysis, probably secondary to an electrocautery injury. This paralysis resolved spontaneously without sequela in less than 6 months.

Lymphoceles

Lymphoceles are a complication of the pelvic lymph node dissection. They can occur even after a transperitoneal approach. When asymptomatic, they should be neglected, but a surgical intervention is necessary when they are infected or cause compression symptoms to adjacent structures (obturator nerve, bladder, colon). Pelvic lymphoceles are treated by percutaneous drainage and/or laparoscopic decompression.

Oncologic results

Oncologic outcomes are based on pathologic examination of the operative specimen and biologic non-progression. Current follow-up of oncology outcomes for laparoscopic prostatectomy are too short; therefore, no definitive advantage between open and laparoscopic prostatectomy can be made.

Pathologic evaluation

The positive surgical margin rate varies widely from one series to another, depending on the population selection, clinical stage, pathologic grade of prostate biopsy, and the experience of the surgeon. In the literature, the overall rate of positive margins after laparoscopic radical prostatectomy ranges between 11.4%[13] and 26.4%.[18]

As demonstrated in other series of radical retropubic prostatectomy,[19] surgical margin status had a significant effect on the biochemical progression-free survival (90% negative vs 67% positive margins at 3 years).[20]

The location of the positive margins with laparoscopic radical prostatectomy is primarily apical (about 50%), as reported in several studies.[20,21]

These rates and locations are comparable to what is already reported in large series of contemporary open retropubic radical prostatectomies, suggesting that it is the disease process itself more than the surgery that is involved in these locations.[22,23]

Biochemical evaluation

Preoperative prostate-specific antigen (PSA), pathologic stage, surgical margin status, and Gleason score in the postoperative specimen are factors for cancer recurrence after radical prostatectomy.

The data on the prognostic factors in the laparoscopic series are similar to those previously published for the open retropubic approach. If pathologic characteristics of the surgical specimens are comparable, definitive cure by the two techniques is similar.

At present, the data available for laparoscopic radical prostatectomy calculated overall progression-free survival rate of 90.5% at 3 years (PSA < 0.1 ng/ml). According to the pathologic stage, the progression-free survival rate was

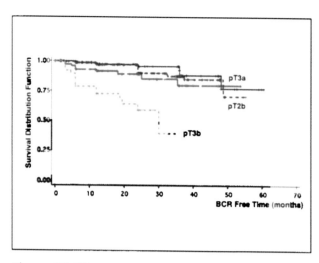

Figure 20.17
Percentage of biochemical progression-free survival (progression = PSA > 0.1 ng/ml) according to pathologic stage.[20]

91.8% for pT2aN0/Nx, 88% for pT2bN0/Nx, 77% for pT3aN0/Nx, 44% for pT3bN0/Nx, and 50% for pT1-3N1 ($p = 0.001$, Figure 20.17).

Clinical evaluation: trocar/ operative site tumor seeding

The question of an additional oncologic seeding related to the laparoscopic technique is controversial but needs to be considered. The majority of prostate tumors are organ-confined. Thus, with no direct tumor contact with the pneumoperitoneum, there is little to no risk of tumor dissemination. With this knowledge, the risk of cutaneous tumor seeding is very low in regard to the number of laparoscopic radical prostatectomies performed for prostate cancer throughout the world. This correlates with no reports of seeding from laparoscopic prostatectomy in the world literature.[24]

The question of trocar/operative site tumor seeding from laparoscopy has been extensively examined for renal cancer by many laparoscopic surgeons.[25,26] The risk for tumor seeding to these sites is similar to traditional open renal surgery. Currently, trocar/operative site seeding has not been reported for laparoscopic radical prostatectomy. An incidence of trocar site seeding was reported after laparoscopic pelvic lymphadenectomy for prostate cancer.[24] In this case a large mass of necrotic prostate cancer was inadvertently entered with gross tumor spillage.

Urinary function

To assess continence rates after radical prostatectomy, a self-administered questionnaire is completed by the patient at home.[27] At present, only preliminary urinary continence outcomes are available secondary to short-term follow-up. Moreover, refinement and evolving operative technique would not allow for long-term follow-up. However, the experiences of our first group of patients undergoing laparoscopic prostatectomy have sufficient follow-up to access long-term outcomes.

In order to evaluate continence as objectively as possible, we have prospectively evaluated the recovery of urinary control in 530 patients operated upon between January 1998 and December 2002. All patients were followed for a minimum of 12 months. Twenty-three patients were excluded from the analysis due to failure to precisely determine the continence status postoperatively. In 263 patients (53%), the puboprostatic ligaments were partially incised during apical dissection and preserved in the remaining patients according to the surgeon's preference. Urinary control was assessed by the International Continence Society (ICS) male questionnaire completed by patients 6 months postoperatively and reviewed by an independent research specialist. Patients were considered continent when they did not require any protection to keep them dry. Patients who used pad(s) even only for few drops were considered incontinent. At 12 months after laparoscopic radical prostatectomy, 79% of patients ($n = 401$) recovered complete urinary control and 92% of patients ($n = 466$) were either totally continent or using only one pad per day. Median time to achieve continence was 1.5 months (range 1–18). Patients younger than 70 years were more likely to achieve total urinary control than older patients ($p < 0.001$). Clinical and pathologic tumor stage ($p = 0.8$ and $p = 0.7$, respectively), preoperative PSA ($p = 0.2$), prior surgery for benign prostatic hyperplasia (TURP or transvesical prostatectomy) ($p = 0.4$), and the development of an early anastomotic leak ($p = 0.2$) did not influence the postoperative continence status. Neither the surgical technique used, with or without puboprostatic ligament preservation, nor the quality of neurovascular bundle preservation, affected the continence recovery or time to achieve continence. We assessed the difficulty of the surgery by blood loss, patient BMI, and the specimen's weight. The specimen's weight was the only significant factor associated with postoperative incontinence ($p = 0.02$).

Thus, the continence rate on the basis of this definition was 79%, while 13% of patients were using only one pad, which corresponds to a so-called 'social continence' rate of 92%, which is comparable to the continence rate usually found in the literature after the open retropubic[27,28,29] or laparoscopic approach.[30]

Sexual function

The evaluation of potency is a very difficult task: no scale is appropriate to evaluate sexual function with respect to and taking into account the multiple medical factors.

The nerve-sparing technique is now performed in every case where it is oncologically feasible.

Interposition sural nerve grafting during radical prostatectomy provides a potential pathway to restoring autonomic innervation while providing excellent oncology control of the cancer. Published data have shown a 75% initial success rate after bilateral sural nerve graft interposition, and recovery after unilateral graft interposition with contralateral nerve preservation appears comparable to recovery with bilateral nerve preservation.[31] Tuerk et al. demonstrated the technical feasibility of sural nerve grafting laparoscopically.[32] Furthermore, laparoscopy provides the important advantages of optical magnification with improved visualization in a bloodless field.

Between 2000 and 2002 in our series, 116 patients with a mean age of 59 (44–70) years and with normal preoperative sexual activity were selected for a nerve-sparing procedure and assessed postoperatively with a self-questionnaire. The rate of erection obtained without any medical assistance ranged from 60 to 80%, and the rate of sexual intercourse, achieved eventually with the assistance of oral drugs, ranged from 33% to 74%, for uni- or bilateral nerve-sparing surgery, respectively. Among the 92 patients with bilateral preservation of the vascular bundle, 52% recovered a potency that allowed satisfactory intercourse in the first 3 months. Some other series confirmed equivalent rates of sexual function when bilateral nerve sparing was technically successful.[21,33]

Since sexual preservation is a critical point, hopefully this rate will improve with time and the quality of erections will allow patients to resume a satisfactory sex life.

This experience supports the fact that anatomic and functional nerve-sparing surgery is technically feasible through a laparoscopic approach with satisfactory results.

Conclusion

Radical prostatectomy can be performed via laparoscopy in an uncompromising manner. Certainly the laparoscopic technique demands advanced technical skill, knowledge of laparoscopic prostate anatomy, an expertise in prostate oncology, and the support of a whole team involved in the care of patients with prostate cancer.

Laparoscopy offers the patient two kinds of benefits. The first benefit is common to all laparoscopic procedures, i.e. a low intra- and postoperative morbidity, with a shortened convalescence. The second benefit is correlated to the magnified vision and the accuracy of the surgery, which provides good and promising functional results in regards to continence and potency. But most importantly, these advantages are supported by equivalent oncologic outcomes to open retropubic radical prostatectomies. These data, obtained from a few centers, must be confirmed by larger prospective series. If confirmed, laparoscopy will become the approach of choice to perform radical prostatectomy effectively with less morbidity. Like all surgical procedures, laparoscopic radical prostatectomy is still evolving and improving. The present status is the basis for future questions. Therefore, laparoscopy is a step towards improving our knowledge of surgery in the care of patients with prostate cancer.

References

1. Schuessler W, Schulam P, Clayman R, et al. Laparoscopic radical prostatectomy: initial short-term experience. Urology 1997; 50:854–7.

2. Griffith D, Schuessler W, Nickell K, et al. Laparoscopic pelvic lymphadenectomy for prostatic adenocarcinoma. Urol Clin North Am 1992; 19:407–15.

3. Bader P, Burkhard F, Markwalder R, Sutuder UE. Is a limited lymph node dissection an adequate staging procedure for prostate cancer? J Urol 2002; 168:514–18.

4. Guillonneau B, Vallancien G. Laparoscopic radical prostatectomy: initial experience and preliminary assessment after 65 operations. Prostate 1999; 39:71–5.

5. Bollens R, Vanden Bossche M, Roumeguere T, et al. Extraperitoneal laparoscopic radical prostatectomy. Results after 50 cases. Eur Urol 2001; 40:65–9.

6. Raboy A, Ferzli G, Albert P. Initial experience with extraperitoneal endoscopic radical retropubic prostatectomy. Urology 1997; 50:849–53.

7. Gill IS, Zippe CD. Laparoscopic radical prostatectomy: technique. Urol Clin North Am 2001; 28:423–36.

8. Rassweiler J, Sentker L, Seemann O, et al. Laparoscopic radical prostatectomy with the Heilbronn technique: an analysis of the first 180 cases. J Urol 2001; 166:2101–8.

9. Hoznek A, Salomon L, Rabii R, et al. Vesicourethral anastomosis during laparoscopic radical prostatectomy: the running suture method. J Endourol 2000; 14:749–53.

10. Abbou CC, Hoznek A, Salomon L, et al. Laparoscopic radical prostatectomy with a remote controlled robot. J Urol 2001; 165:1964–6.

11. Pasticier G, Rietbergen JB, Guillonneau B, et al. Robotically assisted laparoscopic radical prostatectomy: feasibility study in men. Eur Urol 2001; 40:70–4.

12. Tewari A, Peabody J, Sarle R, et al. Technique of da Vinci robot-assisted anatomic radical prostatectomy. Urology 2002; 60:569–72.

13. Dahl DM, L'esperance JO, Trainer AF, et al. Laparoscopic radical prostatectomy: initial 70 cases at a U.S. university medical center. Urology 2002; 60:859–6.

14. Tuerk I, Deger S, Winkelmann B, et al. Laparoscopic radical prostatectomy. Technical aspects and experience with 125 cases. Eur Urol 2001; 40:46–52.

15. Guillonneau B, Rozet F, Cathelineau X, et al. Perioperative complications of laparoscopic radical prostatectomy: the Montsouris 3-year experience. J Urol 2002; 167:5 1–6.

16. Guillonneau B, Gupta R, El Fettouh H, et al. Laparoscopic management of rectal injury during laparoscopic radical prostatectomy. J Urol 2003; 169:1694–6.

17. Bishoff JT, Allaf ME, Kirkels W, et al. Laparoscopic bowel injury: incidence and clinical presentation. J Urol 1999; 161:887–90.

18. Salomon L, Levrel O, de la Taille A, et al. Radical prostatectomy by the retropubic, perineal and laparoscopic approach: 12 years of experience in one center. Eur Urol 2002; 42:104–10.

19. Ohori M, Wheeler TM, Kattan MW, et al. Prognostic significance of positive surgical margins in radical prostatectomy specimens. J Urol 1995; 154:1818–24.

20. Guillonneau B, El-Fettouh H, Baumert H, et al. Laparoscopic radical prostatectomy: oncological evaluation after 1,000 cases at Montsouris Institute. J Urol 2003; 169:1261–6.

21. Eden CG, Cahill D, Vass JA, et al. Laparoscopic radical prostatectomy: the initial UK series. BJU Int 2002; 90:876–82.

22. Fromont G, Guillonneau B, Validire P, Vallancien G. Laparoscopic radical prostatectomy. Preliminary pathologic evaluation. Urology 2002; 60:661–5.

23. Sofer M, Hamilton-Nelson KL, Schlesselman JJ, Soloway MS. Risk of positive margins and biochemical recurrence in relation to nerve-sparing radical prostatectomy. J Clin Oncol 2002; 20:1853–8.

24. Bangma C, Chadia W, Schröder F. Cutaneous metastasis following laparoscopic pelvic lymphadenectomy for prostatic carcinoma. J Urol 1995; 153:1635.

25. Barrett PH, Fentie DD, Taranger L. Laparoscopic radical nephrectomy with morcellation for renal cell carcinoma: the Saskatoon experience. Urology 1998; 52:23–8.

26. Castilho LN, Fugita OEH, Mitre AI, Arap S. Port site tumor recurrences of renal cell carcinoma after video laparoscopic radical nephrectomy. J Urol 2001; 165:519.

27. Sebesta M, Crespedes RD, Luhman E, et al. Questionnaire-based outcomes of urinary incontinence and satisfaction rates after radical prostatectomy in a national study population. Urology 2002; 60:1055–8.

28. Eastham JA, Kattan MW, Rogers E, et al. Risk factors for urinary incontinence after radical prostatectomy. J Urol 1996; 156:1707–13.

29. Geary ES, Dendinger TE, Freiha FS, Stamey TA. Incontinence and vesical neck strictures following radical retropubic prostatectomy. Urology 1995; 45:1000.

30. Olsson LE, Salomon L, Nadu A, et al. Prospective patient-reported continence after laparoscopic radical prostatectomy. Urology 2001; 58:570–2.

31. Kim ED, Nath R, Kadmon D, et al. Bilateral nerve graft during radical retropubic prostatectomy: 1 year follow-up. J Urol 2001; 165:1950–6.

32. Tuerk I, Deger S, Morgan WR, et al. Sural nerve graft during laparoscopic radical prostatectomy. initial experience. Urolog Oncol 2002; 7:191–4.

33. Katz R, Salomon L, Hoznek A, et al. Patient reported sexual function following laparoscopic radical prostatectomy. J Urol 2002; 168:2078–82.

21

Laparoscopic robotic-assisted radical prostatectomy

Jeffrey Evans, Ashutosh Tewari, Robert Moore, and Mani Menon

Introduction

Prostate cancer surgical therapy has evolved dramatically since Young's pioneering radical perineal prostatectomy almost 100 years ago. Millin introduced the radical retropubic approach in 1947, but it was not used commonly until the 1970s secondary to complications with hemorrhage, impotence and incontinence. Since that time, significant advances in the understanding of neurovascular anatomy by pioneers such as Walsh have dramatically improved the mortality and morbidity of the procedures. Walsh states that the three goals of the surgeon, in order of importance, are cancer control, preservation of urinary control, and preservation of sexual function.[1] Many urologic surgeons have proposed a fourth, albeit less important consideration, a minimally invasive approach to the operation that would provide a faster recovery with decreased postoperative discomfort.

In efforts to achieve the above stated goals, Schuessler et al described the first laparoscopic radical prostatectomy in 1992.[2] Subsequent efforts have been undertaken by experienced French laparoscopic urologists Guillonneau and Vallancien[3] and others. Unfortunately, these and other authors have reported a very difficult learning curve and positive margin rates of approximately 20%.[3,4] However, they have found that patients treated with this technique have enjoyed similar continence and erectile function rates, with arguably less postoperative discomfort and quicker recovery times.[3-7] The risk of perioperative complications is similar to the open technique.[8,9]

Robots have been utilized to perform repetitive tasks in many industries. Recently, robotic technologies have been adapted for surgery. This technology offers the surgeon the ability to perform complex operative maneuvers, improves surgical precision, optics and camera control, and makes techniques such as suture placement and intracorporeal knotting easier with minimal operative experience. Thus, using minimally invasive surgical robots potentially enables the surgeon to make a smoother transition from an open surgical technique to a minimally invasive one. Robotic assistance offers an open surgeon sophisticated tools to perform complex laparoscopic surgery. This chapter leaves the discussion of standard laparoscopic radical prostatectomy and the use of robotics in urology to other chapters in this book and focuses on the technique of robotic radical prostatectomy using the da Vinci Surgical System (Intuitive Surgical, Inc., Sunnyvale, California). The technique and results reported here are largely based on the experience of the surgical team at the Vattikuti Urological Institute, Henry Ford Hospital. We will also discuss the controversy of such intervention and the feasibility of telesurgery.

Indications

It is well established that patients with nodal or metastatic disease do not benefit from operative intervention.[10] Patients with locally advanced disease have a significantly worse prognosis and it is imperative that negative surgical margins are obtained. Given the preceding statements, we encourage considering a minimally invasive approach in patients who are suspected of having organ-confined disease based on prostate-specific antigen (PSA), Gleason score, and digital rectal examination. Men with Gleason score > 5 prostate cancers with a Charlson comorbidity score of < 3 are candidates for this procedure.

Patients should be questioned regarding previous abdominal surgery, peritonitis, and orthopedic or neurologic ailments. A history of stroke or cerebral aneurysm is a relative contraindication because the patient will be in pronounced Trendelenburg position for several hours. Previous abdominal surgery is not a contraindication.

da Vinci Surgical System

The da Vinci Surgical System comprises the surgeon's control console and the surgical arm unit (Table 21.1 and Figure 21.1).

Table 21.1 *Components of da Vinci Surgical System*

Surgeon's control console:
- Three-dimensional video screen with one monitor for each eye
- Handles/surgical master (adjustment of motion scale: 2:1, 3:1, 5:1)
- Foot controls (camera control, electrocautery/harmonic scalpel, clutch function)

Surgical arm unit:
- Two robotic arms matched to surgical master via 8 mm port (EndoWrist technology with six degrees of freedom)
- One robotic arm for endoscopic camera via 12 mm port (two high-intensity light sources with two charge-coupled three-chip cameras in a single 0° or 30° instrument)

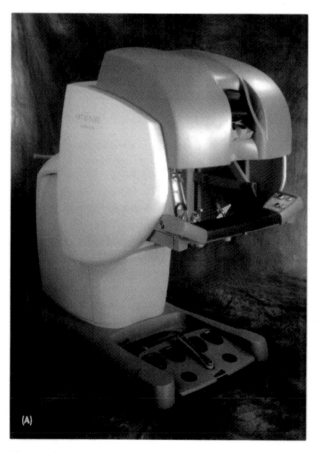

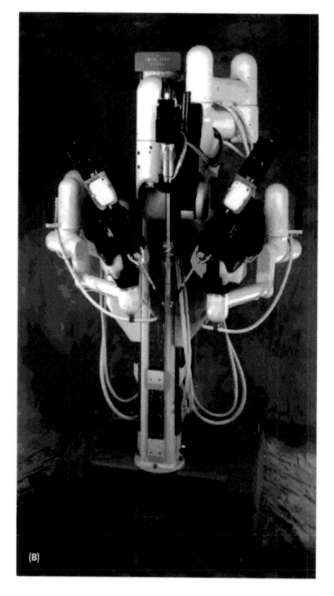

Figure 21.1

(A) Surgeon's control console and (B) surgical arm unit.

Surgeon's control console

The purpose of the console is to provide the surgeon with a sensory experience that is similar to the open surgical approach (Figure 21.1). This is accomplished using a three-dimensional video screen and handles known as the master controls and foot controls.

The optics of the device provide information that is a significant advance over that of the two-dimensional information provided by standard laparoscopy. The endoscope consists of two high-intensity illuminators and two camera devices to provide a high-resolution, three-dimensional image that allows a 5–10 × magnification, which is determined by the distance of the camera to the object (Figure 21.2).

The camera has 0 and 30° lenses. The 30° lens can be oriented upward or downward for adequate visualization.

Foot pedals at the console lock and unlock the camera. The hand controls allow precise movement of the camera when the foot pedal is in the unlocked position. Refocusing can also be accomplished with the foot pedals.

Surgical arm unit

The surgical arm unit consists of three individual devices that control two surgical instruments and the endoscope via input from the hand controls and foot pedals from the surgeon's control console. A variety of surgical instruments are available and are easily interchanged from the surgical arms by the assistants at the operative site (Figure 21.3).

Every motion of the master handles has a response from the 'slave manipulators'. The movements are detected by high-resolution sensors that transfer the movement based on an adjustment motion scale of 2:1, 3:1, or 5:1. This allows for very precise movements by the robot. Additionally, the end effectors of the device increase the degrees of freedom allowed by standard laparoscopy from four to six, aided by the EndoWrist technology, which simulates the action of the human wrist. This can be extremely useful when addressing problematic portions of the operation such as sparing the neurovascular bundles, ligation of the dorsal vein and, most importantly, suturing the urethrovesical anastomosis.

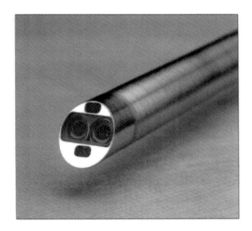

Figure 21.2
A 30° endoscopic camera.

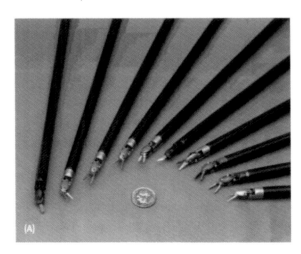
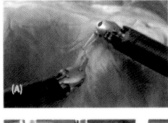
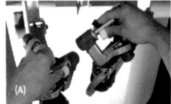
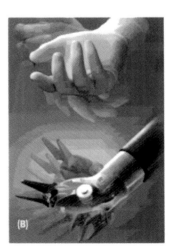

Figure 21.3
(A) Multiple instruments are available to be interchanged with the surgical arm unit. These are controlled via the surgical master handles. (B) EndoWrist technology allows increased flexibility and six degrees of freedom.

Procedure[11,12]

Position

It is imperative to position the patient properly prior to initiating the procedure. The patient is placed in the supine position with adequate padding of the pressure points and shoulder, back, legs, and arms. We use gel pads for the patient's back. Cotton pads are used to protect the axilla and other pressure points. The arms are tucked along the patient's torso and the hands are protected with egg crate foam padding.

The surgical arm unit is quite bulky and must be placed at the foot of the bed for adequate port placement. The length of the arms necessitates either bringing the unit in with the legs splayed laterally or deflecting the legs toward the floor. Care must be taken to adequately pad the lower extremities. The patient is placed in maximal Trendelenburg position to allow the intestines to retract cephalad and provide better pelvic exposure.

Port placement

Proper port placement is critical to this procedure. Three robotic ports and two standard ports are placed in an infraumbilical position after pneumoperitoneum is achieved with a Veress needle introduced through an upper left abdominal quadrant or umbilical puncture. The da Vinci instruments are placed medially. The 12 mm port for the camera is placed at the umbilicus. The remainder of the ports are placed with the 30° up lens to visualize the abdominal wall. The two 8 mm ports are placed caudal and lateral to the camera to avoid interference. They are inserted approximately 10 cm from the midline on a line joining the anterosuperior iliac spine to the umbilicus. The assistants should place their ports superior and lateral to the da Vinci 8 mm ports. Two additional ports are placed in the right side for retraction, suture placement, and suction purposes by the first assistant. The lateral assistant port is 10 mm and the medial one is 5 mm. A sixth 5 mm assistant port may be placed lateral and slightly inferior to the left robotic port. The last laparoscopic cannula is not essential but facilitates retraction, and forces a sometimes unwilling assistant to participate in the operation.

Space within the narrow male pelvis can be quite limited. It is important to place the ports as high within the abdomen as possible where the abdominal surface is broad. Conversely, it is necessary to ensure that the end effectors can adequately reach the distal-most portion of the prostate where the critical portions of the operation occur such as ligation of the dorsal venous complex, dissection of the prostatic apex, and formation of the urethrovesical anastomosis. The authors feel that this is one of the more difficult portions of the learning curve to master. A gestalt of where to place the instruments, based on the patient's length and pelvic structure, must evolve with each procedure performed.

Assistants and telesurgery

Communication between the surgeon and the assistants is imperative. Because the surgeon is displaced from the operative field, he is unaware of what is occurring on the operative field and back table. His only sensory input is via the console. His assistants must be vocal. Conversely, the surgeon must direct his assistants clearly. A microphone system is available to the surgeon so that he can be clearly heard without vocal strain. It can be quite frustrating for the surgeon to maneuver around his assistants' instruments in the limited operative field. Also, he depends on the assistants to rapidly change his end effectors and camera smoothly, place suture material into the surgical field, provide adequate suction–irrigation, and for retraction of the bladder and prostate.

Communication is one of the most critical portions of the operation, but it becomes paramount when telesurgery is being contemplated. Remote robotic prostatectomy has not been performed to date, but other remote procedures such as laparoscopic cholecystectomy have been performed with success.[13] This is a tremendous feat of advanced telecommunications with real-time responses from the surgical arm via a remote console. The skills of the surgical assistants in this setting are even more critical, as port placement and possible conversion to an open procedure are mandatory when performing this surgical modality.

Surgical steps

Creation of the working space

We begin the dissection anteriorly using the 30° lens, looking up. The parietal peritoneum covers the bladder anteriorly and the rectum posteriorly. Between these two structures lie the vasa deferentia, the pelvic vessels, and the distal ureters. The operating surgeon holds the da Vinci long-tip grasper in the dominant hand, and the hook electrocautery in the nondominant hand. The broad, sweeping moves of traditional laparoscopy must be abandoned in favor of fine, finger control. The initial incision is made just above the pubic symphysis. The incision should be low as possible, but high enough to avoid entering the dome of the bladder. It may be useful to start the incision on either side of the medial umbilical ligaments, and to end with urachal transection. The incision is carried down vertically to the vasa, and up to the iliac bifurcation if a lymphadenectomy is being performed. The extraperitoneal space is developed and the bladder is 'dropped' posteriorly.

Lymph node dissection

A standard pelvic lymphadenectomy is performed using the 30° down lens for visualization. We prefer to use a wide field of vision so that the major vessels are always in the field. A 1:3 scaling is used so that the dissection is more precise.

Exposure of the prostatic apex

We use the 0° lens and a 1:3 nonscaling mode for this part of the operation. The tissue is swept away from the pubic symphysis, exposing the endopelvic fascia and puboprostatic ligaments. The levator fibers are mobilized off the prostate to clear a space around the apex. Several venous tributaries may be encountered in this region and should be controlled with bipolar cautery. We leave the puboprostatic ligaments intact and limit the urethra dissection prior to placement of the dorsal vein stitch. This approach has improved our early continence results, with 90% of our patients being free of pads at 8 weeks.

Dorsal vein stitch

The 0° or 30° up lens are used for the dorsal vein stitch without scaling. We use laparoscopic-length suture (6 inch) on a CT-1 needle (0 braided, polyglactin suture with a 36 mm taper needle; Ethicon, Somerville, New Jersey) to control the dorsal venous plexus with two simple stitches over the urethra and at the mid prostate. The prostatic stitch is placed primarily for traction and rotation of the prostate during posterior dissection, not to decrease back-bleeding.

Bladder neck transection

The 30° 'down' lens gives the surgeon the ability to precisely dissect the bladder neck. The prostatovesical junction is usually at the point at which loose fat can no longer be swept off the prostate. With experience, one can identify a shallow groove between the prostate and bladder and the horizontally oriented detrusor fibers. Sometimes the prostatovesical junction is demarcated better laterally than at the midline. Using the electrocautery hook, the bladder neck is incised to expose the Foley catheter. There should be no oozing at this stage of the operation. If bleeding is present, the surgeon may be in the prostate. The balloon is deflated and pulled anteriorly toward the ceiling by the assistant to expose the posterior bladder neck. The

posterior bladder neck should be incised precisely, maintaining a clear detrusor margin for the subsequent urethrovesical anastomosis. After transecting the posterior bladder neck, the anterior layer of Denonvilliers' fascia is transected. The vas deferens is dissected for about 3 inches and then transected, coagulating its vascular supply. The seminal vesicles are dissected out. The deferential artery and seminal vesicle pedicles (at the tip) are controlled using a wristed da Vinci bipolar forceps. Care is taken to avoid using excessive electrical currents, because the neurovascular bundles lie very close to the tips of the seminal vesicles. The remaining attachments between the bladder and prostate are divided with electrocautery to expose the lateral pedicles of the prostate.

Lateral pedicle control and preservation of neurovascular bundles

Using both blunt and sharp dissection, we expose the lateral prostatic pedicles. Early on in our experience, we controlled the pedicles with ligating clips. However, we have seen 4 patients in whom there was delayed migration of the clips into the urethra. Therefore, the pedicles are dissected until we identify the urethral branches of the prostatic artery. These run into the base of the prostate and are individually coagulated, preserving the capsular artery. If nerve sparing is planned, we enter the plane between the layers of prostatic fascia and dissect away the neurovascular bundle. We use the articulated robotic scissors to incise the lateral prostatic fascia anterior and parallel to the neurovascular bundles. Once the correct plane is entered, most of the dissection occurs in a relatively avascular plane. Appropriate traction of the prostate is important to identify the correct plane of dissection. This dissection is carried out as far downward as possible and lateral to the convexity of the prostate.

Dissection behind the prostate

Once both the vas deferens and seminal vesicles have been dissected free, they are pulled upward by the left-sided assistant. This maneuver places the Denonvilliers' fascia on tension, and a faint plane between the rectum and prostate is visible. The posterior dissection plane, at least at the prostatovesical junction, is within layers of Denonvilliers' fascia. In this location, the magnified field shows that there are multiple layers of fascia. In conventional radical prostatectomy, this dissection is carried out behind all layers of Denonvilliers' fascia, and between the rectum and the fascia. We were concerned that we may have a high incidence of positive margins with dissection between the planes; however, this has not been the case. Therefore, we continue to dissect in between the layers of Denonvilliers' fascia because it leaves an added protective fascial layer over the rectum. The distal limit of this dissection is the prostatic apex.

Apical dissection of the prostate

We use a 0° lens with 1:3 scaling to incise the dorsal venous complex and urethra. Using an electro-hook or scissors, the prostatic end of the puboprostatic ligaments and the dorsal vein complex are incised perpendicular to the urethra. To minimize the possibility of a positive apical margin, the anterior wall of the urethra is transected with the scissors 5–10 mm distal to the apex of the prostate. The posterior wall of the urethra and the rectourethralis muscle are transected. The freed specimen is then placed in an EndoCatch1 (US Surgical Corp., Norwalk, Connecticut) specimen retrieval bag.

In our series, as well as in most open radical prostatectomy series, the most common location of positive margins is at the apex.[14] The articulated scissors and three-dimensional visualization allow precise periurethral biopsies without sacrificing urethral length. These biopsies are sent for frozen section. In the rare instance (5% in our series) that they are found to be positive, additional biopsies are taken from the appropriate location. The above approach decreases positive apical margins significantly.

Urethrovesical anastomosis

The tails of a 6 inch dyed and a 6 inch undyed RB1 (3-0 braided, Monocryl suture on a 17 mm taper needle; Ethicon, Somerville, New Jersey) suture are tied together to create a single 12 inch suture with a knot in the middle and a needle at either end. Using the dyed end, the anastomosis is started by passing the needle from outside in at the 4 o'clock position on the bladder and inside out on the urethra. We continue suturing clockwise until the 10 o'clock position. The assistant holds the stitch taut. We then start the undyed end of the suture, passing it outside in on the urethra and then inside out on the bladder. This suture is run counterclockwise until the 11 o'clock position. The needles are cut off, and the free dyed and undyed ends are tied together. This stitch allows completion of the entire urethrovesical anastomosis with a single intracorporeal knot. Importantly, the anastomosis is watertight. A drain is seldom necessary.

Preliminary results

Data collection is complete on 200 of the first 250 patients who underwent surgery by Dr Menon. Table 21.2 summa-

rizes some of the variables. A Gleason score of ≥ 7 for cancer was noted in 57% of patients. The average body mass index (BMI) was high (28); 86% patients had pathologic stage pT2a to pT2b, and the remaining patients were classified as pT3. The mean operative time was 160 min and the mean blood loss was 153 ml. No patient required intraoperative blood transfusion and the mean postoperative hematocrit value was 39%.

Table 21.2 also lists the perioperative complications. The port-site hernias and ileus were seen in our earlier cases. We have had 1 ileus and no hernias in the last 150 cases. The return of sexual function was also evaluated. We noted that at 6 months, 82% men who were < 60 years old had return of sexual function and 64% had sexual intercourse. Additionally, 96% of patients were either free of having to wear pads or were using a liner for security reasons, and 4% were using ≥ 1 pads. Patients who were dry or using a liner were 'mostly satisfied' to 'delighted' with the quality of life because of urinary symptoms, whereas those wearing pads were 'mostly dissatisfied' or 'unhappy' with the quality of life. Forty patients were discharged within 4–6 hours after surgery.

Discussion

The advances in treating prostate cancer over the last 100 years are astounding. Many feel that robotic prostatectomy is the next evolution in surgical therapy of this condition. There is no debate that significant advances have been made in robotic technology, and that this procedure is technically feasible and possibly comparable to the open technique in regards to outcome. However, some argue that the expense involved, difficult learning curve, and arguably modest benefit in hospital stay make this modality unnecessary.[15–17] Some people consider robotic prostatectomy is nothing more than a marketing scheme.[17] We acknowledge the concerns of these authors, but we and other authors feel that this technique holds promise and warrants more investigation.[18–24] The enhanced visual acuity, precision movements afforded by the adjusted motion scaling, six degrees of freedom available with EndoWrist technology, and ability to aid practitioners with less experience from a remote location are very attractive features of any robotic procedure. Prospective randomized trials of open, standard laparoscopic and robotic prostatectomy will answer this controversy, but we are doubtful that they will ever be done, given patient and surgeon emotions. Perhaps a prospective cohort study of results obtained by expert surgeons, using a common approach to evaluate outcomes, may prove to be a surrogate for randomized trials.

Table 21.2 *Baseline, operative, oncologic, and postoperative variables (single team's experience of first 200 cases)*

Variable	Value
Age (years), mean ± SD (range)	59.9 ± 7.1 (42–76)
BMI, mean ± SD (range)	27.7 ± 2.8 (19–38)
Serum PSA (ng/ml), mean ± SD (range)	6.4 ± 2.47 (0.6–41)
Clinical Stage, n (%):	
T1c	80 (49.7)
T2a	17 (10.6)
T2b	64 (39.6)
Gleason score (biopsy), n (%):	
6	135 (66.5)
7	56 (27.6)
8	8 (3.9)
9	4 (1.9)
Pathologic stage, n (%):	
T2a	28 (14.7)
T2b	137 (72.1)
T3a	13 (6.8)
T3b	12 (6.3)
Gleason score (histopathologic specimen), n (%):	
6	86 (43)
7	92 (46)
8	16 (8)
9	6 (3)
Specimen weight (cm³)	45.3 ± 12.3 (18–122)
Percentage cancer, mean ± SD (range)	19 ± 9.8 (1–80)
Node status (%)	0.5
Positive margins (%):	6
Focal	5
Extensive	1
Operative time (min), mean ± SD (range)	160 ± 28 (71–315)
Intraoperative blood loss (ml)	153
Blood tranfusions (%)	0
Mean hemoglobin at discharge (g/dl)	13
Pain score on first postoperative day	3

Table 21.2 *Continued*

Variable	Value
Catheterization time (days)	7
Hospital days	1.2
Undetectable postoperative PSA at 6months (%)	92
Discharge within 24 hours (%)	93
Complications (*n*)	
Port hernia	3/200
Ileus	3/200
Delayed bleeding	1/200
DVT	1/200
Potency after VIP using an EPIC quality of life instrument:	
Any sexual activity (%):	
Men < 60 years old:	
3 months	65
6 months	82
Men > 60 years old:	
3 months	50
6 months	75
Sexual intercourse (%):	
Men < 60 years old:	
3 months	25
6 months	64
Men > 60 years:	
3 months	10
6 months	38

BMI, body mass index; PSA, prostate-specific antigen; DVT, deep vein thrombosis. VIP, Vattikuti Institute Prostatectomy; EPIC, expanded prostate cancer index composite.

References

1. Walsh P. Anatomic radical retropubic prostatectomy. In: Walsh PC, Retik AB, Vaughan ED, et al, eds. Campbell's urology, 8th edn. Philadelphia: WB Saunders, 2002; Chapter 90: 2565–88.

2. Schuessler WW, Kavoussi LR, Clayman RV, et al. Laparoscopic radical prostatectomy: initial case report. J Urol 1992; 147: 246A.

3. Guillonneau B, Vallancien G. Laparoscopic radical prostatectomy: the Montsouris technique. J Urol 2000; 163:1643–9.

4. Guillonneau B, Cathelineau X, Doublet JD, Vallancien G. Laparoscopic radical prostatectomy: the lessons learned. J Endourol 2001; 15(4):441–5.

5. Rassweiler J, Sentker L, Seemann O, et al. Laparoscopic radical prostatectomy with the Heilbronn technique: an analysis of the first 180 cases. J Urol 2001; 166(6):2101–8.

6. Olsson LE, Salomon, Nadu A, et al. Prospective patient-reported continence after laparoscopic radical prostatectomy. Urology 2001; 58(4):570–2.

7. Vallancien G, Cathelineau X, Baumert H, et al. Complications of transperitoneal laparoscopic surgery in urology: review of 1,311 procedures at a single center. J Urol 2002; 168(1):23–6.

8. Lepor H, Nieder AM, Ferrandino MN. Intraoperative and postoperative complications of radical retropubic prostatectomy in a consecutive series of 1,000 cases. J Urol 2001; 166(5):1729–33.

9. Guillonneau B, Rozet F, Cathelineau X, et al. Perioperative complications of laparoscopic radical prostatectomy: the Montsouris 3-year experience. J Urol 2002; 167(1):51–6.

10. Gervas LA, Mata J, Easley JD, et al. Prognostic significance of lymph node metastasis in prostate cancer. J Urol 1989; 142:332–6.

11. Menon M, Tewari A, Peabody J, members of the VIP team. Vattikuti Institute: prostatectomy techniques. J Urol 2003; 169(6):2289–92.

12. Monon M, Tewari A, members of the Vattikuti Institute. Prostatectomy team. Urology 2003; 61(Suppl, 4A): 15–20.

13. Kim VD, Chapman WH, Albrecht RJ, et al. Early experience with telemanipulative robot-assisted laparoscopic cholecystectomy using da Vinci. Surg Laparosc Endosc Percutan Tech 2002; 12(1):33–40.

14. Epstein JI. Pathologic assessment of the surgical specimen. Urol Clin North Am 2001; 28:567–94.

15. Kavoussi LR. Laparoscopic radical prostatectomy: irrational exuberance? Urology 2001; 58(4):503–5.

16. Cadeddu JA, Kavoussi LR. Laparoscopic radical prostatectomy: is it feasible and reasonable? Urol Clin North Am 2001; 28(3):655–61.

17. Gallucci M, Vincenzoni A. Laparoscopic radical prostatectomy: a marketing or surgical strategy? Curr Opin Urol 2001; 11:305–8.

18. Abbou CC, Hoznek A, Salomon L, et al. Laparoscopic radical prostatectomy with remote controlled robot. J Urol 2001; 165(6 Pt 1):1964–6.

19. Abbou CC, Hoznek A, Salomon L, et al. Remote laparoscopic radical prostatectomy carried out with a robot. Report of a case. Prog Urol 2000; 10(4):520–3.

20. Binder J, Kramer W. Robotically-assisted laparoscopic radical prostatectomy. BJU Int 2001; 87(4):408–10.

21. Pasticier G, Rietbergen JB, Guillonneau B, et al. Robotically assisted laparoscopic radical prostatectomy: feasibility study in men. Eur Urol 2001; 40(1):70–4.

22. Samadi DB, Nadu A, Olson E, et al. Robot assisted laparoscopic radical prostatectomy – initial experience in eleven patients. J Urol 2002; 167(4) Suppl: 390(1445).

23. Abbou C, Hoznek A, Ollson L, et al. Telerobotic laparoscopic radical prostatectomy. J Urol 2002; 167(4), Suppl: 180(721).

24. Menon M, Shrivastava A, Baize B, et al. Robot-assisted anatomic subperitoneal prostatectomy: a stereoscopic video. J Urol 2002; 167(4), Suppl: 180(722).

22

Brachytherapy for treatment of prostate cancer

Serdar Deger

Brachytherapy is defined as any local application using radioactive isotopes. About 1901, Pierre Curié was the first to have the vision of using a radioactive source for local treatment of malignancies. Paschkis, Pasteau, Degrais, and Denning were the pioneers between 1910 and 1922 who used radium in the urethra.[1–3] Barringer inserted radium needles into the prostate in 1915.[4] In the mid 1950s, low-energy radioisotopes were developed. In 1952, Flocks injected colloidal gold into the prostate. In 1970, the Sloan Memorial Kettering Cancer Center (MSKCC) started to test iodine 125 for prostate cancer.

In the 1990s, technical changes made brachytherapy an attractive treatment alternative for lower tumor stages.

There are two defined brachytherapy categories: low dose rate (LDR) and high dose rate (HDR) brachytherapy. The two differ in dose rates of radioisotopes and treatment strategies. Common radioisotopes for LDR brachytherapy are iodine-125 (I^{125}) and palladium-103 (Pd^{103}), whereas gold-198 (Au^{198}) and iridium-192 (Ir^{192}) are radioisotopes for HDR treatment.

Table 22.1 shows the radiobiologic differences between these isotopes.

Low dose rate brachytherapy
Iodine-125 and palladium-103

Iodine-125 was introduced in 1970 by Hilaris and Whitmore using an open retropubic approach (Figure 22.1). As a radioisotope with a long half-life of 60 days, which allowed a continuous irradiation, at first it evoked euphoria.[5,6] Unfortunately, data between 1970 and 1980 clarified that iodine was not suitable for patients who had capsule invasive disease and/or undifferentiated cancer.

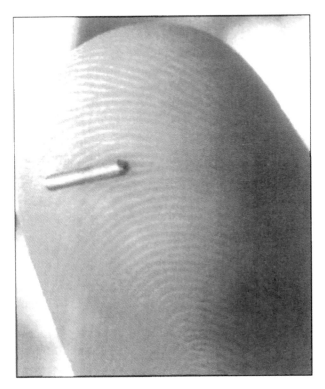

Figure 22.1
An I^{125} seed. Reproduced with permission from New perspective in prostate cancer, 2nd edn., Belldegrun A, Kirby RS, Newling DWW, eds. Oxford: Isis Medical Media Ltd., 2000; 184, Figure 17.1.

Table 22.1 *Radiobiologic features of commonly used radionuclides*

Source	Half-life (days)	Energy (kEV)	Initial dose rate (cGy/h)
Permanent			
I^{125}	60.2	28	5.8
Pd^{103}	17	21	15.3
Au^{198}	2.7	412	21.4 – 27
Temporary			
Ir^{192}	74.2	380	60–90

Palladium-103 (Pd[103]) was introduced in 1987. Characteristics of Pd[103] are similar to I[125]. It emits a low-energy photon with an average energy of 21 keV, and has a half-life of 17 days.[7,8] The first consideration was that tumors with an increased proliferative rate should respond better to Pd[103] and tumors with low doubling rate should respond better to I[125]. However, there have been no clinical trials to verify this consideration.[9]

In the early 1990s technical improvements, such as 3-D computer planning systems with online planning modalities and transrectal ultrasound (TRUS), led to an increase of LDR treatments in patients with prostate cancer.

The introduction of prostate-specific antigen (PSA) enabled prostate cancer to be diagnosed in the early stages, which allowed a better patient selection. Patients were separated in different risk groups (low-, intermediate-, and high-risk groups) and dose descriptions were adapted to those.

In 1995, the American Association of Physics and Medicine Task Group No. 43 (TG-43) recommended an algorithm for calculating the doses of I[125] and Pd[103].[10] The American Brachytherapy Society (ABS) recommended adaptation of these doses for Pd[103] and revised the dose of I[125] to unify LDR dosimetry. Patients with I[125] implants were to receive 144 Gy, and patients with Pd[103] implants were calculated to receive 115–120 Gy using the point source approximation.[11–13]

According to the ABS recommendations, candidates for an LDR monotherapy are stage T1–T2a, Gleason score 2–6, and PSA < 10 ng/ml. Patients with clinical stage T2b–T2c or Gleason score 8–10 or PSA > 20 ng/ml need an additional external radiotherapy. LDR was relatively contraindicated for patients with increased risk factors to develop complications, such as a high AUA (American Urological Association) symptom score, a large median lobe, history of multiple pelvic surgery, previous pelvic irradiation, technical difficulties which may result in inadequate dose coverage, severe diabetes with healing problems, previous transurethral resection of the prostate (TURP), gland size more than 60 ml at the time of implantation, and positive seminal vesicles.[13]

Between 1970 and 1985, 1013 patients with stage T2–T3 lesions were treated with pelvic lymph node resection and I[125] implantations at MSKCC. The approach consisted of an open exploration of the prostate.[6] All rectal and urinary complications resolved spontaneously.[14] The 15-year overall local disease-free survival was 60% in patients with stage T2 and T3 tumors and negative nodes who received a peripheral dose of 140 Gy or more.[15]

Kuban et al defined clinically progression-free survival as no evidence of disease (NED) (in the absence of PSA value).[16] Other study groups, e.g. Peschel et al and Rohloff et al, demonstrated similar results.[17,18]

Radge and Korb published data of 152 patients who were treated with I[125] implants: 98 patients with low-grade/low-stage disease received monotherapy; 54 patients received an additional 45 Gy external radiation. The 10-year disease-free survival (PSA < 0.5 ng/ml) was 60% for the group who received monotherapy and 76% for the combined therapy group.[9]

Beyer and Priestley reported on 489 T1–T2 patients in 1997, with median PSA of 7.3 ng/ml, treated with I[125] monotherapy.[19] The 4-year biochemical disease-free rate was 88% for patients with Gleason score ≤ 4, and 60% for those with Gleason score ≥ 5.

Blasko et al[20] published results of Pd[103] monotherapy (N = 230 patients) with clinical stage T1–T2 tumors (56.1% of the patients had a T2a lesion, 28.3% a T1c lesion). The initial PSA level in 75.7% of the patients was < 10 ng/ml, 40% of the patients had a Gleason score ≥ 7, and the overall biochemical control rate at 9-year follow-up was 83.5% of patients. Failures were local in 3.0%, distant in 6.1%, and PSA progression was observed in 4.3% of patients. Failure was defined as a PSA progression of two consecutive rises in serum PSA. This was different from the ASTRO (American Society of Therapeutic Radiology and Oncology) Consensus Conference definition,[21] which required three rises as definition for failure.

In 2000, Beyer and Brochman published data of 1527 and 695 patients with T1 or T2 Nx–N0M0 prostate cancer treated between December 1988 and December 1995 with either external beam radiation therapy (EBRT) or brachytherapy (BT), respectively. EBRT and BT appeared to be equally efficacious for low-risk patients with T1/T2 tumors and Gleason scores 6 and PSA < 10 ng/dl at 5 years. Patients with Gleason scores 8–10 or PSA between 10 and 20 ng/dl appeared to fare worse with BT alone compared with EBRT. Neither EBRT nor BT were particularly effective for patients presenting with a PSA over 20 ng/dl.[22]

Critz et al combined EBRT with LDR treatment for the early stages of prostate cancer. They reported on about 689 patients treated between 1992 and 1996. Disease-free status was defined as the achievement and maintenance of a PSA nadir of 0.2 ng/ml or less. Median follow-up was 4 years (range 3–7 years). None of these men received neoadjuvant or adjuvant hormonal therapy. Overall 5-year disease-free survival was 88%. Multivariate analysis revealed that pretreatment PSA was the strongest indicator of subsequent disease-free status in regard to Gleason score or clinical stage.[23]

Dattolli et al treated 124 patients with unfavorable risk factors, such as T3 tumor, Gleason score > 6, PSA > 15 ng/ml, with Pd[103] plus external irradiation of 41 Gy. Biochemical progression-free survival was 79% at 3-year follow-up; potency protection was 77%.[24]

Looking at the literature, there are several studies published in regards to LDR brachytherapy, with different definitions of patient risk and biochemical failure. Mostly, patients with a PSA ≤ 10 ng/ml, Gleason score < 7, and stage ≤ T2a were defined as low-risk patients. For these patients, biochemical control was between 50 and 100%. Biochemical failure was defined as a PSA between 0.5 and 1 or, in some series, > 4 ng/ml, or a two-time continuous rise.[19,25–29] In moderate-risk patients, defined as those with a PSA value between 10 and 20 ng/ml, biochemical survival ranged from 45% to 82%.[19,20,28–32] In high-risk patients, characterized by a PSA > 20 ng/ml or a Gleason score > 7, the 5-year biochemical control rates of 30–65% proved unsatisfactory.[19, 20, 29–32]

Combining ERBT with implants improved the 10-year biochemical survival from 64 to 76% (PSA failure definition was PSA > 0.5 ng/ml).[26,33]

The main interest of patients asking for LDR brachytherapy is preservation of potency. Stock et al showed clearly the dosage dependence of sexual potency preservation. Erectile function was assessed using the scoring system of:

- 0 – complete inability to have erections,
- 1 – able to have erections but insufficient for inter-course,
- 2 – can have erections sufficient for intercourse but considered suboptimal and
- 3 – normal erectile function.

In 313 patients with potency score 2 or greater before therapy the no decrease in erectile function score was experienced by 64% and by 30% at 3- and 6-year follow-up. The preservation of potency was 79% and 59% at 3 and 6 years, respectively. Two factors had a significant negative effect on potency in univariate and multivariate analyses. These were high implant dose (D90 > 160 Gy for I[125] and D90 > 100 Gy for Pd[103]) and a pretreatment erectile dysfunction. The rate of potency preservation after brachytherapy was high, but decreased from 3 and 6 years after treatment.[34]

In combination with EBRT, the sexual potency rate dropped in different groups.[27, 35, 36]

Potters et al reported that potency was preserved in 311 of 482 patients, with a 5-year actuarial potency rate of 52.7%. The 5-year actuarial potency rate for patients treated with LDR-brachytherapy as monotherapy was 76%, and for those treated with additional EBRT was 56%. Patients treated with neoadjuvant androgen deprivation (NAAD) had a 5-year potency rate of 52%, whereas those with combination EBRT + LDR brachytherapy + NAAD had a potency rate of 29%. Of 84 patients treated with sildenafil, 52 (62%) had a response.[36]

Rectal complications were rare but grade 3–4 complications (e.g. rectal ulceration, bowel obstruction, fistula formation, proctitis requiring blood transfusion, etc.) were seen. Radiation proctitis following LDR brachytherapy alone occurred in 1–5%.[19,32] Adding EBRT, the rate increases to 7–21%, mostly grade 2–3 complications. Rectal fistula occurred in 1–2.4%.[29, 37–39]

It is difficult to analyze the data for each isotope, due to the absence of prospective randomized trials. The benefit of neoadjuvant-adjuvant hormonal treatment and/or additional EBRT is not documented; data indicate no difference in outcome between I[125] and Pd[103].[29,31,40]

High dose rate brachytherapy
Gold-198

In 1952, Flocks et al introduced gold-198 for the treatment of prostate cancer. Because of a half-life of 2.7 days and penetration depth of 3 mm, gold-198 was ideal for an operative field. In T3 disease, Flocks et al injected 100 mCi of colloidal gold-198 after radical prostatectomy into the pedicles.[41] Complication rate in these patients ($n = 345$) was low; 4.4% of patients had local progression of disease. Progression-free survival in patients with no lymphatic involvement was 74% after 5 years, 66.7% after 10 years, and 27.5% after 15 years treatment.[42]

Colloidal gold-198 was not available after the mid 1970s. Then, gold seeds were implanted into the pedicles after radical prostatectomy. Between 1977 and 1988, 80 patients were treated with this adjuvant radiation therapy (73.8% of them had T3 disease). Ten-year progression-free survival was 84.4% for pT2 tumors and 79.1% for pT3 tumors.[43] In 1997, Loening published long-term follow-up data of patients who were treated with gold seed implantation as primary therapy between 1984 and 1995. The median follow-up was 4 years, and cancer-specific survival was 100% for T1 and T2a, 90% for T2b, and 76% for T3 tumors. The negative biopsy rate 5 years after treatment was 80%. The overall complication rate was low; however, 2 patients developed rectal ulceration, with 1 requiring a colostomy.[44]

Butler et al reported in 1997 the Baylor College experience based on 510 patients, treated between 1965 and 1980. Gold-198 was implanted as boost to an additional EBRT. The implantation was performed by an open retropubic approach. Mean total dose was 69 Gy (45–105 Gy). In this study 23% of the patients had T3 tumor and 30% of patients had lymphatic metastases. Survival rates for all stages were 83 ± 3% after 5 years, 53 ± 5% after 10 years, and 25 ± 10% after 15 years.[45]

The Baylor College group treated 54 patients between 1992 and 1996; 40.7% of these patients had a T1, 50% had a T2 and only 7.4% of them had a T3 lesion. The total dose delivered averaged 71 Gy (59–85 Gy). Additional EBRT was given in 9 patients only. Single acute toxicity was reported in 22 patients and multiple acute toxicity in 20 patients. Toxicity according to the RTOG (Radiation Therapy Oncology Group) toxicity criteria included proctitis in 50.9%, urethritis in 39.5%, and cystitis in 37.7% of patients. Late rectal toxicity occurred in 6.3% and radiation cystitis occurred in 16.7%. No grade III or IV acute or late toxicity was seen. Eighty-one percent of patients with an initial PSA level > 4–10 ng/ml reached a PSA nadir of less than 1 ng/ml, while only 65% with an initial PSA level > 10 ng/ml achieved a PSA nadir < 1 ng/ml. Median follow-up was between 12.5 to 21.6 months.[45] Table 22.2 summarizes progression-free survival data using gold-198.

Iridium-192

The activity of iridium-192 is 16 times higher than that of cobald-60. The half-life of iridium-192 is 74.4 days. Delivered electron energy is between 0.097 and 0.67 MeV. Because of the low gamma energy, radioprotection is much better than with radium: 5 cm lead or 2.6 cm uranium provide enough effective protection.[48] Iridium is used primarily for temporary implant because of its high dose performance. It is used as an LDR and also as an HDR technique.[49,50]

Iridium-192 in an LDR technique has been used since 1977.[51] Tumor control rates of 90–95% were demonstrated, using clinical criteria for failure with follow-up from 1 month to 60 months.[52–60] Because PSA levels are lacking in these studies, the data are currently not useful.

Syed et al published their results on 200 patients who were treated between 1977 and 1985. The open surgical approach was used for placing iridium-192. In addition, 30–40 Gy of external irradiation were given. Local tumor control rates were between 90 and 95.5% and 4–11% of patients had complications such as proctitis and urethral strictures. A significant correlation was found between complications and previously performed TURP. One patient required a colostomy.[61]

In 1986, Porter et al described a transperineal open surgical application with a device called the Micro-Selectron. The MicroSelectron had a plastic ribbon connected to a storage container. Ribbons were fed into a control channel, where they were moved remotely and cut to the desired length. The ribbons were attached to leaders, which were coupled to the MicroSelectron drive system. The system was attached to a patient through a coupling adapter under continuous monitoring.[59] The era of the afterloading technique began with the MicroSelectron system. The advantage of this system is the safety to radiation exposure. Khan et al reported results in 321 patients. The delivered interstitial dose was 3100 cGy to a total dose of 6500 cGy. According to the RTOG system, grade II complications, such as mild dysuria, diarrhea, and proctitis were observed in 0.6–6.5% of the patients, whereas grade III complications were seen in 3 patients. The 5-year local tumor control was 95% for T1c, 93% for T2a, 83.6% for T2b, and 73.1% for T3 tumors.[62]

The establishment of the afterloading technique, based on a treatment plan adapted to the actual geometry of the prostate using computer algorithms to allow a more homogeneous dose within the implant for better tumor coverage, were milestones of modern HDR brachytherapy.

The aim of HDR brachytherapy is to deliver the maximal radiation dose into the prostate while minimizing the radiation dose to the surrounding tissue. Hsu et al published the critical volume tolerance analysis to estimate the potential for further dose escalation using HDR brachytherapy as boost. Dose–volume histograms were plotted for comparison of 7 field conformal EBRT and HDR brachytherapy techniques. Dosage to the normal structures was calculated. The HDR delivered higher doses into the prostate and less to the bladder and rectum.[63]

Different study groups have used HDR brachytherapy in the treatment of localized prostate cancer since the mid 1990s.[64–69] Most data were published by four study groups: the Charité Hospital in Berlin, Germany;[70] the Christian Albert University in Kiel, Germany;[71] the Göteborg-Sahlgrenzka University Hospital in Göteborg, Sweden;[67]

Table 22.2 *The 5- and 10-year progression-free survival using gold-198*

Main author	Progression free survival (%)					Follow-up (years)
	T1		T2		T3	
Loening[44]	100		90		76	5
Butler[45]	76±12	T2a 61±12		T2b 53±16	34±14	10
Carey[46]			60		63	7
Gutierrez[47]			85		43	10
Lannon[49]	83	T2a 91.3		T2b 64.4	50.5	10

and the William Beaumont Hospital (WBH) in Royal Oak, Michigan.[72] Interstitial doses were between 8.25 and 15 Gy in all institutions. Follow-up was between 30 and 98 months. Tumor stages were almost identical, with T3 disease between 13 to 32%. The percentage of T3 disease of the Charité group was 58%: the Charité group performed laparoscopic staging lymph node dissection in all patients. The Sahlgrenzka University Hospital group did a staging lymphadenectomy in only 20 patients. Patients of the William Beaumont Hospital and Christian Albert University had no surgical lymph node staging. Five-year biochemical survival (according to ASTRO criteria[21] with three times rising PSA value, except at Sahlgrenzka University Hospital) as shown in Table 22.3, and ranged from 67% to 84%.

Late grade 2–3 (RTOG) rectal complications were seen in 11% and grade 2–3 urinary complications in 6% of the patients at the Christian Albert University.[71] Late grade 3–4 complications at the Charité occurred in 12.2%, urethral strictures occurred in 7.4%, and 3% of patients suffered from grade 2–3 incontinence; 4 patients developed a rectourethral fistula after rectal ulceration requiring a colostomy. Therefore, the interstitial radiation dose at the Charité was reduced after December 1993 from 10 Gy to 9 Gy per session.[70]

HDR brachytherapy has also been used as monotherapy. In this technique, the template was fixed to the perineum and fractioned interstitial doses of 6 Gy were delivered. The total dose was 48–54 Gy.[73]

Low dose rate technique

Since the introduction of LDR brachytherapy, seed placement was performed with the guidance of a preplanned implantation technique. The preplanned method had a number of disadvantages such as patient positioning and setup, and images taken during the actual implant procedure had to be matched with those obtained during the preimplant planning study. The latter was occasionally difficult to reproduce in the operating room (OR). Alterations in the prostate volume and shape occurred during the interval between preplanning and implantation because of changes in patient position and relaxation of pelvic musculature induced by anesthesia or as a result of hormonal therapy. These changes had caused inaccuracies in an implant based solely on the preplanned images. The preplanning requires a separate TRUS imaging study, which is cumbersome and sometimes difficult to schedule. Furthermore, a separate pubic arch obstruction evaluation study is required in some preplanning techniques.[74]

The ABS reported in 2001 that the preplanned technique for permanent prostate brachytherapy had limitations that could be overcome by an intraoperative planning. They proposed the following terminology in regard to the prostate planning process, with five levels of prostate brachytherapy:

1. Preplanning – creation of an operative plan a few days or weeks before the implant procedure.
2. Intraoperative preplanning – creation of a plan in the OR just before the implant procedure, with immediate execution of the plan.
3. Intraoperative planning (treatment planning in the OR) – the patient and transrectal ultrasound probe are not moved between the volume study and the seed insertion procedure.
4. Interactive planning – stepwise refinement of the treatment plan using computerized dose calculations derived from image-based needle position feedback.
5. Dynamic dose calculation – constant updating of dose distribution using continuous deposited seed position feedback.

The elements of an intraoperative planning system should include the following steps:

- treatment planning in the OR
- image acquisition
- target definition
- organ segmentation (draw contours manually)

Study	No.	Age (years)	Initial median PSA (ng/ml)	Single interstitial dose (Gy)	External dose (Gy)	Follow-up (months)	5-year PFS[a] (%)
Michigan/USA[72]	161	69	9.9	8.25–10.5	46	30	67
Göteborg/Sweden[67]	50	63	–	10	50	45	84[b]
Kiel/Germany[71]	144	68	12.15	9	50	98.4	77.2
Charité/Germany[70]	230	67	12.8	9–10	45–50.4	40.2	69

Table 22.3 *Patient characteristics of high dose rate groups*

[a] Progression-free survival.
[b] Prostate-specific antigen (PSA) 1 ng/ml.

- identification of needle position in relation to prostate
- intraoperative optimization based on imaged needle location
- estimation of seed positions from imaged needle position
- updating of dose calculation based on imaged needle location
- auto organ segmentation
- capturing deposited seed positions in real time
- optimization based on deposited seed location
- dynamic updating of dose calculation based on actual seed position
- account for motion of prostate during placement
- account for intraoperative edema
- postimplant dose calculation at time of surgery
- account for postoperative edema.

Intraoperative preplanning eliminates the preplanning patient visit. Therefore, the approximate number of seeds to be ordered has to be determined from a nomogram or table based on the prostate volume obtained from a computed tomography (CT) scan or an ultrasound (Figure 22.2). TRUS is performed in the OR, and the images are imported in real time into the treatment planning system (Figure 22.3). The target volume, rectum, and urethra are contoured on the treatment planning system either manually or automatically, and a treatment plan is generated. The seeds are implanted into the prostate according to the plan.

Intraoperative preplanning makes two separate TRUS procedures as required in the two-step preplanned method as well as reproducing patient positioning, and setup unnecessary. However, intraoperative preplanning does not account for intraoperative changes in prostate geometry or deviations of needle position from the preplan.[75]

An optimized treatment plan is then performed, the dose–volume histogram (DVH) is generated, and the plan is examined. Seeds can be added or deleted manually, and the new isodose distributions and DVH displays are regenerated if necessary (Figure 22.4). The needles can now be inserted as per plan. In interactive planning, it is critical that the dose calculation is updated based on estimated seed positions derived from actual needle positions. The needles need to be repositioned, or needle positions can be changed in the plan if there are adverse dosimetric consequences. The dose calculation is then updated, based on the actual needle location. The interval at which the dose distribution is recalculated is operator-dependent.

Various interactive planning systems exist: some are commercially available, whereas others are institution-based systems.[74] Commercially available systems include the Interplant system (Burdette Medical System, Champaign, Illinois), PIPER (RTek, Pittsford, New York), SPOT (Nucletron Corporation, Veenandaal, The Netherlands), Strata (Rosses Medical Systems, Columbia,

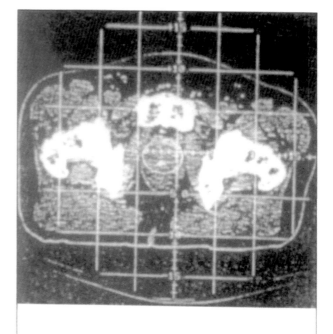

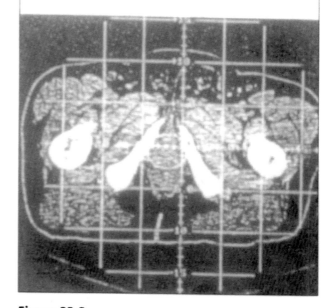

Figure 22.2

Pretreatment CT scans with the traced prostate. Note the relationship between the prostate and pubic arches. Reproduced with permission from New perspective in prostate cancer, 2nd edn., Belldegrun A, Kirby RS, Newling DWW, eds. Oxford: Isis Medical Media Ltd., 2000; 187, Figure 17.2.

Maryland), and VariSeed (Varian Medical Systems, Palo Alto, California). The institution-based systems include those at the MSKCC and Brigham and Women's Hospital in Boston.

In the technique of Stock and Stone et al[76–79] the implantation begins with the insertion of needles, 1 cm apart, into

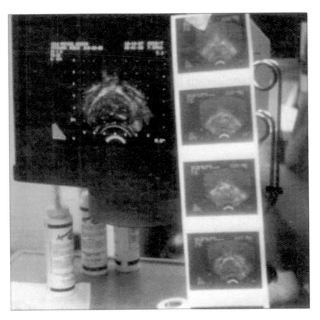

Figure 22.3
Intraoperative transrectal ultrasound images with grid overlay. Reproduced with permission from New perspective in prostate cancer, 2nd edn., Belldegrun A, Kirby RS, Newling DWW, eds. Oxford: Isis Medical Media Ltd., 2000; 188, Figure 17.3.

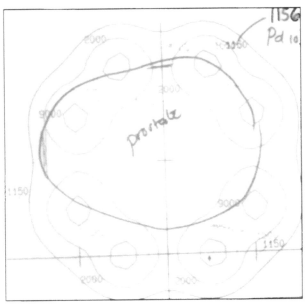

Figure 22.4
A dose–volume histogram of the prostatic apex. The dose drops in the center of the gland. Reproduced with permission from New perspective in prostate cancer, 2nd edn., Belldegrun A, Kirby RS, Newling DWW, eds. Oxford: Isis Medical Media Ltd., 2000; 188, Figure 17.4.

the periphery of the gland at the level of the largest TRUS transverse diameter cut as a guide. The position of the needles is determined on the TRUS images by identifying the echo bright markings, the so-called 'acroflash', of the implanted needles. Seventy-five percent of the seeds are then implanted through these peripheral needles using a Mick applicator. The seed positions are marked on the planning system along the needle track, and isodoses are generated. The remaining 25% of the seeds are implanted using about 6–8 needles in the prostate interior such that they remain 0.5–1 cm from the urethra and cover the periphery of the base and apex. The needle positions in the interior are optimized to limit dose action on normal structures (urethra and rectum) and minimize cold or hot areas within the prostate.

The MSKCC technique[80, 81] relies on an inverse planning optimization program, which uses a genetic algorithm optimization system,[82–85] that attempts to find seed positions on a grid of available or potentially available points. It sites that satisfy the dose constraints for the normal organs, such as the urethra and rectum, while maintaining maximal target coverage with the prescription dose to the prostate. This interactive optimization process analyzes more than 106 possible seed locations to achieve the ideal fit and solution and requires approximately 5–10 min for completion in the operating program. The computer determines the ideal seed location that meets the predetermined dose constraints for the urethra and rectum, and

the target dose. The seeds are loaded using a Mick applicator according to the seed-loading pattern dictated by the plan.

Lo, et al[86] compared the dosimetry results intraoperatively to CT-based evaluation performed 1-month post-implant. They reported a good correlation between intraoperative and postimplant results using intraoperative planning. The mean D90 results intraoperatively compared to those seen postimplant were 178 Gy vs 188.5 Gy for iodine-125 implants and 98 Gy vs 98.5 Gy for boost palladium-103 implants, respectively.

Zelefsky et al demonstrated excellent dose coverage of the prostate with the use of interactive planning.[80] They also showed in a comparative dosimetric analysis of three implant techniques used at MSKCC that lower maximal urethral doses were observed significantly more frequently with the intraoperative computer-generated conformal plan in comparison to a CT preplan approach or an intraoperative ultrasound manually optimized approach.[80,81] Postimplant dosimetric analysis is standard practice following temporary brachytherapy procedures. Its role following permanent implants is less well established. Previous surveys have shown wide variation in dosimetric methods.[87, 88] The ABS organized a panel to develop guidelines for the performance and analysis of postimplant dosimetry.[89] Because the treatment plan and the actual implantation are completed at the time of postimplant analysis, the rationale for its use needs elucidation. The first issue arises from the fact that brachytherapy is an imperfect modality and, certainly, the permanent ultrasound-guided prostate implant technique is no exception. The dose distributions following implantation are not the same as those planned prior to the implant.[90–95] Consequently, it is important to document the actual dose that the prostate and normal adjacent tissues will receive over the life of the implant for evaluating the outcome. Significant underdosing can lead to treatment failure. In this case, additional seed implantation or supplementary EBRT is necessary to achieve the dose.[96] CT-based evaluation of the prostate implant appears to best satisfy the requirements of seed localization target and normal structure delineation and seed-target registration. Because of the possibility of seed migration, the number of implanted seeds may not be the same as the number of seeds present in the prostate at the time of the postimplant CT scan. Therefore, a better approximation of the number of seeds may be obtained by using plane radiographs. The CT technique recommended by the ABS should include the prostate, all the seeds within and around the prostate, and any critical structures for which the dose is to be reported. To accomplish this, it is suggested that a minimum of 2-cm margin be added to the superior and inferior extent of the prostate. A reduced field of view that completely encompasses the volumes and structures of interest, but offers a finer resolution in the plane of the implant, should be used. This reduces the error associated with seed localization and prostate boundary definition. Contiguous axial slices are recommended to reduce the chance of missing seeds between scans. The slice thickness and spacing should not be greater than 5 mm. A catheter placed in the bladder and filled with contrast medium serves to localize the urethra and internal bladder wall. The geometry of the implant, and therefore the dosimetry, is derived directly from the CT images themselves. In some CT scans, the images may contain distortions (such as unequal x and y scaling), and it is important that means of identifying and accounting for such scaling variations be in place.

The TG-43 formalism is recommended for both the pre- and postimplant dosimetry.[98–101] Calculations should be performed using a matrix with resolution limited to 2 mm or less[102] in an effort to minimize the effects of the large dose gradients inherent in a brachytherapy procedure. Normal structures of interest that can be defined by using CT include the urethra and the rectum. The entire prostatic urethra should be defined. Of the rectum only the anterior rectal wall is considered to be a structure of interest.

The values of D100, D90, and D80 represent the doses that cover 100%, 90%, and 80% of the prostate, respectively. The values of V200, V150, V100, V90, and V80 stand for the fractional volume of the prostate that receives 200%, 150%, 100%, 90%, and 80% of the prescribed dose, respectively. The total volume of the prostate (in ml) is

obtained from postimplant dosimetry. The number of days between implantation and the date of the imaging study is used for dosimetric reconstruction. The urethral and rectal doses have to be reported to allow adequate evaluation of postimplant dosimetry and to allow correlation with clinical outcome according to ABS recommendations.

Summary

In summary, brachytherapy for prostate cancer is an alternative treatment. Patient selection is important for choosing the accurate technique. LDR monotherapy seems to be appropriate for patients with low-risk disease (T1–T2a tumor, PSA < 10 ng/ml, and Gleason score < 7).

Looking at advanced disease, dose escalation seems to be necessary. There is no doubt that patients receiving radiation doses exceeding 72 Gy had significantly better biochemical and clinical disease-free survival rates.[103] Advanced disease may benefit from dose escalation with or without synergistic treatment combinations such as interstitial hyperthermia or neoadjuvant-adjuvant antiandrogen therapy.[104–107]

References

1. Pasteau O. Traitment du cancer de la prostate par le Radium. Rev Mal Nutr 1911; 363–7.

2. Pasteau O, Degrais P. The radium treatment of cancer of the prostate. Arch Roentgen Ray (London) 1914; 18:396–410.

3. Denning DL. Carcinoma of the prostate, semin vesicles treated with radium. Surg Gynecol Obstet 1922; 34:99–118.

4. Barringer BS. Radium in the treatment of carcinoma of the bladder and prostate: review of one year's work. J Am Med Assoc 1917; 68:1227–30.

5. Whitmore WF. Interstitial radiation therapy for carcinoma of the prostate. Prostate 1980; 1:157–68.

6. Hilaris BS. Brachytherapy in cancer of prostate: an historical perspective. Semin Surg Oncol 1997; 13:399–405.

7. Nath R, Meigooni AS, Melillo A. Some treatment planning considerations for ^{103}Pd and ^{125}I permanent interstitial implants. Int J Radiat Oncol Biol Phys 1992; 22:1131–8.

8. Bice WS, Prestidge BR, Prete JJ, Dubois DF. Clinical impact of implementing the recommendations of AAPM Task Group 43 on permanent prostate brachytherapy using ^{125}I. Int J Radiat Oncol Biol Phys 1998; 40:1237–41.

9. Radge H, Korb L. Brachytherapy for clinically localized prostate cancer. Semin Surg Oncol 2000; 18:45–51.

10. Nath R, Anderson LL, Luxton G, et al. Dosimetry of interstitial brachytherapy sources: recommendations of the AAPM Radiation Therapy Committee Task Group No. 43. Med Phys 1995; 22:209 –33.

11. Luse RW, Blasko J, Grimm PA. Method for implementing the American Association of Physicists in Medicine Task Group-

43 dosimetry recommendations for 125 I transperineal prostate seed implants on commercial treatment planning systems. Int J Radiat Oncol Biol Phys 1997; 37:737–41.

12. Bice WS, Prestidge BR, Prete JJ, Dubois DF. Clinical impact of implementing the recommendations of AAPM Task Group 43 on permanent prostate brachytherapy using 125 I. Int J Radiat Oncol Biol Phys 1998; 40:1237–41.

13. Nag S, Beyer D, Friedland J, et al. American Brachytherapy Society (ABS) recommendations for transperineal permanent brachytherapy of prostate cancer. Int J Radiat Oncol Biol Phys 1999; 44:789–99.

14. Sogani PC. Pelvic lymphadenectomy: techniques and complications. In: Hilaris BS, Batata MA, eds. Brachytherapy oncology – advances in prostate and other cancers. New York: Memorial Sloan-Kettering Cancer Center, 1983; 79–82.

15. Fuks Z, Leibel SA, Wallner KE, et al. The effect of local control on metastatic dissemination in carcinoma of the prostate: long-term results in patients treated with 125 I implantation. Int J Radiat Oncol Biol Phys 1991; 21:537–47.

16. Kuban DA, El-Mahdi AM, Schellhammer PF. I 125 interstitial implantation for prostate cancer, what have we learned 10 years after? Cancer 1989; 63:2415–20.

17. Peschel RE, Fogel TD, Kacinski BM, et al. I 125 implants for carcinoma of the prostate. Prog Clin Biol Res 1987; 243:177–95.

18. Rohloff R, Tauber R, Schätzl M, et al. Ergebnisse nach interstitieller Strahlentherapie mit J-125 Seeds bei der Behandlung des Prostatakarzinoms. Strahlentherapie und Onkologie 1988; 164:195–201.

19. Beyer DC, Priestley JB Jr. Biochemical disease-free survival following 125 I prostate implantation. Int J Radiat Oncol Biol Phys 1997; 37:559–63.

20. Blasko JC, Grimm PD, Sylvester JE, et al. Palladium-103 brachytherapy for prostate carcinoma. Int J Radiat Oncol Biol Phys 2000; 46:839–50.

21. American Society of Therapeutic Radiology and Oncology. Consensus statement: guidelines for PSA following radiation therapy. Int J Radiat Oncol Biol Phys 1997; 37:1035–41.

22. Beyer DC, Brachman DG. Failure free survival following brachytherapy alone for prostate cancer: comparison with external beam radiotherapy. Radiotherapy and Oncology 200; 57:263–7.

Ling CC, Li WX, Anderson LL. The relative biological effectiveness of I-125 and Pd-103. Int J Radiat Oncol Biol Phys 1995; 32:373–8.

23. Critz FA, Williams WH, Levinson AK, et al. Simultaneous irradiation for prostate cancer. Intermediate results with modern techniques. J Urol 2000; 164:738–43.

24. Dattoli M, Wallner K, Sorace R, et al. ^{103}Pd brachytherapy and external beam irradiation for clinically localized, high-risk prostatic carcinoma. Int J Radiat Oncol Biol Phys 1996; 35:875–9.

25. Stock RG, Stone NN. Permanent radioactive seed implantation in the treatment of prostate cancer. Hem Oncol Clin North Am 1999; 13:489–501.

26. Ragde H, Elgamal AA, Snow PB, et al. Ten year disease free survival after transperineal ultasonography-guided iodine 125 brachytherapy with or without 45 Gy external beam irradiation in the treatment of patients with clinically localized, low to high Gleason grade prostate carcinoma. Cancer 1998; 83:989–1001.

27. Dattoli MJ, Wallner KE, Cash JC, et al. Palladium 103 brachytherapy for clinical T1/T2 prostate carcinoma. Int J Radiat Oncol Biol Phys 1997; 39 (Suppl 1):221.

28. Sharkey J, Chovnick SD, Behar RJ, et al. Outpatient ultrasound-guided palladium 103 brachytherapy for localized adenocarcinoma of the prostate: a preliminary report of 434 patients. Urology 1998; 51:796–803.

29. Grado GL, Larson TR, Balch CS, et al. Actuarial disease-free survival after prostate cancer brachytherapy using interactive techniques with biplane ultrasound and fluoroscopic guidance. Int J Radiat Oncol Biol Phys 1998; 42:289–98.

30. Stokes SH, Real JD, Adams PW, et al. Transperineal ultrasound-guided radioactive seed implantation for organ-confined carcinoma of prostate. Int J Radiat Oncol Biol Phys 1997; 37:337–41.

31. Stock RG, Stone NN. The effect of prognostic factors on therapeutic outcome following transperineal prostate brachytherapy. Semin Surg Oncol 1997; 13:454–60.

32. Wallner K, Roy J, Harrison L. Tumor control and morbidity of following transperineal iodine 125 implantation for stage T1/T2 prostatic carcinoma. J Clin Oncol 1996; 14:449–53.

33. Critz FA, Levinson AK, Williams WH et al. The PSA nadir that indicates potential cure after radiotherapy for prostate cancer. Urology 1997; 49:322–6.

34. Stock RG, Kao J, Stone NN. Penile erectile function after permanent radioactive seed implantation for treatment of prostate cancer. J Urol 2001; 165:436–9.

35. Potters L, Torre T, Fearn PA, et al. Potency after permanent prostate brachytherapy for localised prostate cancer. Int J Radiat Oncol Biol Phys 2001; 50:1235–42,

36. Merrick GS, Butler WM, Galbreath, et al. Erectile function after permanent prostate brachytherapy. Int J Radiat Oncol Biol Phys 2002; 52: 893–902.

37. Zeitlin SI, Sherman J, Raboy A, et al. High dose combination radiotherapy for the treatment of localized prostate cancer. J Urol 1998; 160:91–5.

38. Critz FA, Tarlton RS, Holladay DA. Prostate specific antigen-monitored combination radiotherapy for patients with prostate cancer. I-125 implant followed by external-beam radiation. Cancer 1995; 75:2383–91.

39. Stone NN, Stock RG. Complications following permanent prostate brachytherapy. Eur Urol 2002; 41:427–33.

40. Cha CM, Potters L, Ashley R, et al. Isotope selection for patients undergoing prostate brachytherapy. Int J Radiat Oncol Biol Phys 1999; 45:391–5.

41. Flocks RH, Kerr D, Elkins HB, Culp D. Treatment of carcinoma of the prostate by interstitial radiation with radioactive gold 198: a preliminary report. J Urol 1952; 68:510–22.

42. Flocks RH. The treatment of stage C prostatic cancer with special reference to combined surgical and radiation therapy. J Urol 1974; 109:461.

43. Kwon ED, Loening SA, Hawtrey CE. Radical prostatectomy with adjuvant radioactive gold seed placement: results of treatment at 5 and 10 years for clinical stages A2, B1 and B2 cancer of the prostate. J Urol 1991; 145:524–31.

44. Loening SA. Gold seed implantation in prostate brachytherapy. Semin Surg Oncol 1997; 13:419–24.

45. Butler EB, Scardino PT, Teh BS, et al. The Baylor College of Medicine experience with gold seed implantation. Semin Surg Oncol 1997; 13:406–18.

46. Carey PO, Lippert MC, Constable WC, et al. Combined gold seed implantation and external radiotherapy for stage B2 or C prostate cancer. J Urol 1988; 139:989–94.

47. Gutierrez AE, Merino OR. Adenocarcinoma of the prostate: radioactive gold seed implantation plus external irradiation. Int J Radiat Oncol Biol Phys 1988; 15(6):1317–22.

48. Brix F, Bertermann H. Interstitielle Strahlentherapie mit Iridium 192. In: Sommerkamp H, Altwein JE, eds Prostatakarzinom, Spektrum der kurativen Therapie. München: Karger Verlag, 1989; 84–115.

49. Martinez AA, Edmundsen GK, Cox RS, et al. Combination of external beam radiation and multi-site perineal applicator (MUPIT) for the treatment of locally advanced or recurrent prostatic, anorectal and gynecologic malignancies. Int J Radiat Oncol Biol Phys 1985; 11:391–8.

50. Puthawala AA, Syed AM, Tansey L. Temporary iridium 192 implant in the management of carcinoma of prostate. Endocurietherap/Hypertherm Oncol 1985; 1:25–33.

51. Court B, Chassagne C, Savatovski I. Irradiation interstitielle par fils d'iridium 192 des cancers de la prostate. J d'Urol Néphrol 1977; 83:113–5.

52. Khan K, Crawford ED, Johnson EL. Transperineal percutaneous iridium 192 implant of the prostate. Int J Radiat Oncol Biol Phys 1983; 9:1391–5.

53. Miller LS. After-loading transperineal iridium-192 wire implantation of the prostate. Radiology 1979; 131:527–8.

54. Syed AM, Puthwala A, Tansey LA. Management of the prostatic carcinoma. Combination of pelvic lymphadenectomy, temporary Ir-192 implantation, and external irradiation. Radiology 1983; 149:829–33.

55. Tansey LA, Shanberg AM, Syed AMN. Treatment of prostatic carcinoma by pelvic lymphadenectomy, temporary iridium-192 implant and external irradiation. Urology 1983; 21:594.

56. Bosch PC, Forbes KA, Prassvinichai S. Preliminary observations on the results of combined temporary iridium 192 implantation and external beam irradiation for carcinoma of the prostate. J Urol 1986; 135:722–5.

57. Brindle JS, Benson RC, Martinez A. Acute toxity and preliminary therapeutic results of pelvic lymphadenectomy, combined with transperineal implantation of iridium 192 and external beam radiotherapy for locally advanced prostate cancer. Urology 1985; 25:23.

58. Klein K, Ali MM, Hackler RH. Bilateral pelvic lymphadenectomy, transperineal interstitial implantation of Ir 192 and external beam radiotherapy for advanced localized prostatic carcinoma: toxicity and early results. Endocurie Hypertherm Oncol 1986; 2:23–7.

59. Porter AT, Scrimger JW, Pocha JS. Remote interstitial afterloading in cancer of the prostate: preliminary experience with the MicroSelectron. Int J Radiol Oncol Biol Phys 1988; 14:571–5

60. Koren H, Dollezal P. Interstitielle Iridium Therapie des lokoregionalen Prostatakarzinoms mittels maschinellem Afterloading. In: Hammer, Kärcher, eds. Fortschritte in der interstiellen und intrakavitären Strahlentherapie. München: Zuckschwerdt Verlag 1988; 167–8.

61. Syed AM, Puthwala A, Tansey LA, et al. Temporary iridium 192 implant in the management of carcinoma of the prostate. Cancer 1992; 69:2515–24.

62. Khan K, Thompson W, Bush S, Stidley C. Transperineal percutaneous iridium 192 interstitial template implant of the prostate: results and complications in 321 patients. Int J Radiat Oncol Biol Phys 1992; 22:935–9.

63. Hsu CJ, Pickett B, Shinohara K et al. Normal tissue dosimetric comparison between HDR prostate implant boost and conformal external beam radiotherapy boost: potential for dose escalation. Int J Radiat Oncol Biol Phys 2000; 46:851–8.

64. Martinez A, Gonzalez J, Stromberg J, et al. Conformal prostate brachytherapy: initial experience of a phase I/II dose-escalating trial. Int J Radiat Oncol Biol Phys 1995; 33:1019–27.

65. Kovács G, Wirth B, Bertermann H, et al. Prostate preservation by combined external beam and HDR brachytherapy at node negative prostate cancer patients – an intermediate analysis after 10 years experience. Int J Radiat Oncol Biol Phys 1996; 36:198.

66. Paul R, Hofmann R, Schwarzer JU. Iridium 192 high-dose-rate brachytherapy: a useful alternative for localized prostate cancer? World J Urol 1997; 15:252–6.

67. Borghede G, Hedelin H, Holmäng S, et al. Combined treatment with temporary short-term higher dose rate iridium-192 brachytherapy and external beam radiotherapy for irradiation of localized prostatic carcinoma. Radiother Oncol 1997; 44:237–44.

68. Dinges S, Deger S, Koswig S, et al. High-dose rate interstitial with external beam irradiation for localized prostate cancer – results of a prospective trial. Radiother Oncol 1998; 48:197–202.

69. Mate TP. High dose-rate afterloading 192 Iridium prostate brachytherapy: feasibility report. Int J Radiat Oncol Biol Phys 1998; 41: 525–33.

70. Deger S, Boehmer D, Turk I, et al. High dose rate brachytherapy of localized prostate cancer. Eur Urol 2002; 41:420–6.

71. Galalae RM, Kovacs G, Schultze J, et al. Long-term outcome after elective irradiation of the pelvic lymphatics and local dose escalation using high-dose-rate brachytherapy for locally advanced prostate cancer. Int J Radiat Oncol Biol Phys 2002; 52:81–90.

72. Kestin LL, Martinez AA, Stromberg JS, et al. Matched-pair analysis of conformal high-dose-rate brachytherapy boost versus external-beam radiation therapy alone for locally advanced prostate cancer. J Clin Oncol 2000; 18:2869–80.

73. Yoshioka Y, Nose T, Yoshida K, et al. Intraoperative planning and evaluation of permanent prostate brachytherapy: report of the American Brachytherapy Society. Int J Radiat Oncol Biol Phys 2001; 51:1422–30.

74. Beaulieu L, Aubin S, Taschereu R, et al. Dosimetric impact of the variation of the prostate volume and shape between preplanning and treatment procedure. Int J Radiat Oncol Biol Phys 2002; 53:215–21.

75. Cormack RA, Tempany CM, D'Amico AV. Optimizing target coverage by dosimetric feedback during prostate brachytherapy. Int J Radiat Oncol Biol Phys 2000; 48:1245–9.

76. Stone NN, Ramin SA, Wesson MF, et al. Laparoscopic pelvic lymph node dissection combined with real-time interactive transrectal ultrasound guided transperineal radioactive seed implantation of the prostate. J Urol 1995; 153:1555–60.

77. Stock RG, Stone NN, Wesson MF, et al. A modified technique allowing interactive ultrasound-guided three-dimensional transperineal prostate implantation. Int J Radiat Oncol Biol Phys 1995; 32:219–25.

78. Stone NN, Stock RG, DeWyngaert JK, et al. Prostate brachytherapy: improvements in prostate volume measurements and dose distribution using interactive ultrasound guided implantation and three-dimensional dosimetry. Radiat Oncol Investig 1995; 3:185–95.

79. Stock RG, Stone NN, Lo TC. Intraoperative dosimetric representation of the real-time ultrasound-guided prostate implant. Tech Urol 2000; 6:95–8.

80. Zelefsky MJ, Yamada J, Cohen G, et al. Postimplantation dosimetric analysis of permanent transperineal prostate implantation: improved dose distributions with an intraoperative computer optimized conformal planning technique. Int J Radiat Oncol Biol Phys 2000; 48:601–8.

81. Zaider M, Zelefsky MJ, Lee EK, et al. Treatment planning for prostate implants using magnetic resonance spectroscopy imaging. Int J Radiat Oncol Biol Phys 2000; 47:1085–96.

82. Sloboda RS. Optimization of brachytherapy dose distributions by simulated annealing. Med Phys 1992; 19:955–64.

83. Yu Y, Schell MC. A genetic algorithm for optimization of prostate implants. Med Phys 1996; 23:2085–91.

84. Silvern D, Lee EK, Gallagher RJ, et al. Treatment planning for permanent prostate implants: genetic algorithm versus integer programming. Med Biol Eng Comput 1997; 35:850.

85. Lee EK, Gallagher RJ, Silvern D, et al. Treatment planning for brachytherapy: an integer programming model, two computational approaches and experiments with permanent prostate implant planning. Phys Med Biol 1999; 44:145–65.

86. Lo YC, Stock RG, Hong S, et al. Prospective comparison of intraoperative real-time to post-implant dosimetry in patients receiving prostate brachytherapy. Int J Radiat Oncol Biol Phys 2000; 48(Suppl 1):359–60 (Abstract).

87. Prete JJ, Prestidge BR, Bice WS, et al. A survey of physics and dosimetry practice of permanent prostate brachytherapy in the United States. Int J Radiat Oncol Biol Phys 1998; 40:1001–5.

88. Nag S, Baird M, Blasko J, et al. American Brachytherapy Society (ABS) survey of current clinical practice for permanent brachytherapy of prostate cancer. J Brachyther Int 1997; 13:243–51.

89. Nag S, Bice W, DeWyngaert K, et al. The American Brachytherapy Society recommendations for permanent prostate brachytherapy postimplant dosis analysis. Int J Radiat Oncol Biol Phys 2000; 46:221–30.

90. Yu Y, Waterman FM, Suntharalingam N, et al. Limitations of the minimum peripheral dose as a parameter for dose specification in permanent ^{125}I prostate implants. Int J Radiat Oncol Biol Phys 1996; 34:717–25.

91. Waterman FM, Yue N, Corn BW, et al. Edema associated with I-125 or Pd-103 prostate brachytherapy and its impact on post-implant dosimetry: an analysis based on serial CT acquisition. Int J Radiat Oncol Biol Phys 1998; 41:1069–77.

92. Willins J, Wallner K. CT-based dosimetry for transperineal I-125 prostate brachytherapy. Int J Radiat Oncol Biol Phys 1997; 39:347–53.

93. Bice WS, Prestidge BR, Grimm PD, et al. Centralized multi-institutional post-implant analysis for interstitial prostate brachytherapy. Int J Radiat Oncol Biol Phys 1998; 41:921–7.

94. Dawson JE, Wu T, Roy T, et al. Dose effects of seed placement deviations from pre-planned positions in ultrasound guided prostate implants. Radiother Oncol 1994; 32:268–70.

95. Narayana V, Roberson PL, Winfield RJ, et al. Optimal placement of radioisotopes for permanent prostate implants. Radiology 1996; 199:457–60.

96. Roberson PL, Narayana V, McShan DL, et al. Source placement error for permanent implant of the prostate. Med Phys 1997; 24:251–7.

97. Stock RG, Stone N, Tabert A, et al. A dose-response study for I-125 prostate implants. Int J Radiat Oncol Biol Phys 1998; 41:101–8.

98. Williamson J, Coursey B, DeWerd L, et al. Dosimetric prerequisites for routine clinical use of new low energy photon interstitial brachytherapy sources. Med Phys 1998; 25:2269–70.

99. Luse RW, Blasko J, Grimm P. A method for implementing the American Association of Physicists in Medicine Task Group-43 dosimetry recommendations for ^{125}I transperineal prostate seed implants on commercial treatment planning systems. Int J Radiat Oncol Biol Phys 1997; 37:737–41.

100. Nath R, Anderson LL, Luxton G, et al. Dosimetry of interstitial brachytherapy sources: recommendations of the AAPM Radiation Committee Task Group No. 43. Med Phys 1995; 22: 209–34.

101. Bice WS, Prestidge BR, Prete JJ, et al. Clinical impact of implementing the recommendations of AAPM Task Group 43 permanent prostate brachytherapy using ^{125}I. Int J Radiat Oncol Biol Phys 1998; 40:1237–41.

102. Anderson LL. Brachytherapy planning and evaluation. Endocurie Hyperther Oncol 1991; 7:139–46.

103. Nakamura S, Shimamoto S, Inoue T. High-dose-rate interstitial brachytherapy as a monotherapy for localized prostate cancer: treatment description and preliminary results of a phase I/II clinical trial. Int J Radiat Oncol Biol Phys 2000; 48:675–81.

104. Kupelian PA, Mohan DS, Lyons J, et al. Higher than standard radiation doses (> or = 72 Gy) with or without androgen deprivation in the treatment of localized prostate cancer. Int J Radiat Oncol Biol Phys 2000; 46:567–74.

105. D'Amico AV, Schultz D, Loffredo M, et al. Biochemical outcome following external beam radiation therapy with or without androgen suppression therapy for clinically localized prostate cancer. JAMA 2000; 284:1280–3.

106. Deger S, Böhmer D, Turk I, et al. Interstitial hyperthermia using self-regulating thermoseeds combined with conformal radiation therapy. Eur Urol 2002; 42:147–53.

107. D'Amico AV, Schultz D, Loffredo M, et al. Biochemical outcome following external beam radiation therapy with or without androgen suppression therapy for clinically localized prostate cancer. JAMA 2000; 284:1280–3.

23

High-intensity focused ultrasound for the treatment of prostate cancer

Christian G Chaussy and Stefan Thüroff

Introduction

Since 1989, high-intensity focused ultrasound (HIFU) has been utilized to treat prostate cancer. Preclinical in-vitro and in-vivo studies have established that cancerous tissues may be destroyed with HIFU through coagulative necrosis,[1–3] without cell spread.[4]

The transrectal approach for HIFU administration was validated on a canine model.[5]

In 1992, the first human HIFU study was used to treat benign prostatic hyperplasia (BPH). With the study, the feasibility of the transrectal HIFU for the destruction of prostate tissue was successfully demonstrated.[6] The clinical development of HIFU for prostate cancer has been carried out from 1993 to the present. An overview of the results observed with the Ablatherm prototypes and the standard device is provided in the following sections.

Materials and methods

Clinical studies

During the clinical development, the feasibility to target and to treat the prostate, the histology of the HIFU lesion, and the clinical outcomes were assessed in several different clinical trials.

The Pilot Studies I and II (1993–95), monocentric clinical trials with the first device prototype, were performed in patients with prostate cancer, and $n = 15$ and $n = 11$ patients were included, respectively.[7] These investigations confirmed that it was possible to target the prostate and to destroy cancerous cells. In addition, this preliminary study led to the implementation of several device safety features, which are discussed in a later section.

The European Multicentric Study[8] (1995–2000 for the completion of the patient recruitment) is being conducted in six investigational sites, with a total of $n = 652$ prostate cancer patients being treated. Outcomes are being assessed for HIFU treatment safety and efficacy. This clinical study is still ongoing for the long-term assessment of outcomes.

In parallel, the Nijmegen Study (1997–98) evaluated the histology finding after partial HIFU treatment of the gland in 17 patients who subsequently underwent a radical prostatectomy within 2 weeks of transrectal HIFU therapy.[9–11]

All these clinical investigations are prospective, open-labeled, single-arm clinical trials. They were performed in accordance with the Declaration of Helsinki, the European Standard EN 540, and the local regulations for clinical trials. The studies were approved by local Ethics Committees, and all the patients signed an informed consent form prior to their enrollment.

Devices

All the patients were treated using the Ablatherm device (EDAP S.A., Lyon, France).

Components

The components of the HIFU device are described below:

- an *endorectal probe* composed of two ultrasonic transducers – a high-energy therapy transducer and an imaging transducer
- an *ultrasound scanner* connected to the endorectal probe enables imaging of the target tissue on a monitor

- a *treatment module*, consisting of a patient treatment table, a motorized endorectal probe positioning unit, a high-frequency generator to power the transducer, and a computer to control device operation and built-in safety features.

From the initial HIFU prototype (Figure 23.1) to the current HIFU model, CE mark (January 2000), (Figure 23.2), safety devices have evolved.

Safety features

As a result of the first clinical investigation, safety features were progressively added to protect the patient and improve treatment application. These features are described below:

- *A-mode scanning:* to continuously monitor the distance between the transducer and the rectal wall in order to ensure the proper distance is maintained in order to prevent injury to the rectum. The software blocks active firing in the event of unsafe distances between the transducer and rectal wall.
- *Safety ring:* installing a safety ring around the therapy transducer makes it possible to maintain the constant position of the probe, in relation to the rectal wall, as it rotates between the imaging and treatment modes.
- *Software to identify rectal wall:* this specialized software is used to assist the operator by identifying the position of the rectal wall and automatically aligning the targeted lesions 3–6 mm ahead of it. The software also limits the rotational movements of the treatment head, which, if excessive, could cause the rectum to move away from the therapy transducer.
- *Anticavitation coupling liquid:* a degassed, anticavitation liquid is used as a coupling liquid to prevent any bubbles from forming in the path of the ultrasound (which could interfere with rectal distance measurement).

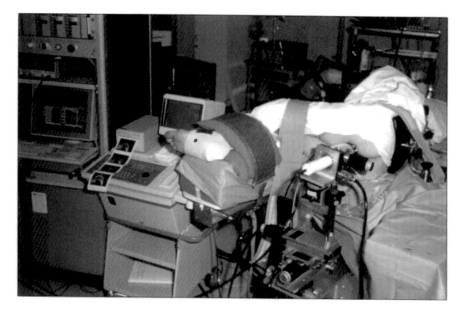

Figure 23.1
First device prototype (1992).
(Courtesy of EDAP S.A., Lyon, France.)

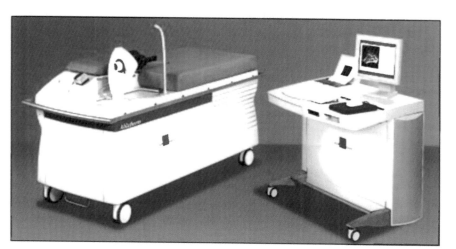

Figure 23.2
Standard device (CE mark). (Courtesy of EDAP S.A., Lyon, France.)

- *Cooling system:* continuously circulates cooling fluid to protect the superficial rectal mucosa from thermal injury.
- *Patient movement alarm:* an audible alarm warns the operator in the event of inadvertent significant patient movement during treatment, and automatically stops HIFU firing.

The primary goal of the above safety features is to preserve surrounding tissues, i.e. the protection of the rectal wall as the posterior part of the prostate is treated.

Technical parameters

Technical parameters evolved in parallel with safety features in order to improve the HIFU performance in treating localized prostate cancer. The HIFU frequency progressively increased from 2.25 MHz to 3.0 MHz, while the shot duration lengthened from 4 to 5 s, and 4.5 s for retreatments (i.e. after previous HIFU, previous external beam radiation therapy, or previous radical surgery). In all cases, a 5 s time interval is maintained between HIFU firings.

The energy is delivered via an endorectal probe, which includes both the imaging (Figure 23.3) and the firing transducer (Figure 23.4). The high-energy ultrasound waves propagate through the rectal wall (Figure 23.5) and are focused on the prostate, generating intense heat and causing the ablation of prostate tissue within the focal area.

Each firing creates a large and reproducible lesion, which spans from the anterior to the posterior prostate capsule. The transducer movements allow for accurate positioning of the focal point and for defining the appropriate lesion depth (dynamic focusing) to match the prostate shape. Continuous firings are delivered repeatedly (Figure 23.6) to obtain a complete treatment of the whole gland while preserving the rectal wall and the surrounding tissues.

Clinical procedure

From 1993 to 1997, patients were systematically treated in two sessions, i.e. one session per lobe. The time interval

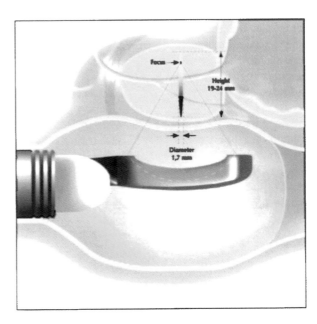

Figure 23.5
HIFU principle. (Courtesy of EDAP SA, Lyon, France.)

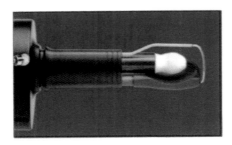

Figure 23.3
Transrectal probe – imaging mode. (Courtesy of EDAP S.A., Lyon, France.)

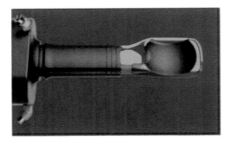

Figure 23.4
Transrectal probe – firing mode. (Courtesy of EDAP S.A., Lyon, France.)

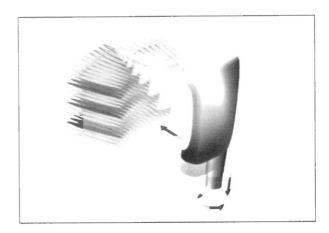

Figure 23.6
Firing sequence for the treatment of the targeted volume. (Courtesy of EDAP S.A., Lyon, France.)

between these two sessions was 1–3 months. However, since 1998, the HIFU treatment of both prostatic lobes has been performed in a single session.

During the follow-up, HIFU retreatments were performed on individuals with residual or recurrent intraprostatic tumors as documented by follow-up prostatic biopsies.

In order to preserve the external sphincter, an adequate safety margin for the (apex) treatment of the apical region was also further defined. Below this safety margin, the portion of the apical prostate not directly targeted receives treatment via heat diffusion from adjacently treated tissue.

Standard procedure

The standard procedure is now defined, and generally aims at treating the entire prostate gland in one 2–3 hour treatment session, although, if needed, a second treatment session can be performed at a minimum interval of 6 months after the first treatment session. The treatment is usually performed under spinal anesthesia. The patient is positioned on the treatment module and the endorectal probe is inserted. Ultrasound imaging is used to detect the contours of the prostate and the targeted treatment volume is defined on the computer screen. Under computer control, the device positions and successively repositions the treatment transducer and delivers HIFU energy according to consecutive treatment blocks defined by the user until all sectors of the prostate have been treated.

Efficacy results
Histologic results: the Nijmegen Study

In this study, to confirm the histologic efficiency of HIFU, 17 patients scheduled for radical prostatectomy for localized prostate cancer underwent a partial treatment (one lobe in which the carcinoma was located) an average of 8 days (range 4–12 days) prior to surgery.[9–11] The excised prostatectomy specimen was then evaluated histopathologically to evaluate the effects of the treatment. Pathologic evaluation revealed that HIFU effects could be accurately recognized macroscopically as a dark red discoloration, with an abrupt transition to pink-white colored, nontreated tissue. This discoloration correlated very well with the coagulative and hemorrhagic necrosis seen on microscopy, with a sharp delineation between treated and nontreated tissue.

In 5 patients, viable tumor was found in the dorsal part of the prostate, and in 11 cases, viable tumor was present in the ventral part of the prostate, out of reach of the HIFU

energy. In no patients was a viable tumor present in the treated area. In most cases, the carcinoma was still visible but not viable. In 3 cases out of 9 where biopsies of the pelvic floor were taken, clear-cut necrosis was seen, the other 6 showing only undisturbed muscular tissue. This indicated that, in some cases, the HIFU effect could extend a few millimeters beyond the targeted area.

This study also demonstrated that radical prostatectomy could be performed soon after HIFU treatment, although potentially there might be an increased risk of stenosis or stress incontinence. During the post-HIFU prostatectomy procedures, the periprostatic tissue appeared edematous but did not cause any serious intraoperative problems.

Following these study results, the treatment duration was increased to 5 s, in order to lengthen the lesion in the posterior part of the prostate where tumors are probably located.

European Multicentric Study

This clinical study started in November 1995, and involved six investigational sites. Patient recruitment was completed in October 2000, with $n = 652$ patients entered and treated. Patient follow-up is still ongoing.

An interim analysis was performed on all the patients included and treated up to November 1999. In total, $n = 559$ patients were analyzed, 402 of them being treated as primary treatment for localized prostate cancer.[8]

For the localized prostate cancer population ($n = 402$), patient baseline characteristics were (mean ± SD): age 69.3 ± 7.1 years, prostate volume 28.0 ± 12.7 ml, prostate-specific antigen (PSA) 10.9 ± 8.7 ng/ml (Table 23.1). Patient distribution according to the disease-related risk level is presented in Table 23.2, using the following definitions:

- low-risk patients: T1–T2a *and* PSA ≤ 10 ng/ml *and* Gleason score ≤ 6
- intermediate-risk patients: T2b *or* PSA ≤ 20 ng/ml *or* Gleason score = 7
- high-risk patients: T2c *or* PSA > 20 ng/ml *or* Gleason score ≥ 8.

At the time of the data analysis, the mean follow-up was 407 days (range 0–1541, Q1 135 days, median 321 days, Q3 598 days). For the biopsy assessment purpose, any positive core in biopsies performed after the last treatment session led to a 'positive biopsy' classification of the patient.

According to the above definitions, the observed negative biopsy rate was 87.2% in the localized prostate cancer population. When stratified according to the risk level, the negative biopsy rates were 92.1% in the low-risk subgroup, 86.4% in the intermediate-risk subgroup, and 82.1% in the high-risk subgroup.

Table 23.1 *Patient baseline characteristics (European Multicentric Study)*

	Age (years)	Prostate volume (ml)	PSA (ng/ml)	Gleason score
n	396	389	397	369
Mean	69.3	28.0	10.9	6.0
SD	7.1	12.7	8.7	1.3
Q1	65.0	19.0	5.8	5.0
Median	70.0	25.0	8.9	6.0
Q3	75.0	34.0	41.0	7.0
Minimum	51.0	4.2	0.1	2.0
Maximum	88.0	120.0	78.0	9.0

PSA, prostate-specific antigen.

Table 23.2 *Patient distribution according to the disease-related risk level (European Multicentric Study)*

Risk level	*n*	Percent
Low risk	114	28.4
Intermediate risk	193	48.0
High risk	95	23.6
Total	402	100.0

Biochemical relapse rate is not presented here. Indeed, most of the patients were enrolled in 1998–99, and at least 1 year of follow-up is needed for a first assessment of PSA stability according to the American Society of Therapeutic Radiology and Oncology (ASTRO) definition (time to nadir + at least 3 successive PSA measurements performed at least 3 months apart).

Long-term results

Gelet and associates evaluated long-term outcomes.[12,13] Indeed, this case series includes all the patients treated on his site since the first pilot study for HIFU in prostate cancer.

In a recent presentation of his series, results were summarized for a population considered as potentially curable, i.e. presenting with a baseline PSA level ≤ 10 ng/ml.[14] These patients (*n* = 94) were treated with the successive prototypes of the device, as a primary therapy for localized prostate cancer (T1-2N0-xM0). Patients characteristics before HIFU treatment are presented in Table 23.3. The mean follow-up of the population was 24 months, but included patients with up to 80 months of follow-up.

Table 23.3 *Patient baseline characteristics for Gelet series with baseline PSA ≤ 10 ng/ml and stage T1–T2*

Characteristic	Mean ± SD
Sample size	*n* = 94
Age (years)	71.8 ± 5.4
PSA level (ng/ml)	5.84 ± 2.48
PSA density (ng/ml)	0.20 ± 0.13
Prostate volume (ml)	34.6 ± 16.9
Gleason score	
2–6	*n* = 58
7–10	*n* = 36

PSA, prostate-specific antigen.

In this population, an 86% negative biopsy rate was observed, including all the control biopsies performed after HIFU treatment. A PSA nadir < 0.5 ng/ml was observed in 70% of the patients. After HIFU treatment, the mean prostate volume was reduced to 17.6 ± 9.8 ml, almost half of the pretreatment volume. In addition, survival curves were calculated with the Kaplan–Meier method, the event being defined as a combination of the biochemical and histologic results: any positive core in control sextant biopsy (whatever the PSA level) or, any biochemical evidence of three consecutive rising PSA levels, or a PSA velocity > 0.75 ng/ml/year with or without positive biopsy. According to this definition, the overall disease-free rate was 77.5% at 4 years, the curve evidencing a plateau from 20 months follow-up (Figure 23.7).

When results were stratified according to the Gleason score, an 85% disease-free rate was observed in patients

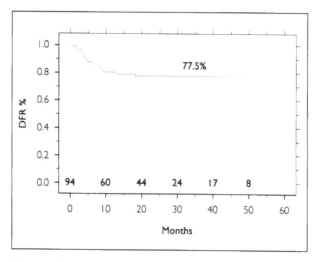

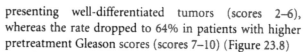

Figure 23.7
Kaplan–Meier survival curve for disease-free rate (DFR) for HIFU treatment of low-risk localized prostate cancer. Gelet series with baseline PSA ≤ 10 ng/ml, stage T1–T2 with an assessment criteria combining both the histologic and the biochemical patient outcome. (Courtesy of EDAP S.A., Lyon France.)

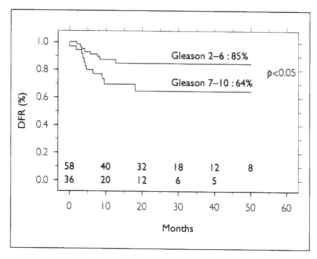

Figure 23.8
Kaplan–Meier survival curves for disease-free rate (DFR) according to the pretreatment Gleason score for HIFU treatment of low-risk localized prostate cancer. Gelet series with baseline PSA ≤ 10 ng/ml, stage T1–T2 with an assessment criteria combining both the histologic and the biochemical patient outcome. (Courtesy of EDAP S.A., Lyon, France.)

presenting well-differentiated tumors (scores 2–6), whereas the rate dropped to 64% in patients with higher pretreatment Gleason scores (scores 7–10) (Figure 23.8)

Gelet also recently presented the results observed in a larger series ($n = 145$),[15] still considering localized prostate cancer patients treated with the Ablatherm as a primary therapy, but with a baseline PSA level up to 30 ng/ml. The patient baseline characteristics are presented in Table 23.4. As previously described, patients were assessed with criteria combining both the histology and PSA stability results. Results were stratified according to the disease-related risk level (definition given in 'European Multicentric Study' section), and survival curves were calculated using the Kaplan–Meier method (Figure 23.9). At 4-year follow-up, the observed disease free rates are 84%, 68%, and 47.5% in the low-, intermediate-, and high-risk subgroups, respectively. In all subgroups, the plateau was achieved at 20 months post-treatment.

Standard device performances

Since 1996, Chaussy and Thüroff have also been involved in the HIFU Ablatherm clinical development. From 1996 to 1999, they treated 184 patients for localized prostate cancer. Follow-up in this population documented an 80% negative biopsy rate and a normalization of the PSA level in 97% of the patients, including 61% of the patients reaching a PSA nadir of < 0.5 ng/ml.[16–18]

Since 2000, Chaussy and Thüroff have utilized the standard device: 3 MHz for 5 s for the firing (shots) duration. A total of 144 patients (stage T1-2N0-xM0 without any previous prostate cancer treatment) were treated with the standard device: 65 patients had 12–18 months follow-up, and were assessable for biopsy results and for PSA stability according to the ASTRO definition. Patient baseline characteristics are presented in Table 23.5. During follow-up, control biopsies were systematically performed (mean, 2.25 sextant biopsy set/patient), as well as PSA

Table 23.4 *Patient baseline characteristics (Gelet series with baseline PSA ≤ 30 ng/ml)*

Characteristic	Mean ± SD
Sample size	$n = 145$
Age (years)	71.9 ± 5.4
PSA level (ng/ml)	9.2 ± 5.8
Prostate volume (ml)	34.6 ± 17.0
Risk level:	
Low risk	$n = 40$ (27.6%)
Intermediate risk	$n = 64$ (44.1%)
High risk	$n = 41$ (28.3%)

PSA, prostate-specific antigen.

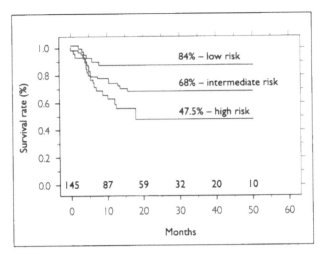

Figure 23.9
Disease-free rates stratified according to the risk level. Gelet series with baseline PSA ≤ 30 ng/ml: Kaplan–Meier survival curve, with an assessment criteria combining both the histologic and the biochemical patient outcome. (Courtesy of EDAP S.A., Lyon, France.)

Table 23.5 *Patient baseline characteristics (Chaussy and Thüroff series)*

Characteristic	Mean (range)
Sample size	n = 65
Age (years)	68.5 (51–81)
Initial PSA level (ng/ml)	12.6 (1–35)
Prostate volume (ml)	22.7 (9–55)
Gleason score	
2–6	45.5%
7	50.0%
8–10	4.5%

PSA, prostate-specific antigen.

measurements every 3 months. Biopsy assessment evidenced an 85.7% negative biopsy rate. Nadir PSA level was generally obtained within 3 months post-HIFU. Median nadir PSA was 0.1 ng/ml, and 92.6% of the patients were still presenting with a stable PSA level at that short-term follow-up. There was a 2% retreatment rate.[19]

Other prostate cancer indications

The HIFU treatment is currently under investigation for special subgroups of patients, particularly patients presenting with local recurrence after previous treatment (external radiation therapy, previous radical prostatectomy, and hormonal ablation), and for tumor debulking in locally advanced stages. Results in these subgroups of prostate cancer are too preliminary to draw a conclusion.

In *n* = 25 radiation-failure patients, Gelet et al[20] presented a high post-HIFU negative biopsy rate of 92%, whereas in only 67% of the patients no disease progression was detected at 12 months mean follow-up (range: 3–63 months). While local control of the cancer seems to be easily achieved for these patients, they are often understaged and present with subclinical disease spread, especially in patients with high Gleason grades. It should be mentioned that these patients are at higher risk for HIFU-related adverse effects, such as urinary incontinence or rectal burn.

Similarly, Chaussy and Thüroff presented small series of patients treated with the above indications.[21] In patients with recurrence after external radiation, after surgery, or after hormonal ablation, they also observed promising local control of the disease, with 78%, 72%, and 79% negative biopsy rates, respectively. They also noted an increased treatment-related morbidity in patients who had undergone a previous local treatment, i.e. in patients treated with HIFU after surgery or external radiation, but not in patients who had been first treated with hormones.

For patients with locally advanced prostate cancer, Chaussy and Thüroff also presented the local HIFU results observed in 24 patients.[22] After a single HIFU session, 50% of the patients presented with negative biopsies, while the tumor mass was reduced by 80% in patients with residual local cancer post-HIFU. The use of HIFU as a palliative local treatment of the primary cancer site to delay disease progression and defer hormone treatment (potentially delay hormone resistance) is nevertheless open to debate.

Safety results

HIFU-related morbidity has also evolved through successive device prototypes, while we have simultaneously optimized the treatment procedure.

During the Pilot Study II, urethrorectal fistulas due to direct rectal burn occurred, and this adverse effect was considered not acceptable for a minimally invasive treatment. As a consequence, additional safety features were progressively implemented, as previously described.

In parallel with the device evolution, the operators also optimized the treatment procedure, in order to minimize the second most severe risk: the occurrence of stress incontinence due to injury of the external sphincter. For this purpose, a safety margin was defined for the apical treatment, leading to a decrease in the occurrence of stress incontinence without an increase in (apical) residual cancer in this region.[16–18]

In 2000, Chaussy and Thüroff described the impact of this device evolution.[23] All patients were systematically assessed post-HIFU with a 50-item questionnaire, which included all the theoretically possible treatment-related complaints or adverse effects. The results described for the 'last 100 patients' are summarized in Table 23.6. The most frequently observed side-effects are the absence of ejaculation, which is generally not a concern in an elderly population, and the immediate post-treatment urinary retention. This post-treatment retention is first due to the edema of the gland, then may be prolonged in the case of prostate tissue sloughing.

To reduce the catheter time after HIFU, and to improve the patient comfort in the immediate follow-up, Vallancien performed a transurethral resection of the prostate (TURP) immediately prior to the HIFU treatment, under the same anesthesia. He demonstrated that TURP does not affect the treatment performance. According to this strategy, Vallancien observed that the mean catheter time went from 9.1 days to 3.3 days.[13,24] The impact of a combined TURP + HIFU treatment was also studied by Thüroff and Chaussy,[25] who observed a reduction of the suprapubic catheter time from 37 days in mean after HIFU to 7 days after TURP + HIFU. The pre- and post-treatment IPSS scores remained unchanged after HIFU (before 5, after 5, in mean), but were improved after TURP + HIFU (before 5, after 2). It should be noted that the patient morbidity after the combined TURP + HIFU treatment was similar to that after a standard (classical) TURP.

Chaussy and Thüroff[16–18] recorded that, after a complete treatment of the gland, two-thirds of the previously potent patients will develop erectile dysfunction. When the prostate cancer seems to involve only one lobe, they proposed a nerve-sparing treatment, excluding 5 mm rim of tissue on the contralateral side near the neurovascular bundle. Utilizing this technique the incidence of erectile dysfunction dropped to one-third of the cases. However, a 15% higher cancer recurrence rate developed in these patients. In these cases, an HIFU retreatment may be performed. It should be noted that these potency results were observed in a population with a mean age of 72 years old.

In conclusion, it can be stated that due to the improvements in the device and in the clinical procedure, severe side-effects such as fistula and grade III stress incontinence did not occur when treating a patient with HIFU as a primary therapy for prostate cancer.

Table 23.6 *Treatment related adverse effects*	
Type of side-effect	Occurrence in the last 100 patients
Death (intra- and post-operative)	0
Fistula	0
Rectal wall burn	0
Hemorrhoidal pain	1
Stress incontinence:	
Grade I (average 27 days)	9
Grade II (average 32 days)	2
Grade III (after TURP)	1
Urge incontinence	0
Urgency	7
Urinary tract infections	13
Significant hematuria	0
Immediate post-treatment retention	100
Total erectile dysfunction	22
Absence of ejaculation	100

TURP, transurethral resection of the prostate.

Discussion and Conclusion

Overall, these HIFU Ablatherm results are often considered difficult to interpret because different device prototypes, different technical parameters, and different clinical procedures were used during the treatment's development period. On the other hand, all these changes were progressive optimization, without sharp modifications, and should be considered as fine tuning. This has led to a standardized device as well as a standardized treatment procedure.

The main advantages of the HIFU treatment may be summarized as follows:

- The learning curve is short for a urologist experienced in transrectal ultrasound (approximately 10 patients according to the experience of the new user sites).
- As a minimally invasive treatment, HIFU may be performed under spinal anesthesia. The HIFU-related morbidity is low, and the post-treatment management is easy. The evening after the HIFU session, the patient returns to normal food, does not need any analgesic medication, and may be discharged the day after with a catheter in place, or a few days later without catheter.
- The nadir PSA is generally obtained within 3 months after HIFU treatment.
- The HIFU treatment may be performed in patients with previous TURP.
- The HIFU treatment may be repeated during patient follow-up. For safety aspects, at least a 6-month

interval is recommended between the two HIFU sessions.

- The HIFU treatment may be performed for local recurrence after previous prostate cancer therapy.
- In the case of local recurrence after HIFU, the patient may still receive a potentially curative treatment (second HIFU session or external beam radiotherapy).

The CE mark, the Ablatherm device, is indicated for the treatment of localized prostate cancer, as a primary therapy in T1–T2 patients, or for the treatment of local recurrence after external beam radiation or after prostatectomy.

In our practice, patients selected for the HIFU Ablatherm treatment are:

- patients who are not candidates for surgery due to their age or comorbidities
- patients who are poor candidates for surgery due to the local conditions (history of prostate surgery or radiation) or with a risk for positive margins
- patients refusing invasive surgery.

As of June 2002, more than 2000 patients have been treated with HIFU for prostate cancer in Europe.

References

1. Chapelon JY, Margonari J, Vernier F, et al. In vivo effects of high intensity ultrasound on prostatic adenocarcinoma Dunning R3327. Cancer Res 1992; 52:6353–7.

2. Gelet A, Chapelon JY. Effet des ultrasons focalisés. J Urol 1993; 99:350.

3. Chapelon JY, Margonari J, Theillère Y, et al. Effects of high-energy focused ultrasound on kidney tissue in the rat and the dog. Eur Urol 1992; 22:147–52.

4. Oosterhof GON, Cornel EB, Smits GAHJ, et al. Influence of high intensity focused ultrasound on the development of metastases. Eur Urol 1997; 32:91–5.

5. Gelet A, Chapelon JY, Margonari J, et al. Prostatic tissue destruction by high intensity focused ultrasound: experimentation on canine prostate. J Endourol 1993; 7:249–53.

6. Gelet A, Chapelon JY, Margonari J, et al. High intensity focused ultrasound experimentation on human benign prostatic hypertrophy. Eur Urol 1993; 23(Suppl 1):44–7.

7. Gelet A, Chapelon JY, Bouvier R, et al. Treatment of prostate cancer with transrectal focused ultrasound: early clinical experience. Eur Urol 1996; 29:174–83.

8. Chaussy C, Thüroff S, Vallancien G, et al. HIFU for the treatment of localized prostate cancer: efficacy results of the European Multicentric Study. J Urol 2001; 165(5 Suppl):388 (Abstract).

9. Beerlage HP, van Lenders GJ, Oosterhof GO, et al. High-intensity focused ultrasound (HIFU) followed after one to two weeks by radical retropubic prostatectomy: results of a prospective study. Prostate 1999; 39:41–6.

10. Beerlage HP, Thüroff S, Debruyne FMJ, et al. Transrectal high intensity focused ultrasound using the Ablatherm device in the treatment of localized prostate carcinoma. Urology 1999; 54:273–7.

11. Van Lenders GJLH, Beerlage HP, Ruijter ET, et al. Histopathological changes associated with high intensity focused ultrasound (HIFU) treatment for localised adenocarcinoma of the prostate. J Clin Pathol 2000; 53:391–4.

12. Gelet A, Chapelon JY, Bouvier R, et al. Transrectal high-intensity focused ultrasound: minimally invasive therapy of localized prostate cancer. J Endourol 2000; 14:519–28.

13. Gelet A, Chapelon JY, Bouvier R, et al. Transrectal high intensity focused ultrasound for the treatment of localized prostate cancer: factors influencing the outcome. Eur Urol 2001; 40:124–9.

14. Gelet A, Chapelon JY, Bouvier R, et al. Cancer localisé de la prostate avec PSA ≤ 10 ng/ml: efficacité du traitement par ultrasons focalisés transrectaux. Progrès en Urologie 2001; 11(Suppl 1):52A (Abstract).

15 Gelet A, Chapelon JY, Bouvier R, et al. Long-term outcome after high-intensity focused ultrasound (HIFU) therapy for localized prostate cancer. J Urol 2002; 167(4 Suppl):392 (Abstract).

16. Chaussy C, Thüroff S. High-intensity focused ultrasound in prostate cancer: results after 3 years. Mol Urol 2000; 4:179–82.

17. Chaussy C, Thüroff S. Results and side effects of high-intensity focused ultrasound in localized prostate cancer. J Endourol 2001; 15:437–40.

18. Thüroff S, Chaussy C. Therapie des lokalen Prostatakarzinoms mit hoch intensivem fokussiertem Ultraschall (HIFU). Urologe (A) 2001; 40:191–4.

19. Chaussy C, Thüroff S. PSA stability after high-intensity focused ultrasound (HIFU) in prostate cancer. J Urol 2002; 167(4 Suppl):347 (Abstract).

20. Gelet A, Chapelon JY, Bouvier R, et al. Récidive locale après radiothérapie externe pour cancer de la prostate: efficacité du traitement par ultrasons focalisés transrectaux. Progrès en Urologie 2001; 11(Suppl 1):52A (Abstract).

21. Chaussy C, Thüroff S. High-intensity focused ultrasound (HIFU) in local recurrence of prostate cancer. J Endourol 2001; 15(Suppl 1): A33 (Abstract).

22. Thüroff S, Chaussy C. High-intensity ultrasound (HIFU) in locally advanced prostate cancer. J Endourol 2001; 15 (Suppl 1): A32 (Abstract).

23. Thüroff S, Chaussy C. High-intensity focused ultrasound: complications and adverse events. Mol Urol 2000; 4:183–7.

24. Jayet C, Guillonneau B, Vallancien G. Traitement du cancer localisé de la prostate par ultrasons focalisés de haute intensité (HIFU) associé à une résection endoscopique de la prostate (TURP). Progrès en Urologie 2001; 11(Suppl 1):26A (Abstract).

25. Thüroff S, Chaussy C. High intensity ultrasound (HIFU) and adjuvant transurethral resection (TURP) – experience with over 100 cases. Eur Urol 2002; 1 (Suppl 1):47 (Abstract).

24

Cryosurgical ablation for treatment of prostate cancer

Moritz Braun, Stefan Wolter and Udo H Engelmann

Introduction

Therapy for localized adenocarcinoma of the prostate is currently undergoing a marked transformation. In addition to retropubic prostate vesiculectomy, the standard operation for many years, perineal and laparoscopic prostatectomy have established themselves recently as alternative treatments. Unfortunately, preoperative diagnostics, especially with regard to imaging, have not kept pace with the development of these new surgical techniques. This means that a complete removal of the entire tumor is possible from a curative point of view, even if this entails serious side-effects (e.g. incontinence). Moreover, in the face of demographic changes in the population of the Western industrialized nations, the quality of life of older people is increasingly becoming a focus of attention. One aspect of quality of life is the maintenance of sexual function. But current therapeutic surgical procedures are often accompanied by the loss of erectile capability, especially since it is impossible to foresee the exact anatomic situation prior to an operation and thus to guarantee maintenance of postoperative sexual function.

For these reasons, other forms of therapy have been sought that entail a lesser degree of side-effects. Technical improvements in radiation therapy, enabling the establishment of external and/or internal radiation – brachytherapy and high dose rate (HDR) afterloading – have made these viable curative therapeutic procedures options to surgery. However, these are subject to strict limitations with regard to the spread and histologic differentiation of the prostate carcinoma. Furthermore, due to the high amount of radiation energy applied, the procedures cannot be repeated. Failure rates ranging from 10 to 30% have been variously cited in the literature.[1–3] Especially for these 'radiation therapy failures', cryotherapy constitutes a valid therapy alternative.

Mechanism of action

In cryotherapy an interstitial application of cold leads to the necrosis of prostate cells. The extracellular water crystallizes, followed by a hyperosmolar cellular dehydration. As a result, the cells shrink as the membranes and other cell compartments are destroyed. Within a few minutes the increased intracellular electrolyte concentration is high enough to induce cell decline. This procedure is known as 'solution effect injury' and usually leads to the death of the affected cells. A further functional mechanism that always leads to cell necrosis is intracellular crystal formation. Both processes are brought about in the course of cryoablation, depending on the speed with which freezing takes place. Whereas intracellular crystallization appears with a sudden and extreme drop in temperature ($-40°C$), the 'solution effect injury' is induced by higher temperatures (from $0°C$) and a slower freezing speed.[4–8]

History

In principle, cryoablation is a relatively old therapeutic procedure. James Arnott in England had already reported on its use as early as 1865. Around 1960 the first generation of cryoablation devices were introduced for treatment of the prostate; they were used to treat benign prostatic hyperplasia (BPH). They used liquid nitrogen for freezing the tissue. Due to the serious side-effects, however, cryotherapy eventually fell into disuse. Then, in the early 1990s, the second generation of devices came onto the market. These work according to the 'Joule–Thomson principle' (gas expansion) and enable significantly better control of the freezing process. In the earlier devices the relatively large needle diameter had made an exact control of the freezing process and the generation of a uniform temperature field virtually impossible.[9]

Today the third generation of devices is being introduced onto the market. With this new technique, similar to that used in interstitial radiation, many fine needles (about 20) are placed perineally, with the exact placement monitored via ultrasound. Temperature probes are used to ensure that neighboring organs (urethra, rectum) are protected from injury, while a consistent low-temperature field can be created to freeze the prostate carcinoma effectively[10,11] (Figure 24.1).

Indications and contraindications

Indications

Generally, cryotherapy is indicated in cases of localized adenocarcinoma of the prostate (pT1/2, Gleason score ≤ 6). The prostate volume should be under 40 ml. Metastatic spread should be excluded.

A distinction is made between primary and secondary indications.

A primary indication exists for those patients who, due to severe comorbidities or a previous treatment (e.g. radiation of a rectal carcinoma), cannot undergo surgery. An indication is also given for patients who refuse surgical intervention and express explicit preference for this kind of curative therapy, always on the condition that the above-mentioned criteria are fulfilled.

Now that various curative radiation options have been introduced (brachytherapy, high dose of radiation (HDR) afterloading, etc.) the possibility of a secondary indication for cryotherapy has taken on a new importance. Depending on which literature is consulted, local failure rates following radiation therapy range between 10 and 30%.[1-3] Because of the HDR employed, repeated treatment is usually out of the question, making cryotherapy a valid treatment option in such cases. Patients are classified as radiation therapy failures who show on three consecutive PSA (prostate-specific antigen) measurements a rise and histopathologic evidence of vital tumor cells by means of a prostate biopsy.

Contraindications

In addition to evidence of metastasis or an unfavorable histopathologic classification (e.g. Gleason score > 6), a previous prostate operation, such as transurethral resection of the prostate (TURP) or suprapubic adenomectomy of the prostate (SPE), should also be viewed as a

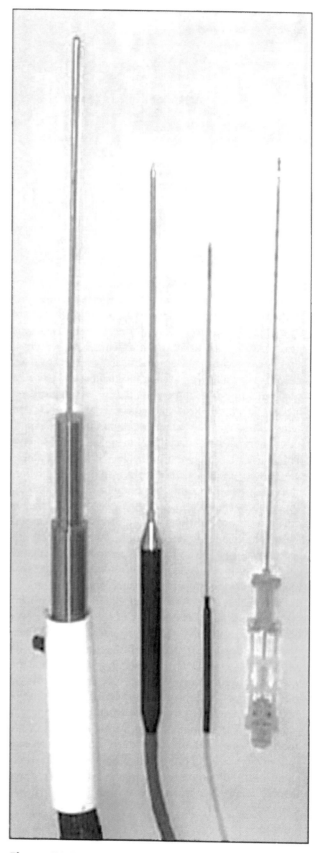

Figure 24.1
The development of cryoprobes.

contraindication for cryotherapy treatment, since the resulting small prostate volume to be expected in such cases (< 20 ml) and postoperative adhesions do not allow for reliable protection of the rectum.

Furthermore, patients with a urothelial carcinoma should not undergo cryotherapy, since this could cause unnecessary complications if a cystectomy should be required at a later date. In such cases it should be determined whether, in light of a histologically unfavourable urothelial carcinoma in combination with a localized prostate carcinoma, primary cystoprostatectomy might be the method of choice.

Since cryotherapy cannot be expected to yield any improvement in micturition, we also exclude patients with marked obstructive micturition difficulties (including patients on catheter drainage). In these cases we introduce primarily an antiandrogen therapy and monitor voiding patterns after at least 3 months of treatment. If at this time, post-void residual volume is low, cryotherapy can be carried out.

In our own clinic we have defined a few additional relative contraindications: here we were guided by safety considerations, so as not to bring discredit to a new, not yet fully established therapeutic procedure. Hence they are relative not absolute contraindications, and must be assessed on an intra- and inter-individual basis:

- inflammatory intestinal diseases
- prior operations in the small pelvis
- bladder diverticula
- coagulopathies (including iatrogen-based).

Preoperative diagnostics

Preoperative diagnostics must first document adenocarcinoma of the prostate by means of a prostate fine-needle biopsy. Histopathologic differentiation (Gleason score) should not be higher than 6. Transrectal ultrasonography is used to determine prostatic volume, usually during the prostate biopsy. A volume of 40 ml should not be exceeded. Further general diagnostic tests follow, including computer tomography (CT) of the abdomen and small pelvis, as well as a bone scan. We also carry out pelvic lymphadenectomy (laparoscopic or minilap) on men with PSA $\geq$ 15 ng/ml, Gleason score $\geq$ 8 disease, or TNM (tumor–node–metastasis) stage T2b or greater. If any metastasis is observed, cryotherapy is not carried out.

Preoperative preparation and execution

Preoperative preparations are not any different from those conducted for brachytherapy or HDR afterloading patients.

Cryoablation of the prostate is undertaken as a one-time or, rarely, two-time operation under general or regional anesthesia, based on the technique described by Onik in 1989 and 1993.[12,13] During the operation the patient is in the dorsal lithotomy position. To prevent infection, ciprofloxacin 2 × 200 mg daily is applied both during and after the procedure. The operation begins with a cystoscopy for orientation. The bladder is then filled with at least 250 ml NaCl 0.9% and a suprapubic catheter is inserted. In our experience any pre-existing obstructive problem is likely to increase in the first postoperative weeks due to reactive swelling, making the suprapubic catheter a necessity during this phase to ensure that the bladder remains free of any residual urine.

After the cystoscope is removed, a transurethral heat catheter is placed in order to protect the prostatic urethra from any cold-induced damage. This allows for a significant reduction in the rate of complications with regard to excretion of necrosic urethral particles or subvesical obstructions. A pump system constantly circulates body temperature fluid through the transurethral heat catheter, serving to ward off coldness in areas that should be protected. Methylene blue solution may be added to this irrigation fluid. A blue coloration of the urine leaving the suprapubic catheter would then show the surgeon that the heat catheter had been damaged in the course of the prostate biopsy. In order to reduce the risk of a catheter defect, it is recommended that the heat catheter first be blocked when the prostate puncture is complete.

A transrectal ultrasound (TRUS) probe is fixed in place. Precise measurements of the prostate are taken and the correct insertion of the puncture needles planned. Monitoring the procedure continually via ultrasound, a puncture aid (template) is used to help place up to 20 echogenous puncture needles perineally in the prostate tissue. The hyperechogenous needles are then brought into the desired position and their placement checked via ultrasound in the sagittal and transversal planes. The probes should be placed from anterior to posterior, in order to enable an optimal sonographic visualization (Figures 24.2–24.4). Several separate thermoprobes can be placed inside or outside the gland in order to facilitate more precise control of the freezing process (Figure 24.5). In addition to allowing the surgeon to make sure the required temperature is maintained for a complete cold-induced necrosis (monitoring of effectiveness), this also helps to prevent rectal fistulae and protects the vasomotor nerve bundle responsible for maintaining erectile ability.

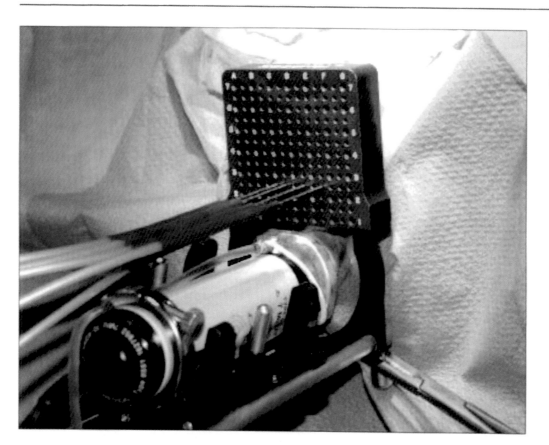

Figure 24.2
Placement of the upper cryoprobe row.

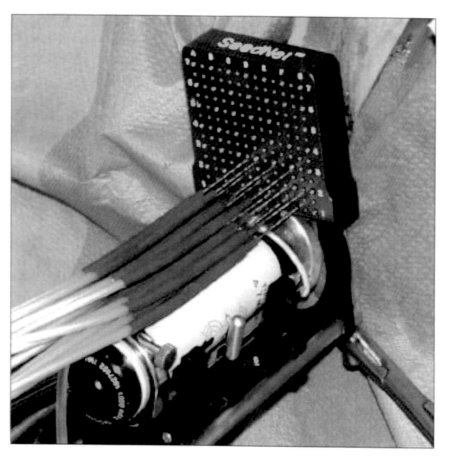

Figure 24.3
All cryoprobes placed.

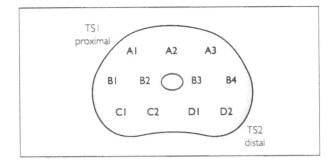

Figure 24.4
Schematic placement of the cryoprobes (A–D), and possible position of the thermosensors (TS).

Technical advances in cryotherapy techniques have made it possible to freeze or thaw individual or grouped cryoprobes independently of one another, allowing for a high degree of localized temperature control.

Once all cryoprobes have been placed, they are activated sequentially from anterior to posterior, so that the resulting ice balls melt together. As the therapeutic tissue temperature zone of −40°C is reached, it is possible to monitor the growing ice ball exactly by means of the high-resolution TRUS and based on the temperature readings from the thermoprobes. The freezing phase is maintained for about 10–15 min.

The hyperechogenous boundary of the ice ball can be followed on the ultrasound image, while the thermoprobes register temperatures in the area of the prostate capsule. The rectal wall can usually be monitored quite well sonographically. Upon completion of the 15 min freezing cycle, the cryoprobes are switched off for about 10 min – initiating the thawing process. The cryoprobes are not warmed actively for the thawing phase, in order to achieve slower, more natural thawing. A second freezing cycle is carried out in the same way to complete the 'double freeze' procedure. Depending on the length of the prostate, the cryoprobes are then pulled out somewhat and the 'double freeze' process is repeated apically. Experience shows that time can be saved by first carrying out the freezing process basally and then apically, and then repeating the process. Thus, the time required for natural basal thawing is used for apical freezing, and vice versa (Figure 24.6).

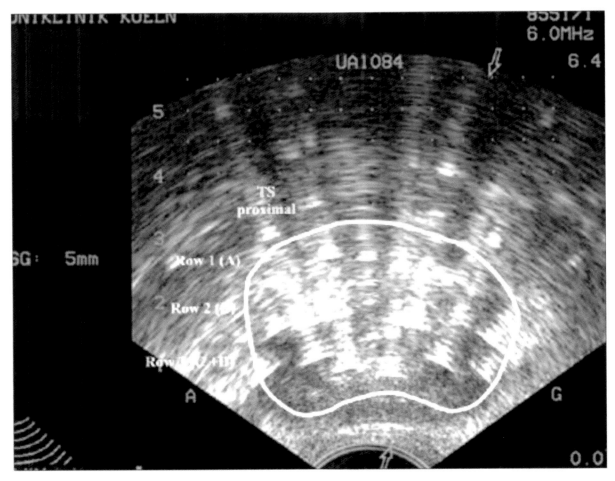

Figure 24.5
Ultrasound after placement of all cryoprobes.

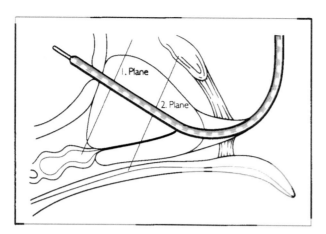

Figure 24.6
Placement of the cryoprobe tips for proximal (1. Plane) and distal (2. Plane) treatment.

After cryoablation is completed, the probes are removed. The transurethral heat catheter should remain in situ for an additional 15 min. Manual compression of the perineum and subsequent application of a compression bandage helps to prevent the development of hematomas.

Technical equipment

Currently, three different companies manufacture cryoablation devices. All instruments are equipped with a thawing device so that the ablation can be executed in multiple cycles, enhancing its effectiveness. At present we are using the SeedNet system produced by the Galil Medical, together with multifrequent, biplanar TRUS for three-dimensional visualization of the prostate. This system contains needles with a smaller diameter (17-gauge), so that more needles can be used to effect a more even distribution of temperature. In addition, it is possible, for protecting sensitive structures (e.g. the rectum), to place thawing needle(s). The ultrasound probe is fixed onto a stepper unit with a 17-gauge template. Ultrasound technology is the area that currently offers most room for progress in the treatment technique. Now that three-dimensional ultrasound is possible, anatomic idiosyncrasies of the prostate can be seen more easily, leading to more individualized planning of the cryotherapy procedure.[14] Combining ultrasound with a Doppler signal would be even more helpful in identifying possible carcinoma growth beyond the confines of the prostate itself, as well as in localizing the periprostatic neurovascular bundle.[15]

Operative access and helpful tips

Operative access

As already described above, now that TRUS is available, perineal access makes the most sense. In some exceptional cases, when for primary treatment a radical perineal prostatectomy is attempted, but during the operation a locally too advanced tumor stage is found (apex or neurovascular bundle infiltration, etc.), an 'open' cryoablation may be performed.

Neoadjuvant antiandrogen treatment

The size of the prostate is an important criterion in determining whether cryotherapy is indicated. In one study, 26 of 43 patients who underwent cryotherapy were treated preoperatively with a complete androgen blockade. The indication for this treatment was a prostate volume of > 40 ml. The androgen blockade was carried out for 3 months prior to the operation and the volume changes monitored by means of regular ultrasound checks. Postoperatively, these patients demonstrated comparable oncologic results to those who did not undergo androgen therapy.[16] Our results were similar to those achieved by Bahn et al. They also observed a significant reduction in volume (33.3 to 21.3 ml), with a progression rate of 13.3%.[17] In their group of 119 patients, Cohen and coworkers were able to demonstrate an advantage for those receiving preoperative therapy.[18,19] In summary, it can be stated that preoperative antiandrogen treatment expands the possibilities of cryotherapy. Whether or not this creates a survival advantage for these patients needs to be evaluated in the course of further studies.

Enhancing effectiveness

The reduction in size of the cryoneedles used not only offers the advantage that with a larger number of needles a more even temperature field can be generated but it also harbors the danger of an incomplete ablation.[20] The injection of antifreezing proteins (AFP) might prove helpful here. In an experiment using animals, Muldrew and coworkers were able to demonstrate that subcutaneous injection of AFP prior to cryoablation led to a significant improvement in ablation results.[21]

Intra- and postoperative complications

Incontinence

Postoperative incontinence is certainly a parameter for the patient's continued quality of life. There are diverse claims with regard to this factor in the literature. While in our study group 69% of previously radiated patients were incontinent, we found that only 1% of the patients receiving cryotherapy as primary treatment suffered from this complaint.[22] Long and coworkers had similar results.[23] The explanation probably lies in the cumulative injury to the sphincter externus. For such patients the preoperative performance of a sextant biopsy (if this has not already been done) is to be recommended. Histopathologic examination of the biopsy specimen close to the apex should preferably show no infiltration of the known prostate adenocarcinoma. This would allow for a larger safety margin protecting the sphincter region during cryoablation.

Patients who manifest marked obstructive voiding symptomatic preoperatively will under some circumstances experience an aggravation of these symptoms postoperatively, even to the point of dysuria. This represents a dilemma for the physician: on the one hand, an indication for the performance of cryotherapy exists; on the other hand, one will probably need to perform a TURP postoperatively, involving a high risk for incontinence. The physician has no choice here but to perform this subsequent surgery after an interval of 3 months, and to carry out the operation sparingly. In the interim, the patient needs a suprapubic catheter, maintaining a micturition log and documenting amounts of residual urine.

Injury to the rectum

One problem feared in association with cryotherapy is the possibility of injury to the rectum, accompanied by the development of a rectourethral fistula. The probability of this occurring is relatively high in those patients with locally advanced tumor growth or those who have undergone radiation. As a preventive measure, the injection of saline solution into Denonvilliers' fascia is recommended. This increases the distance between rectum and prostate, thus minimizing the risk of rectal injury. Onik was able to demonstrate on more than 200 patients that this commonly dreaded complication could thus be avoided.[24] In 25 other patients who experienced a relapse following radiation, this technique also served to preclude any rectal injuries.[25]

Using needles with small diameter, it is possible to place two of them in (or beside) the rectum wall. We are also able to avoid rectal fistulas with active thawing, during the freezing circle. This also works in already-radiated men.

Impotence

The loss of potency following cryotherapy is relatively frequent. Various authors have reported impotence rates of around 80–90%.[26–28] This is one of the major disadvantages of cryotherapy, compared to radical nerve-sparing prostatectomy. When cryotherapy is carried out thoroughly and completely with regard to tumor control, the paraprostatic tissues are inevitably affected, and with them the corresponding vasomotor nerve bundles. Hence, some authors define a postoperative loss of potency as an expression of a successful ablation, especially in cases of large tumor volume with possible paraprostatic extension. Even if nerve regeneration appears to be a possibility in some cases, physicians have recently begun to search for ways of performing a more 'nerve-sparing cryotherapy'. An important role will probably be played here, as mentioned above, by the improvement of sonographic representation. The introduction of three-dimensional sonography enables a better visualization of the prostate and therefore a more precise placement of the cryoprobes.[29] It would thus seem to be possible to identify the vasomotor nerve bundles and safeguard them as required.

In a small group of 9 patients, Onik and co-workers were able to maintain erectile ability in 7 patients solely by protecting the vasomotor nerve bundle on the side opposite the tumor. Their selection criteria for a 'nerve-sparing cryotherapy' are:

- unilateral tumour invasion
- small tumour volume.

They were thus able to avoid compromising their oncologic results.[30]

Injury to the urethra

Prior to the introduction of the urethral heat catheter, problems with postoperative changes in the urethra, in combination with marked dysuria and urethral excretion of tissue fragments were frequent concerns. The heat system has been in use since 1996, serving to protect the urethral mucosa and prevent necroses from forming there. This has rapidly reduced urethral complications, without however precluding them altogether (33% in our patients). De la Taille and Katz left the heat catheter in situ for a further 2 hours and were thus able to completely eliminate urethral complications.[31]

Results

In our own study we were able to demonstrate that the postoperative PSA value for 58% (28/48) of patients was under 0.5 ng/ml 6 months after the cryoablation, and 79% (38/48) of the patients had a negative follow-up biopsy. In this same patient group, treatment success could also be shown to be dependent on tumor stage as well as on tumor differentiation.[32]

Our results are essentially in keeping with those of others who have investigated this therapy, even at a time when we were still using a second-generation cryoablation device[8,28,33,34] (Table 24.1). Overall, one can state that our initially good results have been confirmed, even after long-term observation (up to 5 years). It can thus be established that, from the standpoint of oncology, cryotherapy in patients with primary indications yields results comparable to those achieved through surgical procedures or brachytherapy. As to postoperative morbidities, our patient group showed the following results: impotence could be observed after 6 months in 77% (27/35 preoperatively potent men) of patients. Interestingly enough, during further follow-up, 3 of these men regained erectile potency adequate for normal sexual intercourse, without receiving any sort of erection-promoting therapy. Thirty-three percent (19/57) of the men suffered from postoperative dysuria in combination with 'sloughing'. A further 13 of the 57 patients (22%) experienced prolonged urine retention, which had to be treated in 6 patients (10%) using TURP. Incontinence developed in 9% (5/57) of the patients, traceable in 2 of the patients to a sphincter injury; the other patients were treated satisfactorily by conservative management. Fortunately, we observed no rectourethral fistulae. This spectrum of postoperative complications is comparable with that evaluated by Long and co-workers in their large-scale multicenter study. They compared the frequency of complications with those following radiation therapy and found a similar distribution[28] (Table 24.2).

A special importance can be attributed to studies of 'salvage cryotherapy', i.e. as therapy for secondary indica-

tions. Two decisive aspects come into play here. For one thing, after radiation therapy has failed, the patient finds himself in a difficult predicament. An operation is often not an option, either because the patient himself has refused surgical intervention as primary therapy or because accompanying illnesses originally precluded more extensive surgery. Now, either a much more difficult operation ensues, or, as an alternative, a long course of palliative androgen-blocking medication. This often does not correspond with the patient's own wishes, however, and is also a poor solution economically; compared with the high costs of long-term medication, the expense of performing cryotherapy will be amortized within 2 years. Studies of patients who received prior treatment show that in these cases results can be achieved that are just as good as those in patients for whom cryotherapy represents the primary intervention [35–38] (Table 24.3). Therefore, for our clinic, where cryotherapy is not used as often as radiation (external or interstitial), the secondary indication is actually the main indication. Even if the rate of postoperative morbidity seems to be somewhat higher, this should surely be regarded as acceptable in view of the excellent oncologic outcomes.

Table 24.2 *Postoperative morbidity: multicenter study (cryotherapy) vs literature overview (radiation)*

Symptom	External radiation	Brachytherapy	Cryotherapy
Incontinence	0–13%	0–5%	7.5%
Impotence	37–70%	10–40%	93%
TURP	0–3%	0–4%	13%
Rectourethral fistula	1–9%	0–7%	0.5%

Source: reproduced with permission from Long et al.[28]

Table 24.1 *Cryosurgical ablation series of prostate cancer for primary indications*

Main author	Number of patients	PSA < 0.5 ng/ml	Negative postoperative biopsy
Bahn[33]	590	63.3%	87%
Leibovici[11]	12	66.6%	n.i.
Long [28]	975	36–60%[a]	82%
Ellis [34]	75	n.i.	84%

[a]According to risk group (low, medium, high). n.i. = not investigated.

Table 24.3 *Cryosurgical ablation series of prostate cancer for secondary (salvage) indications*

Main Author	Number of patients	PSA < 0.5 ng/ml	Negative postoperative biopsy
Ghafar[35]	38	74%	n.i.
Chin[36]	118	96%	94.1%
Izawa[37]	145		79%
de la Taille[38]	43	n.i.	66%

Source: reproduced with permission from Long et al.[28] n.i. = not investigated.

Conclusion

Based on the results of clinical studies carried out by the US Health Care Financing Administration (HCFA), cryotherapy has been approved for primary and secondary (radiation failure) therapy of adenocarcinoma of the prostate in the United States. For the same indications cryotherapy got the FDA (Food and Drug Administration) Approval. Hence, it can no longer be regarded as an experimental therapeutic procedure.

Apart from the fact that cryotherapy represents a valid curative therapy option for localized tumors, answering the justifiable desire of many patients for a minimally invasive form of treatment, cryotherapy also makes sense from an economic standpoint. When radiation therapy fails, often the only solution that has to be discussed is antiandrogen treatment with, at best, a palliative expectation.

In our view cryotherapy of the localized prostate carcinoma is still no substitute for radical prostatectomy, which remains the standard therapy for this condition. Because of the long progression time for prostate cancer (up to 15 years), a balanced assessment can only be made following further studies. An important adjunct requirement for this therapy is that all cryotherapy patients be monitored in accordance with standardized parameters over long periods of time following treatment.

With regard to radiation, cryoablation can already today be considered a genuine alternative. This procedure is particularly interesting for clinics and medical centers that do not offer radiation therapy and have no license to handle radioactive substances, but still wish to offer their patients a promising semi-invasive therapeutic procedure.

In the form of salvage therapy (for secondary indications), cryotherapy represents a treatment alternative that is of great value to patients; also, from an economic point of view, it should be actively endorsed.

References

1. Coen JJ, Zietman AL, Thakral H, Shipley WU. Radical radiation for localized prostate cancer: local persistence of disease results in a late wave of metastases. J Clin Oncol 2002; 20(15):3199–205.

2. Rosser CJ, Chichakli R, Levy LB, et al. Biochemical disease-free survival in men younger than 60 years with prostate cancer treated with external beam radiation. J Urol 2002; 168(2):536–41.

3. Hurwitz MD, Schnieder L, Manola J, et al. Lack of radiation dose response for patients with low-risk clinically localized prostate cancer: a retrospective analysis. Int J Radiat Oncol Biol Phys 2002; 53(5):1106–10.

4. Mazur P, Miller RH. Survival of frozen-thawed human red cells as a function of the permeation of glycerol and sucrose. Cryobiology 1976; 13(5):523–36.

5. Gage AA, Guest K, Montes M, et al. Effect of varying freezing and thawing rates in experimental cryosurgery. Cryobiology 1985; 22(2):175–82.

6. Orpwood RD. Biophysical and engineering aspects of cryosurgery. Phys Med Biol 1981; 26(4):555–75.

7. Rabin Y, Steif PS, Taylor MJ, et al. An experimental study of the mechanical response of frozen biological tissues at cryogenic temperatures. Cryobiology 1996; 33(4):472–82.

8. Hoffmann NE, Bischof JC. The cryobiology of cryosurgical injury. Urology 2002; 60(2 Suppl 1):40–90.

9. Homasson JP, Thiery JP, Angebault M, et al. The operation and efficacy of cryosurgical, nitrous oxide-driven cryoprobe. I. Cryoprobe physical characteristics: their effects on cell cryodestruction. Cryobiology 1994; 31(3):290–304.

10. Rabin Y, Julian TB, Wolmark N. A compact cryosurgical apparatus for minimally invasive procedures. Biomed Instrum Technol 1997; 31(3):251–8.

11. Leibovici D, Zisman A, Siegel YI, Lindner A. Cryosurgical ablation for prostate cancer: preliminary results of a new advanced technique. Isr Med Assoc J 2001; 3(7):484–7.

12. Onik G. Transperineal prostatic cryosurgery under transrectal ultrasound guidance. Sem Intervent Radiol 1989; 6:90–6.

13. Onik GM, Cohen JK, Reyes GD, et al. Transrectal ultrasound-guided percutaneous radical cryosurgical ablation of the prostate. Cancer 1993; 72(4):1291–9.

14. Ghanei A, Soltanian-Zadeh H, Ratkewicz A, Yin FF. A three-dimensional deformable model for segmentation of human prostate from ultrasound images. Med Phys 2001; 28(10):2147–53.

15. Potdevin TC, Moskalik AP, Fowlkes JB, et al. Doppler quantitative measures by region to discriminate prostate cancer. Ultrasound Med Biol 2001; 27(10):1305–10.

16. Derakhshani P, Neubauer S, Braun M, et al. Cryoablation of localized prostate cancer. Experience in 48 cases, PSA and biopsy results. Eur Urol 1998; 34(3):181–7.

17. Bahn DK, Lee F, Solomon MH, et al. Prostate cancer: US-guided percutaneous cryoablation. Work in progress. Radiology 1995; 194(2):551–6.

18. Cohen JK, Miller RJ, Rooker GM, Shuman BA. Cryosurgical ablation of the prostate: two-year prostate-specific antigen and biopsy results. Urology 1996; 47(3):395–401.

19. Cohen JK, Rooker GM, Miller RJ Jr, Merlotti L. Cryosurgical ablation of the prostate: treatment alternative for localized prostate cancer. Cancer Treat Res 1996; 88:167–86.

20. Moore Y, Sofer P. Successful treatment of locally confined prostate cancer with the seed net system: preliminary multicenter results. Clin Applic Notes 2001.

21. Muldrew K, Rewcastle J, Donnelly BJ, et al. Flounder antifreeze peptides increase the efficacy of cryosurgery. Cryobiology 2001; 42(3):182–9.

22. Derakhshani P, Zumbe J, Neubauer S, Engelmann U. Cryoablation of localized prostate cancer: neoadjuvant downsizing of prostate cancer with LH-RH analogue depot before cryosurgery. Urol Int 1998; 60(Suppl 1):2–8.

23. Long JP, Fallick ML, LaRock DR, Rand W. Preliminary outcomes following cryosurgical ablation of the prostate in patients with clinically localized prostate carcinoma. J Urol 1998; 159(2):477–84.

24. Onik G. Image-guided prostate surgery: state of the art. Cancer Control 2001; 8(6):522–31.

25. Onik G, Narayan P, Brunelle R. Saline injection into Denovilliers's fascia during prostate cryosurgery. J Min Ther Relat Tech 2000; 9:423–7.

26. Badalament RA, Bahn DK, Kim H, et al. Patient-reported complications after cryoablation therapy for prostate cancer. Arch Ital Urol Androl 2000; 72(4):305–12.

27. Robinson JW, Dufour MS, Fung TS. Erectile functioning of men treated for prostate carcinoma. Cancer 1997; 79(3):538–44.

28. Long JP, Bahn D, Lee F, et al. Five-year retrospective, multi-institutional pooled analysis of cancer-related outcomes after cryosurgical ablation of the prostate. Urology 2001; 57(3):518–23.

29. Chin JL, Downey DB, Mulligan M, Fenster A. Three-dimensional transrectal ultrasound guided cryoablation for localized prostate cancer in nonsurgical candidates: a feasibility study and report of early results. J Urol 1998; 159(3):910–14.

30. Onik G, Narayan P, Vaughan D, et al. Focal 'nerve-sparing' cryosurgery for treatment of primary prostate cancer: a new approach to preserving potency. Urology 2002; 60(1):109–14.

31. de la Taille A, Katz AE. Cryosurgery: is it an effective option for patients failing radiation? Curr Opin Urol 2000; 10:409–13.

32. Sommer F, Derakhshani P, Zumbé J, Engelmann U. Die Bedeutung der Kryotherapie beim lokalisierten Prostatakarzinom. Urologe A 2001; 48(3):185–90.

33. Bahn DK, Lee F, Badalament R, et al. Targeted cryoablation of the prostate: 7-year outcomes in the primary treatment of prostate cancer. Urology 2002; 60(2 Suppl 1):3–11.

34. Ellis DS. Cryosurgery as primary treatment for localized prostate cancer: a community hospital experience. Urology 2002; 60(2 Suppl 1):34–9.

35. Ghafar MA, Johnson CW, De La Taille A, et al. Salvage cryotherapy using an argon based system for locally recurrent prostate cancer after radiation therapy: the Columbia experience. J Urol 2001; 166(4):1333–7; discussion 1337–8.

36. Chin JL, Pautler SE, Mouraviev V, et al. Results of salvage cryoablation of the prostate after radiation: identifying predictors of treatment failure and complications. J Urol 2001; 165(6 Pt 1):1937–41; discussion 1941–2.

37. Izawa JI, Perrotte P, Greene GF, et al. Local tumor control with salvage cryotherapy for locally recurrent prostate cancer after external beam radiotherapy. J Urol 2001; 165(3):867–70.

38. de la Taille A, Hayek O, Benson MC, et al. Salvage cryotherapy for recurrent prostate cancer after radiation therapy: the Columbia experience. Urology 2000; 55(1):79–84.

25

Hyperthermia in the treatment of prostate cancer

Serdar Deger

Prostate cancer is the fourth most common cancer in men worldwide. In the United States it is the most common cancer diagnosis and the second most common cause of cancer-related mortality.[1] The treatment of prostate cancer creates considerable controversy due to the vast array of different options currently available. Radical prostatectomy effectively eliminates cancer in a large number of patients. However, experience in the last decade has shown that the radical surgery does not always result in local tumor control in patients with capsule invasive prostate cancer.[2] Major advances in the radiotherapeutic treatment of prostate cancer have been realized with the development of linear accelerators, conformational techniques, transrectal ultrasound imaging, and insertion of radioactive materials directly into the prostate.[3–5] In spite of the improved radiation therapy tumor control of locally advanced disease, under 70% of T2c–T3 tumors with Gleason score less than 6 are not adequately treated.[6]

The uncertain results and possible side-effects of current treatment options have created fertile ground for innovative strategies in the treatment of prostate cancer.

Normal tissue tolerates temperatures of 41–44°C. The absence of regulatory mechanisms in malignant tissue can result in tissue damage from necrosis if the same temperature range is used. The exact cause of cell death from hyperthermia is not yet completely understood. Changes in cell metabolism that relate directly to the Krebs cycle, lipid metabolism, oxidative phosphorylation, and glycolysis may be involved. In addition, an inhibition of cellular repair mechanisms, an enhanced direct cytotoxicity in radiation-resistant phases of the cell cycle (G2 and S phases), and damage to the cell membrane and the cytoskeleton have been postulated as possible mechanisms of action.[7] Raaphorst et al first reported cytotoxic effects of hyperthermia in mammalian cell lines in 1979. The extent of the hyperthermic cytotoxicity depends on the thermal dose, which is a function of the amount of heat administered and the duration of exposure to heat.[8,9]

Hyperthermia has been demonstrated to improve clinical outcomes, including survival, in several phase III trials for different types of malignancies.[10–14] The effects of irradiation can be enhanced by hyperthermia of tissues due to its additional cytotoxicity (from 42.5 to 43°C) and sensitization (from 40.5 to 41°C). Cytotoxicity induced by hyperthermia appears to be enhanced under microenvironmental conditions such as reduced perfusion, acidosis, and reduced cell metabolism.[15,16]

Mittelberg et al reported synergy between hyperthermia and radiation. They did not observe radiation resistance due to thermotolerance in a prostate cancer cell model. They suggested that injury to heated and irradiated prostate cancer cells was possibly due to separate mechanisms working simultaneously.[17]

Peschke et al used three different sublines of a Dunning rat prostate carcinoma R3327 model (anaplastic, moderately differentiated, and well differentiated) to show that local tumor hyperthermia alone induced growth delay in both differentiated tumors, while the anaplastic tumor subline did not respond. Combining hyperthermia with radiation, cell damage in anaplastic tumors improved.[18,19] This study group also worked on radiation dose rate, sequence, and frequency of heating, and found a clear thermal enhancement of low dose rate irradiation, with maximal sensitization when hyperthermia was given just before irradiation.[20]

Li and Franklin studied apoptosis in irradiated and heated PC-3 prostate cancer cells. They found that apoptosis was an important mode of death in heated cells, but not in irradiated cells. No significant apoptosis was observed when cells were heated at 42°C for 240 min. Thus, a heating temperature of 43°C and above may be required to induce significant apoptosis in a clinically feasible duration of time. They concluded that apoptosis-inducing modalities such as hyperthermia may supplement radiation therapy in the future management of prostate cancer.[21]

Different heat delivery systems for the prostate have been described. Achieving therapeutic temperatures in the prostate is difficult. Because of their acute toxicity non-invasive techniques such as radiofrequency phased arrays limit the amount of heat that can be applied.[22]

The combination of hyperthermia with radiation therapy to treat prostate cancer has been investigated since the 1970s, but several study results have been disappointing.[23–25] Anscher et al[23] combined 44–46 Gy EBRT (external beam radiation therapy) with regional hyperthermia of ≥ 42°C and reported 3-year disease-free survival rates of only 25% in patients with stage T3–T4, mean PSA value of 69 ng/ml, and mean Gleason scores ranging from 7 to 9.

One way to overcome some of the limitations of external heating systems for the prostate is by direct heating of the prostate through interstitial hyperthermia. Advantages of the interstitial invasive techniques of hyperthermia application compared with noninvasive approaches include:

1.   defined energy application in the tumor with protection of rectum and bladder
2.   more effective local therapy
3.   homogeneous energy distribution and better temperature distribution.

One strategy of interstitial heating systems is transrectal hyperthermia. In the early 1990s, a transrectal ultrasound device was developed, especially for prostate hyperthermia.[26,27] A phase I trial combining transrectal hyperthermia with EBRT (standard radiotherapy to the prostate and periprostatic tissues, using a four-field approach with 1.8–2 Gy daily fractions applied 5 times/week to a total dose of 67–70 Gy) was performed at the University of Arizona by Fosmire et al.[28] The ultrasound power was delivered from a water-cooled 16-element partial-cylindrical intracavitary array. Fosmire et al reported that transrectal ultrasound hyperthermia was well tolerated by the patients. However, the average temperature (measured using thermocouples inserted into the prostate) was only 41.9 ± 0.9°C over 30 min. Using this device, a phase II trial of hyperthermia and EBRT with or without hormonal therapy for locally advanced prostate cancer was performed by Hurwitz et al on 9 patients with clinical T2b–T3b prostate cancer.[29] The total radiation dose delivered was 6660 cGy ± 5% of the prescribed target volume using a three-dimensional conformal technique. A four-field technique was used for all patients. Two hyperthermia treatments are administered at least 1 week apart during the first 4 weeks of radiation. Five patients also received hormonal therapy. Median temperature for each treatment was 40.8°C. Mean cumulative equivalent minutes, for which 43°C temperatures were measured, was 3.4 min (0.5 ± 13.1 min). Rectal wall temperature was maintained at ≤ 40°C. Treatment duration was limited in three of 17 sessions due to positional discomfort. Using the National Cancer Institute Common Toxicity Criteria, acute toxicity was limited to grade 1. No excess toxicity was noted with a full course of radiation therapy ± hormonal therapy. Using this described method in 2002,[30] this study group reported about 30 patients having rectal toxicity. A cooling water bolus was maintained between 33°C and 37°C to keep the maximum rectal wall temperature within treatment guidelines. Rectal toxicity was correlated with maximum allowable rectal wall temperature of > 40°C (7 of 11 patients had an acute grade 2 proctitis).

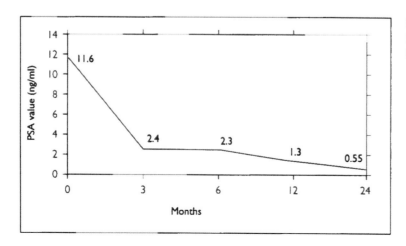

Figure 25.1
PSA (prostate-specific antigen) value follow-up of the Charité Group.

Using the same ultrasound device, Raaymakers et al[31] reported no additional long-term toxicities with the combination of hyperthermia and radiation for treatment of prostate cancer in 26 patients with stage T3 or N+ prostate cancer with median follow-up of 71 months. Similar to the Hurwitz trial, all patients received EBRT using a four-field technique. The median radiation dose was 68 Gy in 2 Gy fractions. The thermal treatment goal in this initial study was to obtain temperatures of 42.5°C within the prostate for 30 min for either one or two hyperthermia treatments. The disease-free survival rate was 39%. The median pretreatment prostate-specific antigen (PSA) level was 29 ng/ml (range, 6–104 ng/ml).

Another interstitial hyperthermia technique is multi-electrode current source (MECS) interstitial hyperthermia. Adequate hyperthermia has proven difficult to achieve with regional radiofrequency technology.[25] Regional radiofrequency systems resulted in relatively low tumor temperatures during treatment.[31] The MECS interstitial hyperthermia system uses segmented radiofrequency electrodes. Each individual electrode controls the locally measured tissue temperature.[32,33]

As early as 1994, a phase I study was reported comprising 36 patients with prostate cancer (5 with locally recurrent, 15 with a T2, and 16 with T3 stage prostate cancer), treated with radiofrequency-induced hyperthermia and iridium-192 brachytherapy from 1987 until 1992.[34] In this study, two-dimensional, steered 0.5 MHz radiofrequency-induced interstitial hyperthermia was administered in combination with 50 Gy external radiation for 5 weeks, followed by 30 Gy iridium-192 interstitial brachytherapy. Two hyperthermia sessions for 45 min were planned, immediately before and after brachytherapy. Between 7 and 32 1.5 mm steel trocar hyperthermia electrodes were positioned transperineally in the prostate.

Van Vulpen et al[35] published a feasibility study of interstitial hyperthermia for prostate carcinoma using the MECS interstitial hyperthermia system on 12 patients with prostate cancer (T3NxM0), who were treated between July 1999 and January 2001. Conformal radiation therapy using a three-field technique with 6 and 18 MV photons delivered 70 Gy in 2 Gy fractions to the prostate and seminal vesicles. The average overall patient temperature measured on the heating catheters was 44.3°C. The bladder and rectal temperatures were below 40°C. The authors reported that an MECS interstitial hyperthermia treatment in combination with radiation was well tolerated. During the hyperthermia sessions, no side-effects occurred. In the combined treatments, no toxicity above grade 2 was seen for urinary, rectal, constitutional, and sexual complaints. In both publications[34,35] long-term survival data was not included.

An innovative therapeutic approach for the treatment of prostate cancer is interstitial hyperthermia in combination with percutaneous radiation therapy, using implantable ferromagnetic thermoseeds, which generate heat by induction in a magnetic field. Ferromagnetism is based on the quantum mechanical nature of the inner electrons of a material and leads to the generation of a dipole. At the so-called Curie temperature, the material loses its magnetic dipole momentum. Paramagnetism occurs when the temperature of the alloy rises above this value. If ferromagnetic material is exposed to a surrounding field, atomic dipoles straighten out, and, when the field oscillates, heat is generated. The material heats up until the Curie temperature is reached and the ferromagnetic characteristics are lost. The selection of alloys with a known Curie temperature allows for a self-regulating system. Based on these specifications, thermoseeds with a defined Curie point can be chosen.[36–38] Since the ferromagnetic implants remain in the prostate, hyperthermia induction can be repeated as often as necessary.

Several investigators have described animal models using ferromagnetic thermoseeds for prostate treatment.[39–41] Deger et al[42] used ferromagnetic cobalt–palladium alloy thermoseeds for interstitial hyperthermia in combination with ERBT for prostate cancer patients. This study group examined several alloys such as nickel–copper before evaluating the optimal biocompatibility. Cobalt–palladium was the most promising alloy,[38,43,44] while other investigators also reported on palladium–nickel and ferrite core/metallic sheath thermoseeds.[45,46]

To achieve interstitial hyperthermia, Deger et al[42,47] used thermoseeds with a Curie temperature of 55°C. They added a three-dimensional conformal radiotherapy of 68.4 Gy, given simultaneously with hyperthermia in daily fractions of 1.8 Gy. A patented coil system (50 kHz) was utilized to establish the magnetic field. Six 60-min hyperthermia treatments were conducted in all patients at an interval of 1 week. Using thermocouples, the measured intraprostatic temperatures were found to be between 42°C and 48°C. During treatment the urethral and rectal temperatures were measured to be between 38°C and 43°C and between 37°C and 39.5°C, respectively.[48] No seed migration was observed on follow-up X-rays. At a mean follow-up time of 15 months, 5% (3/57) patients showed progression of disease at an average time of 20.3 months. Initial mean PSA value of these patients was 34 ng/ml; all had T3 disease. Two patients had local and 1 patient had systemic progression. PSA follow-up data of this patient group were comparable to the data of the patients treated with a high dose rate brachytherapy[49] and better than those of the patients who received conformal radiation therapy in the same institution.

Currently, the literature does not provide enough oncologic data on the use of hyperthermia for the treatment of prostate cancer. Most studies describe feasibility and toxicity. Nevertheless, interstitial hyperthermia in combination with conformal radiotherapy may be a powerful new method of improving the results of EBRT for localized prostate cancer. In addition, the combination of hyperthermia with chemotherapeutics[50,51] or thermo- or radiosensitizing modalities[52-54] may offer further potential in improving the treatment of localized prostate cancer with lower morbidity than current treatment options.

References

1. Ries LA, Wingo PA, Miller DS, et al. The annual report to the nation on the status of cancer, 1973–1997, with a special section on colorectal cancer. Cancer 2000; 88:2398–424.

2. Zietman AL, Shipley WU, Willet CG. Residual disease after radical surgery or radiation therapy for prostate cancer – clinical significance and therapeutic implications. Cancer 1993; 71:959–69.

3. Hanks GE, Lee WR, Schultheiss TE. Clinical and biochemical evidence of control of prostate cancer at five years after external beam radiation. J Urol 1995; 154:456–9.

4. Hanks GE, Schultheiss TE, Hunt MA, Epstein B. Factors influencing incidence of acute grade 2 morbidity in conformal and standard radiation treatment of prostate cancer. Int J Radiat Oncol Biol Phys 1995; 31:25–9.

5. Schultheiss TE, Hanks GE, Hunt MA, Lee WR. Incidence of and factors related to late complications in conformal and conventional radiation treatment of cancer of the prostate. Int J Radiat Oncol Biol Phys 1995; 32:643–50.

6. Hanks GE, Hanlon AL, Schultheiss TE, et al. Conformal beam treatment of prostate cancer. Urology 1997; 50:87–92.

7. Seegenschmiedt MH, Sauer R. The current role of interstitial thermoradiotherapy. Strahlenther Onkol 1992; 168:119–140.

8. Raaphorst GP, Romano SL, Mitchell JB, et al. Intrinsic differences in heat and/or X-ray sensitivity of seven mammalian cell lines cultured and treated under identical conditions. Cancer Res 1979; 39:396–401.

9. Sapareto SA, Dewey WC. Thermal dose determination in cancer therapy. Int J Radiat Oncol Biol Phys 1984; 10:787–800.

10. Valdagni R, Amichetti M. Report of long-term follow-up in a randomized trial comparing radiation therapy and radiation therapy plus hyperthermia to metastatic lymph nodes in stage IV head and neck patients. Int J Radiat Oncol Biol Phys 1994; 28:163–9.

11. Overgaard J, Gonzalez Gonzalez D, Hulshof MC, et al. Hyperthermia as an adjuvant to radiation therapy of recurrent or metastatic malignant melanoma. A multicentre randomized trial by the European Society for Hyperthermic Oncology. Int J Hyperthermia 1996; 12:3–20.

12. Vernon C, Hand J, Field S, et al. Radiotherapy with or without hyperthermia in the treatment of superficial localized breast cancer: results from five randomized controlled trials. International Collaborative Hyperthermia Group. Int J Radiat Oncol Biol Phys 1996; 35:731–44.

13. Sneed PK, Stauffer PR, McDermott MW, et al. Survival benefit of hyperthermia in a prospective randomized trial of brachytherapy boost +/− hyperthermia for glioblastoma multiforme. Int J Radiat Oncol Biol Phys 1998; 40:287–95.

14. Van der Zee J, Gonzalez Gonzalez D, van Rhoon GC, et al. Comparison of radiotherapy alone with radiotherapy plus hyperthermia in locally advanced pelvic tumours: a prospective, randomised, multicentre trial. Dutch Deep Hyperthermia Group. Lancet 2000; 355:1119–256.

15. Seegenschmiedt MH. Interstitiale thermoradiotherapie. Onkologie 1996; 1:87–94.

16. Ryu S, Brown SL, Khil MS, et al. Preferential radiosensitization of human prostatic carcinoma cells by mild hyperthermia. Int J Radiat Oncol Biol Phys 1996; 34:133–8.

17. Mittelberg KN, Tucker RD, Loening SA, Moseley P. Effect of radiation and hyperthermia on prostate tumor cells with induced thermal tolerance and the correlation with HSP70 accumulation. Urol Oncol 1996; 2:146–51.

18. Peschke P, Hahn EW, Wenz F, et al. Differential sensitivity of three sublines of the rat Dunning prostate tumor system R3327 to radiation and/or local tumor hyperthermia. Radiat Res 1998; 150:190–4.

19. Peschke P, Klein V, Wolber G, et al. Morphometric analysis of bromodeoxyuridine distribution and cell density in the rat Dunning prostate tumor R3327–AT1 following treatment with radiation and/or hyperthermia. Histol Histopathol 1999; 14:461–9.

20. Peschke P, Hahn EW, Wolber G, et al. Interstitial radiation and hyperthermia in the Dunning R3327 prostate tumour model: therapeutic efficacy depends on radiation dose-rate, sequence and frequency of heating. Int J Radiat Biol 1996; 70:609–16.

21. Li WX, Franklin WA. Radiation- and heat-induced apoptosis in PC-3 prostate cancer cells. Radiat Res 1998; 150(2):190–4.

22. Anscher MS, Samulski TV, Leopold KA, Oleson JR. Phase I/II study of external radio frequency phased array hyperthermia and external beam radiotherapy in the treatment of prostate cancer: technique and results of intraprostatic temperature measurements. Int J Radiat Oncol Biol Phys 1992; 24:489–95.

23. Anscher MS, Samulski TV, Dodge R, et al. Combined external beam irradiation and external regional hyperthermia for locally advanced adenocarcinoma of the prostate. Int J Radiat Oncol Biol Phys 1997; 37:1059–65.

24. Emami B, Scott C, Perez CA, et al. Phase III study of interstitial thermoradiotherapy compared with interstitial radiotherapy alone in the treatment of recurrent or persistent human tumors. A prospectively controlled randomized study by the Radiation Therapy Group. Int J Radiat Oncol Biol Phys 1996; 34:1097–104.

25. Myerson RJ, Scott CB, Emami B, et al. A phase I/II study to evaluate radiation therapy and hyperthermia for deep-seated tumours: a report of RTOG 89–08. Int J Hyperthermia 1996; 12:449–59.

26. Diederich CJ, Hynynen K. The development of intracavitary ultrasonic applicators for hyperthermia: a design and experimental study. Med Phys 1990; 17:626–34.

27. Hynynen K. Ultrasound heating technology. In: Thermoradiotherapy and thermo-chemotherapy, Vol 1. Seegenschmiedt MH, Fessenden P, Vernon CC, eds. Berlin: Springer-Verlag 1995; 253.

28. Fosmire H, Hynynen K, Drach GW, et al. Feasibility and toxicity of transrectal ultrasound hyperthermia in the treatment of locally advanced adenocarcinoma of the prostate. Int J Radiat Oncol Biol Phys 1993; 26(2):253–9.

29. Hurwitz MD, Kaplan ID, Svensson GK, et al. Feasibility and patient tolerance of a novel transrectal ultrasound hyper-

thermia system for treatment of prostate cancer. Int J Hyperthermia 2001; 17:31–7.

30. Hurwitz MD, Kaplan ID, Hansen JL, et al. Association of rectal toxicity with thermal dose parameters in treatment of locally advanced prostate cancer with radiation and hyperthermia. Int J Radiat Oncol Biol Phys 2002; 53:913–18.

31. Raaymakers BW, Van Vulpen M, Lagendijk JJ, et al. Determination and validation of the actual 3D temperature distribution during interstitial hyperthermia of prostate carcinoma. Phys Med Biol 2001; 46:3115–31.

32. Lagendijk JJW, Visser AG, Kaatee RSPJ, et al. Interstitial hyperthermia and treatment planning: the 27 MHz multi-electrode current source method. Activity Special Rep 1995; 6:83–90.

33. van der Koijk JF, Crezee J, Kotte ANTJ et al. The influence of vasculature on temperature distributions in MECS interstitial hyperthermia: importance of longitudinal control. Int J Hypertherm 1997; 13:365–85.

34. Prionas SD, Kapp DS, Goffinet DR, et al. Thermometry of interstitial hyperthermia given as an adjuvant to brachytherapy for the treatment of carcinoma of the prostate. Int J Radiat Oncol Biol Phys 1994; 28:151–62.

35. van Vulpen M, Raaymakers BW, Lagendijk JJ, et al. Three-dimensional controlled interstitial hyperthermia combined with radiotherapy for locally advanced prostate carcinoma – a feasibility study. Int J Radiat Oncol Biol Phys 2002; 53:116–26.

36. Tucker RD, Ehrenstein T, Loening SA. Thermal ablation using interstitial temperature self regulating cobalt–palladium seeds. A new treatment alternative for localized prostate cancer? In: Schnorr D, Loening SA, Dinges S, Budach V, eds. Lokal fortgeschrittenes Prostatakarzinom, Berlin: Blackwell, 1995: 221–40.

37. Case JA, Tucker RD, Park JB. Defining the heating characteristics of ferromagnetic implants using calorimetry. J Biomed Mater Res 2000; 53:791–8.

38. Le UT, Tucker RD, Park JB. The effects of localized cold work on the heating characteristics of thermal therapy implants. J Biomed Mater Res 2002; 63:24–30.

39. Tompkins DT, Vanderby R, Klein SA, et al. Temperature-dependent versus constant-rate blood perfusion modelling in ferromagnetic thermoseed hyperthermia: results with a model of the human prostate. Int J Hyperthermia 1994; 10:517–36.

40. Tompkins DT, Vanderby R, Klein SA, et al. The use of generalized cell-survival data in a physiologically based objective function for hyperthermia treatment planning: a sensitivity study with a simple tissue model implanted with an array of ferromagnetic thermoseeds. Int J Radiat Oncol Biol Phys 1994; 30:929–43.

41. Paulus JA, Tucker RD, Loening SA, Flanagan SW. Thermal ablation of canine prostate using interstitial temperature self-regulating seeds: new treatment for prostate cancer. J Endourol 1997;11:295–300

42. Deger S, Bohmer D, Roigas J, et al. Interstitial hyperthermia using thermoseeds in combination with conformal radiotherapy for localized prostate cancer. Front Radiat Ther Oncol 2002; 36:171–6.

43. Ferguson SD, Paulus JA, Tucker RD, et al. Effect of thermal treatment on heating characteristics of Ni–Cu alloy for hyperthermia: preliminary studies. J Appl Biomater 1993; 4:55–60.

44. Paulus JA, Parida GR, Tucker RD, Park JB. Corrosion analysis of NiCu and PdCo thermal seed alloys used as interstitial hyperthermia implants. Biomaterials 1997; 18:1609–14.

45. Meijer JG, van Wieringen N, Koedooder C, et al. The development of PdNi thermoseeds for interstitial hyperthermia. Med Phys 1995; 22:101–4.

46. Cetas TC, Gross EJ, Contractor Y. A ferrite core/metallic sheath thermoseed for interstitial thermal therapies. IEEE Trans Biomed Eng 1998; 45:68–77.

47. Deger S, Boehmer D, Turk I, et al. Interstitial hyperthermia using self-regulating thermoseeds combined with conformal radiation therapy. Eur Urol 2002; 42:147–53.

48. Tucker RD, Loening SA, Huidobro C, Larson T. The use of permanent interstitial temperature self regulating rods for the treatment of prostate cancer. Radiat Oncol 2000; 55(Suppl 1):132 (Abstract).

49. Deger S, Boehmer D, Turk I, et al. High dose rate brachytherapy of localized prostate cancer. Eur Urol 2002; 41:420–6.

50. Roigas J, Wallen ES, Loening SA, Moseley PL. Effects of combined treatment of chemotherapeutics and hyperthermia on survival and the regulation of heat shock proteins in Dunning R3327 prostate carcinoma cells. Prostate 1998; 34:195–202.

51. Roigas J, Wallen ES, Loening SA, Moseley PL. Estramustine phosphate enhances the effects of hyperthermia and induces the small heat shock protein HSP27 in the human prostate carcinoma cell line PC-3. Urol Res 2002; 30:130–55.

52. Lee YJ, Lee H, Borrelli MJ. Gene transfer into human prostate adenocarcinoma cells with an adenoviral vector: hyperthermia enhances a double suicide gene expression, cytotoxicity and radiotoxicity. Cancer Gene Ther 2002; 9:267–74.

53. Asea A, Mallick R, Lechpammer S, et al. Cyclooxygenase inhibitors are potent sensitizers of prostate tumours to hyperthermia and radiation. Int J Hyperthermia 2001; 17:401–14.

54. Asea A, Ara G, Teicher BA, et al. Effects of the flavonoid drug quercetin on the response of human prostate tumours to hyperthermia in vitro and in vivo. Int J Hyperthermia 2001; 17:347–56.

26

Surgical robotic applications in minimally invasive uro-oncology surgery

Dan Stoianovici, Robert Webster, and Louis R Kavoussi

Introduction

Surgical robots have begun to appear on the market in the last few years and have started to populate the operating rooms in large medical centers. These systems have already established their ability to augment a surgeon's dexterity in minimally invasive procedures and have the potential to improve patient outcome, even though, for the moment, their cost is prohibitively high for widespread application. As surgeons become increasingly aware of the clinical benefits of these systems and costs are driven down by technological advance and availability, we foresee that robots will become standard operating room tools. Initial use of a handful of robots has already demonstrated their surgical potential. As technology evolves, robots may not only improve performance in minimally invasive procedures but may also enhance the performance of other existing procedures or even make possible entirely new kinds of operations.

This chapter outlines the current capabilities and limitations of several commercially available and experimental surgical robots. Local and telesurgical systems and procedures are discussed together with a forecast of future development. We provide an overview of surgical robotic technology, terminology, and classification, as well as a short history of their evolution, highlighting the potential of these systems, before proceeding to discuss several specific surgical systems.

Overview of surgical robotics

Computer-integrated surgical systems are a new class of 'intelligent' surgical tools which may include surgical robots. The robotic manipulator itself is just one element of a larger system that includes preoperative planning based on medical images, intraoperative registration (matching the patient to the presurgical images) and a combination of robotically assisted and manually controlled tools for carrying out the plan, as well as patient verification and follow-up.

The chief advantages of robotic manipulation of surgical tools are generally:

- accurate registration of patient's body to medical images
- consistent movement, free of fatigue and tremor
- the ability to work in imaging environments unfriendly to human surgeons
- the ability to reposition instruments quickly and accurately through complex trajectories or onto multiple targets.

In surgical robotics the task may either be predefined by the surgeon based on preoperative/interventional data or, for more complex procedures, be defined as the surgery progresses in the operating room. On the basis of this distinction, surgical robots may be classified into two main groups: image-guided and surgeon-driven systems. These categories both make use of the complementary skills/advantages of the surgeon and the robot, but they do so in different ways.

Image-guided robotic systems excel at precisely reaching a target specified by the surgeon. In radiologic interventions such as percutaneous needle access, these systems are used to guide and sometimes to insert a needle, instrument, or probe. Their purpose is to act as a trajectory-enforcement device, correctly aligning the needle based on images from ultrasound, C-arm or biplanar fluoroscopy units, computed tomography (CT) or even magnetic resonance imaging (MRI) scanners.[1] Image-guided systems take advantage of the capability of robotic systems to register the medical image to the patient more easily and accurately than humans can. The robot can then precisely manipulate instruments to reach the locations in the patient space that are selected in the medical image. The system complements the planning and decision-making skills of the surgeon by actualizing his intention.

With surgeon-driven robots, the surgeon directly controls the motion of the instruments held by the robot. These systems combine the fine manipulation capabilities of robotic systems with the surgeon's perception and judgment, performing scaled-down, steady, tremor-free motion. These robots enable increased resolution of movement and vision, and make laparoscopic tools more dexterous. The laparoscopic robot 'hands' emulate the movement capability of human hands and wrists much better than do the traditional laparoscopic tools. Additionally, robotic systems can fuse radiographic and three-dimensional (3D) data to real-time surface data, providing better visualization of the target tissue or structures that need to be avoided.

When performing surgery with a robotic system, the surgeon is often located distal to the operating field. Robotic tools allow easier access to confined spaces in minimally invasive procedures and also enable the doctor to be at a distance from the patient and, thus, perform telesurgery.[2] Future developments may allow the computer to sense joint and muscle movements in the operator's hands, arms, head and neck, and to respond accordingly. A prototype system currently under development senses the electrical signals in the operator's biceps, and flexes or extends a robotic arm accordingly.[3] Increased public demand for minimally invasive surgery is not being satisfied by a sufficient number of experienced, qualified surgeons.[4] Telemedicine provides the unique advantage of allowing specialists in remote locations to assist and train local surgeons. Robotic tools enable the remote surgeon not only to offer advice but also to participate directly in the operation. This has been successfully done intercontinentally, as described later.

Robotic systems have profound implications when applied to training. Robotic and computer training simulations can enable some surgical training activities to be carried out in virtual reality or simulated environments without risk and/or harm to an animal or human patient. Further, these devices may one day allow surgical learning progress to be measured quantitatively and tracked over time.

Robotic surgery is a fascinating and quickly evolving field of medicine as doctors and engineers collaborate to develop innovative new procedures and the technology that makes them possible. While patients will grow to appreciate the accuracy of robots, they will always want the judgment of a human doctor in control of the robot. Robotic technology will never replace the doctor, but it represents a new type of tool with promising capabilities.

History of urologic robots

Robotic-assisted devices in medicine were first used in rehabilitation before making their way into the operating room.[5] Surgical robotics pioneered in the 1980s in the fields of orthopedics and neurosurgery with predefined-task robots.[6] Because of the difficulty of building robots to operate on soft tissue organs with their higher deformability and mobility, urology robotics (URobotics) was slower to develop. Although these difficulties delayed development of URobotics, innovative research has produced several systems either applicable to, or purposely designed for, urology.

The first URobot was the PROBOT, introduced in 1989 by a group at the Imperial College in London for performing robot-assisted transurethral resection of the prostate (TURP).[7,8] The robot serially cored the periurethral prostatic tissue, while hemostasis was achieved manually using electrocautery after completion of the tissue resection. The device never achieved widespread use; however, since then, many minimally invasive techniques for the treatment of benign prostatic hyperplasia have been introduced, thus confirming the desire to replace the standard TURP with a less-invasive strategy. Transrectal ultrasound (TRUS) is used in many of these new techniques for intraoperative monitoring and image-guided robot assistance.

In 1994, Potamianos et al investigated a robotic system to assist the urologist with intraoperative percutaneous renal access.[9] They employed a passive, encoded arm equipped with electromagnetic brakes, mounted onto the operating table. The access needle was manually positioned as prescribed by a computer, which triangulated the calyx location from multiple C-arm X-rays.[10] In-vitro experiments evaluating system performance demonstrated a targeting accuracy within 1.5 mm or less.

In 1995, a research group headed by Russell Taylor at IBM developed the remote center of motion (RCM) concept and implemented it on the LARS robot.[11,12] The RCM is a component of nearly all medical robotic systems today. LARS was used in our institution for experimental percutaneous renal access.[13] These experiments revealed areas for improvement and led our URobotics research group to create the PAKY-RCM (Percutaneous Access of the Kidney) robot.[14]

The use of robots in laparoscopy is yet another step in the evolution of minimally invasive techniques and has been successfully applied in several centers in Europe and the USA. The first robots used to control laparoscopic tools in urologic surgery were manipulator arms such as the Automated Endoscopic System for Optimal Positioning (AESOP; Computer Motion, Inc., Goleta, California). Such laparoscopic systems are quite recent, having been developed in the late 1990s and cleared by the FDA (Food and Drug Administration) within the past few years.

The entire history of robots in surgery is rather short, but in this brief period, the technology has matured sufficiently to prove its worth. Systems developed thus far seem to be adaptable to specific architectures and characteristics imposed by the stringent surgical environment.

Common components of surgical robotic systems

Perhaps the most important and specific component of the surgical robot is the manipulator. Surgical manipulators are electromechanical arms equipped with sensors and actuators responsible for holding and precisely moving the surgical instrument under computer control. The most common kinematic architecture of surgical manipulators has thus far been the RCM, which is a specific characteristic of surgical robots as opposed to industrial types.

The RCM is a mechanism used by the surgical manipulator to enable and facilitate the pivoting motion of instruments about a fixed point in space, normally located on the instrument itself. This mechanism enables minimally invasive instruments to preserve a consistent entry point, or port, throughout the entire procedure. This technique was developed by observing the surgeon's natural motion in manual laparoscopy. The RCM is a mechanism that accomplishes the same task. Following the insertion of the instrument, the RCM causes it to pivot about a fixed point in space – the point where it enters the body. Different robots use more or less sophisticated means of implementing the RCM, but there are very few surgical systems not using this principle today. In fact, all commercially available surgical robots are RCM-based robots.

Another important general component of medical robotic systems is the image acquisition device. This may generally be any medical imaging device (video, infrared, ultrasound, X-ray, or MRI), although imager compatibility issues exist, especially for the class of MRI scanners. Minimally invasive surgery utilizes intraoperative video and/or infrared cameras to provide the surgeon with a view of the surgical area. Since laparoscopy is highly dependent on the quality of the image the surgeon sees, there has been considerable recent attention paid to progress in optimizing laparoscopic imaging. Presently in use, stereo endoscopes allow for 3D visualization of the surgical field.[15] This increases surgical performance by facilitating more precise dissection between delicate anatomical planes and razor-sharp precision when handling sutures and minute tissue layers.[16,17] Unfortunately, many of the current technologies for 3D imaging are bulky and difficult to use. High-definition (HD) imaging is now available, although not in widespread use. HD camera chips produce more than 2 million pixels of resolution (or approximately 4 times better than the best traditional camera chips). It is estimated that the current cost of a complete HD video system for the operating room ranges between US$250,000 and US$500,000.[15] Although cost presently prohibits many laparoscopic centers from using HD technology, as the technology matures and costs drop, it is only a matter of time before HD technology becomes standard operating room technology.

The computer is the third general component of the surgical robotic system. Surgical robots bring computers into the operating room in a new way, providing a link between the 'data world' of medical images, sensors, and databases, and the physical world of surgical actions. This combination makes it possible to plan and execute surgical interventions precisely and predictably by fusing real-time and presurgical information about the patient. This information can then be used to improve surgical decision making and real-time control of surgical instruments. As robotic systems continue to incorporate real-time control and sensing, interventions will become more consistent and accurate than freehand interventions.

Furthermore, the computer inherently has the ability to acquire and retain a great deal of information about each intervention. For example, how much force was applied? For how long? Where, exactly, was a suture placed? Many such questions have yet to be quantitatively understood. Currently, the analysis of such log data attracts a good deal of attention within the medical robotics research community. As research progresses, we expect that lessons will be learned and additional experience will be acquired by surgeons through the use of these new 'smart' tools. This will, in turn, improve surgical quality and outcomes, in much the same way that similar uses of data have improved manufacturing quality and flight safety.

Image-guided robotic systems

The idea behind image-guided robotic systems is to allow the surgeon to 'point and click' on a medical image of a location within an organ, approve his or her selection and cause a robot to place a tool (a needle for example) at the physical equivalent of the position selected on the medical image. The first example of such a system was the work of Potamianos et al described previously.

The Johns Hopkins URobotics Laboratory[18] has developed several robotic components for image-guided percutaneous access. PAKY is an active and radiolucent needle driver.[19] Originally held by a passive arm, the needle in the needle driver was manually positioned under C-arm guidance. It was then locked in place and the needle inserted automatically under the surgeon's joystick control.[20] The next step was automation of the needle orientation procedure, which was accomplished with the addition of the RCM module.[14] The RCM supports and orients the PAKY driver while maintaining the fixed location of the needle tip. The combination of the two robotic systems enables the surgeon to place the needle automatically at a target specified on the computer screen by the urologist, on the basis of fluoroscopic images.[21] The PAKY-RCM offers an unquestionable improvement in needle placement accuracy and lowers procedure time while reducing radiation exposure to the patient and the urologist.[22]

Clinically, the PAKY-RCM system was tested in local as well as in several transatlantic telesurgical cases.[23] The PAKY-RCM system was also used under CT guidance with the Laser-Based CT/MR Registration.[24] This method of registering the patient to the image makes use of the laser markers readily available on any CT scanner. Once registered in this manner, the organ of interest can be targeted precisely. The procedure has been successfully used for biopsies and radiofrequency (RF) ablation of targets on the kidney and spine, as well as for nephrostomy tube placements.[25]

The newest robotic system from the Johns Hopkins URobotics Laboratory is called Tracker (Figure 26.1). It is mounted on the CT table and enters the scanner along with the patient.[26] Percutaneous access is achieved in the confined space of the imager without interfering with imager functionality. Tracker has undergone final laboratory evaluations and is now under clinical trial.[27,28]

The imaging method that yields perhaps the best-quality soft tissue images is MRI. Unfortunately, this is also the imaging method most difficult to use with a traditional (metal) robot. The high magnetic fields of the MRI cause forces equal to 27 times gravity on ferromagnetic metal objects, as well as heating them and causing other undesirable effects. Despite these difficulties, there is strong motivation for building an MRI-compatible robot because of the imaging capabilities of this technology. While CT scans are becoming more accurate, even spiral CT cannot provide as much information as MRI for many pathologies and organ systems. Using a CT scan, it is often possible to see small, suspicious areas in the prostate, but have extreme difficulty in accurately targeting them with the biopsy needle while relying on printed images and simultaneous TRUS. It can certainly be frustrating to see a lesion without having the option to locate it outside the scanner. The ideal solution is to be able to perform a biopsy under the real-time guidance of MRI images.

Several research groups are currently examining this problem. One MRI-compatible system for noninvasive surgery has been developed by Hynynen et al.[29] Another MRI-compatible device, a needle insertion manipulator using ultrasonic actuation, has been built by Masamune et al at the University of Tokyo[30] and tested on phantoms. Yet another system is currently under investigation at Brigham and Women's Hospital, Boston, Massachussetts. This is a robot with two long arms that extend into the imaging field by entering the space between sections of a specially designed 'double donut' MRI scanner.[31] The system can be used as an image-guided surgical assistant, integrating preoperative planning and intraoperative MRI images. The Johns Hopkins URobotics Laboratory is also working on a multi-imager-compatible robot with MRI capability for precise prostate access that incorporates a new kind of harmonic and planetary motor.[32] While there is much current research aimed at building MR-compatible robots, there are no clinically applicable systems of this type on the market at the present time.

Another interesting system, under investigation by an Italian group, uses a different strategy to improve the link between medical images and reality. The group have developed and evaluated an ultrasound-guided robot for use in transperineal biopsies.[33,34] This system uses four real-time video cameras and integrates this information with data gathered from the TRUS to position the robot for sample collection. Although the system has demonstrated target accuracy of 1–2 mm, expense and set-up time presently hinder feasibility.

A system for prostate brachytherapy with TRUS guidance is under development in the Johns Hopkins URobotics Laboratory in collaboration with the CISST Engineering Research Center and Burdette Medical Systems, Inc. Recently, a first evaluation has been successfully completed on phantom models[35] (Figure 26.2), and a specifically designed robot, which will integrate with the Burdette brachytherapy stand and dosimetry algorithms, is currently under development. This system will take advantage of advances in ultrasound technology that enable the TRUS alone to be sufficiently precise to hit targets accurately without the need for a cooperative, concurrent imaging modality.

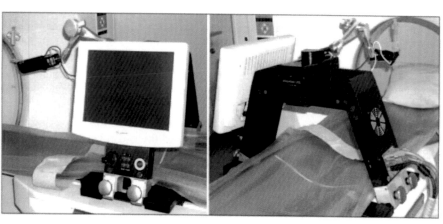

Figure 26.1
Tracker robot for CT-guided interventions. (Courtesy of Johns Hopkins URobotics Laboratory, Johns Hopkins Medical Institutions (JHMI).)

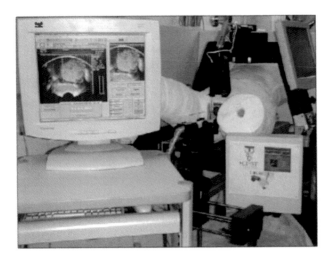

Figure 26.2
System for ultrasound-guided robotic brachytherapy. (Courtesy of Johns Hopkins URobotics Laboratory and Burdette Medical Systems, Inc.)

Surgeon-driven robotic systems

In contrast to image-guided robots, which automatically manipulate instruments under the prescription of the physician based on the digital image information, surgeon-driven systems take the surgeon's input continuously and, in real time, translate it to corresponding instrument manipulation. Surgeon-driven robots augment the manipulation capabilities of the physician in ways that passive, classic instruments cannot. They can decrease tremor, scale motion, aid in manipulation of tissues in confined spaces, and have the potential to provide remote haptic (tactile and force) feedback. They thereby enable decreasingly invasive operations to be performed.

The first surgeon-driven surgical assistant to receive FDA clearance was the AESOP, a robotic, laparoscopic camera holder. The AESOP has six degrees of freedom (DOF), two of which are passive (meaning they are positioned by hand and do not have motors actuating them). AESOP is easily mounted on the operating room table and can be conveniently stored away, mounted on a special cart. The function of AESOP is to hold and orient a laparoscopic camera under hand, foot or voice control.[36] The two passive joints protect against lateral forces on the abdominal wall during camera manipulation.

Perhaps the primary reason for AESOP's success is that it is simple to operate and, at the same time, reliable and safe. Additionally, the robot is easy to disconnect intraoperatively in the (highly unlikely) event that problems should arise. It is routinely used at several institutions and in many surgical disciplines, including a variety of laparoscopic urologic procedures.[37–39] The camera is significantly steadier under robot control and neither operative set-up

nor breakdown time is increased with the use of a robotic assistant.[40]

A surgeon-driven system to manipulate instruments designed for open surgery has been developed at the Stanford Research Institute (SRI), Menlo Park, California. The surgeon operates the two-armed robot equipped with high-mobility grippers from a remote console. Bowersox and Cornum have used the system for in-vivo porcine nephrectomies and repair of bladder and urethral injuries.[41]

Perhaps the most successful surgeon-driven robot thus far is the daVinci Surgical System for laparoscopy (Intuitive Surgical, Inc., Mountain View, California). The system was tested in early 2000 in Europe by cardiovascular surgeons performing laparoscopic cardiac bypass operations without using an extracorporeal cardiopulmonary bypass.[42] The daVinci Surgical System consists of a three-armed robot connected to a remote surgeon console (Figure 26.3). The surgeon operates the system while seated at the nonsterile console. The vision system is controlled using foot pedals and displays a 3D image of the surgical field similar to that seen in the open surgery case. The surgeon's movements are translated in real time to movements of the pencil-sized instruments in the surgical field. These enter the patient through small ports (on the order of 5–10 mm, depending on the tool). Two of the robotic arms are used for manipulating the surgical instruments, while the third arm manages the laparoscope. The instruments (needle holders, scissors, dissectors, scalpel, etc.) have seven DOF including rotation, and are maneuvered by a robotic wrist.

Using the daVinci Surgical System, one can potentially bypass much of the long learning curve traditionally associated with minimally invasive surgery. This is because the device automatically orients tool motion with respect to the camera view. Move your hand up and the tool moves up in the image, regardless of whether this lies physically in the same direction. Thus, the difficult, inverted, counterintuitive movements of conventional laparoscopy are eliminated and replaced by natural hand-eye coordination. Also possible is the reorienting of the surgeon's hands to more comfortable positions. With traditional laparoscopic tools, it is sometimes necessary to work with arms uncomfortably contorted in order to reach an object with the tools at the proper orientation. Using the daVinci Surgical System, the surgeon can move the tools to the proper location and orientation, press a button to hold them in place while he moves his controls to a comfortable position and then resume control of the tools. The daVinci Surgical System was cleared by the FDA in mid-2001 and is already in use at many centers throughout the USA in several surgical disciplines. Robot-assisted urologic surgery has already been successfully performed for partial/total and donor nephrectomies, pelvic lymphadenectomy, pyeloplasties, cryoablation procedures, diagnosis and treatment of cryptorchidism, as well as for radical prostatectomy and retroperitoneal procedures.[43–47]

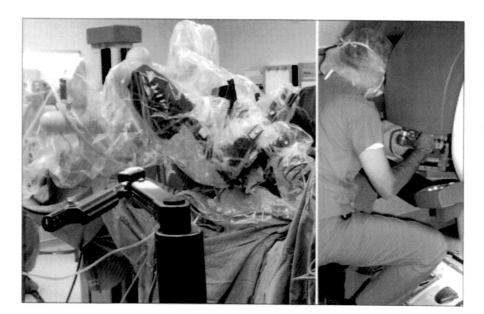

Figure 26.3
AESOP arm (foreground – left) and daVinci Surgical System (background – left, and surgeon's console – right) in a laparoscopic prostatectomy case at Johns Hopkins Medical Institutions (JHMI).

A competitor system is the Zeus system from Computer Motion, Inc., Goleta, California (the makers of AESOP). Similar to the daVinci Surgical System, the Zeus consists of the combination of three robot arms and a surgeon's control console. The system uses one AESOP for the laparoscope and the other two arms hold surgical instruments. Compared to the daVinci Surgical System, Zeus appears safer and requires significantly less preoperative setup. On the other hand, until recently, Zeus had exhibited lower dexterity of the tools within the patient. However, the company seems to have addressed this with the MicroWrist line of end-effector tools. Zeus received FDA clearance as a general laparoscopic tool in September 2002. The system has been used experimentally in a number of operations, including urology cases.[46,48] Most recently, Dr Peter Schulam at UCLA has used the system for reconstructing the kidney's draining system.[49]

Although very precise, present robotic systems lack the capability of completely reproducing tactile sensation (known as haptics). Some systems, such as Zeus, include partial force feedback,[50] but realistic, general haptic feedback is still a research topic. While the daVinci Surgical System does have some haptic feedback capability, this is usually disabled when the robot is used, because it does not provide a realistic feel. This is primarily because the forces are sensed from outside the patient, causing forces generated at the port to have a predominant effect, disturbing the sensation of forces experienced at the tip of the instrument. Haptics is an active research topic within the engineering community.[51,52] A good deal of work has been done investigating new kinds of tactile sensors.[53–57] There are also theoretical questions as yet unanswered about how best to display haptic information and there are a number of technical obstacles to overcome in hardware develop-

ment, signal processing, and systems integration before general haptic feedback will be possible.[56–58]

Telemedicine, telementoring, and telesurgery

The real-time data exchange of medical information between physicians in different locations is known as telemedicine. Telementoring describes the assistance of an experienced surgeon in a remote operation, while telesurgery implies his active involvement in the operation, manipulating instruments through the use of remotely controlled robots. The increasing accessibility of telecommunication systems, ranging from simple telephone lines to high-bandwidth fiberoptic and satellite transmissions,[59] allows physicians to communicate with their peers over any terrestrial distance. Teleconferences, broadcast surgeries, and consultations of specialists are common today, along with the worldwide exchange of medical images and data through the Internet. Surgical teleconsulting has been demonstrated to improve medical decision making, patient outcomes, and medical training.[60] Instead of being forced to travel long distances to other countries, specialists can now be available at any desired location for conferences or meetings while they sit at their office desks. Telemedicine has been successfully carried out over long distances between hospitals in the USA and Europe. Initial reports of telementoring and telesurgery were published as early as 1994 by Kavoussi et al.[39,61] and followed by a variety of intercontinental operations .[62–68]

In most cases, the surgeon remotely operated one or two robots, assisting the surgical team at the local hospital. The surgery begins with the local team setting up the operation: inserting the trocars and positioning the robots. Then, the remote surgeon controls only the laparoscope held by the robot to obtain a view of the surgical field. He also, in some cases, uses a telestrator to illustrate incision lines, anatomic structures, or critical areas visually to the local team.[69] The lag times for transmission of data have all been reported to be less than 200 ms and are hardly noticed during the procedure.[61,69,70]

By using an additional robot like the PAKY-RCM, the remote surgeon can actively retract organs or insert needles. The first transatlantic, assisted telerobotic surgery using two robots was successfully performed between Baltimore, Maryland, and Munich, Germany, in April 2001.[71] The remote surgeon controlled the laparoscope from his house via the AESOP robot, as well as a laparoscopic retractor with the PAKY-RCM robot. Active involvement in the operation was achieved by managing the gas inflation, telestration and electrocautery (Figure 26.4). For the transmission of the audio and video signal as well as robot control, a total of 512 kilobits per second (kbps) was needed, delivered by four ISDN lines at 128 kbps each. Although the remote expert was half a world away from the patient, his active involvement in the operation, along with the live visual and audio displays, gave the feeling of the expert's being in the operating room.

The most profound example of telesurgery thus far is known as Operation Lindbergh. This surgery was carried out using the Zeus robotic system between New York (remote location) and Strasbourg, France (patient loca-tion). The procedure was a complete laparoscopic chole-cystectomy, and was performed in September 2001. The surgery was carried out by Dr M Gagner (remote surgeon) under the local supervision of Professor J Marescaux, and was a complete success.[67] The event achieved worldwide recognition[63,64] in popular and scientific media.

One of the future goals of telesurgery is to deliver health care in medically underserved areas and thereby limit patient transportation.[65] Additionally, telesurgery has applications in armed conflicts where qualified medical care may not be readily accessible. This scenario was successfully investigated with telementoring via satellite connection between an aircraft carrier and a medical center in the USA.[72] In the long term, telesurgery could also be used in the longlasting, manned space missions of the future.

Before these goals become a reality, however, several issues must be addressed. Telemedicine of any kind is dependent on continuous and high-quality signal trans-mission.[59] Although local setup does not theoretically require a surgeon, experienced surgeons must be on hand at the patient's location, ready to take over the operation in case of system or transmission failure. Additionally, because of the necessary technical assistance in both loca-tions, coordination of such efforts, especially across several time zones, has proved challenging.

Another source of difficulty is the fact that medical tech-nology currently is advancing too rapidly for legislation to keep pace. Among the issues requiring attention are interstate and international licensure regulations, billing,

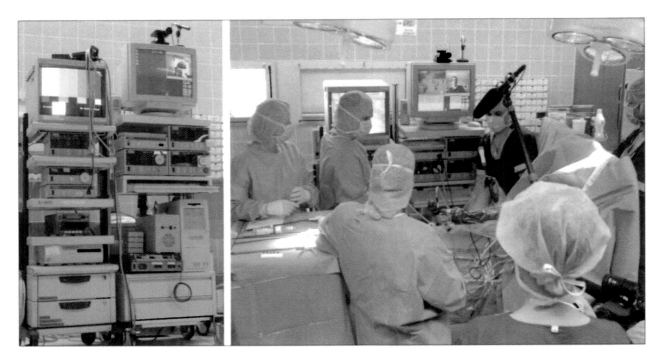

Figure 26.4
Remote controlled instrumentation and Munich operating room in telesurgery case.

informed consent, and malpractice insurance. It may be necessary to institute committees to set international standards, rules, regulations, and safety measures for the protection of the patient. The stringent technical requirements and costs of telesurgery are currently satisfied only by specialized centers throughout the world. However, the field is expected to expand in the future through wider distribution of robotic systems, and as reliable low-cost communication systems become more readily available.

Training devices for minimally invasive techniques

As mentioned earlier, there is currently a worldwide demand for laparoscopic specialists in many fields of surgery. Since an insufficient number of qualified training programs exists, surgeons currently attend training courses or observe procedures at specialized centers. While initial direct experiences with experts are very important, a constant exposure to the experience of laparoscopic manipulation is mandatory to keep and expand the acquired skills.[63] In a comparison of surgeons who attended a laparoscopic course, See et al[73] found the complication rate for surgeons who did not continually perform minimally invasive procedures three times greater than that of their course colleagues who did.[73,74] It is therefore crucial not only to train qualified laparoscopic surgeons in certified programs but also to ensure ongoing practice and mentoring.

Laparoscopy can be efficiently taught and tested using robotic devices, allowing instruments to be manipulated while various techniques and difficult situations are simulated. With these tools, tutoring by experienced minimally invasive surgeons as well as self- or computer-guided, hands-on training can be performed in a stress-free environment.

A 3-step laparoscopy training system is near completion in our URobotics Laboratory.[18] The first of these devices allows the trainee to become accustomed to the inverted manipulation of laparoscopic tools under direct (3D) vision. Using this system, the trainee inserts instruments through ball-joint trocar ports and operates on phantom or animal specimens. The Step 2 trainer is a closed box with similar entry ports for training under 2D visualization. The Step 3 trainer, presently in the experimental stages, replaces the opaque box used in the Step 2 trainer with a high-fidelity synthetic torso (Figure 26.5) which follows the male anatomy of the Visual Human Project of the National Library of Medicine (NLM). This Step 3 trainer closely simulates true human laparoscopy and reduces the need for surgical training on animals. The torso allows for the in-situ inclusion of abdominal animal organs, presents a disposable abdominal wall that can be

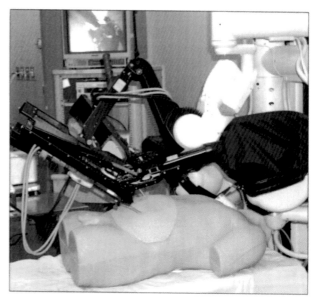

Figure 26.5
High-fidelity synthetic torso for urologic laparoscopy training. (Courtesy of Johns Hopkins URobotics Laboratory, Johns Hopkins Medical Institutions (JHMI).)

pressurized, and also includes respiratory simulation by connecting the torso to a respirator.

The ideal laparoscopy training method would be virtual reality (VR) based. In surgery, VR trainers provide the opportunity to learn through interacting with a simulated 3D environment. The VR student can perform in many different scenarios and create diverse teaching modules.[75] VR training can provide performance feedback and, perhaps someday, provide certification standards for training urologists.[76,77]

A VR flexible ureteroscopy simulator (HT Medical, Inc., Rockville, Maryland) allows surgeons to practice navigating through, and evaluating, the urinary collection system. Perhaps the most advanced VR simulators in urology thus far have been created by Dr Manyak's research group at George Washington University. The GWU team uses the Visible Human dataset for generating surface-based geometric data. Their systems are specialized VR trainers that provide a realistic experience of the lower urinary tract in endoscopic procedures.[78] The group has developed and continues to expand a computer-based surgical simulator that incorporates a surgical tool interface with anatomic detail and haptic feedback.

The use of VR in training has demonstrated that more-experienced laparoscopic surgeons perform surgical tasks with greater accuracy and efficiency than less-experienced surgeons.[79] Improvements in collision detection and graphics, among other things, are presently being tested. Clearly, the widespread distribution of realistic training devices has the potential to improve the skill of laparoscopic urologists worldwide.

Conclusion

New tools such as surgical robots provide diverse and promising possibilities for improving existing surgical techniques and for developing new ones. Among many other advantages, robots are often able to improve the dexterity and precision with which minimally invasive surgery is carried out.

Several surgical robotic systems have been developed, tested, and cleared by the FDA. Some of these have already demonstrated powerful clinical utility within urology. With continued technological improvements and the emphasis of both sides on strong partnerships between doctors and engineers, surgical robotics will continue to broaden horizons in the practice of urology.

Acknowledgments

Some of the research included in this presentation from our URobotics Laboratory was partially supported by grant No. 1R21CA088232–01A1 from the National Cancer Institute (NCI) and by grant No. PHD0103 from the American Foundation of Urologic Disease (AFUD). Robert Webster is supported by a fellowship from the National Defense Science and Engineering Graduate Fellowship (NDSEG). The contents of this chapter are solely the responsibility of the authors and do not necessarily represent the official views of NCI, AFUD, or NDSEG.

Disclosure

Under a licensing agreement between Image Guide and the Johns Hopkins University, Dr Stoianovici and Dr Kavoussi are entitled to a share of royalty received by the University on sales of some products described in this chapter. Dr Stoianovici, Dr Kavoussi, and the University own Image Guide stock, which is subject to certain restrictions under University policy. The terms of this arrangement are being managed by the Johns Hopkins University in accordance with its conflict of interest policies.

References

1. Stoianovici D, Cadeddu JA, Kavoussi LR. Urologic application of robotics. American Urological Association – 1999 AUA Update Series. Vol. XVIII, 1999; Lesson 25:194–200.

2. Caddedu JA, Stoianovici D, Kavoussi LR. Telepresence and robotics: urology in the 21st century. Contemp Urol 1997; 9:86–97.

3. Suryanarayanan S, Reddy NP, Gupta V. An intelligent system with EMG-based joint angle estimation for telemanipulation. Stud Health Technol Inform 1996; 29:546–52.

4. Mack MJ. Minimally invasive and robotic surgery. JAMA 2001; 285:568–72.

5. Cadeddu JA, Stoianovici D, Kavoussi LR. Robotics in urologic surgery. Urology 1997; 49:501–7.

6. Buckingham RA, Buckingham RO. Robots in operating theatres. BMJ 1995; 311:1479–82.

7. Davies BL, Hibberd RD, Coptcoat MJ, Wickham JE. A surgeon robot prostatectomy – a laboratory evaluation. J Med Eng Technol 1989; 13:273–7.

8. Davies BL, Hibberd RD, Ng WS, et al. The development of a surgeon robot for prostatectomies. Proc Inst Mech Eng [H] 1991; 205:35–8.

9. Potamianos P, Davies BL, Hibberd RD. Intra-operative imaging guidance for keyhole surgery: methodology and calibration. International Symposium on Medical Robotics and Computer Assisted Surgery, Pittsburgh, PA, 1994.

10. Potamianos P, Davies BL, Hibberd RD. Intra-operative registration for percutaneous surgery. International Symposium on Medical Robotics and Computer Assisted Surgery, Baltimore, MD, 1995.

11. Taylor RH, Funda J, Eldridge B, et al. A telerobotic assistant for laparoscopic surgery. IEEE Engineering in Medicine and Biology Magazine 1995; 279–87.

12. Taylor RH, Funda J, Grossman DD, et al. Remote center-of-motion robot for surgery. 5,397,323, Mar. 14

13. Bzostek A, Schreiner S, Barnes A, et al. An automated system for precise percutaneous access of the renal collecting system. In: CVRMed-MRCAS, ed. Lecture notes in computer science. Springer-Verlag, 1997:1205–99.

14. Stoianovici D, Whitcomb L, Anderson J, et al. A modular surgical robotic system for image-guided percutaneous procedures. In: Lecture notes in computer science, medical image computing and computer-assisted interventions, Cambridge, Mass, October 11–13, 1998, Vol. 1496, Springer-Verlag.

15. Kourambas J, Preminger GM. Advances in camera, video, and imaging technologies in laparoscopy. Urol Clin North Am 2001; 28:5–14.

16. Babayan RK, Chiu AW, Este-McDonald J. The comparison between 2-dimensional and 3-dimensional laparoscopic video systems in a pelvic trainer. J Endourol 1993; 7: S195.

17. Chiu AW, Babayan RK. Retroperitoneal laparoscopic nephrectomy utilizing three-dimensional camera. Case report. J Endourol 1994; 8:139–41.

18. Stoianovici D. URobotics – urology robotics at Johns Hopkins. Comput Aided Surg 2001; 6:360–9.

19. Stoianovici D, Kavoussi LR, Whitcomb LL, et al. Friction transmission with axial loading and a radiolucent surgical needle driver. United States Patent 6,400,979, June 4, 2002.

20. Stoianovici D, Cadeddu JA, Demaree RD, et al. An efficient needle injection technique and radiological guidance method for percutaneous procedures. In: Lecture notes in computer science, medical robotics and computer-assisted surgery, Grenoble, France, March, 1997, Vol. 1205. Springer-Verlag.

21. Patriciu A, Stoianovici D, Whitcomb L, et al. Motion-based robotic instrument targeting under C-Arm fluoroscopy. In: Lecture notes in computer science, medical image computing and computer-assisted interventions, Pittsburgh, PA, October 11–14, 2000, Vol. 1935. Springer-Verlag.

22. Cadeddu JA, Stoianovici D, Chen RN, et al. Stereotactic mechanical percutaneous renal access. J Endourol 1998; 12:121–5.

23. Bauer J, Lee BR, Stoianovici D, et al. Remote percutaneous renal access using a new automated telesurgical robotic system. Telemed J E Health 2001; 7:341–6.

24. Patriciu A, Solomon SB, Kavoussi LR, Stoianovici D. Robotic kidney and spine percutaneous procedures using a new laser-based CT registration method. In: Lecture notes in computer science, medical image computing and computer-assisted interventions, Utrecht, Netherlands, October 14–17, 2001, Vol. 2208. Springer-Verlag.

25. Solomon S, Patriciu A, Masamune K, et al. CT guided robotic needle biopsy: a precise sampling method minimizing radiation exposure. Radiology 2001; In Press.

26. Stoianovici D, Cleary K, Patriciu A, et al. AcuBot: a robotic system for radiological interventions. IEEE Trans Robotics and Automation 2003: 3,19:926–30.

27. Cleary K, Stoianovici D, Patriciu A, et al. Robotically assisted nerve and facet blocks: a cadaveric study. Acad Radiol 2002; 9:821–5.

28. Cleary K, Onda S, Banovac F, et al. CT-directed robotic biopsy testbed: user interface and coordinate transformations. Comput Ass Rad Surg 2001; Elsevier: 171–77.

29. Hynynen K, Darkazanli A, Unger E, Schenck JF. MRI guided noninvasive ultrasound surgery. Med Phys 1992; 20:107–16.

30. Masamune K, Kobayashi E, Masutani Y, et al. Development of an MRI-compatible needle insertion manipulator for stereotactic neurosurgery. J Image Guid Surg 1995; 1:242–8.

31. Chinzei K, Miller K. Towards MRI guided surgical manipulator. Med Sci Monit 2001; 7:153–63.

32. Stoianovici D, Kavoussi LR. Planetary – Harmonic Motor. United States Provisional Patent 60/411,906, Filed 9/19/02.

33. Rovetta A. Tests on reliability of a prostate biopsy telerobotic system. Stud Health Technol Inform 1999; 62:302–7.

34. Rovetta A. Computer assisted surgery with 3D robot models and visualisation of the telesurgical action. Stud Health Technol Inform 2000; 70:292–4.

35. Fichtinger G, DeWeese TL, Patriciu A, et al. System for robotically assisted prostate biopsy and therapy with intraoperative CT guidance. Acad Radiol 2002; 9:60–74.

36. Mettler L, Ibrahim M, Jonat W. One year of experience working with the aid of a robotic assistant (the voice-controlled optic holder AESOP) in gynaecological endoscopic surgery. Hum Reprod 1998; 13:2748–50.

37. Partin AW, Adams JB, Moore RG, Kavoussi LR. Complete robot-assisted laparoscopic urologic surgery: a preliminary report. J Am Coll Surg 1995; 181:552–7.

38. Sackier JM, Wang Y. Robotically assisted laparoscopic surgery. From concept to development. Surg Endosc 1994; 8:63–6.

39. Kavoussi LR, Moore RG, Partin AW, et al. Telerobotic assisted laparoscopic surgery: initial laboratory and clinical experience. Urology 1994; 44:15–19.

40. Kavoussi LR, Moore RG, Adams JB, Partin AW. Comparison of robotic versus human laparoscopic camera control. J Urol 1995; 154:2134–6.

41. Bowersox JC, Cornum RL. Remote operative urology using a surgical telemanipulator system: preliminary observations. Urology 1998; 52:17–22.

42. Chitwood WR Jr, Nifong LW. Minimally invasive videoscopic mitral valve surgery: the current role of surgical robotics. J Card Surg 2000; 15:61–75.

43. Binder J, Jones J, Bentas W, et al. [Robot-assisted laparoscopy in urology. Radical prostatectomy and reconstructive rectroperitoneal interventions]. Urologe A 2002; 41:144–9.

44. Hemal AK, Menon M. Laparoscopy, robot, telesurgery and urology: future perspective. J Postgrad Med 2002; 48:39–41.

45. Rassweiler J, Frede T, Seemann O, et al. Telesurgical laparoscopic radical prostatectomy. Initial experience. Eur Urol 2001; 40:75–83.

46. Breda G, Nakada SY, Rassweiler JJ. Future developments and perspectives in laparoscopy. Eur Urol 2001; 40:84–91.

47. Rassweiler J, Binder J, Frede T. Robotic and telesurgery: will they change our future? Curr Opin Urol 2001; 11:309–20.

48. Schuessler WW, Schulam PG, Clayman RV, Kavoussi LR. Laparoscopic radical prostatectomy: initial short-term experience. Urology 1997; 50:854–7.

49. UCLA. Robots in surgery: no longer science fiction. Clark Urological Center Newsletter, Vol. 14, 2002:1–2.

50. Reichenspurner H, Damiano RJ, Mack M, et al. Use of the voice-controlled and computer-assisted surgical system ZEUS for endoscopic coronary artery bypass grafting. J Thorac Cardiovasc Surg 1999; 118:6–11.

51. Gerovichev O, Marayong P, Okamura AM. The effect of visual and haptic feedback on manual and teleoperated needle insertion, medical image computing and computer assisted intervention (MICCAI). Lecture Notes in Computer Science, 2002, Vol. 2488.

52. Kitagawa M, Bethea BT, L GV, et al. Analysis of suture manipulation forces for teleoperation with force feedback, medical image computing and computer assisted intervention (MICCAI). Lecture Notes in Computer Science 2002; 2488: 155–162.

53. Wellman PS, Dalton EP, Krag D, et al. Tactile imaging of breast masses: first clinical report. Arch Surg 2001; 136:204–8.

54. Pawluk DT, Howe RD. Dynamic contact of the human fingerpad against a flat surface. J Biomech Eng 1999; 121:605–11.

55. Pawluk DT, Howe RD. Dynamic lumped element response of the human fingerpad. J Biomech Eng 1999; 121:178–83.

56. Howe RD, Peine WJ, Kontarinis DA, Son JS. Remote palpation technology for surgical applications. IEEE Engineering in Medicine and Biology Magazine. Vol. 14, 1995:318–23.

57. Howe RD. Tactile sensing and control of robotic manipulation. Adv Robotics 1994; 8:245–61.

58. Stoianovici D. Robotic surgery. World J Urol 2000; 18:289–95.

59. Broderick TJ, Harnett BM, Merriam NR, et al. Impact of varying transmission bandwidth on image quality. Telemed J E Health 2001; 7:47–53.

60. Demartines N, Mutter D, Vix M, et al. Assessment of telemedicine in surgical education and patient care. Ann Surg 2000; 231:282–91.

61. Lee BR, Caddedu JA, Janetschek G, et al. International surgical telementoring: our initial experience. Stud Health Technol Inform 1998; 50:41–7.

62. Ballantyne GH. Robotic surgery, telerobotic surgery, telepresence, and telementoring. Surg Endosc 2002; 16;1389–1402.

63. Clayman RV. Transatlantic robot-assisted telesurgery. J Urol 2002; 168:873–4.

64. Larkin M. Transatlantic, robot-assisted telesurgery deemed a success. Lancet 2001; 358:1074.

65. Link RE, Schulam PG, Kavoussi LR. Telesurgery. Remote monitoring and assistance during laparoscopy. Urol Clin North Am 2001; 28:177–88.

66. Malassagne B, Mutter D, Leroy J, et al. Teleeducation in surgery: European Institute for Telesurgery experience. World J Surg 2001; 25:1490–4.

67. Marescaux J, Leroy J, Gagner M, et al. Transatlantic robot-assisted telesurgery. Nature 2001; 413:379–80.

68. Frimberger D, Kavoussi LR, Stoianovici D, et al. Telerobotic Surgery zwischen Baltimore und München. Urologe A 2002; 41:489–492.

69. Micali S, Virgili G, Vannozzi E, et al. Feasibility of telementoring between Baltimore (USA) and Rome (Italy): the first five cases. J Endourol 2000; 14:493–6.

70. Fabrizio MD, Lee BR, Chan DY, et al. Effect of time delay on surgical performance during telesurgical manipulation. J Endourol 2000; 14:133–8.

71. Frimberger D, Kavoussi LR, Stoianovici D, et al. Telerobotische Chirurgie zwischen Baltimore und München. Der Urologe [A] 2002; 41:489–92.

72. Cubano M, Poulose BK, Talamini MA, et al. Long distance telementoring. A novel tool for laparoscopy aboard the USS Abraham Lincoln. Surg Endosc 1999; 13:673–8.

73. See WA, Cooper CS, Fisher RJ. Predictors of laparoscopic complications after formal training in laparoscopic surgery. JAMA 1993; 270:2689–92.

74. Colegrove PM, Winfield HN, Donovan JF Jr, See WA. Laparoscopic practice patterns among North American urologists 5 years after formal training. J Urol 1999; 161:881–6.

75. Satava RM, Jones SB. Preparing surgeons for the 21st century. Implications of advanced technologies. Surg Clin North Am 2000; 80:1353–65.

76. Arnold P, Farrell MJ. Can virtual reality be used to measure and train surgical skills? Ergonomics 2002; 45:362–79.

77. Laguna MP, Hatzinger M, Rassweiler J. Simulators and endourological training. Curr Opin Urol 2002; 12:209–15.

78. Manyak MJ, Santangelo K, Hahn J, et al. Virtual reality surgical simulation for lower urinary tract endoscopy and procedures. J Endourol 2002; 16:185–90.

79. Taffinder N, Sutton C, Fishwick RJ, et al. Validation of virtual reality to teach and assess psychomotor skills in laparoscopic surgery: results from randomised controlled studies using the MIST VR laparoscopic simulator. Stud Health Technol Inform 1998; 50:124–30.

27

Complications of uro-oncology laparoscopic surgery

Sam B Bhayani and Louis R Kavoussi

Introduction

Over the past decade, urologic laparoscopy has evolved from an experimental technique to an efficacious and popular surgical modality. As the field has matured, investigators have recognized the complications of performing urologic laparoscopy. Although many complications are an inevitable part of practice, risks can be decreased by the informed laparoscopist. The surgeon who offers minimally invasive surgery must be prepared to manage or avoid these complications when subjecting patients to laparoscopic procedures. Overall, the complication rate of urologic laparoscopic procedures is 3.5–11.9%. Reoperation is required in 0.08–1.1% of cases, and the mortality rate is approximately 0.09%.[1–5] Although these results have largely been published by experienced laparoscopists, they demonstrate that the knowledgeable surgeon can safely offer laparoscopic alternatives to major open surgeries. As with open surgery, complications are more prevalent in complex procedures and are more common earlier in the learning curve. Hence, initial cases should be highly selected, and open instruments should be readily available. As the surgeon's comfort level and experience grow, more complex procedures can be attempted.

To recognize, manage, and ultimately minimize complications, the laparoscopist must be familiar with laparoscopic physiology and laparoscopic surgical anatomy. Additionally, the surgeon must have an intimate knowledge of the complex equipment used in performing the operations. Also, given the limited operative view, the surgeon must strive to understand not only what is in the operative field but also what is in the nonvisualized visceral structures. Finally, when discussing risks of laparoscopic surgery, the patient should be informed of the possibility of open conversion in all cases.

Complications may arise at any point in the procedure, from positioning of the patient to postoperative management. The operating room (OR) team must be vigilant in recognizing potential problems at any time during the case. Effective communication between the surgeon, assistants, anesthesiologist, and staff is desirable. All OR personnel should be familiar with laparoscopic and open surgical equipment and monitors.

Complications from positioning

Laparoscopic procedures are sometimes longer than their open counterparts. Also, extremes in table movement may be needed so that the bowel can be moved out of the operative field. Consequently, proper padding of the patient's pressure points is necessary. Neuromuscular injuries are infrequent, but may contribute to patient morbidity. A recent multi-institutional study of 1651 patients undergoing urologic laparoscopic procedures revealed a 2.7% incidence of neuromuscular injury.[6] Injuries were more common with upper retroperitoneal procedures (3.1%) than with pelvic laparoscopy (1.5%). Patients in the full flank position were found to be more prone to neuromuscular injury than those in the partial flank position. Rhabdomyolysis occurred in 6 patients (0.4%); all had undergone upper retroperitoneal laparoscopy, were heavier, and underwent longer procedures. Institutions with higher volumes of laparoscopic procedures had a lower incidence of complications.

Neuromuscular injuries can be minimized by close attention to padding and positioning of the patient. Heavier patients undergoing retroperitoneal procedures should be informed of their increased risk of these injuries. Hidden pressure points, such as the axilla, legs, and arms, should be carefully checked after all manipulations of the OR table. Patients with little body fat are at risk for rhabdomyolysis. Therefore, hard surfaces such as a beanbag should be avoided. Rhabdomyolysis should be considered in patients with low urine output, extensive muscle pain, or darkened urine. A serum creatine kinase level will be elevated, and urine myoglobin may be increased. Treatment is largely supportive; volume expansion and urinary alkalinization are recommended, and diuretics can be used to maintain urine output. Acute renal failure may require consultation with a nephrologist and temporary dialysis. In the majority of cases, renal function will improve.

Neuromuscular problems may also affect the surgeon. After performing laparoscopic procedures, urologists reported pain in their necks, shoulders, backs, wrists, and hands at frequencies of 17–67%.[6] Some surgeons required professional consultation for their injuries. To minimize these injuries, the surgeon must be positioned for comfort and efficiency. Monitors must all be within the surgeon's sight, and pedals for dissecting instruments should be placed in an ergonomic fashion. The table height must be adjusted to the surgeon's comfort level to minimize fatigue. Standing stools are commonly used. Additionally, various laparoscopic OR environments have been engineered to enhance surgeon comfort and control (OR1, Karl Storz, Tuttlingen, Germany; Hermes, Stryker: Endoscopy, San Jose, California). These systems include highly mobile video monitors and voice or touchscreen control of lighting and insufflation.

Complications with access and insufflation

Access to the peritoneal cavity may be achieved with Veress needle insufflation and blind trocar placement ('closed technique'), or an open incision through the fascia, with placement of a blunt Hasson trocar under direct vision ('open technique'). Newer optical access trocars incorporate a laparoscope into the initial trocar so the path of access may be visualized. All three techniques are widely used, but open access has a slightly lower complication rate in large retrospective series.[7,8] However, smaller prospective randomized trials have not shown a difference in major complications between closed-access and open-access techniques.[9] Optical access has not been as widely evaluated as the other two techniques, but may be safer than closed access, since the path of access is visualized.[10,11] Nevertheless, there are reports of bowel injury with the use of optical access trocars. Access-related complications most commonly involve preperitoneal insufflation, injury to visceral vessels or bowel, and abdominal wall hemorrhage.

Preperitoneal insufflation occurs if the Veress needle is placed superficial to the peritoneal cavity. Limited insufflation of this potential space results in the peritoneum being pushed away from the abdominal fascia, and may make subsequent trocar placement difficult. One indicator of preperitoneal insufflation is high pressure at low volume of insufflated carbon dioxide. If a trocar is placed, preperitoneal fat will be visualized, and the abdomen may appear asymmetrical. Management of this complication usually necessitates open trocar access with a direct cutdown into the peritoneal cavity. Preperitoneal insufflation also may result in significant subcutaneous emphysema. Finally, the peritoneal space may not fully expand after proper access is achieved, thus limiting visualization in portions of the operative field. Preperitoneal insufflation can be avoided by performing a 'drop test'; saline is injected into the Veress needle, and if it freely flows into the abdomen under gravity, the Veress needle is most likely properly placed. However, this test is not perfect, and the pressure and flow monitors should be closely watched during initial insufflation. If high pressure and low flow are achieved at low volume, then the Veress needle is likely not placed properly, and preperitoneal insufflation is a possibility.

Major vascular injury during access must be recognized immediately in order to avoid catastrophic sequelae. Vascular placement of the Veress needle is apparent when aspiration reveals blood in the syringe. Although the needle can be safely withdrawn in many cases, some instances have required open surgical repair, and death has been reported from an aortic puncture.[12] An alternative is to leave the needle in place, and directly examine the puncture from an access point. The needle can be withdrawn under direct vision, and appropriate hemostatic measures can be instituted. If a major injury is suspected, laparotomy should be performed. Laparoscopic vascular repair is possible, but should be undertaken only by an experienced surgeon.

Trocar injury to the aorta, vena cava, or major pelvic vessels may occur during access. Brisk blood return will be noted with removal of the obturator or during laparoscope insertion. The obturator should be returned to the cannula to tamponade the hemorrhage. Immediate laparotomy should be considered, and the trocar should be left in place as it can guide the surgeon to the site of injury. The laparoscopist may need the assistance of a vascular specialist to obtain control of the injured vessel, and the anesthesiologist should be active in resuscitation of the patient. If the trocar has been displaced from the injury, the laparoscope may be inserted into the abdomen to visualize the site of hemorrhage. Nevertheless, laparotomy should not be postponed in patients with major vessel injury from trocar placement, as these patients have substantial morbidity and mortality.[13] Delayed recognition has been reported several times, as the injury may be outside of the operative field, or hemorrhage may be confined to the retroperitoneum or pelvis.[14,15]

The Veress needle may also be placed into the small or large intestine. Upon aspiration, enteric contents may be noted in the syringe. Access should be made at a second site, and the area can be inspected for enteric leak. If necessary, the injury can be oversewn laparoscopically, or if a large defect is noted, laparotomy and formal repair may be needed. If the misplaced Veress needle is not recognized, insufflation of the bowel will reveal high pressures at low volumes. Flatus or asymmetrical distention of the abdomen may be noted. In patients with suspected abdominal adhesions, an open-access technique may be used to minimize this complication.

Trocar injury to the bowel requires repair. Upon insertion of the laparoscope, the inner mucosa of the bowel may be visualized, thus securing the diagnosis. Injury may also be noted after insertion of the secondary trocars, revealing more extensive injuries on the path of the initial access port. Laparotomy for repair of the injury may be necessary. The entire bowel should be examined circumferentially, as 'through and through' injury may have occurred. Laparoscopic repair of an isolated injury is possible for surgeons experienced with intracorporeal suturing or stapling.

Abdominal wall injury during access may be a cause of hemorrhage. The most significant vessels causing this complication are the inferior epigastric vessels, which may be injured from lateral trocar placement. Usually, a constant dripping of blood from the trocar indicates injury to abdominal wall vessels. A hematoma may develop at the site of injury. Transillumination of the abdominal wall will help to avoid superficial vessels, but the inferior epigastric pedicle usually will not be seen.

The epigastric vessels usually lie at the margin of the rectus sheath, and trocars should be placed lateral to this site. Handheld intraoperative ultrasound has been used to localize the epigastric vessels intraoperatively with great success, but may not be practical in most cases.[16]

If abdominal wall hemorrhage is suspected, the area should be inspected externally and laparoscopically. The bleeding vessel can be cauterized if it is visualized. If not seen well, a variety of suture techniques can be used to control the hemorrhage. The Carter–Thomason fascial closure device (Inlet Medical Inc., Eden Prairie, Minnesota) can be used to create circumferential control of the vessel. Alternatively, a Keith needle may be passed through the skin on one side of the vessel. The needle is grasped with laparoscopic forceps, guided back through the skin and around the vessel, and tied over a bolster. If suturing is not possible, a Foley catheter can be passed into the site, inflated, and retracted against the abdominal wall, thus tamponading the vessel. This technique is probably safe for small venous tears, but control of arterial bleeders may be variable. Importantly, all port sites should be examined at the conclusion of the operation as the trocars are withdrawn. A trocar may occlude a torn vessel, which may reopen upon withdrawal of the trocar from the port site. Newer radially dilating and nonbladed trocars may reduce the incidence of abdominal wall injuries, but further studies need to confirm these theoretical benefits.[11, 17]

Gas embolism

Gas embolism is a rare but devastating complication. Although CO_2 is currently the insufflant of choice because of its high solubility in blood, gas embolism may still occur with its use. Embolism commonly occurs in initial access, during which a punctured vein is insufflated. It may also occur at high intraperitoneal pressure, as gas may be forced into an open vein. Gas embolism is usually recognized when there is rapid cardiovascular collapse. Signs of this complication include a mill wheel murmur, bradycardia or arrhythmia, mydriasis, decreases in oxygen saturation, hypotension, or arrest. End-tidal CO_2 is classically decreased, but may be increased with smaller emboli.[18–20]

Gas embolism occurs when a CO_2 bolus enters the peripheral venous circulation, passes through the right ventricle, and obstructs the outflow of the right heart. These events lead to a decrease in circulatory flow to the left ventricle, decreased cardiac output, and profound cardiovascular collapse.[19,20] Emergent treatment of this complication is necessary; the patient should be placed in the left lateral decubitus position with the head down. Cardiopulmonary resuscitation with appropriate pressors is often necessary, and an attempt may be made to percutaneously aspirate the embolus by guiding a central line into the right heart. Several deaths have been reported from gas embolism, and vigilant cardiac monitoring during the procedure is essential to recognition of this entity.

Gas embolism may also occur with the argon beam coagulator. This instrument is often used during laparoscopic partial nephrectomy to assist with hemostasis of the incised renal parenchyma.[21–24] The flow rate of the argon beam coagulator may be as high as 6 liters/min, often forcing pneumoperitoneum pressures above 40 mmHg. This high-pressure environment, coupled with actively bleeding venules, can produce an environment in which argon embolism is conceivable. Additionally, argon is 17 × less soluble than carbon dioxide. Avoidance of this complication centers on maintaining safe pressures during argon beam coagulation. The CO_2 insufflant may be turned down to lower pressure, and most importantly, a vent can be opened on a trocar to permit rapid gas escape. If argon embolism does occur, treatment is similar to that for CO_2 embolism. Cardiac arrest and death have been reported with the device.[25–27]

Complications related to the pneumoperitoneum

The pneumoperitoneum can alter the patient's physiologic homeostasis. Since the detailed physiology of the pneumoperitoneum is covered in a previous chapter, only the major adverse consequences will be discussed here. As most of the complications are pressure dependent, the laparoscopist should attempt to use the lowest pressure possible during the operation. Most surgeons work between 10–15 mmHg, with higher pressures used transiently to limit bleeding in the field.

The cardiodepressant effects of the CO_2 pneumoperitoneum are well documented.[28,29] Patients generally will experience increased vascular resistance, impaired venous return, and decreased cardiac output. Although these changes may not affect the otherwise healthy individual, patients with compromised cardiac function may be sensitive to these effects, particularly at higher pressures. Patients with severe cardiac dysfunction may require invasive monitoring with central venous catheters or Swan–Ganz lines.

Transperitoneal absorption of CO_2 can lead to hypercarbia and acidosis.[28,29] Usually this effect is countered by increasing minute ventilation; however, patients with impaired pulmonary function or obstructive pulmonary disease may not compensate. Generally, lowering the CO_2 pressure can counter the hypercarbia. In severe cases of hypercarbia, the insufflant may be changed to helium, thus eliminating the insulting agent. Helium, however, is markedly less soluble than CO_2, and gas embolism is an inherent risk.[30,31] Nitrous oxide may also be used as an insufflant, and has little effect on end-tidal CO_2.[32]

Urine output is suppressed during laparoscopy,[33] primarily because of decreased renal vein flow and compression of the renal parenchyma. Compression of the ureter has not been implicated, as stenting the patient will not increase urinary flow. The oliguria resolves after the procedure, and no long-term adverse sequelae are known. It is imperative that the anesthesia team be aware of this effect and avoid overhydration of the patient.

The medical effects of the pneumoperitoneum can last for several hours after the procedure ends, as acid–base and ventilatory changes must normalize. Patients with medical comorbidities should be observed closely in the post-anesthesia unit for potential medical complications from the laparoscopic procedure.

Electrosurgical injury

Unlike open surgery, laparoscopic surgery requires the increased use of energy sources to perform tissue/organ ablation. Complications from the use of electrosurgery may arise in this unique operating environment.

Monopolar energy is commonly used in laparoscopic surgery, and a basic understanding of electrosurgical physics is essential to avoiding complications from this energy source. Monopolar energy is transmitted as a complete circuit; the electricity originates at a generator, travels through the surgical instrument to the target tissue, and then spreads over surrounding tissue to the abdominal wall, where a grounding pad re-establishes a connection to the generator. Any break in this electrical loop can injure tissue at the point of disjunction. One mechanism of injury is an insulation defect in the surgical instrument,

leading to energy transmission at the leak point. When an insulation defect occurs and cautery use is attempted, energy transmission will not be seen on the target tissue. Instead, the energy will be transmitted at the leak point. The instrument should be withdrawn immediately, and tissues in the path of the instrument should be examined for electrosurgical injury. The device should be closely examined for cracks and insulation defects.

Direct coupling can also cause electrosurgical injury. In this case, another instrument is in contact with the electrosurgical instrument and current is transmitted to the secondary device. Importantly, this contact between instruments may occur outside the field of view. To avoid direct coupling, trocars and instruments should be separated at a reasonable distance, so that the instruments are prevented from crossing or touching. Of note, direct coupling may occur over metal clips or staples; most newer clips are titanium, but the patient may have metallic clips from a previous procedure.

A rare mechanism of electrosurgical injury occurs secondary to capacitive coupling. This injury occurs if the current cannot be transmitted back to the abdominal wall. Such a situation arises with hybrid cannulae, in which the metal shaft of the trocar is anchored to the skin with a plastic apron. The cannula can accumulate electrical energy, which will be transmitted upon contact with tissue or another instrument. With modern access devices, this complication has not been reported.

Electrosurgical injuries may be limited by using alternative energy delivery systems. Bipolar energy is transmitted through an instrument in which the active electrode and the return electrode are in close proximity. Only the area between the electrodes receives the electrical current; there is not a complete electrical circuit through the patient. The most commonly used instruments can also function as forceps or graspers. An alternative energy source is the harmonic scalpel, which utilizes ultrasonic energy.

Although electrical injuries can be minimized with alternative energy devices, none of these devices is protective against a direct organ insult. All energy sources may directly injure bowel or vascular structures during dissection if they are inadvertently fired in close proximity to the naive tissue. Vascular injuries are usually readily apparent, and can be controlled laparoscopically with sutures or hemostatic tissue sealants. Bowel injury may not be apparent, and surgeons should maintain a high clinical suspicion.

Unrecognized bowel injury and management

Bowel injury may occur at numerous points in any laparoscopic procedure. Bowel may be inadvertently injured during access, dissection, removal or introduction of instruments, and closure. A review of the literature suggests that 69% of injuries are unrecognized at the time of initial laparoscopy.[34] Intraoperative diagnosis may be suggested by blanching of the enteric surface or serosal tears. If a small enterotomy is noted, intraoperative laparoscopic repair is reasonable with intracorporeal suturing. The bowel should be closely examined for multiple injuries, especially if trocar injury is suspected. Bowel resection and reanastomosis is also possible via intracorporeal technique, or extracorporeally through extension of a port site. Open repair should be performed if laparoscopic repair is not feasible.

If unrecognized intraoperatively, the postoperative diagnosis of bowel injury can be difficult. Traditionally, patients with bowel injury present predictably and rapidly with leukocytosis, peritoneal signs, fever, and sepsis. However, laparoscopic bowel injury may not follow this dogma; the presentation is frequently atypical and delayed. The mean time to recognition of bowel injury is 2–4 days after the insult, and may be as late as 2–4 weeks after surgery. Furthermore, patients commonly present with pain at a trocar site, abdominal distention, leukopenia, and diarrhea. Computer tomography (CT) scan can aid in diagnosis, and most patients should undergo open exploration.[34] Mortality is considerable, and may be increased in patients with duodenal injury.[35] After exploration, patients may require intensive care support and parenteral nutrition. Despite the rare occurrence of bowel injury, the clinician should maintain a high level of suspicion for the injury, as the sequelae may be devastating.

Port-site metastases

Laparoscopic surgery is becoming a prevalent treatment modality for various genitourinary malignancies. Therefore, prevention of port-site metastases is necessary to maintain favorable oncologic outcome. The incidence of port-site metastasis after genitourinary oncologic surgery appears to be low; there have been two reports of seeding after radical nephrectomy for renal cell carcinoma and three reports of seeding after treatment of transitional cell carcinoma.[36-39]

The two cases of port-site metastases from renal cell carcinoma are instructive. In one case, the final tumor was a high-grade T3 lesion with sarcomatoid elements. The recurrence of such a tumor at a port-site is analogous to the general surgical literature, in which aggressive cancers such as cholangiocarcinoma have a high rate of port site metastases.[40] The second case occurred after morcellation of a specimen in a patient with ascites; multiple port-site metastases were noted on follow-up. It is unknown if tumor cells were seeded into the ascetic fluid during the dissection or morcellation. These two cases suggest that contamination must be avoided upon specimen extraction. If the surgeon prefers morcellation, an impermeable

tear-proof sac should be used, the field should be doubly draped to prevent exposure of the port site to the specimen, contaminated instruments should be removed, and gloves should be changed at the conclusion of the procedure. The port site should be irrigated thoroughly with heparinized saline. Care is paramount in patients with ascites, as the fluid may transmit the tumor cells throughout the peritoneum.

Port-site hernias

Herniation of bowel or omentum through the trocar sites is a recognized complication of laparoscopy. Generally, 10 mm trocar sites are closed at the fascia level, whereas 5 mm trocar sites are not. In children, 5 mm trocar sites should be closed because they are more prone to development of hernias. Even though most investigators do not close the 5 mm site in adults, there have been rare reports of bowel and omental herniation through the 5 mm site.[41-43] If the 5 mm site is used extensively, the fascia could be weakened, and closure may be favored; ultimately the decision to close these sites is individualized.

New radially dilating trocars make a smaller fascial defect than bladed trocars, and some advocate not closing the 10 mm trocar site if these newer devices are used. These trocars make a fascial defect of 6–8 mm with a 10/12 mm trocar, and the overlying muscle is split instead of incised. Preliminary studies of the radially dilating trocars have not reported herniation, but longer-term and larger studies are needed to verify this outcome.[44, 45]

Individual procedures

Since the first laparoscopic nephrectomy was described by Clayman et al in 1991, surgeons have expanded the use of laparoscopy to several other procedures.[46] Several series have documented the efficacy and safety of operations that were traditionally performed with open techniques. The following sections will review complications which are salient to the more commonly performed laparoscopic urologic procedures. These include nephrectomy (donor, radical, partial, simple), nephroureterectomy, pyeloplasty, adrenalectomy, retroperitoneal lymphadenectomy, and prostatectomy. Most of these procedures have complications which mirror their open counterparts, but laparoscopic management is possible in several instances.

Donor nephrectomy

One unique complication that has been encountered in laparoscopic donor nephrectomy compromises ureteral complications in the recipient. Two groups reported an increase in ureteral complications in their initial experience. Technical modifications have been made to successfully minimize this complication. The ureteral dissection is very limited to preserve the vascular supply to the structure; no dissection is performed lateral to the gonadal vein. The gonadal vein and ureter should be harvested in one large bundle of tissue. This alteration has decreased the ureteral complication rate from 10% to 3%, which is similar to rates in open series.[47, 48]

Radical nephrectomy

Major complications occur in 3–8% of laparoscopic radical nephrectomies.[49–54] Hemorrhage is the most common major complication, and can be controlled with pressure from sponges, identification of the bleeding vessel, and selective use of suture, cautery, fibrin glue, or clips. Conversion to a hand-assisted operation or open operation can also aid in control of bleeding. Other reported complications include injury to the superior mesenteric artery, diaphragmatic injury, pancreatic fistula, and splenic injury.

Dissection of the upper pole of the kidney can result in a diaphragm injury. A small rent may not be apparent, but the anesthesiologist may note an increase in pCO_2. These injuries have been repaired with intracorporeal suturing, synthetic meshes, and tissue glue.[55–58] A residual pneumothorax may be aspirated or a chest tube may be placed to allow lung inflation.

Radical nephroureterectomy

Major complications occur in 8–12% of cases, and hemorrhage is the major cause of conversion.[59–63] Complications may also occur secondary to the management of the distal ureter. There are many methods to resect the distal ureter and intramural tunnel; however, retroperitoneal recurrence has been reported after using the 'pluck' technique.[64]

Partial nephrectomy

Laparoscopic partial nephrectomy is an emerging technique, and can be reasonably undertaken by experienced laparoscopists. In most series, the patients are highly selected, as peripheral and exophytic lesions are more amenable to excision than central or large tumors. In the largest published series, Gill et al note that only 20% of their institutions' partial nephrectomies are approached laparoscopically.[65] Complications occur in up to 20% of

patients, and predominantly include hemorrhage and urine leak.[65–67]

Hemorrhage may be controlled intraoperatively by suturing of the parenchyma, fibrin glue, argon beam coagulation, and/or preoperative ablation with radiofrequency energy. Vascular clamping is an option, as is hand assistance. Ultimately, if these adjunctive measures fail to control hemorrhage, the operation may be converted to an open procedure or to a laparoscopic radical nephrectomy. Postoperative hemorrhage has also been reported and patients can be stabilized with transfusions. Embolization of bleeding vessels or re-exploration should be considered.

Urine leak may occur even if the collecting system appears to be adequately closed. Hemorrhage in the renal bed may also damage the suture line and contribute to collecting system openings. Leaks can be identified intraoperatively by placing an external stent and injecting saline or indigo carmine into the collecting system. Alternatively, leaks may be detected with direct visualization of the collecting system under laparoscopic magnification. A drain should be placed in the retroperitoneum to evacuate excess fluid and prevent urinoma. If a urine leak develops, continue suction drainage for 7–10 days to create a controlled fistula. Then, the drain is taken off suction, and can usually be removed in 48 hours. If a large symptomatic urinoma is present, it may be percutaneously drained.

Laparoscopic pyeloplasty

The major complication has been urinary leakage and ascites, secondary to drain migration.[68] This occurred in 2% of patients in the largest series. This complication may be avoided by placing the drain posterior to the line of Toldt, and posterior to the repair.

Simple nephrectomy

A simple laparoscopic nephrectomy may be more difficult than a radical nephrectomy if the patient has had multiple episodes of pyelonephritis. Tissue planes may be indistinct because of inflammation and scarring. Particular caution is advised in patients with xanthogranulomatous pyelonephritis, in whom the complication rate is very high, and open conversion is required in more than 50%.[69, 70]

Adrenalectomy

A recent review of publications reporting 50 series of laparoscopic adrenalectomy revealed bleeding as the most common complication of laparoscopic adrenalectomy.[71] This complication is more common in the early experience. Bleeding may arise from the renal vein, adrenal vein, vena cava, or renal artery branches. Bleeding also accounts for 30% of conversions. The overall transfusion rate of 2.8% is similar to that in open series. Laparoscopic reexploration for hemorrhage has been successful in 6/7 patients in the reported series.

Retroperitoneal lymph node dissection

Hemorrhage is the major complication of laparoscopic retroperitoneal lymph node dissection for stage I nonseminomatous germ cell tumors.[72–78] Reports of hemorrhage from the vena cava, renal vein, lumbar veins, and gonadal vein have been reported. In most cases hemorrhage can be controlled with pressure, clips, tissue glues, and/or suturing, but conversion should be considered if laparoscopic repair is difficult. The overall conversion rate ranges from 2.6% to 6.9%.

Postchemotherapy laparoscopic retroperitoneal lymph node dissection carries a much higher complication rate than primary lymph node dissection; a similar situation is seen with the corresponding open procedures.[79, 80] In one series chylous ascites occurred in 21% of patients, but resolved in all patients with dietary adjustments. In another series, major complications occurred in 42% of patients, with renal vascular injury being a major cause of morbidity.

Radical prostatectomy

Radical prostatectomy is a challenging laparoscopic procedure, and should be undertaken by an experienced team with intracorporeal suturing abilities. The overall complication rate is 8.9–18.8%. Conversions occur more commonly in the initial experience, and range from 1.2% to 4.4%. Major intraoperative complications include rectal and bowel injury, anastomotic leak, pelvic or intraperitoneal hematoma, and bladder or ureteral injury. Long-term data on potency and continence are still pending.[81–86]

Hemorrhagic complications usually arise from the dorsal venous complex or the prostatic pedicles.[86] The dorsal venous complex can be visualized closely and oversewn or cauterized if necessary. The technique of hemostasis on the pedicles may vary, depending upon the indications for nerve sparing. If nerve sparing is used, the estimated blood loss of the procedure may be increased, and precise vascular control with the bipolar instrument is recommended. A rare cause of hemorrhage is an epigastric

artery injury from a trocar site. Care should be taken to inspect the lateral trocar sites for bleeding, particularly at the time of closure.

Rectal injury may occur during the posterior dissection of the seminal vesicles, or during the apical dissection if Denonvilliers' fascia has not been adequately separated from the apex.[86] Although a rectal bougie may aid in identification of the rectum, it cannot absolutely prevent injury. If recognized intraoperatively, rectal injury can be sutured laparoscopically. However, laparotomy and diversion should be considered in the event of fecal contamination or large injuries.

Bowel injuries have been missed intraoperatively during this operation, and may be related to transmission of current or direct injury from replacement of instruments. As previously stated, presentation may be atypical. General surgical consultation is indicated, and laparotomy is usually necessary.

Ureteral injury may occur if the ureter is mistaken for the vas deferens. Lateral superior identification of the vas can prevent this complication. Ureteral necrosis has also been noted with extensive mobilization of the bladder to release it from the peritoneum. Unrecognized injury may be manifested in urinary ascites and elevated creatinine.

Vesicourethral anastomotic leak occurs in up to 10% of patients.[81–86] Patients may develop an elevated serum creatinine as a result of intraperitoneal urine absorption. Most patients exhibit high pelvic drain output. Decrease of fluid intake, verification of Foley catheter position, and continued drainage have been successful in most cases.

Urinary retention may develop when the Foley catheter is removed on postoperative day 1 or 2. By postoperative day 4, the incidence of this complication is < 5%.

Summary

To minimize complications of urologic laparoscopic procedures, the surgeon should understand laparoscopic physiology and should be experienced with specialized surgical instrumentation. Although complications are of a frequency similar to that of open surgery, the recognition and management of many complications differ. The informed and experienced surgeon can decrease complications and effectively deliver the advantages of minimally invasive urology.

References

1. Cadeddu JA, Wolfe JS Jr., Nakada S et al. Complications of laparoscopic procedures after concentrated training in urological laparoscopy. J Urol 2001; 166:2109.

2. Fahlenkamp D, Rassweiler J, Fornara P, et al. Complications of laparoscopic procedures in urology: experience with 2,407 procedures at 4 German centers. J Urol 1999; 162:765.

3. Thomas R, Steele R, Ahuja S. Complications of urological laparoscopy: a standardized 1 institution experience. J Urol 1996; 156:469.

4. Soulie M, Salomon L, Seguin P, et al. Multi-institutional study of complications in 1085 laparoscopic urologic procedures. Urology 2001; 58:899.

5. Vallancien G, Cathelineau X, Baumert H. et al. Complications of transperitoneal laparoscopic surgery in urology: review of 1,311 procedures at a single center. J Urol 2002; 168:23.

6. Wolf JS Jr., Marcovich R, Gill IS et al. Survey of neuromuscular injuries to the patient and surgeon during urologic laparoscopic surgery. Urology 2000; 55:831.

7. Catarci M, Carlini M, Gentileschi P, et al. Major and minor injuries during the creation of pneumoperitoneum. A multi-center study on 12,919 cases. Surg Endosc 2001; 15:566.

8. Bonjer HJ, Hazebroek EJ, Kazemier G, et al. Open versus closed establishment of pneumoperitoneum in laparoscopic surgery. Br J Surg 1997; 84:599.

9. Jirecek S, Drager M, Leitich H, et al. Direct visual or blind insertion of the primary trocar. Surg Endosc 2002; 16:626.

10. McKernan JB, Finley CR. Experience with optical trocar in performing laparoscopic procedures. Surg Laparosc Endosc Percutan Tech 2002; 12:96.

11. String A, Berber E, Foroutani A, et al. Use of the optical access trocar for safe and rapid entry in various laparoscopic procedures. Surg Endosc 2001; 15:570.

12. Oza KN, O'Donnell N, Fisher JB. Aortic laceration: a rare complication of laparoscopy. J Laparoendosc Surg 1992;2:235.

13. Chapron CM, Pierre F, Lacroix S, et al. Major vascular injuries during gynecologic laparoscopy. J Am Coll Surg 1997; 185:461.

14. Nordestgaard AG, Bodily KC, Osborne RW Jr., et al. Major vascular injuries during laparoscopic procedures. Am J Surg 1995; 169:543.

15. Seidman DS, Nasserbakht F, Nezhat F, et al. Delayed recognition of iliac artery injury during laparoscopic surgery. Surg Endosc 1996; 10:1099.

16. Whiteley MS, Laws SA, Wise MH. Use of a hand-held Doppler to avoid abdominal wall vessels in laparoscopic surgery. Ann R Coll Surg Engl 1994; 76:348.

17. Cuellar DC, Kavoussi PK, Baker LA, et al. Open laparoscopic access using a radially dilating trocar: experience and indications in 50 consecutive cases. J Endourol 2000; 14:755.

18. Mann C, Boccara G, Fabre JM, et al. The detection of carbon dioxide embolism during laparoscopy in pigs: a comparison of transesophageal Doppler and end-tidal carbon dioxide monitoring. Acta Anaesthesiol Scand 1997; 41:281.

19. Cottin V, Delafosse B, Viale JP. Gas embolism during laparoscopy: a report of seven cases in patients with previous abdominal surgical history. Surg Endosc 1996; 10:166.

20. Muth CM, Shank ES. Gas embolism. N Engl J Med 2000; 342:476.

21. Stifelman MD, Sosa RE, Nakada SY, et al. Hand-assisted laparoscopic partial nephrectomy. J Endourol 2001; 15:161.

22. Janetschek G, Daffner P, Peschel R, et al. Laparoscopic nephron sparing surgery for small renal cell carcinoma. J Urol 1998; 159:1152.

23. Winfield HN, Donovan JF, Lund GO, et al. Laparoscopic partial nephrectomy: initial experience and comparison to the open surgical approach. J Urol 1995; 153:1409.

24. Gill IS, Delworth MG, Munch LC. Laparoscopic retroperitoneal partial nephrectomy. J Urol 1994; 152:1539.

25. Kono M, Yahagi N, Kitahara M, et al. Cardiac arrest associated with use of an argon beam coagulator during laparoscopic cholecystectomy. Br J Anaesth 2001; 87:644.

26. Veyckemans F, Michel I. Venous gas embolism from an Argon coagulator. Anesthesiology 1996; 85:443.

27. Fatal gas embolism caused by overpressurization during laparoscopic use of argon enhanced coagulation. Health Devices 1994; 23:257.

28. Wolf JS Jr, Stoller ML. The physiology of laparoscopy: basic principles, complications and other considerations. J Urol 1994; 152:294.

29. Sharma KC, Brandstetter RD, Brensilver JM, et al. Cardiopulmonary physiology and pathophysiology as a consequence of laparoscopic surgery. Chest 1996; 110:810.

30. Wolf JS Jr, Clayman RV, McDougall EM, et al. Carbon dioxide and helium insufflation during laparoscopic radical nephrectomy in a patient with severe pulmonary disease. J Urol 1996; 155:2021.

31. Wolf JS Jr, Carrier S, Stoller ML. Gas embolism: helium is more lethal than carbon dioxide. J Laparoendosc Surg 1994; 4:173.

32. Tsereteli Z, Terry ML, Bowers SP, et al. Prospective randomized clinical trial comparing nitrous oxide and carbon dioxide pneumoperitoneum for laparoscopic surgery. J Am Coll Surg 2002; 195:173.

33. Dunn MD, McDougall EM. Renal physiology. Laparoscopic considerations. Urol Clin North Am 2000; 27:609.

34. Bishoff JT, Allaf ME, Kirkels W, et al. Laparoscopic bowel injury: incidence and clinical presentation. J Urol 1999; 161: 887.

35. El-Banna M, Abdel-Atty M, El-Meteini M, et al. Management of laparoscopic-related bowel injuries. Surg Endosc 2000; 14:779.

36. Otani M, Irie S, Tsuji Y. Port site metastasis after laparoscopic nephrectomy: unsuspected transitional cell carcinoma within a tuberculous atrophic kidney. J Urol 1999; 162:486.

37. Fentie DD, Barrett PH, Taranger LA. Metastatic renal cell cancer after laparoscopic radical nephrectomy: long-term follow-up. J Endourol 2000; 14:407.

38. Castilho LN, Fugita OE, Mitre AI, et al. Port site tumor recurrences of renal cell carcinoma after videolaparoscopic radical nephrectomy. J Urol 2001; 165:519.

39. Ahmed I, Shaikh NA, Kapadia CR. Track recurrence of renal pelvic transitional cell carcinoma after laparoscopic nephrectomy. Br J Urol 1998; 81:319.

40. Paolucci V. Port site recurrences after laparoscopic cholecystectomy. J Hepatobiliary Pancreat Surg 2001; 8:535.

41. Nezhat C, Nezhat F, Seidman DS. Incisional hernias after operative laparoscopy. J Laparoendosc Adv Surg Tech A 1997; 7:111.

42. Eltabbakh GH. Small bowel obstruction secondary to herniation through a 5-mm laparoscopic trocar site following laparoscopic lymphadenectomy. Eur J Gynaecol Oncol 1999; 20: 275.

43. Lajer H, Widecrantz S, Heisterberg L. Hernias in trocar ports following abdominal laparoscopy. A review. Acta Obstet Gynecol Scand 1997; 76:389.

44. Leibl BJ, Schmedt CG, Schwarz J, et al. Laparoscopic surgery complications associated with trocar tip design: review of literature and own results. J Laparoendosc Adv Surg Tech A 1999; 9:135.

45. Liu CD, McFadden DW. Laparoscopic port sites do not require fascial closure when nonbladed trocars are used. Am Surg 2000; 66:853.

46. Clayman RV, Kavoussi LR, Soper NJ, et al. Laparoscopic nephrectomy: initial case report. J Urol 1991; 146:278.

47. Philosophe B, Kuo PC, Schweitzer EJ, et al. Laparoscopic versus open donor nephrectomy: comparing ureteral complications in the recipients and improving the laparoscopic technique. Transplantation 1999; 68:497.

48. Ratner LE, Montgomery RA, Maley WR, et al. Laparoscopic live donor nephrectomy: the recipient. Transplantation 2000; 69:2319.

49. Barrett PH, Fentie DD, Taranger LA. Laparoscopic radical nephrectomy with morcellation for renal cell carcinoma: the Saskatoon experience. Urology 1998; 52:23.

50. Dunn MD, Portis AJ, Shalhav AL, et al. Laparoscopic versus open radical nephrectomy: a 9-year experience. J Urol 2000; 164:1153.

51. Chan DY, Cadeddu JA, Jarrett TW, et al. Laparoscopic radical nephrectomy: cancer control for renal cell carcinoma. J Urol 2001; 166:2095.

52. Portis AJ, Yan Y, Landman J, et al. Long-term followup after laparoscopic radical nephrectomy. J Urol 2002; 167:1257.

53. Gill IS, Meraney AM, Schweizer DK, et al. Laparoscopic radical nephrectomy in 100 patients: a single center experience from the United States. Cancer 2001; 92:1843.

54. Ono Y, Kinukawa T, Hattori R, et al. Laparoscopic radical nephrectomy for renal cell carcinoma: a five-year experience. Urology 1999; 53:280.

55. Gonzalez CM, Batler RA, Feldman M, et al. Repair of a diaphragmatic injury during hand assisted laparoscopic nephrectomy using an onlay patch of polypropylene and polyglactin mesh. J Urol 2002; 167:2512.

56. Potter SR, Kavoussi LR, Jackman SV. Management of diaphragmatic injury during laparoscopic nephrectomy. J Urol 2001; 165:1203.

57. Rehman J, Landman J, Kerbl K, Clayman RW. Laparoscopic repair of diaphragmatic defect by total intracorporeal suturing: clinical and technical considerations. JSLS 2001; 5:287.

58. Bhayani S, Grubb R, Andriole G. Use of gelatin matrix to rapidly repair diaphragmatic injury during laparoscopy. Urology 2002; 60:514.

59. Jarrett TW, Chan DY, Cadeddu JA, et al. Laparoscopic nephroureterectomy for the treatment of transitional cell carcinoma of the upper urinary tract. Urology 2001; 57:448.

60. Landman J, Lev RY, Bhayani S, et al. Comparison of hand assisted and standard laparoscopic radical nephroureterectomy for the management of localized transitional cell carcinoma. J Urol 2002; 167:2387.

61. Shalhav AL, Dunn MD, Portis AJ, et al. Laparoscopic nephroureterectomy for upper tract transitional cell cancer: the Washington University experience. J Urol 2000; 163:1100.

62. Gill IS, Sung GT, Hobart MG, et al. Laparoscopic radical nephroureterectomy for upper tract transitional cell carcinoma: the Cleveland Clinic experience. J Urol 2000; 164:1513.

63. Keeley FX Jr, Tolley DA. Laparoscopic nephroureterectomy: making management of upper-tract transitional-cell carcinoma entirely minimally invasive. J Endourol 1998; 12:139.

64. Elbahnasy AM, Hoenig DM, Shalhav A, et al. Laparoscopic staging of bladder tumor: concerns about port site metastases. J Endourol 1998; 12:55.

65. Gill IS, Desai MM, Kaouk JH, et al. Laparoscopic partial nephrectomy for renal tumor: duplicating open surgical techniques. J Urol 2002; 167:469.

66. McDougall EM, Elbahnasy AM, Clayman RV. Laparoscopic wedge resection and partial nephrectomy – the Washington University experience and review of the literature. JSLS 1998; 2:15.

67. Rassweiler JJ, Abbou C, Janetschek G, et al. Laparoscopic partial nephrectomy. The European experience. Urol Clin North Am 2000; 27:721.

68. Jarrett TW, Chan DY, Charambura TC, et al. Laparoscopic pyeloplasty: the first 100 cases. J Urol 2002; 167:1253.

69. Cadeddu JA, Chan DY, Hedican SP, et al. Retroperitoneal access for transperitoneal laparoscopy in patients at high risk for intra-abdominal scarring. J Endourol 1999; 13:567.

70. Bercowsky E, Shalhav AL, Portis A, et al. Is the laparoscopic approach justified in patients with xanthogranulomatous pyelonephritis? Urology 1999; 54:437.

71. Brunt LM. The positive impact of laparoscopic adrenalectomy on complications of adrenal surgery. Surg Endosc 2002; 16:252.

72. Janetschek G, Hobisch A, Holtl L, et al. Retroperitoneal lymphadenectomy for clinical stage I nonseminomatous testicular tumor: laparoscopy versus open surgery and impact of learning curve. J Urol 1996; 156:89.

73. Janetschek G, Hobisch A, Peschel R, et al. Laparoscopic retroperitoneal lymph node dissection. Urology 2000; 55:136.

74. Janetschek G, Hobisch A, Peschel R, et al. Laparoscopic retroperitoneal lymph node dissection for clinical stage I nonseminomatous testicular carcinoma: long-term outcome. J Urol 2000; 163:1793.

75. Janetschek G, Peschel R, Hobisch A, et al. Laparoscopic retroperitoneal lymph node dissection. J Endourol 2001; 15:449.

76. Nelson JB, Chen RN, Bishoff JT, et al. Laparoscopic retroperitoneal lymph node dissection for clinical stage I nonseminomatous germ cell testicular tumors. Urology 1999; 54:1064.

77. Rassweiler JJ, Seemann O, Henkel TO, et al. Laparoscopic retroperitoneal lymph node dissection for nonseminomatous germ cell tumors: indications and limitations. J Urol 1996; 156:1108.

78. Rassweiler JJ, Frede T, Lenz E, et al. Long-term experience with laparoscopic retroperitoneal lymph node dissection in the management of low-stage testis cancer. Eur Urol 2000; 37:251.

79. Palese MA, Su LM, Kavoussi, LR. Laparoscopic retroperitoneal lymph node dissection after chemotherapy. Urology, 60: 130, 2002

80. Janetschek G, Hobisch A, Hittmair A, et al. Laparoscopic retroperitoneal lymphadenectomy after chemotherapy for stage IIB nonseminomatous testicular carcinoma. J Urol 1999; 161:477.

81. Guillonneau B, Cathelineau X, Doublet JD, et al. Laparoscopic radical prostatectomy: the lessons learned. J Endourol 2001; 15:441.

82. Guillonneau B, Rozet F, Barret E, et al. Laparoscopic radical prostatectomy: assessment after 240 procedures. Urol Clin North Am 2001; 28:189.

83. Guillonneau B, Vallancien G. Laparoscopic radical prostatectomy: the Montsouris experience. J Urol 2000; 163:418.

84. Hoznek A, Salomon L, Olsson LE, et al. Laparoscopic radical prostatectomy. The Creteil experience. Eur Urol 2001; 40:38.

85. Rassweiler J, Sentker L, Seemann O, et al. Laparoscopic radical prostatectomy with the Heilbronn technique: an analysis of the first 180 cases. J Urol 2001; 166:2101.

86. Guillonneau B, Rozet F, Cathelineau X, et al. Perioperative complications of laparoscopic radical prostatectomy: the Montsouris 3-year experience. J Urol 2002; 167:51.

Index

Page numbers in *italics* indicate figures or tables

T - #1061 - 101024 - C408 - 276/216/19 [21] - CB - 9781841845661 - Gloss Lamination